H. Niwa (Supervising Editor)
H. Tajiri, M. Nakajima, K. Yasuda (Editors)
New Challenges in Gastrointestinal Endoscopy

H. Niwa (Supervising Editor)
H. Tajiri, M. Nakajima,
K. Yasuda (Editors)

New Challenges in Gastrointestinal Endoscopy

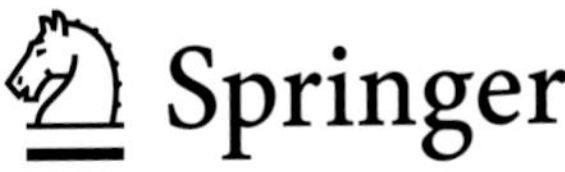

Supervising Editor:
Hirohumi Niwa, M.D.
President, Japan Gastroenterological Endoscopy Society
3-22 Kanda Ogawa-machi, Chiyoda-ku, Tokyo 101-0052, Japan
Professor of Medicine, St. Marianna University School of Medicine
2-16-1 Sugao, Miyamae-ku, Kawasaki 216-8511, Japan

Editors:
Hisao Tajiri, M.D.
Professor, Division of Gastroenterology and Hepatology, Department of Internal Medicine, The Jikei University School of Medicine
3-25-8 Nishishinbashi, Minato-ku, Tokyo 105-8461, Japan

Masatsugu Nakajima, M.D.
President, Kyoto Second Red Cross Hospital
355-5 Kamanza-dori, Maruta-machi-agaru, Kamigyo-ku, Kyoto 602-8026, Japan

Kenjiro Yasuda, M.D.
Director, Department of Gastroenterology, Kyoto Second Red Cross Hospital
355-5 Kamanza-dori, Maruta-machi-agaru, Kamigyo-ku, Kyoto, 602-8026, Japan

Library of Congress Control Number: 2008929897

ISBN 978-4-431-78888-1 Springer Tokyo Berlin Heidelberg New York
e-ISBN 978-4-431-78889-8

Springer is a part of Springer Science+Business Media
springer.com

Printed in Japan

Typesetting: SNP Best-set Typesetter Ltd., Hong Kong
Printing and binding: Kato Bunmeisha, Japan

Printed on acid-free paper

Preface

It goes without saying that recent developments in the field of gastrointestinal (GI) endoscopy have been remarkable. GI endoscopy has now become indispensable in both the diagnosis and treatment of GI disorders. Advances in GI endoscopy have been largely the result of cooperation between endoscopists and endoscopic manufacturers in the development of new instruments and new techniques. In Japan, joint academic and industrial research commenced in this field in 1957. We, the endoscopists of Japan, have continued to actively promote the development and use of new models and clinical applications, and also have put much effort into education and training.

The inaugural Endoscopy Forum Japan (EFJ) was held in August 1999 in Otaru, Hokkaido. Now, in the summer of 2008, it has been 10 years since the first EFJ was held. In that time, a total of 187 leading young endoscopists, including colleagues from Asia, Australia, Europe, and the United States, have participated in this forum, discussing issues at the forefront of the field and inspiring new techniques and original ideas that have spread to other parts of the world. Because EFJ's primary commitment is to internationalization, all presentations and discussions have been conducted in English. An equally important goal is standardization of procedures, therapeutic methods, and related medical instruments. Furthermore, we are actively promoting joint academic and industry research to stimulate further advances in GI endoscopy.

Over these past 10 years, through EFJ, GI endoscopy has yielded many new diagnoses and treatments, including:

1) The establishment of diagnostic significance based on a multicenter randomized study of endoscopic sphincterotomy (EST) and endoscopic papillary balloon dilation (EPBD) for common bile duct stones, metallic stent versus plastic stent for malignant biliary stricture, magnifying endoscopy, narrow band imaging (NBI), autofluorescence endoscopy (AFI), and endocytoscopy (ECS).
2) The expansion of indications, newer devices, and therapeutic methods of endoscopic mucosal resection (EMR) and endoscopic submucosal dissection (ESD) for early GI cancers.
3) The standardization of pancreatobiliary endoscopic ultrasound (EUS), and EUS-guided fine-needle aspiration (EUS-FNA) by the EFJ working group.

The Organizing Committee of EFJ therefore has decided to publish the results we have achieved in this book entitled *New Challenges in Gastrointestinal Endoscopy* in order to disseminate these results to a wider audience of endoscopists, and to contribute to the development of endoscopic medicine all over the world. We believe that the book is a groundbreaking, edifying, and engrossing publication in the field of gastrointestinal endoscopy, and recent advances in endoscopic diagnosis and treatment are precisely described using more than 250 beautiful color photographs. Furthermore, future perspectives of newer technologies are accurately described not only from a medical standpoint but from an engineering one as well.

We express our thanks and appreciation for the generous contributions of time, effort, and, most importantly, superb knowledge and experience to our colleagues who authored chapters; and our eternal gratitude to Professor Hirohumi Niwa, President of the Japan Gastroenterological Endoscopy Society for heartfelt advice and support. Finally, we would also like to express our deep appreciation to Olympus Medical Systems, Tokyo, Japan, for their continued support.

Hisao Tajiri, M.D.
Chairman, Organizing Committee of the Second-Generation EFJ (2004–2008)
Masatsugu Nakajima, M.D.
Chairman, Organizing Committee of the First-Generation EFJ (1999–2003)
Kenjiro Yasuda, M.D.
Secretary General, Organizing Committee of EFJ (1999–2008)

EFJ Organizing Committee

Naotaka Fujita

Masahiro Igarashi

Yoshinori Igarashi

Haruhiro Inoue

Mitsuhiro Kida

Hiroyuki Maguchi

Manabu Muto

Masatsugu Nakajima

Yusuke Saitoh

Hisao Tajiri

Shinji Tanaka

Naohisa Yahagi

Hiroo Yamano

Kenshi Yao

Kenjiro Yasuda

Contents

Barrett's Esophagus

Stomach

Small Intestine

Colon

Cholangioscopy and Pancreatoscopy

EUS

Appendix

History and Future Development of Endoscopy

The History of Digestive Endoscopy

Hirohumi Niwa

Summary. In the early 19th century, elementary attempts were made to observe the larynx, rectum, vagina, and urinary tract using primitive endoscopes. In 1868, Kussmaul attempted to observe the inside of the stomach with a rigid straight tube, achieving no successful results. Around this time, it was discovered that bright light is gained by sending electricity to a platinum wire under cooling with running water. After that, many different types of rigid gastroscopes were developed with this newly discovered system as the light source, which was an incandescent platinum wire at first, then miniature light bulbs. In 1932, Schindler developed a flexible gastroscope with a bending function at the tip. Several experiments were also conducted to make a diagnosis by photographs taken with a miniature camera inserted in the stomach. Lange et al. and other researchers engaged in this approach, but none of their apparatuses could stand practical clinical use. In 1950, completely separately from Lange's experiment, Uji et al. developed the gastrocamera. Although Uji's gastrocamera could not withstand practical use either, Tasaka's group at the First Department of Internal Medicine, Faculty of Medicine, University of Tokyo, had started clinical experiments with the gastrocamera in 1953 and added various improvements to make it a truly practical medical device. In 1957, Hirschowitz made a fiberscope. Based on this technology, the gastrocamera equipped with a fiberscope was developed and disseminated widely throughout Japan. As the technology of fiberscopes advanced, endoscopes for colon, esophagus, and duodenum were developed as well. The videoscope, which has become the mainstream of endoscopes today, was developed as television technology progressed. Image enhancement, image analysis, and narrow-band imaging technology are the hot topics in endoscopy today. Autofluorescence imaging is also one of the recent topics of endoscopy. In this chapter, the author foresees the future advancement of endoscopy.

Key words. Rigid gastroscope, Intragastric photography, Fiberscope, Videoendoscope, Narrow-band imaging (NBI), Autofluorescence imaging (AFI)

Japan Gastroenterological Endoscopy Society, 3-22 Kanda Ogawa-machi, Chiyoda-ku, Tokyo 101-0052, Japan
St. Marianna University School of Medicine, 2-16-1 Sugao, Miyamae-ku, Kawasaki 216-8511, Japan

Early Endoscope Models

It was as early as the times of Hippocrates that people first attempted to observe inside the human body using some form of instrument. Some of these instruments were discovered in the ruins of Pompeii that had been buried under volcanic ejecta in the 1st century. After this time, no remarkable progress was made in endoscopy until the 19th century.

In the early 19th century, several primitive versions of the endoscope such as the instruments by Bozzini (1805), Segalas (1826), Fisher (1827), Bonnafont (1834), Avery (1843), and Désormeaux (1853) appeared. The target organs of these early endoscopes were mainly the larynx, rectum, vagina, and urethra.

Figure 1A portrays Bozzini's light conductor of 1805, which looks like a lantern with a height of 34 cm. The light source was a candle. The insertion part was attached to the opening in the front wall, and the observer looked in from the window in the back. It was possible to observe urethra, rectum, and vagina. This picture appeared in his monograph. Figure 1B shows the original model, which is now preserved in the Nitze-Leiter Museum, Medico-Historical Institute of Vienna University. After World War II, it was taken away by American military personnel when they occupied Vienna. Recently, the American Surgical Society gave it back to Vienna University.

There were various kinds of specula. The speculum in Fig. 1B is equipped with a concave mirror and a flat mirror in the tip. It was possible to observe larynx, pharynx, and upper esophagus, which were impossible to observe with a straight-view speculum. The flat mirror was used for illumination, and a concave mirror was used for observation. Although there was some improvement by Ilg to provide brighter illu-

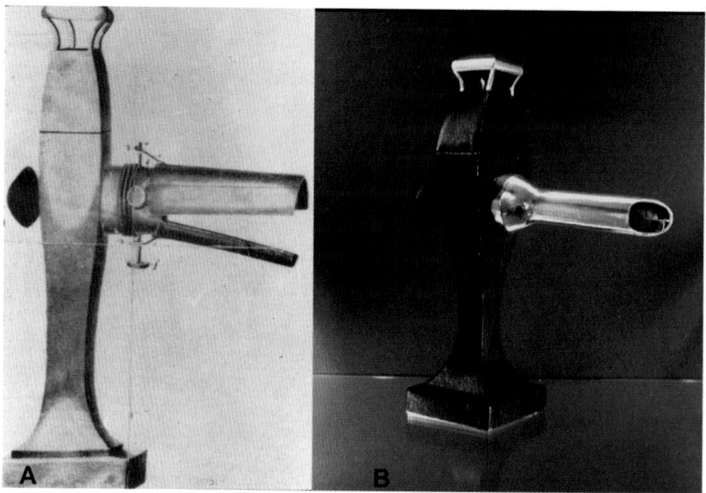

Fig. 1. Bozzini's light conductor

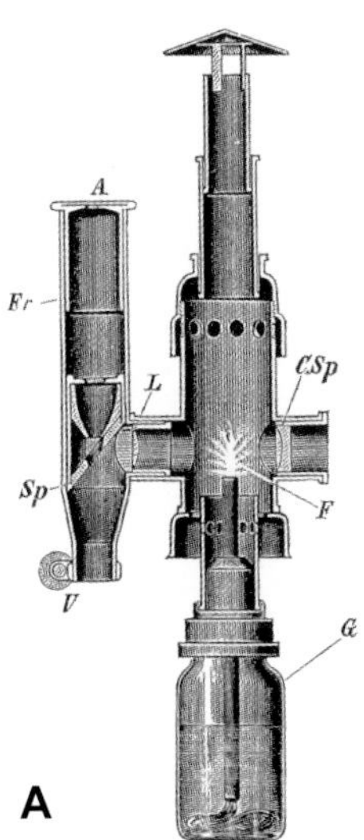

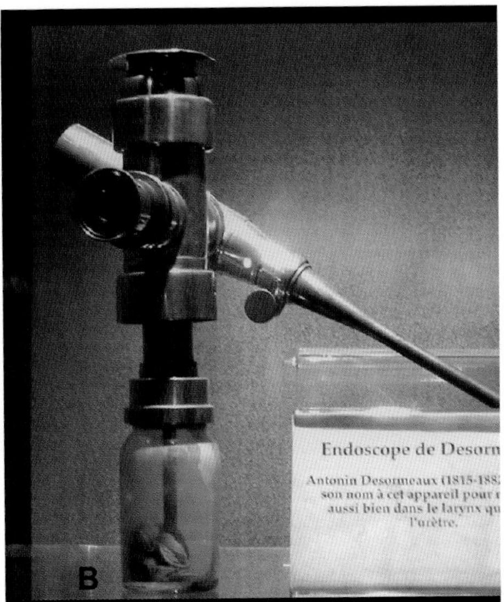

FIG. 2. Désormeaux's device

mination, there was strong objection to the practical application of Bozzini's light conductor from the University of Vienna. There was also a reproach from the Church about the act of observing inside the human body. For these reasons, attempts at observation using this instrument were not continued.

Désormeaux created an apparatus that he named an endoscope in 1853. The left side of the apparatus shown in Fig. 2A is the optical body tube and the right side is the light source. The light source was a lamp fired by a mixture of alcohol and turpentine. Inside the optical tube there is a mirror with a small hole in the center, so the light is reflected within the optical tube. The insertion part is fixed to the lower end of the optical tube. Observation is carried out from the small hole at the upper end of the optical tube. It was possible to move the optical tube while keeping the light source always vertical (Fig. 2, right).

This apparatus was mainly targeted for observation of the urethra and bladder. It was also possible to observe the rectum by replacing the insertion part of the apparatus.

Rigid and Flexible Gastroscopes

Kussmaul was the first person who tried using an endoscope to observe inside the human stomach in 1868. Figure 3 shows a replica of the instrument preserved in Kyusyu University of Japan. Seeing the performance of a sword-swallower, Kussmaul got a hint of the idea that a straight rigid bar could be inserted into the

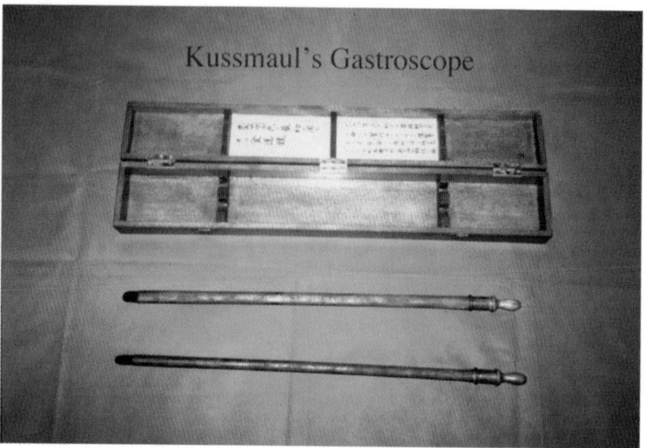

FIG. 3. Kussmaul's gastroscope

stomach. However, it was impossible to observe the stomach except near the cardia.

The biggest problem of early endoscopes was the light source. In the mid-1800s, it had already been discovered that bright light could be obtained by the electric glow of a platinum wire with a water cooling system. This technology was applied to observation of the larynx in the 1860s.

Nitze and Leiter invented an esophagoscope (Fig. 4A) and gastroscope in 1879. The scope consisted of many metal parts, just like the shell of a prawn. The scope was made flexible by loosening the wires and straightened by tightening the wires after insertion. However, its practical value is unknown.

In 1881, Mikulicz invented a rigid gastroscope. The light source was a platinum glow wire with water cooling. To prevent the lens from contamination while passing the esophagus, there was a cover to protect the lens during insertion (Fig. 4B). Mikulicz succeeded in observing gastric cancer and ulcer cases.

A cystoscope with a miniature light bulb mounted was created by Nitze in 1886. After that, various kinds of rigid gastroscopes were invented, as shown in Table 1.

Sussman's gastroscope (1911) is well known. The wire was loosened to bend the gastroscope when inserting it into the body, and then the wire was pulled to straighten the scope when it had reached the stomach (Fig. 5A). However, it is reported that this mechanism caused considerable pain to the patient.

Elsner's gastroscope was developed in 1911 (Fig. 5B). It was a side-viewing scope. When the handle at the controlling part was rotated, the prism in the tip part was pushed to cause it to rise up. Then it was possible to view backward or straight forward by adjusting the prism.

In 1932, Schindler and Wolf developed a flexible gastroscope (Fig. 6). A number of lenses of short focal distance were built into the shaft, relaying the image sequentially to the other end. The image was conveyed even though the gastroscope proper was bent as much as 30°. Use of this device was widespread in Europe and the United States, but in Japan it was used in only a small number of institutions.

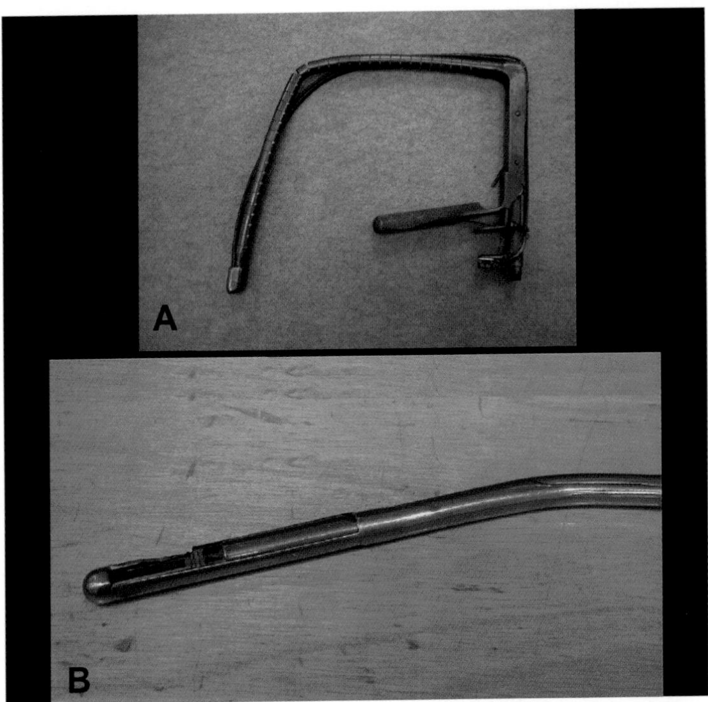

FIG. 4. **A** Nitze and Leiter esophagoscope. **B** Mikulicz's gastroscope

TABLE 1. Rigid gastroscopes

Mikulicz's gastroscope	1881
Kelling's gastroscope	1897
Kuttner's gastroscope	1897
Rosenheim's gastroscope	1895
Jackson's gastroscope	1907
Loening and Stieda gastroscope	1908
Elsner's gastroscope	1909
Sussman's gastroscope	1911
Steinberg's gastroscope	1921
Schindler's gastroscope	1923
Korbsch's gastroscope	1925
Hübner's gastroscope	1926

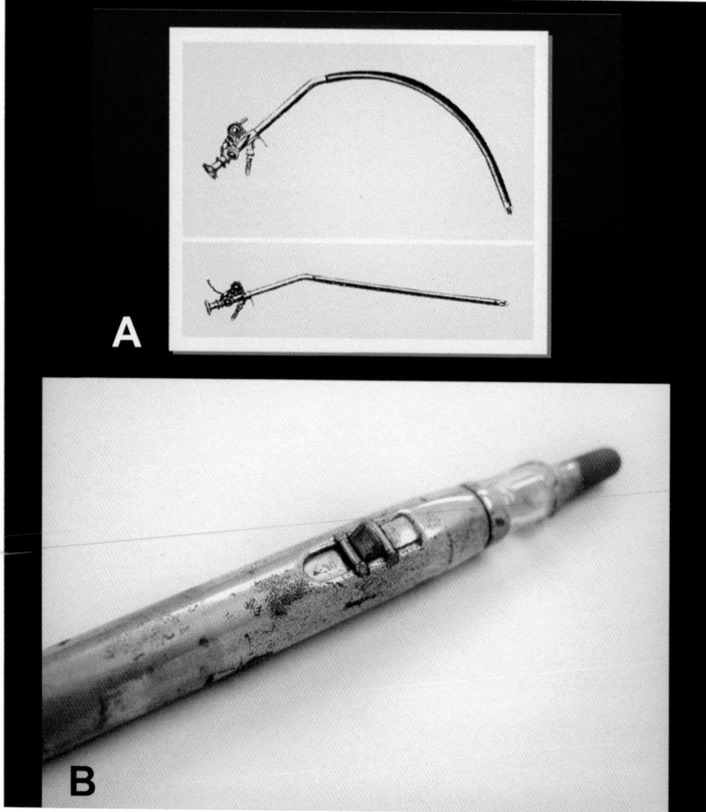

FIG. 5. A Sussman's gastroscope. B Elsner's gastroscope

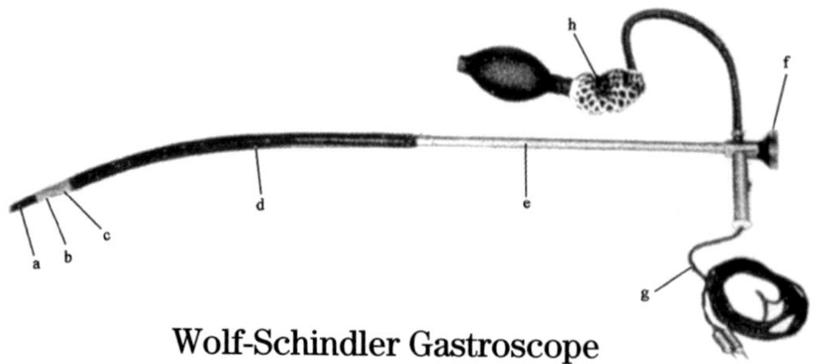

FIG. 6. Wolf–Schindler flexible gastroscope

Intragastric Photography (Gastrocamera)

Intragastric photography is a method to make a diagnosis by inserting a miniature camera into the stomach. Einhorn was the first person who thought of the potential of making a diagnosis by intragastric photography (1889). After that, there were several attempts at intragastric photography.

Schaaf developed his device in 1898, and in the same year, Lange and Meltzing developed their device. Schaaf's device was a direct-forward-view type, and it could take only one picture. With the Lange and Meltzing device and the Porges and Heilpern gastrophotor, it was possible to get many pictures.

Figure 7A shows the construction of the Lange and Meltzing apparatus. The camera, the lamp, and film storage were built into the tip. However, the pictures obtained by this method were very poor because of the long exposure time required by the immature film technology of that time and insufficient depth of insertion. The reason for this latter problem was lack of knowledge of the shape and position of the living stomach because X-ray observation was not yet available. No valuable results were gained with this instrument, and it did not attract further attention.

In 1929, a gastrophotor was invented by Porges and Heilpern in Vienna. It contains 16 sets of a pinhole camera without the lens (Fig. 8A). It was able to produce 8 sets of stereophotographs at a time (Fig. 8B) but was soon abandoned.

Uji, at the Branch Hospital, University of Tokyo, made the intragastric photography apparatus named the gastrocamera in 1950. At the tip were the camera lens, light

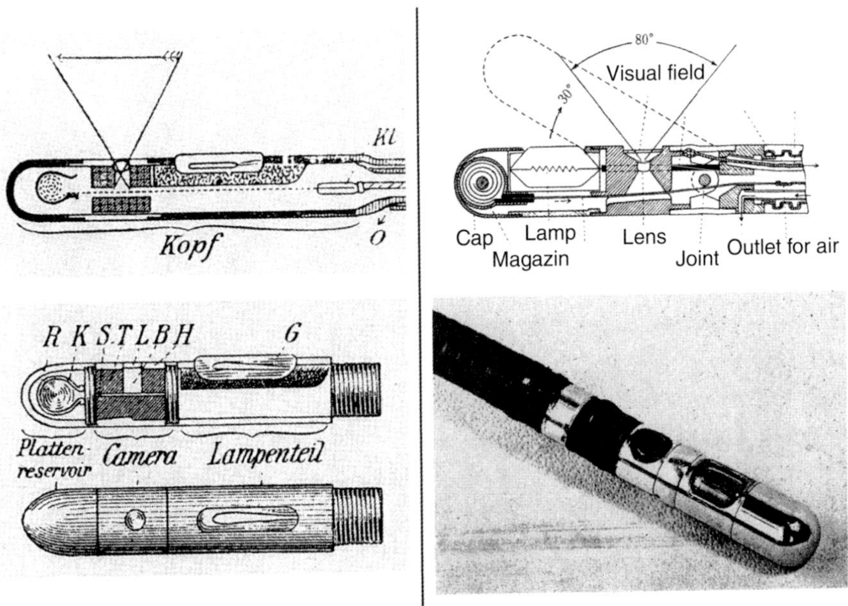

Fig. 7. A Lange and Meltzing device. B Gastrocamera (Uji)

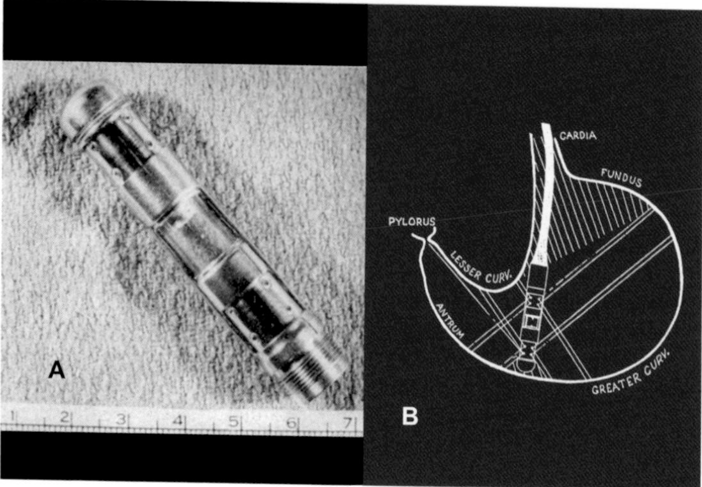

FIG. 8. Gastrophotor

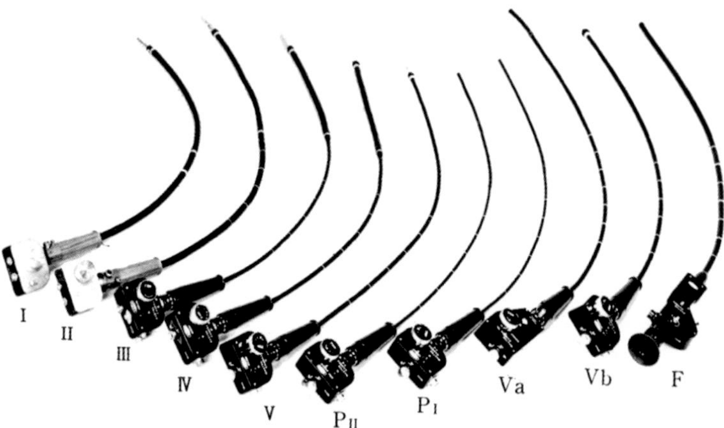

FIG. 9. Progression of gastrocamera (transition). F shows the gastrocamera with fiberscope

bulb, and film cassette (Fig. 7B). It was very similar to the Lange and Meltzing device made about 50 years ago. The gastrocamera was inserted into the stomach and took pictures of the inner surface of the stomach, and diagnosis was made by analyzing these pictures. With the early models, it was very difficult to take good pictures. As a result, there was doubt as to its clinical value.

In 1953, the author's group in the 1st Department of Medicine, University of Tokyo (Sakita, Ashizawa, Utsumi, Niwa, et al.), started clinical study using gastrocamera. It was very difficult to obtain good pictures with the gastrocamera at first. Also, there were frequent mechanical troubles. With repeated improvement of the instruments, establishment of photography technique, and progress in picture interpretation, other hospitals gradually appreciated the value of gastrocamera and adopted it around 1955.

Figure 9 shows the various models starting with the type I gastrocamera. It is clearly shown that the diameter of the apparatus became thinner and thinner with the newer models. The type V gastrocamera (Fig. 10A) was the most popular. Pictures were taken blindly, guided only by the light seen through the abdominal wall. The type Va has a bending part near the tip. Figure 10B is a picture of early gastric cancer taken by a gastrocamera type V. By gathering gastrocamera photographs of early gastric cancer cases from leading nationwide institutes, the basis of early gastric cancer diagnostics was finally established in 1957.

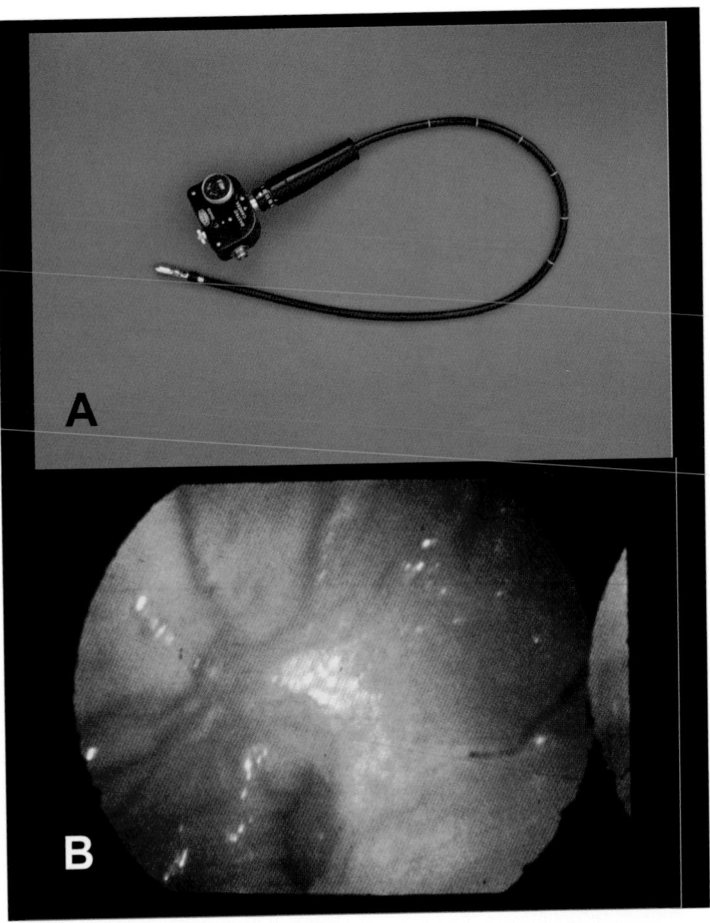

FIG. 10. **A** Type V gastrocamera. **B** Early cancer shown with type V gastrocamera

Fiberscope

Lamm proved the theory of glass fiberoptics by experiments in 1930 when he was still a medical student in Germany. Figure 11A shows his experimental device: the light source, the lens, and a bundle of glass fibers. If an image of a filament of a light bulb is produced on the edge of a glass fiber bundle, the image is transmitted to the other edge of the bundle, although the image is not so clear (Fig. 11B). Lamm recommended that Schindler apply this principle to development of a flexible gastroscope, maintaining that glass fiber would make an easily handled, patient-friendly flexible gastroscope. However, Schindler declined his offer on the grounds that glass fiber was not suitable for a flexible gastroscope.

Hirschowitz developed a prototype of the fiberscope in 1957. Figure 12A shows the original model. Production of the fiberscope in Japan was started in 1963. Olympus

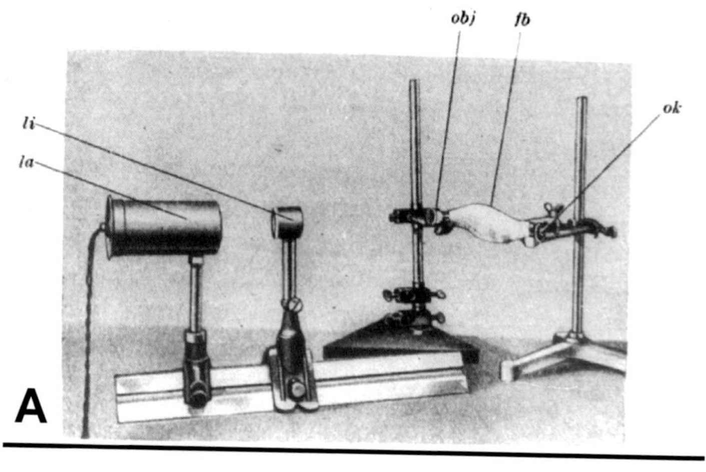

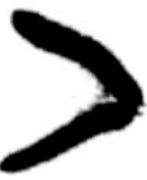

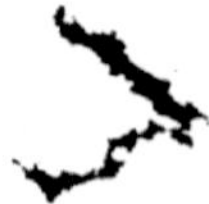

Fig. 11. Lamm's experiment with fiberoptics. **A** Device. **B** Transmission of picture

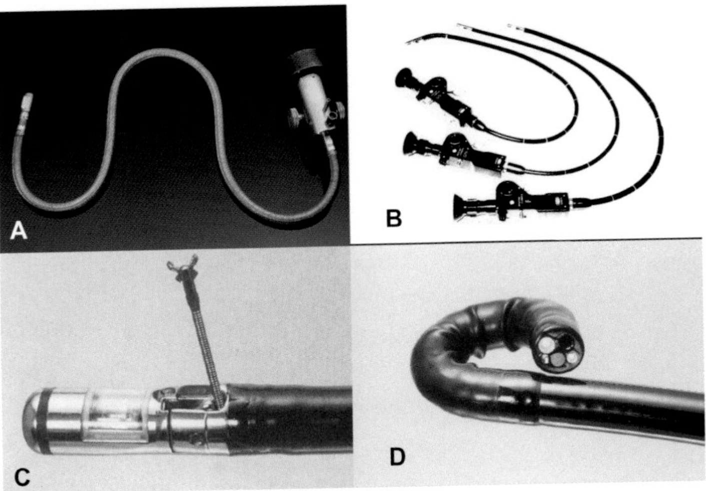

Fig. 12. **A** Prototype fiberscope (Hirschowitz). **B** Gastrocamera with fiberscope. **C** Fiberscope with biopsy function. **D** Direct-forward-view fiberscope

Medical Systems, Tokyo, Japan, developed the gastrocamera with a fiberscope in 1964. The apparatus at the bottom of Fig. 12B is the first model. An angulation mechanism was not adopted. The intragastric camera at the tip was still inevitable because the technology of taking photographs of the images transmitted by a fiberscope was not yet established in those days. Therefore, the photographs taken with the built-in camera were regarded as the main source for diagnosing, while the fiberscope was used as the finder of the camera. In 1966 a thinner model was introduced, which is shown in the middle of Fig. 12B. Then, the model GTF-A with an angulation mechanism (see top of Fig. 12B) was introduced. As technology advanced, a biopsy channel was added (Fig. 12C), and manufacturers started introducing various fiberscopes for the stomach.

The lighting intensity improved with the light source using glass fiber. It had also become possible to take pictures by attaching a camera onto the eyepiece. Models with a direct-forward-viewing system were created in the mid-1970s. Those so-called pan-endoscopes have remarkably advanced observation ability, with a wider view angle, brighter image, and wider angulation range at the tip (Fig. 12D). Models with a direct-forward-view system became widespread after the early 1980s and replaced side-view scopes in the late 1980s.

Colonocamera and Colonofiberscope

As use of the gastrocamera became widespread, attempts began to extend its application to the colon. In 1958, Matsunaga tried to apply the type II gastrocamera for colon examination. This attempt was aimed at recording sigmoidoscopic findings, because

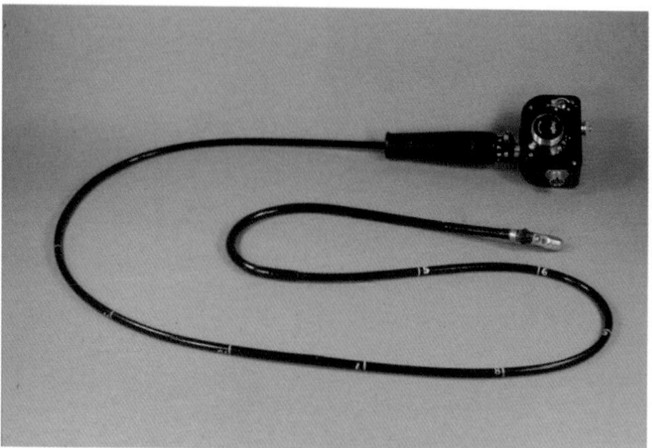

FIG. 13. Colonocamera (Niwa)

it was impossible to take pictures through the sigmoidoscope. The sigmoidcamera was projected from the tip of the rigid proctosigmoidscope to obtain photographic records.

Niwa (1960) developed a colonocamera (Fig. 13), which is an elongated version of the type V gastrocamera, to take pictures of the area of the splenic flexure for the first time. In this colonocamera, the distance between the lens and lamp is very short. It was possible to take pictures near the splenic flexure. However, because of the small numbers of pictures produced, the practical value of this apparatus was quite limited.

As practical application of the gastrofiberscope progressed, attempts were also to apply the technology to colon examination. After 1965, Niwa's group, Matsunaga's group, and Yamagata's group, respectively, worked on the study of colonoscopy. An attempt at colon observation was made by Niwa in 1965 by using a prototype fiberscope with a direct-forward-view optical system (Fig. 14A). The visual angle of this scope was 35°; there was no angulation mechanism. The shaft was very stiff, insertion into the descending colon was very difficult even in the proximal sigmoid colon, and it was not possible to obtain a good image.

The next prototype, developed by Niwa in 1966, could be used as for both forward- and side-viewing by changing the lens (Fig. 14B). However, this prototype also proved to have no practical value. The next prototype by Niwa in the same year had a rotating prism mechanism. A prism was set inside the circumferential glass window, and it could be rotated at the handle of the controlling part (Fig. 14C). However, insertion into the descending colon was difficult with this model also. Based on these experiences, the author ultimately succeeded in developing a short colonofiberscope with Olympus Medical Systems in 1968. The shaft was 67 cm long, with up-and-down angulation (Fig. 14D). The target of observation was mainly set at the sigmoid colon. This device became the basis for the Olympus SB type colonofiberscope.

In contrast, Matsunaga and his coworkers had aimed to observe the right-side segment of the colon. They developed a prototype colonoscope with a working length

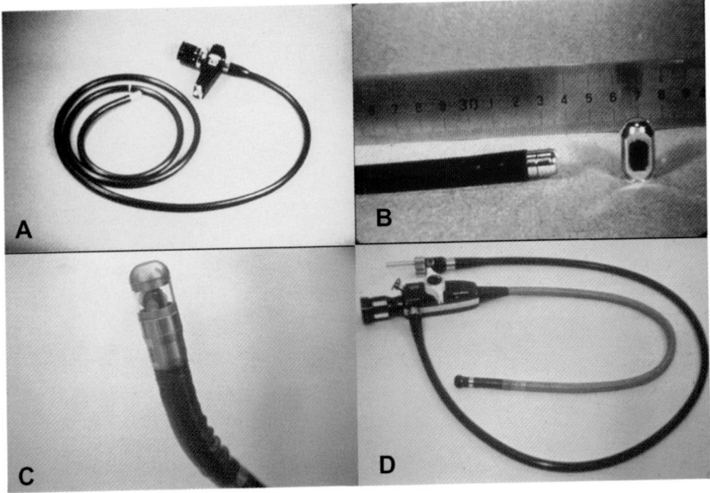

Fig. 14. A Forward-view prototype colonoscope (Niwa). B Forward and side-viewing prototype (Niwa). C Rotating prism system prototype (Niwa). D Prototype of short colonofiberscope (Niwa)

of 120 cm and four-way angulation in 1968, and extended it to 2 m in the following year; this became the basis for the LB-type long colonofiberscope of Olympus Medical Systems. Yamagata's group also developed another type of colonoscope with another company.

In Western countries, Overholt developed a prototype of the sigmoid fiberscope in 1963. He made an improved version of the fiberscope in 1967.

Videoendoscope

Development and practical application of the videoendoscope was realized owing to the progress of television technology.

The attempt to introduce television technology to endoscopy was started with an experiment to attach an image pickup device to the eyepiece of a fiberscope and observe the image formed on a TV monitor. The author started the experiments in 1964 by using three vidicon image pickup vacuum tubes based on the synchronous three-tube system with Columbia Company and Olympus Medical Systems (Fig. 15A). Because illumination was insufficient for the experiment, the author used a brighter light bulb to gain maximum light intensity, cooling with running water. However, the image gained with this device was too dark to have practical value. There was also water leakage in the shaft.

After that, with the cooperation of Victor Company, the author shifted to the frame sequential method using a 3-inch image orthicon and a light guide system for illumination, finally succeeding in development of a practically valuable device in February 1968 (Fig. 15B). The problem with this device was low operability because of direct

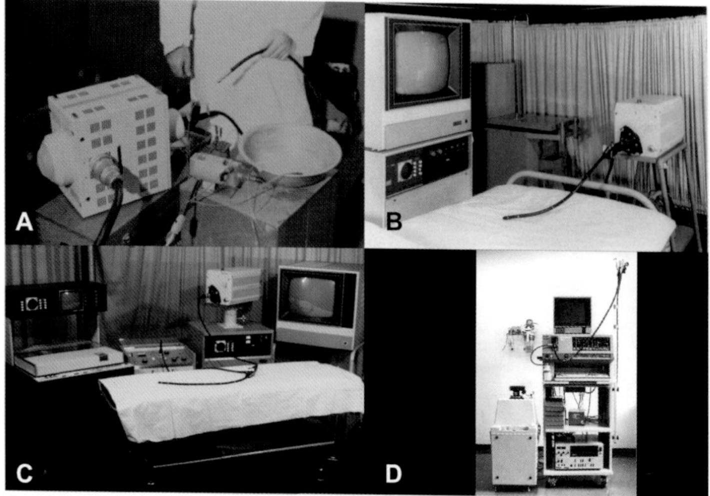

Fig. 15. **A** Synchronous three-tube system prototype (Niwa). **B** Frame sequential system with orthicon (Niwa). **C** With connecting fiber bundle (Niwa). **D** Early model of Olympus videoendoscope

connection of the videoscope to the image pickup device of the television apparatus. Addition of a connecting fiber bundle could improve operability to some extent (Fig. 15C), but the problem was that the esophagoscope was the only type equipped with a light guide system at that time. The image gained with this device was not good, so it was impossible to use for practical clinical purposes.

The CCD, or charge-coupled device, was invented in 1964. Miniaturization of the CCD made it possible to build it into an endoscope. A videoscope equipped with a CCD was first developed by Welch-Allyn Company of the United States in May 1983. Shortly after, several Japanese companies began producing commercially available models. Figure 15D shows the early model of the Olympus videoendoscope. Eventually, replacement of fiberscopes with videoscopes occurred very rapidly.

Figure 16 shows the principle of the color production system of the videoendoscope and color printing. The color production system of the videoendoscope is an additive color process and the color production system of color printing is a subtractive color process. The three primary colors in the video system are red, green, and blue. It is possible to make any color by blending these three primary colors.

There are two types of videoendoscope image reproduction systems. One is called the instantaneous single-plate color chip system (Fig. 17A).The CCD used in this system has three kinds of pixels that are designed to sense the colors of red, blue, and green, respectively. Four pixels of red (1), green (2), and blue (1) constitute a unit, and they work in a group. The other type is the single-plate RGB sequential system (Fig. 17B).

In the sequential system, there is a rotating filter with red, blue, and green colors, through which light is shone to the same CCD pixels to reproduce the three colors in

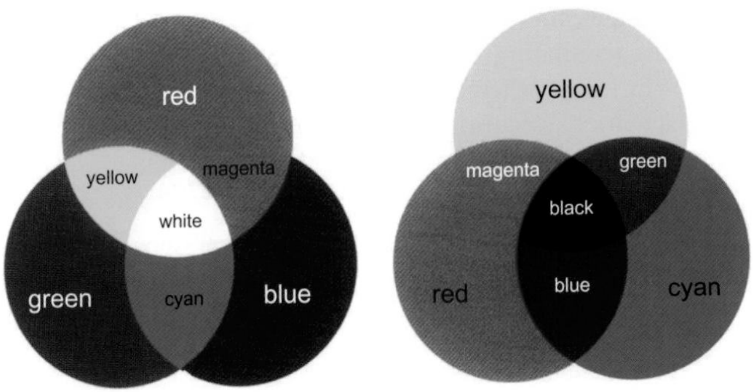

Fig. 16. Principle of color production system

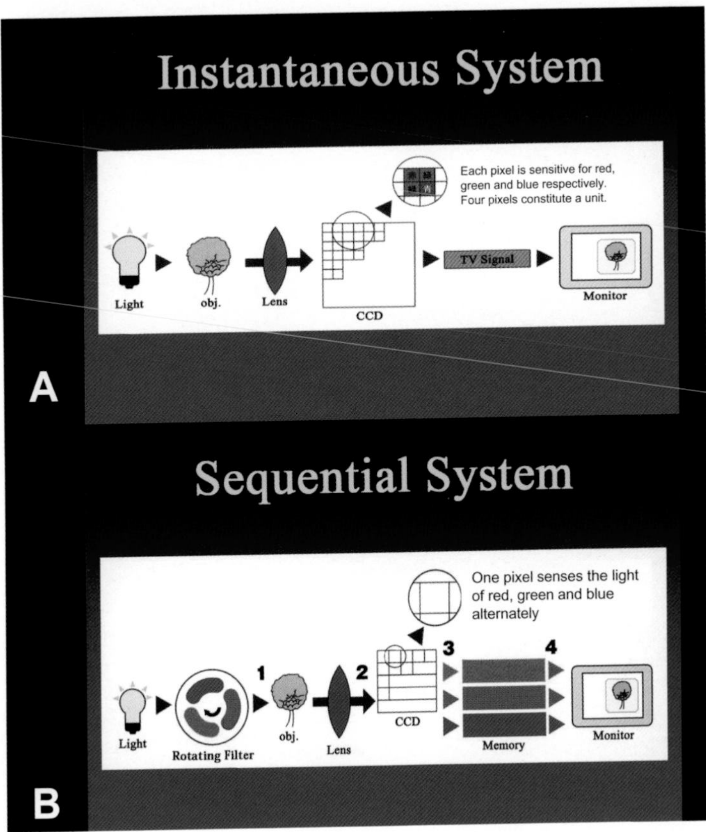

Fig. 17. Image reproduction system of videoscope

sequence. In this system, the three primary colors are sensed by any pixels on the chip by sequentially irradiating red, blue, and green light to them. The sequential system dominates in Japan, whereas the instantaneous system is prevalent in other countries. The sequential system makes more use of the advantages of videoscopes because there are wider ranges of applications. The videoendoscope allows not only picture enhancement but also various types of image processing and analysis. Also, it is also possible to apply infrared ray observation, various measurement techniques, a filing system, and so on.

Hemoglobin Index Color Enhancement

Hemoglobin index (IHb) color enhancement emphasizes color closer to hemoglobin. This system is effective in detecting subtle redness. Figure 18A shows the principle of IHb color enhancement processing. Slight differences of the red part appeared more

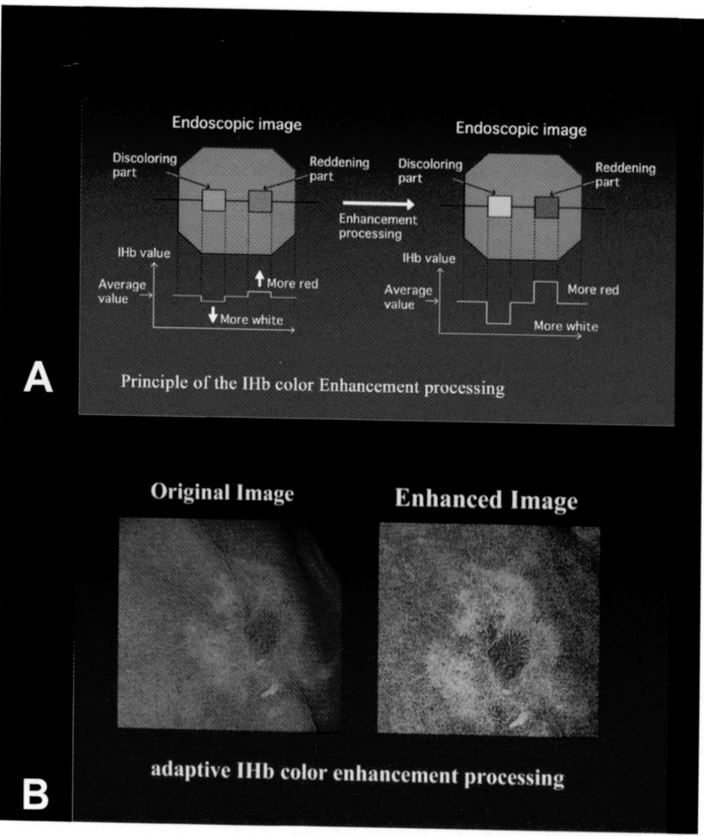

Fig. 18. Hemoglobin index color enhancement

exaggerated, and the discoloring white part appears more whitish. In Fig. 18B, the figure on the left is the original image of the red part of the lesion, and the one on the right is the enhanced image of the same lesion. The contrast of the red lesion and the whitish part appeared more exaggerated.

Adaptive Structure Enhancement

Adaptive structure enhancement emphasizes the high-frequency component wave. Through this process, it is possible to enhance the structure clearly at the obtained distance, while it can be effective to enhance the detailed pattern for close-up observation.

Figure 19A shows the effect of color and structure enhancement, the upper view being the original and the lower views images of this procedure. The contour and

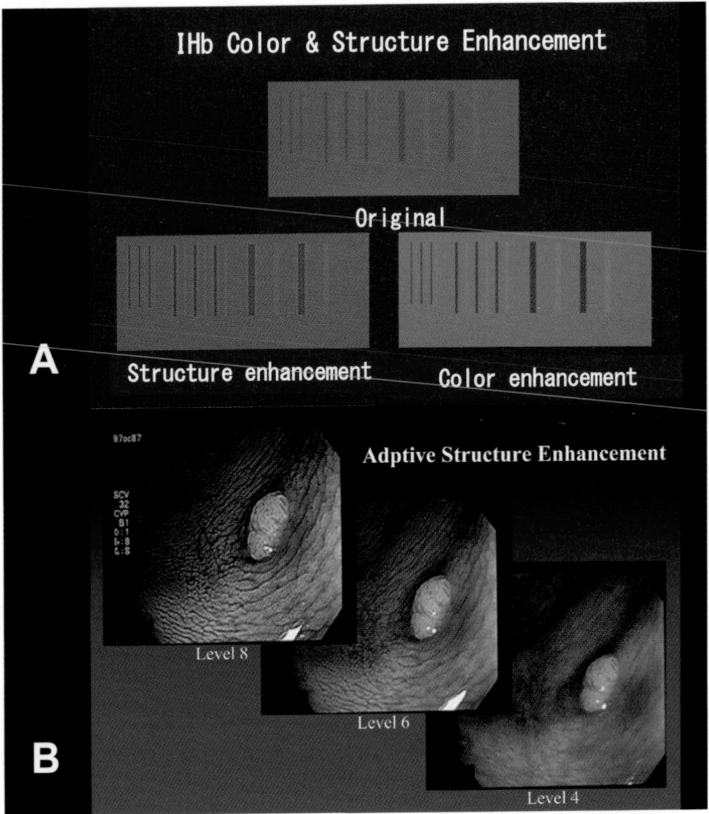

Fig. 19. Adaptive structure enhancement

color of the bars are shown clearly in the processing pictures. Figure 19B shows the images produced by this method. By such processing, the contour of the lesion and the condition of the mucosal surface are clearly revealed with level 8 enhancement.

Infrared Ray Videoendoscope

Figure 20A is a comparison of the human eye and a CCD. The CCD is sensitive not only to visible light but also to infrared ray. Figure 20B shows the difference in light penetration rate through human buccal tissue depending on different wavelengths of light. It shows that light of around 1100 nm penetrates human tissue best.

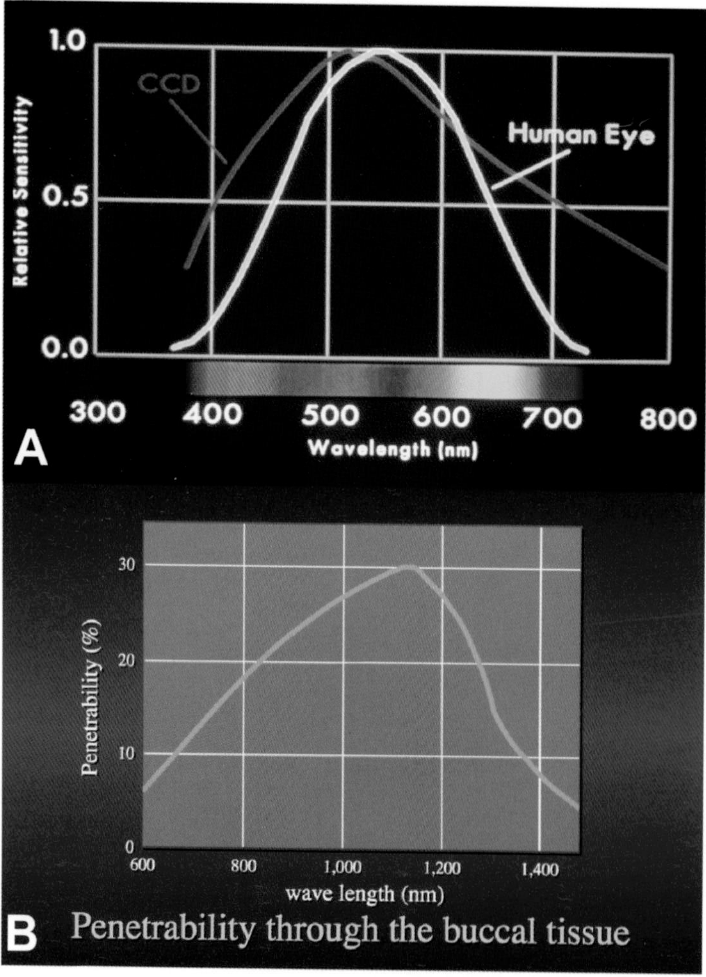

Fig. 20. Comparison of human eye and charge-coupled device (CCD)

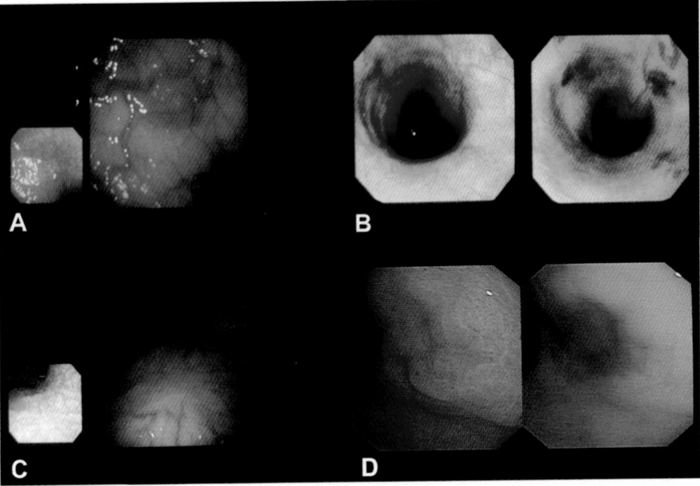

Fig. 21. Infrared ray videoendoscope. **A** Inside of human stomach. **B** Solitary varices of the esophagus. **C** Gastric ulcer scar. **D** Early gastric cancer

The pictures in Fig. 21A show the inside of the stomach. With injection of indocyanine green (ICG), which absorbs infrared rays well, vessels in deeper layers can be described precisely. The picture on the left was taken under ordinary illumination, and the picture on the right was taken under infrared ray. With infrared, it becomes possible to observe blood vessels beneath the mucosa. The liver is also visible. In the case of solitary varices of the esophagus, the varices appear clearly in the infrared pictures (Fig. 21B). Figure 21C pictures an ulcer scar under infrared rays. No blood vessels are observed at the scar area.

It is also known that there are special findings in early cancer cases. The figure on the left in Fig. 21D is an image under ordinary lighting whereas that on the right is an image gained through the infrared ray. The lesion of early cancer appears as a blue area.

Narrow-Band Imaging

Recently, narrow-band imaging has attracted much attention as a new frontier of endoscopy. This is a technology combining the permeation properties of light, which vary depending on the range of wavelength, and false color display.

About 50 years ago, that is, the age of the intragastric gastrocamera, the preliminary experiments using a surgically isolated specimen had been done by the author's group at the University of Tokyo. In Fig. 22A, the photograph on the left was taken under normal light and that on the right by ultraviolet light. The picture taken under ultraviolet light shows details of the border of early gastric cancer, with loss of folds, and the mamillatedsurface of the gastric antrum looks like a formalin-fixed specimen. The

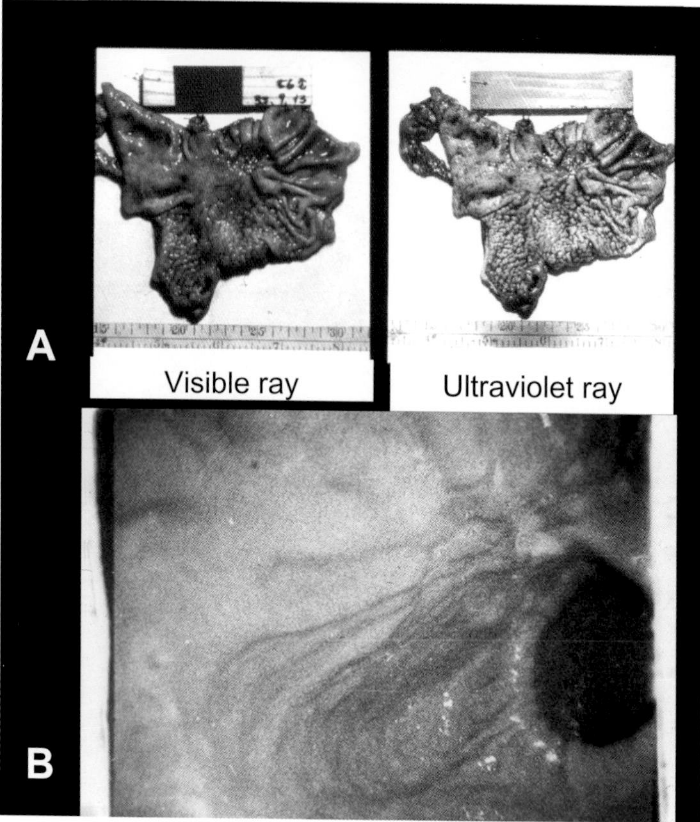

Fig. 22. **A** Effect of ultraviolet ray imaging in resected stomach. **B** Picture taken using ultraviolet ray gastrocamera

ultraviolet ray mostly reflected off the mucosal surface because of its low rate of penetration. Therefore, the fine structure of the mucosal surface is vividly depicted.

Based on these experiments, the author's group developed an intragastric ultraviolet ray gastrocamera. Figure 22B shows an early gastric cancer case recorded by the ultraviolet gastrocamera. The contour of early cancer (IIc) with abrupt cessation of folds is clearly described. However, the ultraviolet ray gastrocamera was discarded because of its high-voltage electricity requirements and also for fear of harm caused to the human body by ultraviolet rays. However, as the dye spray method had not yet been introduced and biopsy technique had not been established, the ultraviolet gastrocamera was an effective method at that time. Therefore, I believe this ultraviolet gastrocamera was the forerunner of narrow-band imaging (NBI).

Observation under blue ray provides information about the shallow layers of mucosa, whereas observation under red rays, which have a high penetration rate to the mucosa, provides information on the deeper layers. NBI was developed with a

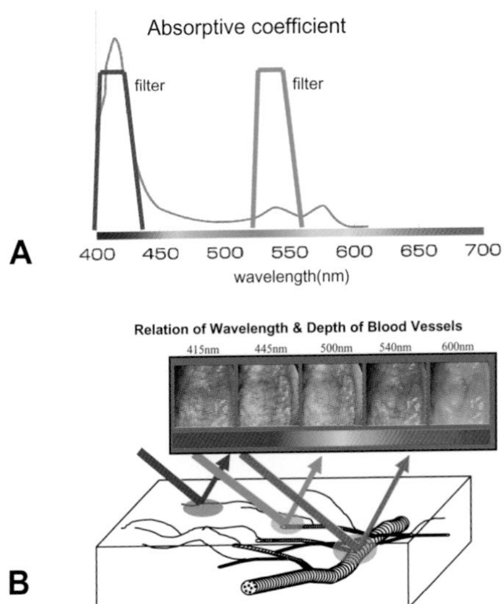

Fig. 23. **A** Absorptive coefficient in various wavelengths. **B** Relationship of wavelength and blood vessels

view to acquire detailed information on mucosal surfaces making use of the nature of short wavelengths of light.

Hemoglobin absorbs wavelengths of 415 nm and 540 nm best among the visible light spectra (Fig. 23A). The rate of scattering of light is dependent on wavelength, and it diminishes as the wavelength becomes longer from the short blue wavelengths to the longer red wavelengths. Therefore, light of a longer wavelength tends to penetrate deeper into body tissue. If the spectrum of the light source is narrowed down to around 415 nm, the light is absorbed efficiently by hemoglobin in capillary vessels in the superficial layer, which enables depicting images of the capillary vessels vividly. On the other hand, if the light source is kept around 540 nm, it is possible to visualize blood vessels in the submucosal layer. Figure 23B shows the relationship of wavelength of light and depth of blood vessels.

The NBI endoscopy devices are equipped with two NBI filters of 415 and 540 nm, respectively, placed between the RGB rotation filter and the light source. When the filters are inserted in the light path, NBI observation becomes available (Fig. 24A). To display an endoscopic image on a TV monitor, the image at 415 nm is allocated mainly to the blue and green channels of the videoscope, and the image at 540 nm is allotted to the red channel to display as a false color.

Today's NBI system is designed to describe the brightness variation of the capillary vessels in the mucosal surface as the contrast patterns of brownish-red color and to describe the blood vessels in a deeper layer as the cyan color gradation. In this case (Fig. 24B), the superficial capillaries appear brown and the submucosal vessels appear blue.

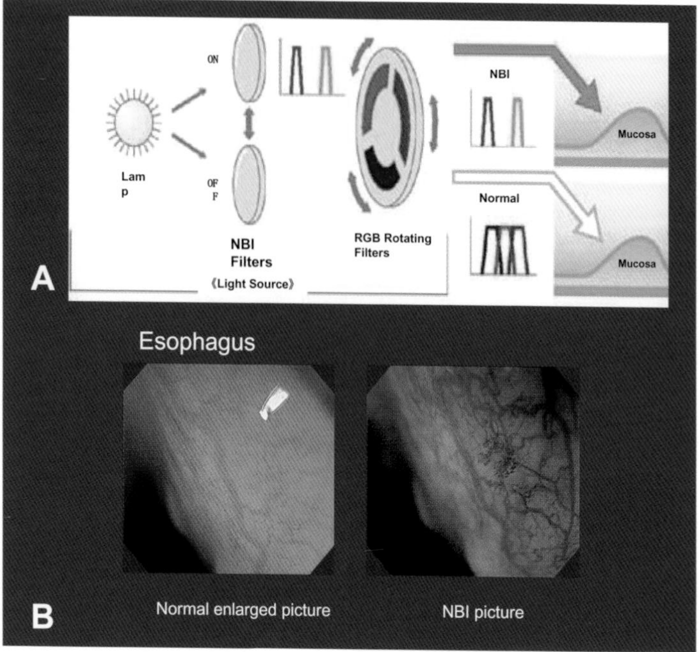

FIG. 24. **A** System of narrow-band imaging (NBI) endoscopy. **B** Picture using NBI endoscopy. (Photograph courtesy of Dr. H. Inoue)

In diagnosis of diseases in the gastrointestinal tract, especially in early cancer cases, abnormalities first appear in the capillary vessels on the mucosal surface. Observation of capillary vessels in the superficial layer is very important for early detection of cancer.

Autofluorescence Imaging

Recently, autofluorescence imaging (AFI) has attracted much attention. Fluorescence is a phenomenon observed when a substance emits a part or the whole of the light energy, so that once it is absorbed, usually the fluorescence wavelength becomes longer than that of the original exciting light.

This technology was already tried by our group using a gastrocamera. In the basic studies by the author using surgically resected specimens (Fig. 25A), autofluorescence appears in pale blue. Fluorescence was not detected in gastric ulcers, erosions, or bleeding areas. On the right in Fig. 25B, taken with a fluorescent gastrocamera, early gastric cancer is seen on the lesser curvature of the gastric angle. No fluorescence is observed in the lesion. The autofluorescence of gastric mucosa being quite weak, and

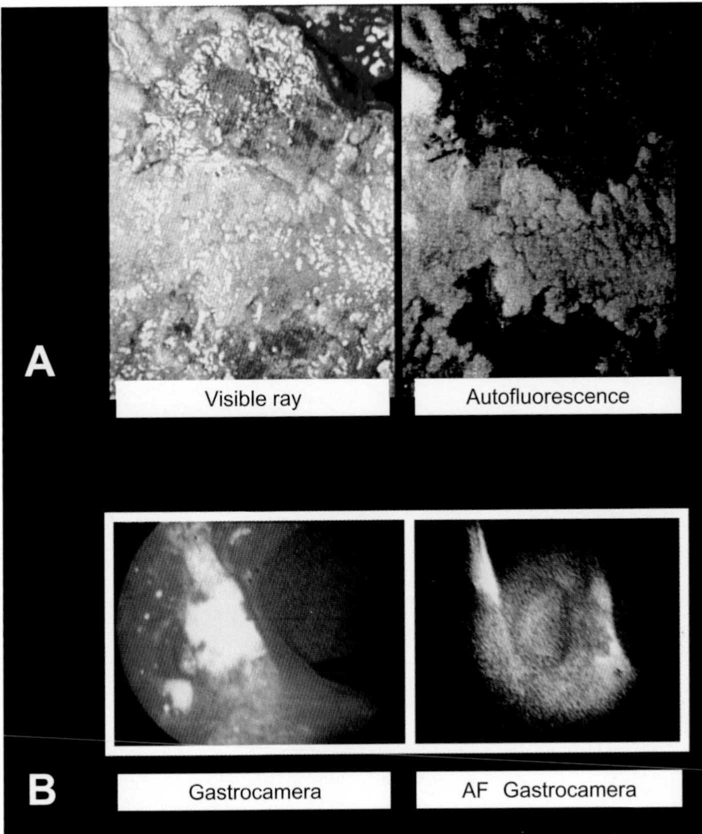

Fig. 25. **A** Autofluorescence in surgically resected stomach compared to visible light. **B** Autofluorescence (*AF*) gastrocamera

sensitivity of the film being low, it required intensifying treatment to obtain this picture, making the picture very rough in resolution. However, it is observed that no fluorescence is seen in the legion of the IIc type early cancer. Autofluorescence imaging of today is based on the same principle.

Figure 26A shows the relationship of illumination and autofluorescence. The left side shows the spectrum of exciting light and on the right is the spectrum of autofluorescence. Fluorescence has a longer wavelength than the exciting light. The upper view is normal tissue and the lower is adenoma of the colon: note that tumor tissue has weak fluorescence compared with normal colon tissue. In recent videoendoscopes, a unit for fluorescence observation has been developed. On the monitor, normal tissue appears green and tumor tissue appears red (Fig. 26B) because tumor tissue has fewer blue color elements as a result of its weak fluorescence.

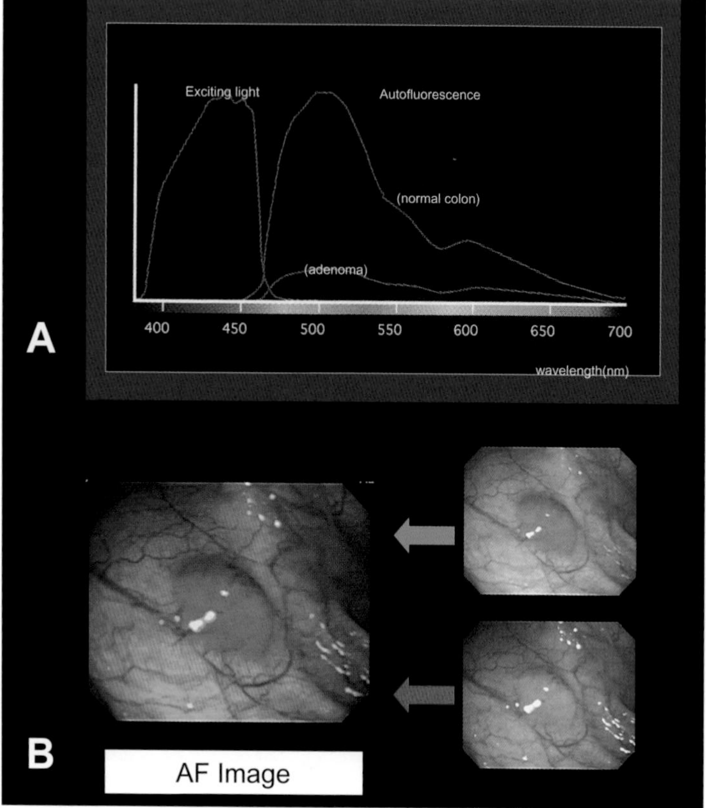

Fig. 26. **A** Relationship of exciting light and fluorescence. **B** Autofluorescence imaging (AFI)

Liquid Crystal Monitor

A Braun tube, as in a TV monitor, is quite large and the depth of the apparatus is very great. Recently, a liquid crystal monitor has appeared. The liquid crystal monitor is thin compared with an ordinary Braun tube monitor. There are many colored small filters on the surface of the liquid crystal monitor. Illumination is accomplished by light through a liquid crystal from the back of the filters. The monitor of the future is probably a liquid crystal monitor instead of a Braun tube.

Future Prospects of Endoscopy

Reviewing the history of development of endoscope, we note that every 30 to 50 years a revolutionary new invention has been seen (Fig. 27). The author presumes the videoscope would continue to take the dominant role in the 21st century. However, a

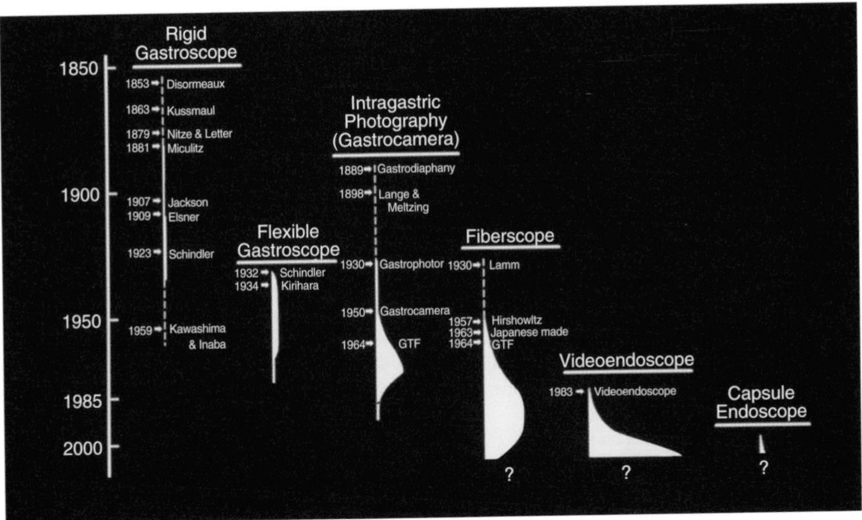

Fig. 27. History of the development of endoscopes

new technology that has potential to replace the videoendoscope in future is capsule endoscopy.

A capsule endoscope for the small intestine was introduced by an Israeli company in 2000. All the published pictures were narrow range and taken very close to the glass surface on the tip. At present, therefore, this device is by no means effective to observe the stomach, although it has been experimentally applied in the colon. However, the author believes the capsule endoscope is the one new technology that has potential to replace the videoscope in future.

Epilogue

In the history of endoscopy, new facts have never appeared suddenly. As old things become improved, new facts are discovered, influenced by development of other fields of technology. The Japanese novelist Yasushi Inoue often quoted a phrase to the effect that nothing can be achieved by forcing its culture, but that accomplishments should be grown gradually just as spring sunshine grows a seed to bud, seedling, leaf, and flower to fruit. I think this is the same in the field of endoscopy.

Looking back at the history of endoscopy, we notice that studies tried by earlier researchers are tried later in different forms over and over again. By refocusing on old studies, new facts are often discovered. The ancient Chinese philosopher Confucius taught the importance of consulting old things to know new things. This wisdom holds true perfectly for endoscopy.

For Further Reading

1. Niwa H (1997) The history of gastrointestinal endoscopy. Nihon Medical Center, Tokyo
2. Edmonson JM (1991) History of the instruments for gastrointestinal endoscopy. Gastrointest Endosc 37:27–56
3. Vilardell F (2006) Digestive endoscopy in the second millennium. Thieme, Stuttgart
4. Schindler R (1950) Gastroscopy: the endoscopic study of gastric pathology, 2nd edn. University of Chicago Press, Chicago
5. Lange F, Meltzing (1898) Die Photographie des Mageninnern. Münch Med Wochenschr 45:1585–1588
6. Heilpern J, Porges O (1930) Ber die Gastrophotogrraphie, eine neue Untersuchungsmethode. Klin Wochenschr 9:15–17
7. Niwa H (1996) The history and future prospects of digestive endoscopic medicine in Japan. Third bulletin. The Asian-Pacific Society for Digestive Endoscopy, Tokyo, Japan, pp 69–80
8. Ashizawa S, Sakita T, Niwa H, et al (1959) Gastrocamera. Ogata-shoten, Tokyo
9. Niwa H, Kaneko E, Umeda N (1975) Endoscopic diagnosis of gastric diseases. Nankodo, Tokyo
10. Niwa H, Utsumi Y, Nakamura T, et al (1966) Endoscopy of the colon. Proceedings of the First Congress of the International Society of Endoscopy, 16–18 Sep, Tokyo, pp 425–431
11. Niwa H, Fujino M, Yoshitoshi Y (1972) Colonic fiberscopy for routine practice. Advances in gastrointestinal endoscopy. Piccin, Padua, pp 549–555
12. Niwa H, Sakai Y, Williams CB (2003) History of endoscopy in the rectum and colon. In: Waye JD, Rex JK, Williams CB (eds) Colonoscopy: principles and practice. Blackwell, Malden, pp 1–20
13. Classen M, Philip J (1984) Electric endoscopy of the gastrointestinal tract. Initial experience with a new type of endoscope that has no fiberoptic bundle for imaging. Endoscopy 16:16–19
14. Niwa H, Kawaguchi A, Miyahara T, et al (1992) Clinical use of new video-endoscopes (EVIS 100 and 200). Endoscopy 24:187–238

Advances in Endoscopic Imaging and Diagnosis: Toward Molecular Imaging

Hisao Tajiri

Summary. Molecular imaging has been formally defined as the detection, spatial localization, and quantification of specific molecular targets and events that form the basis of various pathologies. Cancer is the greatest target in the short-term tasks of molecular imaging, and molecular imaging is important in various aspects of tackling this target. As image-enhanced endoscopy, narrow-band imaging (NBI) can provide morphological data to show changes in the morphology of the target and is particularly useful for obtaining images of the mucous surface layer with enhanced microvascular structures. Autofluorescence imaging (AFI) allows observation of morphological changes in terms of fluorescence intensity. Ultrahigh-magnification endoscopy such as the microscopic or confocal method allows real-time observation and diagnosis of changes in cellular structure within the body. In contrast, endoscopic molecular imaging is a procedure by which changes in quality, in terms of fluorescence intensity, are observed, and which allows acquisition of higher-level information in a simple form. As for endoscopic molecular imaging, exploration of markers, development of probes, and adequate imaging devices are three keys to clinical application. Not only molecular biological findings but also points of contact with various engineering techniques are extremely important for making progress in molecular imaging. Cooperation among the medical, engineering, and industrial fields has been advocated. In addition, cooperation with the fields of pharmaceutical sciences and biology is also necessary.

Key words. Bioendoscopy, Molecular imaging, Narrow-band imaging, Autofluorescence imaging, Near-infrared optical imaging

Introduction

Gastroenterology is a relatively new specialty among the various disciplines in medicine, but it has witnessed tremendous progress over the past 25 years. In the field of endoscopy, remarkable advances in nanotechnology are driving the tendency toward

Division of Gastroenterology and Hepatology, Department of Internal Medicine, The Jikei University School of Medicine, 3-25-8 Nishishinbashi, Minato-ku, Tokyo 105-8461, Japan

minimizing every element and mechanism involved to a microlevel. In the 21st century, capsule-type endoscopes are expected to be developed, to play a significant role in the screening and treatment of various diseases. The age of "bioendoscopy" is also expected to begin in the near future, when endoscopes will be used for evaluation of the pathophysiological features of disease to provide a diagnosis.

Science and technology fields that have produced great innovations in modern medicine include diagnostic imaging and molecular biology. Molecular imaging evolving from these bases is currently attracting considerable attention. Molecular imaging has been formally defined as the detection, spatial localization, and quantification of specific molecular targets and events that form the basis of various pathologies [1]. The scientific field of molecular imaging is broadly divided into the following two categories: ex vivo imaging of cells and tissues and in vivo imaging of organs, small animals, and humans. The latter is concerned with visualization of events taking place in the body, with consideration of medical applications in the future, using mostly medical diagnostic imaging techniques such as magnetic resonance imaging (MRI), single photon emission computed tomography (SPECT), positron emission tomography (PET), and in vivo fluorescence and luminescence imaging techniques.

X-ray, CT, and MRI have provided useful morphological diagnostic approaches for functional diagnosis, and the active stages of SPECT and PET have changed from functional to metabolic diagnosis. The evolution of functional MRI and PET has enabled elucidation of higher brain functions and imaging of molecular functions. It is expected that, by extension, molecular imaging will serve as a fundamental technology for evaluating gene therapy and developing new drugs in the near future.

Purpose of Molecular Imaging

Now that the human genome analysis is almost complete, there will be evolutionary progress toward multiple healthcare technologies consisting of a complex of science and technology in various multidisciplinary fields ranging from the molecular or gene level, with a scale of several dozen nanometers, to the tissue or organ level and to virtual human science at the individual level. Molecular imaging has the potential of achieving direct observation of the expressions of gene functions in gene therapy. In addition, the use of various molecular imaging approaches in specific functional imaging appears to be promising. In the field of clinical medicine, the structure and function of proteins produced by the gene rather than the gene information per se are more likely to yield direct clues to understanding a disease.

Molecular imaging aims to visualize the time course of organic activity at the molecular level by utilizing various imaging techniques and thereby elucidating the meaning of the molecular mechanisms in life science. The data obtained by molecular imaging not only facilitate the elucidation of molecular mechanisms but also form the basis for diagnosis. Molecular imaging can provide findings that serve as seeds for further progress in medical sciences, including the development of new drugs and applications to drug delivery approaches. To obtain tangible molecular images, neural transmission or receptor imaging, antibody/peptide imaging, and gene imaging using antisense or reporter genes have been tried under the concept of molecular imaging as a form of specific functional imaging.

Molecular imaging can progress in the following two directions: (1) visualization of particular targeted molecules in the body, and (2) microscale visualization at the cellular level. Technological development and research should be advanced in both directions. In addition, visualization of time-course changes by dynamic molecular imaging is an important factor.

Conventional radionuclide imaging (particularly PET) is a promising strategy for achieving the first aforementioned goal, and major future tasks may include the development of tracers or other agents rather than imaging techniques. As to the second direction of research just noted, development of imaging techniques themselves is necessary. Instead of the conventional MRI, a new mode of MR, such as magnetic resonance spectroscopic imaging (MRSI), is attracting hopes and expectations.

Advances in Endoscopic Imaging

Detailed observation of the mucosa is an essential component of diagnostic and therapeutic endoscopy. A high-definition (HD)-TV processor (Olympus Medical Systems, Tokyo, Japan) was introduced for this purpose. This new system, in which scopes with a substantially increased number of pixels and a HD-TV signal processing technique are employed, yields very high resolution images. If this processor were used in combination with a HD-TV-compatible monitor, the information obtained could be expected to increase even further, because very clear endoscopic images would be obtained in which even small blood vessels and details of the mucosal surface would be reproduced quite faithfully. "Structural enhancement" and "adaptive index of hemoglobin (IHb) color enhancement" have been employed in endoscopic image analysis. Advances in these processing techniques, as well as the development of other image-processing technologies, may be expected to markedly improve endoscopic diagnosis, almost comparable to histopathological examination. It is expected that these techniques may eventually allow automated endoscopic diagnosis [2].

Magnifying electronic endoscopes currently used clinically have outer diameters and manipulability comparable to those of ordinary electronic endoscopes, have a magnifying power of about ×80 to ×100, and yield information on minute mucosal patterns and capillary abnormalities, which are thought to be reflective of structural atypism [3]. In endoscopic evaluation of the squamous epithelium of the esophagus, magnifying endoscopes have been used for distinguishing malignant tumors from benign diseases, as well as for evaluating the depth of tumor invasion on the basis of the information obtained regarding the morphological changes in the intrapapillary capillary loop (IPCL) [4]. Magnifying endoscopy seems to be particularly useful for the diagnosis of colorectal tumors. These endoscopes allow stereoscopic observation of living tissues and reveal even minute patterns on the gastrointestinal mucosa.

One of the new endoscope systems is the narrow-band imaging (NBI) system (Olympus Medical Systems). We applied this NBI system in combination with magnifying electronic endoscopy to observe the mucosal surface and reported that the visualization of capillary patterns specific to cancer was useful to distinguish minute cancers from benign lesions, to evaluate the histological type and degree of differentiation of cancer, and to precisely determine the extent of cancer [5–7]. Methods of functional imaging and analysis via endoscopes are also developing rapidly. Efforts are ongoing to develop and evaluate fluorescence-based diagnostic technologies for the detection of premalignant and early-stage malignant lesions in many organs. These techniques exploit either naturally occurring autofluorescence (AF) from endogenous fluorophores or fluorescence caused by an exogenously administered fluorescent drug, for example, 5-aminolevulinic acid. We have studied only AF emitted from endogenous fluorophores, and clarified that collagen, which fluoresces in the green wavelength range, is one of the major sources of tissue AF. It is important to take into account tissue changes in addition to changes in gross tissue morphology [8]. These tissue changes may include alterations in local blood volume, tissue metabolic activity, and relative fluorophore concentrations. There is already considerable evidence that AF endoscopy has promise for diagnosis of early carcinomas and premalignant lesions in the gastrointestinal tract as an adjunct to conventional endoscopy [9]. In particular, it has good potential for identifying small or flat tumors and tumor margins, as well as premalignant lesions, and for assessing grade and tumor response to therapy.

Optical coherence tomography (OCT), in which weak infrared rays are applied to the tissue, allows noncontact and noninvasive visualization of the cross-sectional structures of tissues at a precision close to that of loupe images. In contrast to ultrasonography, which uses sound echoes, OCT uses near-infrared rays (1300 nm) for exploration, and a resolution of 10–20 μm can be achieved by utilizing interference. Histological typing of cancer is based on the evaluation of structural atypism and cellular atypism. It is expected that endoscopy using a confocal endomicroscope would yield visual information also useful for the evaluation of cellular atypism. This endoscope, using laser and optical technology, allows living tissues to be visualized at the cellular level, because the scope can yield images as valuable as histopathological findings within the living body [10,11]. With this system, changes in the cell structure can be observed immediately, mitigating the need for histopathological examination of biopsy specimens (Figs. 1, 2). Thus, the lesion can be evaluated in its entirety, even at the microscopic level, during endoscopy, often making qualitative diagnosis possible. This system is changing the conventional concept of endoscopy.

More recently, an endocytoscopy system has been developed that yields magnified optical endoscope images (images magnified 500 to 1000 fold)[12]. This system allows reliable clinical imaging. When combined with methylene blue staining, for example, identification of even cellular nuclei may become possible. Endoscopy using this system has revealed that this system is capable of resolving the characteristics of cancer cells (distorted nuclei and increased N/C ratio) and other visual information indispensable for the evaluation of cellular atypism. Improvement in function, such as confocal endomicroscopy and endocytoscopy, allows practical implementation of intraoperatively histological diagnosis, leading to the integration of diagnosis and treatment [13].

In this closely approaching age of "bioendoscopy," it is expected that, in addition to morphological diagnosis using conventional endoscopes, the pathophysiology of diseases will also be elucidated through endoscopic evaluation of lesions at the cellular level using an ultra-magnifying endoscope, and that functional diagnosis will be made using devices such as a fluorescent endoscope or infrared fluorescent endoscope [14].

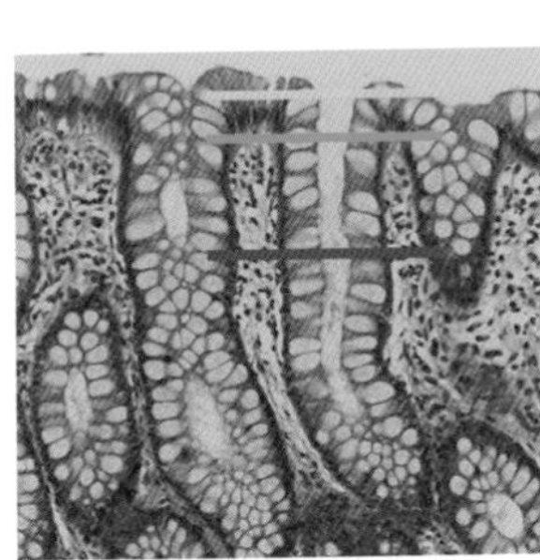

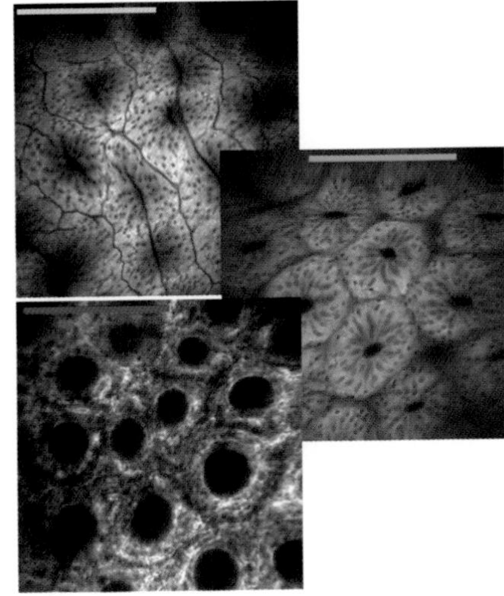

Fig. 1. Confocal endomicroscopy images and light micrograph with hematoxylin and eosin (H&E) staining show surface layer (*yellow*), intermediate layer (*green*), and deep (*blue*) layer in the normal large intestine (FOV = 500 μm)

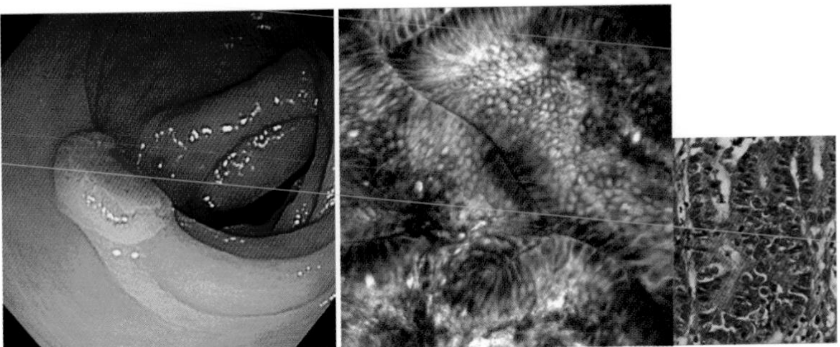

Fig. 2. Conventional endoscopic image (*left*) and confocal endomicroscopy image (*middle*) of early colon cancer. Light micrograph with H&E staining (*right*) shows moderately differentiated adenocarcinoma (FOV = 500 μm)

Recently, endoscopic examinations with new imaging techniques in addition to conventional endoscopic imaging are being performed increasingly, as described earlier. Consequently, various terms have been used for these imaging techniques, causing confusion and misunderstanding. Therefore, we would like to propose the term image-enhanced endoscopy and the new object-oriented classification of endoscopic imaging, as shown in Tables 1 and 2. [15]

Table 1. Object-oriented classification of endoscopic imaging.

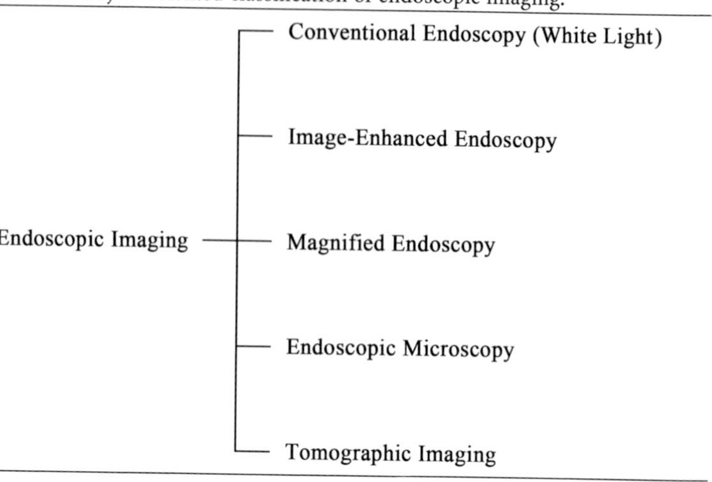

Endoscopic Imaging	Conventional Endoscopy (White Light)
	Image-Enhanced Endoscopy
	Magnified Endoscopy
	Endoscopic Microscopy
	Tomographic Imaging

Table 2. Object-oriented further detailed classification of endoscopic imaging.

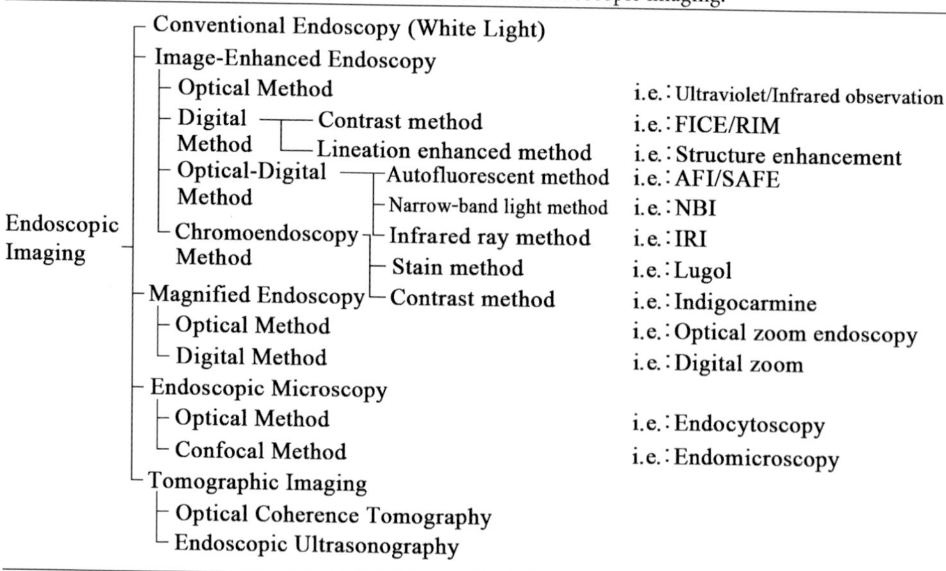

Endoscopic Imaging	Conventional Endoscopy (White Light)			
	Image-Enhanced Endoscopy	Optical Method		i.e.: Ultraviolet/Infrared observation
		Digital Method	Contrast method	i.e.: FICE/RIM
			Lineation enhanced method	i.e.: Structure enhancement
		Optical-Digital Method	Autofluorescent method	i.e.: AFI/SAFE
			Narrow-band light method	i.e.: NBI
			Infrared ray method	i.e.: IRI
		Chromoendoscopy Method	Stain method	i.e.: Lugol
			Contrast method	i.e.: Indigocarmine
	Magnified Endoscopy	Optical Method		i.e.: Optical zoom endoscopy
		Digital Method		i.e.: Digital zoom
	Endoscopic Microscopy	Optical Method		i.e.: Endocytoscopy
		Confocal Method		i.e.: Endomicroscopy
	Tomographic Imaging	Optical Coherence Tomography		
		Endoscopic Ultrasonography		

FICE, Fujinon (flexible) imaging color enhancement; RIM, real-time image mapping, AFI, autofluorescence imaging; IRI, infrared imaging; SAFE, simultaneous autofluorescence endoscopy; NBI, narrow-band imaging

Near-Infrared Optical Imaging

The near-infrared (NIR) region of the electromagnetic spectrum is immediately adjacent to the visible spectrum, which extends from violet to red. NIR imaging offers a number of important advantages. There is less autofluorescence in the NIR compared with visible wavelengths; the decreased background improves visibility (the target-to-background ratio) of exogenously administered fluorochromes [16]. It is also possible to split light across different wavelengths, similar to a prism, allowing true simultaneous imaging of the full spectrum of visible light and NIR light. The anatomic view that surgeons are currently accustomed to using is maintained, while a second camera records fluorescence that is generated by molecular reporters.

The other vital components to molecular optical imaging are the imaging agents. There are three general classes of imaging probes: nonspecific agents, targeted agents, and smart probes. Fluorescent versions of all three have been used extensively in preclinical studies. The smart probes have been particularly promising for lesion detection. This class of optical imaging agents increases fluorescence after interacting with specific proteolytic enzymes, such as cathepsins [17].

Imaging of cathepsin protease activity has resulted in improved detection of neoplasia in preclinical models including models of ovarian cancer and transitional cell carcinoma of the bladder. This approach was also tested for imaging of murine models of intestinal adenomas and demonstrated improved ex vivo detection of noninvasive polyps as small as 50 μm in diameter. NIR light can be separated into several distinct wavelength bands that can independently record distinct molecular activities, each reported by different fluorochromes [18]. Mahmood and Upadhyat [16] have applied this multiparameter approach to evaluate colonic adenomas and adenocarcinomas in terms of protease activity and lesion perfusion, to help noninvasively segregate lesions between these groups. The protease imaging agents and endoscopic systems are both clinically translatable, and clinical trials for colonoscopy are expected to begin in the next few years. Initial preclinical work suggests that the approach may also be effective in detecting adenocarcinomas in the setting of colitis, based on differential protease expression between the sites of neoplasia and inflammation.

Apart from protease-activatable probes, there are a number of other targeted and nonspecific optical probes applicable to the detection and therapy management of colorectal cancer. One notable example is the optical analogue to the intravascular MRI agents. These compounds are fluorescently labeled macromolecules that maintain a long blood half-life. Such fluorescent blood pool agents are especially useful for determining the vascular volume fraction of known tumors. This type of imaging has been shown in preclinical models to noninvasively assess vascular changes after antiangiogenic therapy.

Hama et al. [19] have shown that it is possible to develop a family of imaging probes based on a two-step activation schema in which the first step is the administration of a targeted biotinylated antibody and the second step is the administration of an activatable fluorophore, which remains the same regardless of the targeting antibody. This method benefits from a target amplification effect because approximately ten biotin molecules are anti-HER1 (human epidermal growth factor receptor type 1), and can bind up to 10 NeutrAvidin-conjugated BODIPY-FL (nAv-BDPfl) molecules, greatly amplifying the net fluorescence. Taken together with the 10-fold activation of fluorescence by biotin binding, this method has the potential to achieve a signal-to-background ratio about 100 fold higher compared with the use of a nonbiotinylated antibody–fluorophore conjugate. In addition, this method does not require the enzymatic activation or biological clearance of unbound reagents or internalization of the nAv-BDPfl complex. Thus, this method has the potential to be highly specific and highly sensitive for the detection of tiny cancer deposits.

Goal of Molecular Imaging

Cancer is the greatest target in the short-term tasks of molecular imaging, and molecular imaging is important in various aspects of tackling this target. Although ^{18}F-fluorodeoxyglucose (FDG), which is applicable to human subjects, is currently becoming the gold standard marker in cancer diagnosis, various other procedures are also possible. It is necessary to extend the knowledge obtained in cell biology to imaging technology, leading to the development of a new contrast agent. In connection with metastasis of cancer cells, much remains unclear about in vivo cell–cell association. Successful imaging of the association seems to allow the elucidation of mechanisms of cancer metastasis and progression. In addition, molecular imaging is important for molecular therapy and gene therapy. It is necessary to make full use of reporter genes. There are two methods of molecular imaging using gene expression, that is, the antisense method and the reporter gene method.

If we unite the results of research on genes and newly found receptors with imaging technology, and combine various imaging methods, it becomes possible to visualize dynamic processes in the body. Then, it is expected that information on genes, put to good use, will allow diagnosis and evaluation of various diseases and facilitate observation of the distribution of drugs used for treatment of these diseases.

Optical technologies, particularly those using near-infrared rays, have recently been making remarkable advances. Application of these techniques may allow us to obtain topographic views with the light from substances in the body, and this would facilitate the application of various reporter genes. Although PET is not practical because of the issue of radiation exposure, optical technology enables continuous observation of lasting changes in the subject. PET has the advantage of high sensitivity, whereas MRI has the advantages of superior spatial and temporal resolution and high tissue contrast. On the other hand, optical imaging benefits from high resolution, real-time imaging, and the ability to image multiple molecular targets simultaneously. Moreover, advances in the design of optical molecular probes have paved the way for the application of this technology to detection and monitoring of pathophysiological process such as cancer, atherosclerosis, and inflammation [20].

Toward Realization of Endoscopic Molecular Imaging

As image-enhanced endoscopy, NBI can provide morphological data to show changes in the morphology of the target and is particularly useful for obtaining images of the mucous surface layer with enhanced microvascular structures. Autofluorescence imaging (AFI) allows observation of morphological changes in terms of fluorescence intensity. Ultrahigh-magnification endoscopy, such as the microscopic or confocal method, allows real-time observation and diagnosis of changes in cellular structure within the body. In contrast, endoscopic molecular imaging is a procedure by which changes in quality, in terms of fluorescence intensity, are observed, and which allows acquisition of higher-level information in a simple form. As for endoscopic molecular imaging, exploration of markers, development of probes, and adequate imaging devices are three keys to clinical application (Fig. 3). The currently possible target molecules are those shown in Table 3, and research is progressing rapidly in the context of the current international rivalry.

Not only molecular biological findings but also points of contact with various engineering techniques are extremely important for making progress in molecular imaging. Cooperation among the medical, engineering, and industrial fields has been advocated. Cooperation with the fields of pharmaceutical sciences and biology is also necessary. Thus, we must aggressively work toward research and development of these healthcare technologies that hold the promise of playing important roles for the next generation.

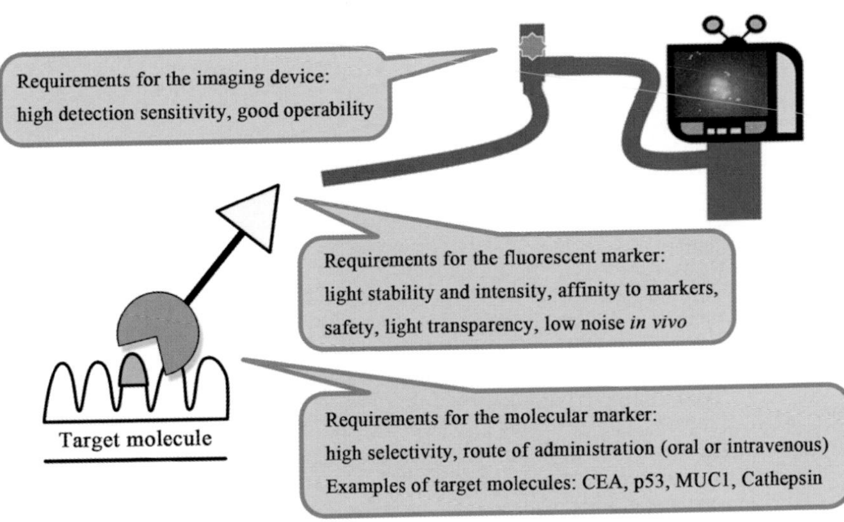

Fig. 3. Conditions of realization of endoscopic molecular imaging

TABLE 3. What molecules should be targeted?

- ◆ Molecules involved in cell proliferation
  Cathepsin B/D
  EGFR (Her2, Her1, etc.)
  Cox-2
  Ki-67
  (Mutation of) K-*ras*/APC
- ◆ Molecules involved in cellular infiltration
  MMP-2/MMP-9
- ◆ Molecules involved in angiogenesis
  VEGFR (VEGR receptor)
  Integrin
- ◆ Molecules involved in apoptosis
  Caspase 3
  Annexin V
- ◆ Molecules involved in hypoxia
  HIF-1α
  Glucose
- ◆ Molecules involved in the level of cellular activity
  Esterase
  Lectin
- ◆ Molecules involved in gene mutation
  ROS (reactive oxygen species)
- ◆ Molecules involved in immortalization of cells
  (Mutation of) P53
  Telomerase

References

1. Weissleder R, Mahmood U (2001) Molecular imaging. Radiology 219:316–333
2. Tajiri H (2005) Future perspectives of gastrointestinal endoscopy and joint academic-industrial research following technological innovation in medical and biological engineering. Dig Endosc 17:S97–S104
3. Tajiri H, Doi T, Endo H, et al (2002) Routine endoscopy using a magnifying endoscope for gastric cancer diagnosis. Endoscopy 34:772–777
4. Inoue H, Kumagai Y, Yoshida T, et al (2000) High-magnification endoscopic diagnosis of the superficial esophageal cancer. Dig Endosc 12:S32–S35
5. Tajiri H, Matsuda K, Fujisaki J (2002) What can we see with the endoscope? Present status and future perspectives. Dig Endosc 14:131–137
6. Nakayoshi T, Tajiri H, Fujisaki J, et al (2004) Magnifying endoscopy with narrow band imaging for gastric cancer. Endoscopy 36:1080–1084
7. Sumiyama K, Kaise M, Tajiri H, et al (2004) Combined use of a magnifying endoscope with a narrow band imaging system and multi-bending endoscope for *en bloc* EMR of early gastric cancer. Gastrointest Endosc 60:79–84
8. Izuishi K, Tajiri H, Fujii T, et al (1999) The histological basis of detection of adenoma and cancer in the colon by autofluorescence endoscopic imaging. Endoscopy 31:511–516
9. Tajiri H (2007) Autofluorescence endoscopy for the gastrointestinal tract. Proc Jpn Acad, Ser: B 83:248–255
10. Poneros JM, Brand S, Bouma BE, et al (2001) Diagnosis of specialized metaplasia by optical coherence tomography. Gastroenterology 120:7–12

11. Kiesslich R, Hoffman A, Neurath MF (2006) Colonoscopy, tumors, and inflammatory bowel disease: new diagnostic methods. Endoscopy 38:5–10
12. Kumagai Y, Monma K, Kawada K (2004) Magnifying chromoendoscopy of the esophagus: in vivo pathological diagnosis using an endocytoscopy system. Endoscopy 36: 590–594
13. Tajiri H (2007) What do we see in the endoscopy world in 10 year's time? Dig Endosc 19:S174–S179
14. Ito S, Muguruma N, Kusaka Y, et al (2001) Detection of human gastric cancer in resected specimens using a novel infrared fluorescent anti-human carcinoembryonic antigen antibody with an infrared fluorescence endoscope in vitro. Endoscopy 233: 849–853
15. Niwa H, Tajiri H (2008) Proposal for a new classification of endoscopy imaging. Clinical Gastroenterology 23:137–141 (in Japanese)
16. Mahmood U, Upadhyat R (2007) Current and future imaging paradigms in colorectal cancer. Semin Colon Rectal Surg 18:132–138
17. Weissleder R, Tung CH, Mahmood U, et al (1999) In vivo imaging of tumors with protease-activated near-infrared fluorescent probes. Nat Biotechnol 17:375–378
18. Mahmood U, Tung CH, Tang Y, et al (2002) Feasibility of in vivo multichannel optical imaging of gene expression: experimental study in mice. Radiology 224:446–451
19. Hama Y, Urano Y, Koyama Y, et al (2007) Activatable fluorescent molecular imaging of peritoneal metastases following pretargeting with a biotinylated monoclonal antibody. Cancer Res 67:3809–3817
20. Sheth RA, Upadhyay R, Weissleder R, et al (2007) Real-time multichannel imaging framework for endoscopy, catheters, and fixed geometry intraoperative systems. Mol Imaging 6:147–155

Further Development of Endoscopic Imaging: "Era of Light" Activities with Optics and Image Processing Technology

Kazunari Nakamura

Summary. The early detection of cancer offers a higher possibility of a cure by laparoscopy or surgery. For proper treatment, the early detection of lesions and an accurate diagnosis are necessary. Endoscope quality has improved as the basis of endoscopic diagnosis.

Over 20 years have passed since the development of the videoscope. Diagnostic imaging today has been further improved by increased resolution, as with HDTV, applying enhancement technology to identify mucosa appearance and subtle color changes, and using magnifying scopes of improved operability.

The absorption and scattering characteristics of tissues differ according to the examination wavelength, resulting in major differences in the information obtained. Using a videoscope that mounts a CCD as a light sensor and selecting a wavelength that is suited to the objective and the characteristics of the tissue, new diagnostic information can be obtained. For this reason, further developments of the endoscope are hoped for.

This chapter looks at the technological developments desired by the many doctors participating in EFJ, and discusses the future possibilities of technological developments from the perspective of a developer.

Key words. Magnifying videoscopes, HDTV system, Structural enhancement, NBI (narrow-band imaging), ECS (endocytoscope system)

Introduction

Since Olympus Medical Systems, Tokyo, Japan, developed the world's first gastrocamera in 1950, we have been developing a fiberoptic endoscope that transmits the image through an image guide made by optical fibers and a video endoscope that mounts a CCD (Charge Coupled Device) chip at the tip of the scope.

Olympus Medical Systems Corp., Research and Development Division 1, Imaging Products Development, 2951 Ishikawacho, Hachioji, Tokyo 192-8507, Japan

Today, the video endoscope has become an essential tool for diagnosis, along with the spread of the esophagogastroduodenoscope, colonoscope, bronchoscope, and ultrasonic endoscope and its improvements. We have been working on improving the image quality as a basis for endoscopic diagnosis by generations from the initial Evis-1 to the fourth Evis Lucera and Lucera Spectrum. We firmly believe that the early detection and accurate diagnosis of cancer are crucial for reliable therapy, since early cancer can be cured by endoscopic treatment or surgery.

This chapter describes the technical aspects of optical and image processing technologies that EFJ has noted or strongly requested.

Basic Configuration of the Video Endoscope

The video endoscope differs from the fiberoptic endoscope largely in terms of the CCD chip mounted on the tip of the endoscope as the image sensing device. As this architecture processes and transmits the electrical signal captured by the CCD device, it is important for obtaining better pictures to improve the CCD device itself, the way of image processing, the signaling system, and how to display the image on a screen.

Also, the determinants of image quality are as wide-ranging as contrast, electrical noise, distribution of light, etc., while the most important factors are resolution and color reproduction.

Technological Development of the CCD for a Video Endoscope

In order to enhance the resolution, it is important to increase the number of pixels in the CCD. However, a CCD with a higher number of pixels becomes larger, and this makes the outer diameter of the video endoscope bigger. On the other hand, a smaller CCD is required to make a thin scope, but then the pixel count and subsequently the resolution decrease. To improve the ease of insertion and operation of the video endoscope, a thinner diameter tip is important, and this greatly depends on the size and shape of the CCD device.

To make a thin video endoscope of good resolution, a smaller sized CCD with a higher pixel count is needed, and the size of an individual pixel must be reduced. However, a finer pixel is not only difficult to make, but it is also difficult to ensure sufficient brightness because of less light reception per pixel. Brighter illumination requires a thicker light guide, and this will also be a factor in making the endoscope thicker. Meanwhile, amplifying the electrical signal to increase the brightness will pull out more noise onto the image.

We have been developing thinner diameter endoscopes with a higher resolution, as shown in Fig. 1, by solving these multiple trade-offs with new technologies and developing high-quality CCDs dedicated to video endoscopy.

Signal Processing System

There are basically two types of imaging system for video endoscopes, the synchronous system and the frame sequential system. The synchronous system video endoscope has mosaic color filters attached to the surface of the CCD pixels. The color filters most generally used are yellow (Y), cyan (Cy), magenta (Mg), and green (G).

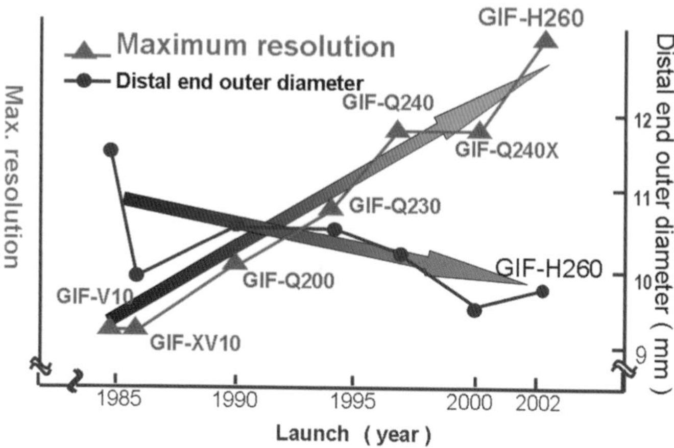

Fig. 1. Improvement in resolution and outer diameter

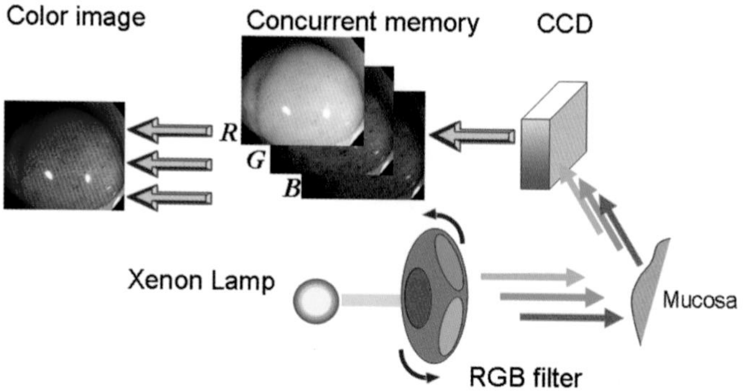

Fig. 2. Signal processing of the RGB system

The frame sequential system CCD has no color filters over the pixels, but picks up red (R), green (G) and blue (B) signals by sequentially illuminated RGB lights, as shown in Fig. 2. The RGB signals will be temporarily cached in the memory and displayed on the monitor at the moment when all three RGB signals are received.

As fundamental features, the frame sequential system will bring vivid color reproduction by using three primary colors, downsize the CCD with a high-quality image by combining three different signals, and minimize color inconsistencies between scopes because the color filters that determine color reproduction are built into the light-source unit.

Moreover, the frame sequential system is suitable for image processing because the number of pixels for each R, G, and B color signal is the same, and that enables us to obtain better resolution.

The frame sequential system has a fundamental shortcoming in that color drift occurs when viewing moving pictures, but the Evis Lucera incorporates an image processing engine that diminishes this drift.

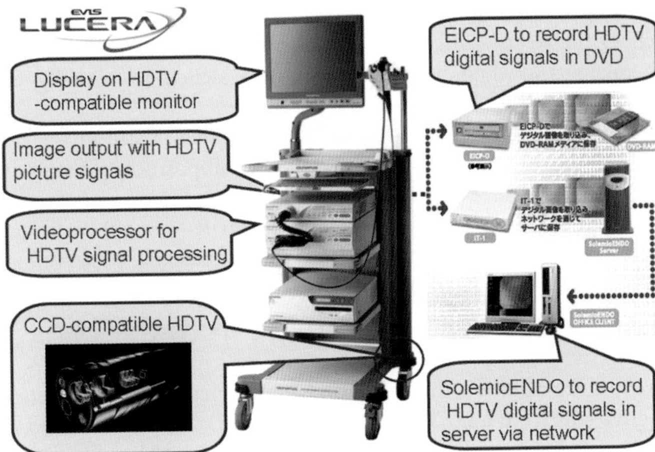

FIG. 3. Configuration of the HDTV endoscope system

HDTV Support

The numerous improvements to the CCDs increased pixel count mean that it reaches the fundamental limit of the widely used NTSC (National Television Standards Committee) system which has 525 scanning lines. HDTV offers over twice the number of scanning lines at 1125, and is considered to be the best video signal format for the next generation of video endoscope systems.

The new Evis Lucera brings a higher image quality to the entire endoscope system by providing complete support for the HDTV format from the CCD, image processing, signal transmission, and display to image recording, as shown in Fig. 3.

Correcting Color Drift in Motion and Still Pictures

Although the frame sequential system has many advantages, it has a fundamental shortcoming in that color drift occurs with moving objects, as described above. The Evis Lucera has a newly developed "color drift correcting feature," and the problem is greatly reduced. This feature activates the algorithm that infers the proper color of each pixel in the color-drifting areas and corrects only the pixels showing color drift in real time. Only as much correction is applied as there is noticeable color drift, and therefore natural color reproduction is available even when viewing objects with strong movements.

On the other hand, even conventional devices had a "color drift preventing freeze" feature that automatically selected the image of least color drift for taking still pictures. However, the timing of the still picture often differed from the physician's intentions because of the time-lag between when the freeze switch was clicked and the best image selected by the video processor. This was particularly noticeable when an object was zoomed in on.

To fix this problem, a "prefreeze" feature that regularly stores the last 60 frames in the memory was incorporated into the Evis Lucera. This automatically selects the best still image from the 60 frames and immediately displays it on the screen when the physician clicks the freeze switch. This enables physicians to check that the best still image was taken, and then operate the release switch to actually capture the picture.

Unlike the "color drift preventing freeze" feature, the best still image can be taken even if the object moves after the physician sets the composition of the picture as long as the freeze switch is pressed within 1 s.

This feature has made it easier to obtain color-drift-free still pictures even with magnified observation by the zoom function, which is usually preferred today.

Greatly Improved Water Drainage from the Lens

In an endoscopic examination, the lens is dirtied by mucus. Therefore water is sprayed on the objective lens from a nozzle mounted nearby to clean the lens. No matter how much progress has been made with image quality enhancement, viewing and taking beautiful images is quite difficult if the surface of the lens is soiled, and there had been a strong demand to improve this feature.

Despite many efforts to address this problem, no obvious improvements were achieved. However, in order to deliver a high-quality image suitable for HDTV systems, this problem had to be corrected somehow, so previous countermeasures were reworked one by one until all the outstanding problems were resolved. The nozzle shape, the spray button, and the pump were improved, and a small ridge was added around the lens to drain water through the edge of the lens and remove droplets instantly, thereby producing clear images. This improvement has been commended by many doctors.

Improvements to the Magnifying Function of Video Endoscopes

Some video endoscopes have a second optical system for enlarging and observing mucosal structures in greater detail (the so-called "zoom video endoscope"), but it has been pointed out that the mechanism of this optical system makes the scope wider and detracts from its maneuverability. For this reason, research has been conducted not only into improvements in the basic performance of enlarged observations, but also into technological developments to make a scope with a thinner diameter but with the same maneuverability as ordinary scopes.

Zoom Video Endoscopes and Magnification

A zoom video endoscope allows a range of viewing, from the distant to the close-up, in a single device. It has an optical mechanism that shifts a movable lens back and forth along the optical axis to change the focal point of the objective and to selectively switch the image between a wide-angle shot (called "wide") and a narrow-angle shot with high magnification (called "tele").

The magnification of video endoscopes is expressed as the ratio of the actual size of the object to the size of the object as it appears on the monitor. The magnification changes as the distance between the object and the scope changes, and it is maximized when the object is positioned at the nearest point within the focal range of the endoscope. The magnification of a video endoscope should be considered at the same time as the size of the monitor, because the displayed size of the object varies according to the size of the monitor. At Olympus Medical Systems, the magnification is defined for an endoscope image projected onto a 14-inch monitor. However, an 18-inch high-resolution LCD monitor is the standard for the CF-H260AZ discussed later, and therefore the magnification in that case is defined based on an image projected onto an 18-inch monitor.

Latest Zoom Video Endoscope

Features of CF-H260AZ for Colonoscopy

Ordinary Thin Diameter Endoscopes. Downsizing the complicated optical system is one of the biggest issues with a zoom video endoscope. No matter how good the image quality is, an endoscope with a larger diameter will not be widely accepted on the market because of the problems of insertion. The tip size of the CF-H260AZ, the latest HDTV-compliant zoom video endoscope, is smaller than that of its predecessor the CF-Q240Z and is comparable to the CF-230.

Better Image Quality and Practical Electronic Zoom via HDTV. Figure 4 shows how much clearer the image of the CF-H260AZ is in comparison with a conventional CF-Q240 when a portion of the image is magnified. Unlike an optical zoom, the electronic zoom does not shift the focal point, yet despite the superior operability, a degraded picture quality was previously an issue. The CF-H260AZ delivers a practical electronic zoom with less degradation of image quality than earlier models, as seen in Fig. 5, by adopting a new high-pixel CCD and digitized processing of HDTV signals. With the 18-inch HDTV LCD monitor, the optical zoom attains a maximum 70× magnification

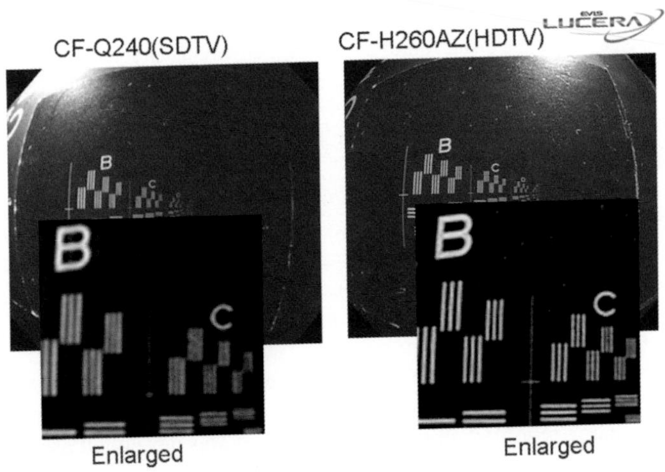

Fig. 4. Comparison of the resolution of a conventional endoscope system and an HDTV endoscope system

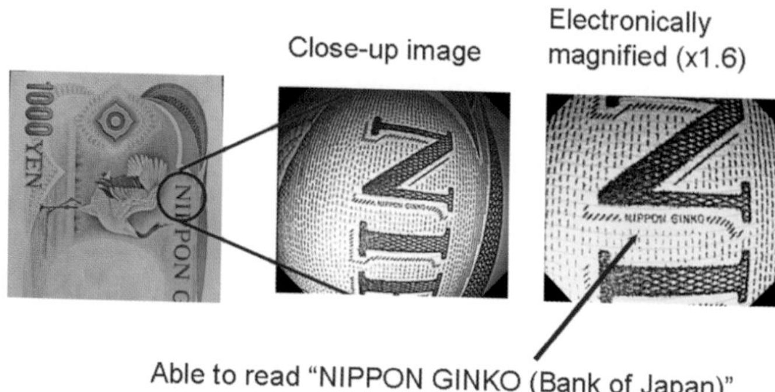

Fig. 5. Enlarged image by an HDTV endoscope system

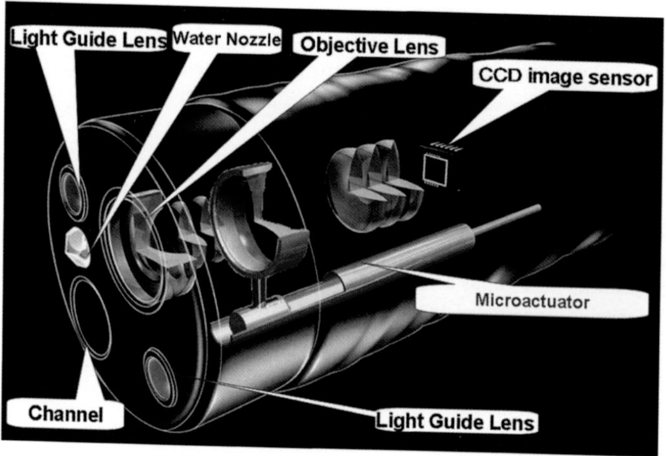

Fig. 6. Basic structure of the distal end of an electric magnifying endoscope

in tele mode, but it can be boosted up to 130× by adding an electronic zoom of 1.4×, 1.6×, or 1.8×.

Wider Field of View. The higher resolution allowed the CF-H260AZ to have a wider field of view in tele mode. The field of view at 100× magnification was only 40° with the CF-Q240Z, and it had been pointed out that the targeted areas of lesions were easily going out of view in tele mode because of its narrow field of view. The CF-H260AZ has a wide 80° field of view in tele mode, since it delivers sufficient resolution at about 70× magnification.

Easy Operation of Magnification using a Motorized Zoom Actuator. As shown in Fig. 6, the CF-H260AZ has the same motorized zoom actuator as the CF-Q240Z. The ultra-small actuator, mounted on the tip of the scope, was developed using micromachine technology and is controlled electrically to slide the movable lens back and forth. This system allows precise control of the lens position, and therefore it is easy to use at an intermediate magnification, for example 60×.

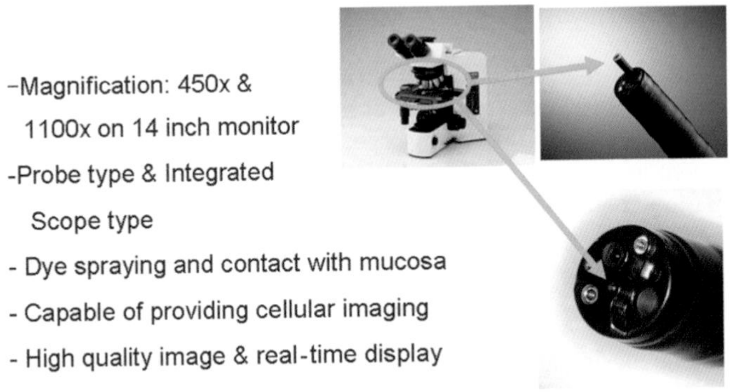

Fig. 7. Super-high-magnification video endoscope

Endoscope for the Upper Digestive Tract

In the latest zoom video endoscope for the upper gastrointestinal (GI) tract, the insertion tube has a slightly bigger outer diameter than the conventional GIF-Q240 and the same diameter at the tip of the scope. It has also an optical system with a variable focal point, as with endoscopes for colonoscopy. However, the mechanism of the zoom function is a nonelectrical type, which has a minimal effect on the size of the outer diameter of the endoscope because downsizing the outer diameter is the first priority for an upper GI tract endoscope.

Ultra-Magnified Viewing Using an Endocytoscope System

The endocytoscope system (ECS), shown in Fig. 7, is an endoscope with an optical system for ultra-magnification at the same level as a microscope. Two prototypes were fabricated: a probe type of 3.2 mm outer diameter for fitting to the instrumental channels of ordinary endoscopes, and an internal type that is built into an ordinary scope. It is expected that it will be possible to obtain images of high contrast by staining cell nuclei with a dye such as methylene blue. It is also expected to give nuclear-level observations at 500× or 1100× beyond those of conventional zoom video endoscopes, and research into optical biopsy has already begun with this device [1].

Improvements via Image Processing

Various improvements have given enhanced resolution, which allows detailed observations of mucosal structure beyond the ability of the naked eye by using the zoom video endoscope. On the other hand, since the early detection of small lesions relies on identifying subtle changes in the appearance or color of mucosa, image processing technologies as well as improved resolution have also been developed in order to make these subtle changes clear and visible.

Structure Enhancement

Unlike conventional edge enhancement, structure enhancement is carried out with a digital filter to enhance information about important mucosal structures such as the pit-pattern seen through a video endoscope. As shown in Fig. 8,1, it keeps the amount of enhancement low in an area of much noise, and high in an area which has important information about the appearance of the mucosal structure which is necessary for endoscopic diagnosis.

Adaptive IHb Color Enhancement

IHb is the acronym for index of hemoglobin. It approximates the membrane blood flow by performing an interframe operation between the R, G, and B images [2]. Using this index, subtle color changes in membranes can be enhanced, as shown in Fig. 8,2, which cannot be obtained by increasing the resolution alone. Flare and brown spots that tend to be overlooked in normal membranes become clear and visible.

Figure 9 shows a test result of using both adaptive IHb color enhancement and structural enhancement on a chart with a subtle color change. By simultaneously using these two types of enhancement processing, both subtle color changes and changes in the membrane appearance become readily identifiable.

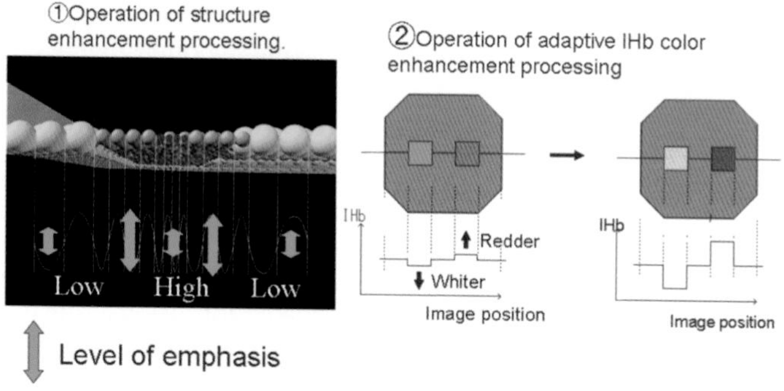

Fig. 8. Operation of image processing

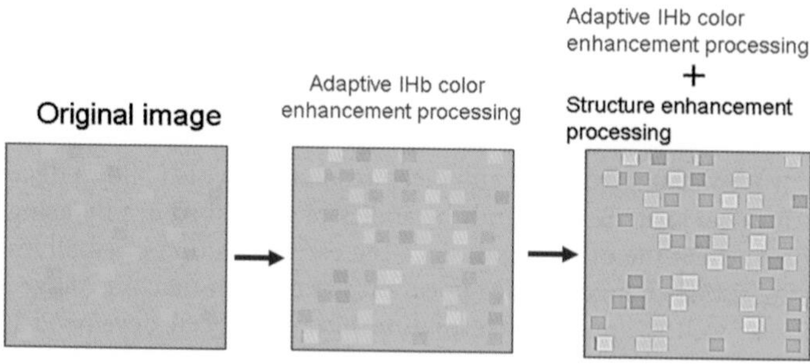

Fig. 9. Effect of the combination of image processing

Obtaining Additional Diagnostic Information by Changing Signal Wavelength

In order to make use of higher resolution technology such as HDTV, various improvements have been made to render high-quality images as if the inside of the body is being observed by the naked eye. Moreover, the new technologies described above, such as the zoom video endoscope, structure enhancement, and adaptive IHb color enhancement, have made it possible to provide images that are, in a certain sense, better than those seen by the naked eye.

Efforts made over about 20 years since the development of the video endoscope have targeted the reproduction of natural and faithful images as a means of improving examinations that serve as the basis for making diagnoses. As a result, the Evis Lucera has attained the target set by the first video endoscope. Of course, it cannot be considered perfect, but as its name suggests (lucera means "era of light"), various demands and issues that were technically difficult until now have been solved, and the video endoscope has given a discrete level of satisfaction. Only a video endoscope incorporating a CCD as an image sensor was able to deliver the possibility of a practical optical diagnostic system that could not be attained with the combination of fiberscopes and the naked eye.

We thought that one other improvement could be made to provide additional information for endoscopic diagnosis and contribute to the advancement of endoscopy, i.e., to select wavelengths according to the characteristics of each tissue.

Obtaining High-Contrast Mucosa Information by Narrow-Band Imaging

Various efforts have been made to increase the resolution, such as to increase the pixel count of CCDs and to provide HDTV support. However, when attention turned to the wavelength characteristics of tissues, the fundamental merits of constructively using light in the short wavelength band, where scattering is high and a peak of absorption exists, were advocated as a means for capturing mucosa surfaces in higher resolution, as shown in Fig. 10. To this end, technological development in narrow-band imaging (NBI) is being promoted [3].

Light penetration can be restricted to the surface layers by using a B filter of the spectral transmittance of the three RGB optical filters used in sequential framing to create a narrow band that cuts light of wavelengths which are longer than the mean wavelength at which hemoglobin absorption is the maximum, as shown in Fig. 11.

Using image processing with narrow-band light, the clarity of minute structures of the mucous surface and capillary networks is improved [4], and this is expected to help improve the early diagnosis of cancer in ways that cannot be achieved by enhancing CCD resolution alone.

Infrared Imaging (IRI) Technology to Make Deep Blood Vessels Visible

Unlike the short wavelength band, the long wavelength band is minimally absorbed and scattered by tissue, and therefore light reaches to greater depths. Moreover,

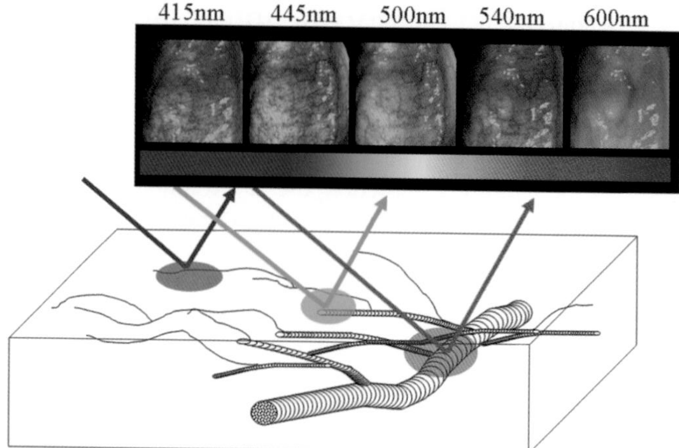

FIG. 10. Differences in endoscopic images of human hypoglottis mucous by different wavelengths

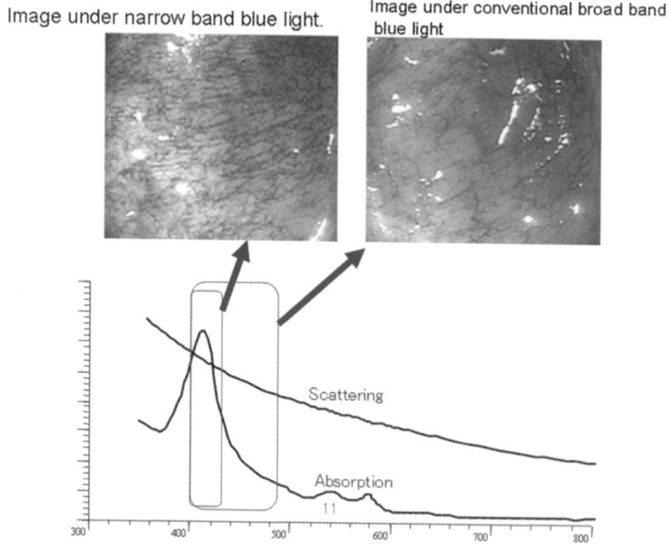

FIG. 11. Clarifying the image by narrowing the band of blue light

because the CCD mounted at the tip of a videoscope is sensitive not only to the visible light band but also to the near infrared band, this near infrared band can be used to observe deep locations that were difficult to see in ordinary examinations [5].

Video endoscope systems for infrared observation filter out the infrared light from the visible light emitted from a xenon lamp to allow users to select between visible light for an ordinary examination and infrared light for an infrared observation.

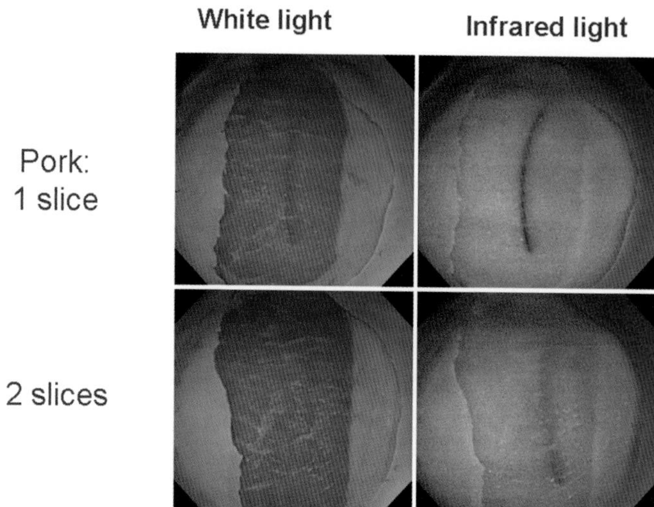

Fig. 12. Comparison of images between white light and infrared imaging (IRI)

In infrared observations, two types of infrared light, of mean wavelength 805 nm and 900 nm, respectively, are put through signal processing so that 805-nm light appears red and 900-nm light appears green or blue. The resulting image is shown in color. Often, the indocyanine green (ICG) contrast medium that is used in liver tests is introduced by intravenous injection to increase the contrast of infrared images. As shown in Fig. 12, locations containing a large amount of ICG are shown in blue because this contrast medium indicates the strong absorption characteristic of 805-mm light. It is expected to improve our diagnostic ability because it now becomes possible to observe deep blood vessels that cannot be seen in ordinary examinations.

Autofluorescence Imaging (AFI) Technology for Viewing Tissue Fluorescence

It is a known fact that tissues fluoresce imperceptibly, but because the light is weak, it is necessary to develop a supersensitive endoscopic system. A video endoscope that allows real-time observation of this fluorescent light was developed by incorporating a super high sensitive CCD, optical filters optimized for fluorescent light observation, and image processing technology dedicated to this new method.

Figure 13 shows the configuration of an autofluorescence imaging (AFI) system. It produces color images from the fluorescent image created by the excitation light (390–470 nm) for exciting the fluorescent substance in the tissue and the reflected light image created at the wavelength (540–560 nm) absorbed by hemoglobin in the blood.

Areas with swollen mucosal surfaces scatter and absorb more excitation light and fluorescent light than normal mucosa, causing the fluorescent light to diminish.

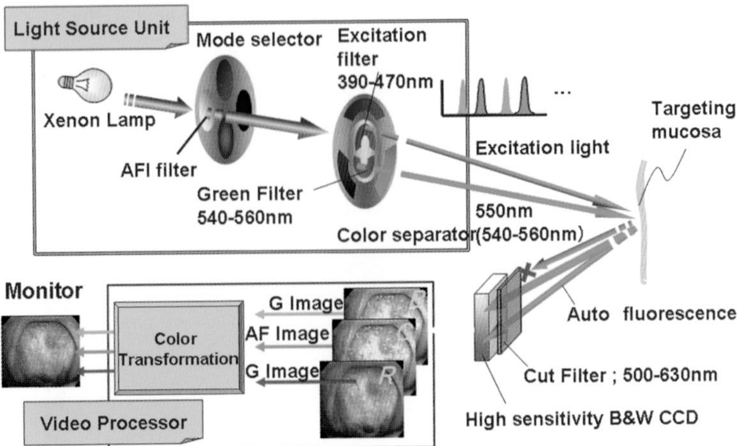

Fig. 13. Scheme of an autofluorescence imaging (AFI) system

However, the reflected light of 540–560-nm wavelength reflects off the mucosa without attenuating.

In hemorrhaged or inflamed locations, the excitation light, fluorescent light, and all reflected light of 540–560 nm diminishes because of absorption by hemoglobin in the blood. In this way, slightly swollen or inflamed locations appear slightly different colors than normal tissue. AFI is a hopeful technology for supporting the early detection of minute lesions such as early cancer by enhancing and displaying tumoric lesions in a different color from normal tissue [6].

To Realize Molecular Imaging

With the cooperation of many doctors in EFJ and elsewhere, the Evis Lucera was commercialized as a new-generation system of hidden potential, as shown in Fig. 14. Next-generation endoscopic systems that not only identify lesions from subtle changes at the tissue level, but also capture cancerous tissue at the cellular level, and eventually at the genetic and protein level, by using cancer-making antigens and fluorescent markers to stain only cancerous cells [7] or mark cancerous genes are no longer just a dream.

For this kind of imaging, chemical agents that stain only early-stage cancerous cells in the near infrared band without adversely affecting the fluorescence of tissue need to be developed as a technology for selectively detecting fluorescent probes of multiple wavelengths at high resolution in the 600–800-nm band in order to obtain molecular information about cancer.

As shown in Fig. 15, the development of these technologies will facilitate the detection of early-stage cancer cells and lead to minimally invasive treatments in stages at low risk of metastasizing to other organs or lymph nodes, hence helping to improve the quality of life (QOL) of patients.

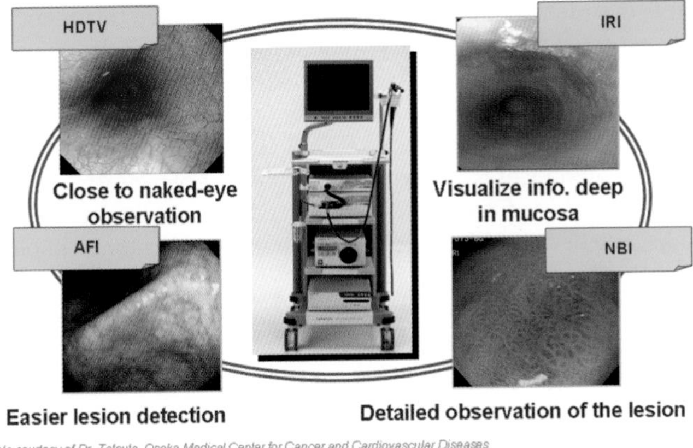

FIG. 14. Goal of the "era of light"

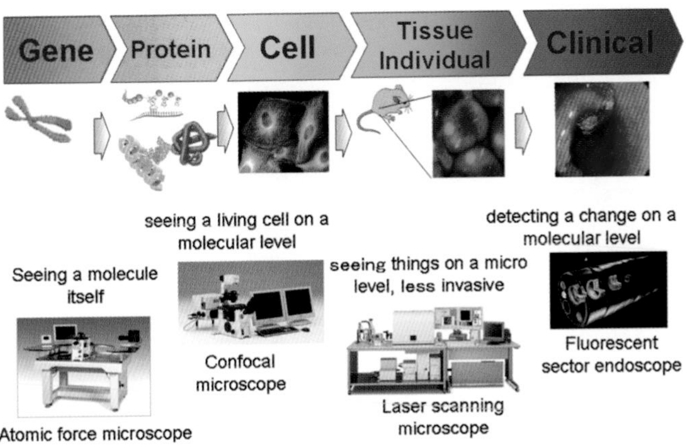

FIG. 15. Molecular imaging from basic research to clinical application

Conclusions

Video endoscopes that aim to improve image quality to the level of observations by the naked eye have reached the point of discussing optical biopsies through the adoption of HDTV systems, improvements in zoom video endoscopes, and super magnification observation over 1000×.

Moreover, it is becoming easier to examine locations which had been difficult to reach with conventional devices thanks to ultrathin video endoscopes, small intestinal endoscopes, capsule endoscopes, etc. Nevertheless, insertion for colonoscopies remains highly difficult even when using a variable-stiffness function or an endoscopic position detection unit (UPD), and improvements such as training systems are still needed.

In addition, in order to improve the quality of endoscopic treatment in general, it is absolutely essential that laboratory management matches the examination flow. Risk management, not only during the examination but also in cleaning, disinfecting, and other processes, is of growing importance.

On the other hand, the development of EMR (Endoscopic Mucosal Resection) and ESD (Endoscopic Submucosal Dissection) techniques is being carried out, and instruments and endoscopes dedicated to endoscopic treatment and cure rates are increasing alongside early detection and accurate diagnoses using new technologies such as the ultrasound endoscope.

The pursuit of easier ways of early detection and accurate diagnosis is meeting the challenge of minimizing the limit of obtaining more natural-looking images, which was the original demand placed on video endoscopes. In addition, endoscope devices that can provide new diagnostic information using light of specific wavelength bands and digital image processing technology are also being developed.

Because of the growing call for innovation in endoscopic treatment environments, EFJ is spearheading cooperative activities between industry and academia, together with numerous doctors and medical professionals. In our aging society, we want to contribute to the realization of patient-friendly, safe, secure, and highly efficient medical care environments that reduce the cost of medical care and enable people to lead healthy rewarding lives.

References

1. Inoue H, Kazawa T, Sato Y, et al. (2004) In vivo observation of living cancer cells in the esophagus, stomach, and colon using a catheter-type contact endoscope, the "endocytoscope system". Gastrointest Endosc Clin N Am 14:589–594
2. Kawano J, Sato N, Tsuji S, et al. (1989) Blood flow analysis by videoscope imaging. Gastroenterol Endosc 1:461–467
3. Mizuno H, Gono K, Takehana S, et al. (2003) Narrow-band imaging technique. Tech Gastrointest Endosc 5:78–81
4. Machida H, Sano Y, Fujii T, et al. (2002) Clinical application of sequential framing scope using narrow-band RGB filter (narrow-band imaging) for colonoscopy. Early-stage colon cancer detection 2002 vol.6 No. 6
5. Mataki N, Nagao S, Kawaguchi A, et al. (2003) Clinical usefulness of a new infrared videoendoscope system for diagnosis of early-stage gastric cancer. Gastrointest Endosc 57:336–342
6. Bergman J (2005) Gastroesophageal reflux disease and Barrett's esophagus. Endoscopy 37:8–18
7. Ito S, Muguruma N, Kimura T, et al. (2003) Principle and clinical application of the infrared fluorescent endoscope. Bio THERM 23:77–97

Future Perspectives for Esophageal and Colorectal Capsule Endoscopy: Dreams or Reality?

Jean-Francois Rey

Summary. Video capsule endoscopy is a breakthrough for small bowel exploration. Of course, other applications such as the esophagus or colon should be considered. In this chapter, we review the potentials, pitfalls, and expectations of capsule endoscopy applied to the esophagus and colon. We also "dream" of further developments of this new technology.

Key words. Video capsule endoscopy, Capsule esophagus, Capsule colon

Introduction

When we were asked to write a paper on future developments in video capsule endoscopy (VCE) of the esophagus and colon, we wondered how to describe the future of this new technology with a realistic perspective on the clinical benefit of our patients—the ultimate goal of all physicians. Should we allude to a well-known movie where travel inside the human body is a compelling dream, that journalists made so much of when Given Imaging introduced capsule endoscopy in 2002, or, more seriously, should we consider the progress in digestive endoscopy in the past 30 years? This thought recalled our own astonishment at an early concept of VCE that was presented at the Olympus Medical Systems, Tokyo, Japan, booth during the 1994 World Congress in Los Angeles. We try, in this chapter, to encompass both approaches: both to envisage the possibilities of this fascinating new device and, on the other hand, to try to assess the clinical benefits of VCE for esophageal or colonic exploration. Our dream could be based on a paper written by David Fleischer in 1994: 2020 Vision [1]. Let us recall just a short extract from Fleischer's forecast:

"We have to GAIN ACCESS. But why in the world would a patient want to do anything as unnatural as swallow a long black tube attached by an umbilical cord to a light system? Such an endoscope will seem as primitive and undignified to the 2020

Hepatology and Gastroenterology Department, Institut Arnault Tzanck, 06700 Saint Laurent du Var, France doctors as the "silver bullet" rigid proctoscope seems to us today. The newer endoscopes will be self-contained disposable units similar to a capsule. The patient will swallow it, just like taking a pill. Impregnated with microsensors, it will be directed through the digestive tract by "endoscopists" sitting at work stations. Using the same remote capabilities by which we manipulate space satellites through distant galaxies, the endoscopist will guide the endoscope from the esophagus to the rectum (or vice versa)."

But our dream must face the realities of modern medicine, that is, more patient oriented and with financial constraints that relate to both the demographic fact of increasing aging populations in developed countries and reduction in the growth of healthcare budgets. Although conventional endoscopy might be the only approach for esophageal exploration, traditional digestive colonoscopy will be challenged by other technologies such as the Aer-O-scope [2]. This new environment for gastroenterologists has been assessed by Cotton and colleagues [3], and we share some of their analysis. The financial and organizational realities are a new approach for physicians and healthcare providers. VCE could be an important tool in changing our gastroenterological practice with the involvement of other colleagues (that is, primary care physicians or nurses) and with the more demanding concepts of patient management. But if VCE has come to be considered, over a few years, to be the gold standard for small-bowel exploration [4], it is important to emphasize that national healthcare providers have been very slow to agree to pay for it. The notable cost of the device is probably one of the reasons, but the negative effect of the considerable coverage in the public media has also probably contributed. In our underfunded healthcare system, health providers are no longer inclined to pay for dreams. This will is even more pertinent for the esophageal or colon capsules, as cost-effective tools are already available.

The Esophageal Capsule

The Device and the Protocol for Capsule Examination

The PillCam ESO is 11 × 26 mm in size with a CMOS sensor at each end. In its latest version, it captures images at a rate of 14 frames per second compared with the 4 frames per second of the usual small-bowel capsule. The image has a 140° field of view and provides a 1:8 magnification, with a depth of view of 1–30 mm [5]. Patients are asked to fast for 8 h before the examination. They are instructed to drink 100 ml water to clear saliva from the esophagus. A special protocol is applied to keep the capsule in the esophageal tract for as long as possible. Patients are in the supine position when they ingest the video capsule with 10 ml water; the patient is then slowly raised to a sitting position over the course of the next 6 min, and during this time patients are required to avoid speaking or moving. An early pilot study was carried out in which a length of string was attached to the capsule. Esophageal data were obtained, at this early stage, by Ramirez et al. [6], but even with a favorable assessment of patient acceptance this method has not been further developed because it caused throat discomfort for the patients.

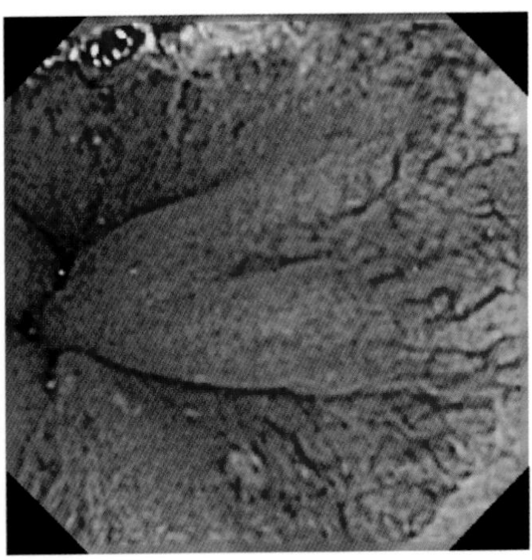

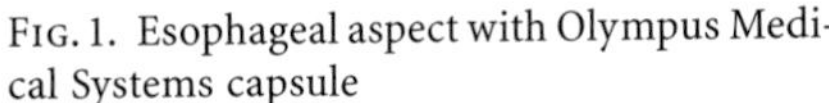

FIG. 1. Esophageal aspect with Olympus Medical Systems capsule

Clinical Trials

Two interesting trials on the evaluation of portal hypertension and varices were published in the same issue of *Endoscopy* in 2006 [7,8]. This indication could be important for the early diagnosis of varices in cirrhotic patients or for the follow-up of patients already treated with ligation. Eisen and colleagues [7] presented data from 32 enrolled patients where VCE was compared with conventional gastroscopy under conscious sedation; 22 of the patients were undergoing screening examinations. The mean VCE esophageal transit time was 134.5 s (range, 5–380 s). Conventional endoscopy identified varices in 23 patients; these were all identified in the capsule examinations, with one false positive in addition. Portal hypertension gastropathy was diagnosed in 19 patients by both endoscopic and capsule examinations. In the other studies, Lapalus et al. [8] enrolled 21 patients, with a mean reading time of 213 s (range, 6–1200 s); the results were slightly less favorable as only 84.2% of the patients endoscopically diagnosed as having varices were identified at the capsule examination. The authors underlined the high acceptability, safety, and potential for increasing compliance with screening recommendations. However, a review of the data shows that one patient in the Lapalus study was unable to swallow the capsule, and that could raise questions about whether the capsule could be described as "highly acceptable." Those early studies should be evaluated to clarify the clinical benefit for the patient and healthcare services. First, conventional esogastroscopy and, even more, nasogastroscopy are well-accepted procedures without complications. Second, at the same time, a minute examination with the latest high-definition technique such as narrow-band imaging (NBI) is possible, together with complete gastric and duodenal examination. Biopsies or endoscopic treatments such as ligation are also possible. Third, "patient-friendliness" is more a marketing concept than a true medical evaluation of tolerance. There is a definite need for further clinical trials with complete reports of upper gastrointestinal examination, especially in cirrhotic patients in whom other abnormalities can be associated with varices.

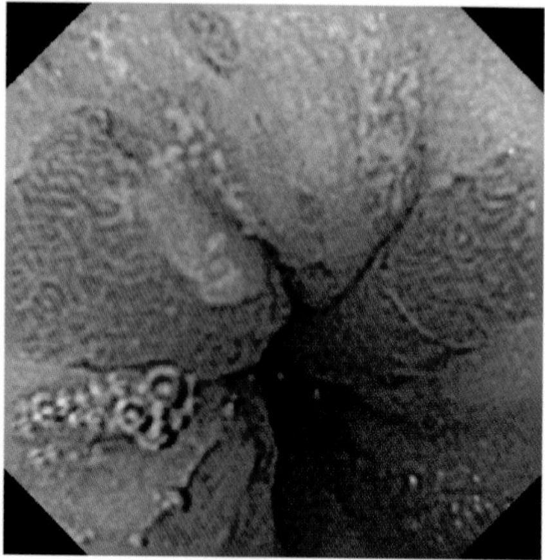

Fig. 2. Barrett esophagus with Olympus Medical Systems capsule

Barrett Esophagus

Gastroesophageal reflux disease (GERD) and Barrett esophagus are other potential indications (Figs. 1, 2). Eliakim and colleagues [5] conducted a study involving seven centers and 106 patients in which they compared VCE with conventional endoscopy; they found a high sensitivity (92%) and specificity (95%) for esophageal abnormalities (Barrett esophagus or GERD). Lin et al. [9], in a series of 96 patients with Barrett's esophagus, found less spectacular results, with a sensitivity of only 67% and specificity of 83% for identifying Barrett esophagus. Sharma et al. [10] enrolled 94 patients and also found less favorable results: the sensitivity was 67% for Barrett esophagus with a specificity of 87% and, for patients undergoing surveillance for Barrett esophagus, the sensitivity was 79% and the specificity 78%. In summary, only the Eliakim study showed results that were favorable for VCE; the others highlighted the necessity for improving both technology and method. This hesitation was also the conclusion of the Gerson and Lin study [11] in which a cost analysis was found in favor of conventional endoscopy versus VCE.

The Colon Capsule

The Device

The Pillcam Colon Capsule has two sensors that enable the device to acquire video images from each end. It is slightly larger than the small-bowel capsule (32 × 11 mm). The optics have a wider field of view (more than twice that of the first Pillcam small-bowel capsule), and an automatic light control avoids overexposure. Pictures are acquired at the rate of 4 frames per second (Fig. 3). After an initial activation and transmission of images for 5 min, the capsule goes into a "sleep" mode for approximately 2 h, after which time it spontaneously recommences image acquisition and transmission [12].

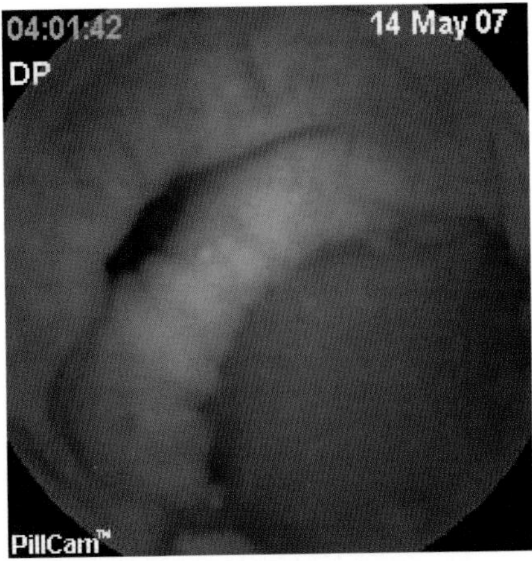

Fig. 3. Colon capsule imaging with Given Imaging capsule

First Clinical Trials

The two first clinical trials were reported in *Endoscopy* by Schoofs et al. (31 patients) and Eliakim et al. (91 patients), with promising results for pilot studies [12,13]. Using a special protocol designed to obtain a clean colon and enhancement of motility, the colon was screened for a mean time of 177 ± 128 min, the wide range being a consequence of the large variation in bowel motility. In the Belgian study the overall sensitivity was 77%, the specificity was 70%, the positive predictive value was 59%, and the negative predictive value was 84%. In the Eliakim study, the results were reported slightly differently, with readings of the colon capsule data by three separate panels in comparison with the conventional colonoscopic result. These overall results are reported in Table 1. We have some questions concerning the Eliakim study: multiple readings, with knowledge of conventional colonoscopy findings, induced some analytical bias. Also, their report that a suspected polyp in the transverse colon was not found at repeat colonoscopy raises a question, as, with high-definition endoscopy and NBI, a polyp located in the transverse colon should not be missed because this is not a very difficult area to examine. The study of Schoofs and colleagues is more convincing, with a blind analysis and more traditional reporting of data. In both studies the miss rates for colon capsule endoscopy and conventional endoscopy are significant. This difference results from the differing technology: colon capsule endoscopy does not have the angling and inflation capabilities of conventional endoscopy, whereas the two capsule sensors can more easily visualize areas behind folds. (It is to overcome that limitation that the latest generation of colonoscopes has a wider angle of view and the Aer-O-scope has 360° coverage.)

Preparation for Colonic Capsule Endoscopy

In all cases, colonoscopic examinations require thorough large-bowel preparation. A limited amount of residue or fluid can be washed and moved during conventional

TABLE 1. Results of colon capsule endoscopy for colonic abnormalities.

		R. Eliakim [12]		
	N. Schoofs [13]	First lecture	Second lecture	Third lecture
Sensitivity	77%	56%	69%	76%
Specificity	70%	69%	81%	100%
Positive predictive value	59%	57%	74%	100%
Negative predictive value	84%	67%	78%	78%

TABLE 2. Preparation for colon capsule endoscopy.

Two days before exam	
All day	Low-residue diet
One day before exam:	
All day	Clear liquids only
1900–2100	2 l polyethylene glycol solution (1 cup every 10–15 min)
Examination day:	
0700–0800	1 l polyethylene glycol solution (1 cup every 10–15 min)
0800	Fast until first dose of oral sodium phosphate + water (except for Tegaserod and PillCam Colon ingestions)
0815	6 mg Tegaserod (with a cup of water)
0830	PillCam Colon ingestion (with a cup of water)
1030	Booster dose 1 of oral sodium phosphate: 30 ml sodium phosphate + 1 l water
1300	6 mg Tegaserod (with a cup of water)
1400	Booster dose 1 of oral sodium phosphate: 15 ml sodium phosphate + 0.5 l water
1500	Optional light snack (low fiber)
	Fast until conventional colonoscopy procedure
1630	10 mg Bisacodyl rectal suppository
1900	Conventional colonoscopy performed

If dose 1 of sodium phosphate was administered during the time period indicated below	...then the booster dose 2 of sodium phosphate was administered at the time indicated below	...and the Bisacodyl suppository was administered at the time indicated below
1030–1130	1400	1630
1130–1300	1500	1630
1300–1400	1600	1700
1400–1500	1700	No suppository given
1500–1600	No booster dose 2 given	No suppository given

No booster doses or suppositories were given if the capsule remained in the stomach after 1600

colonoscopy. Colon capsule endoscopy requires a very demanding protocol to obtain a clean colon and also to enhance bowel motility (Table 2). Residues are also a pitfall and a main drawback in virtual colonoscopy, which is why we consider that talk of a "patient-friendly examination" is overoptimistic. Current practice is based on an oral approach to cleansing. The bowel preparation is one of the main patient concerns as the protocol for colon capsule endoscopy is even more demanding than that routinely used for conventional colonoscopy. Pharmaceutical companies have been very slow to improve the various possibilities. Use of polyethylene glycol (PEG) solution is, in most cases, the best overall preparation, as Phospho-soda gives unreliable results in the ascending colon and has some potential side effects in elderly patients. Bowel preparation will be the main limitation to the large-scale use of colon capsule endoscopy for rectal screening. We also think that it is currently misleading to suggest that colonic capsule endoscopy could be easily carried out at the patient's home. It is necessary for nurses or physicians, using the external viewer, to look for impaired gastric emptying or any abnormalities during the small-bowel transit. It is a common error in some papers on capsule endoscopy to mingle dreams or hopes with clinical realities.

VCE for Colorectal Cancer Screening

In most countries, colorectal screening methods are at present based on fecal occult blood testing (FOBT), sigmoidoscopy, or total colonoscopy, and most experts currently consider conventional colonoscopy to be the best available method for recording images in the detection of colonic disease. High-definition video endoscopy with NBI allows characterization of the detected lesion during the procedure and, in most cases, immediate endoscopic treatment with polypectomy or endoscopic mucosal resection (EMR). Acceptability and tolerability have been improved during the past 5 years, with mechanical improvements (such as variable stiffness, wider angle of view, thinner colonoscopes, and scope guides) leading to reduction in complications, with perforation being unusual in diagnostic colonoscopy. At the same time, the wider use of conscious or deep sedation with propofol has enhanced patient acceptance. As does conventional colonoscopy, colon capsule endoscopy (and also indeed virtual colonoscopy) entails the discomfort of bowel preparation for the patient. When comparing methods in this report, we should use data from the 21st century. In summary, with modern colonoscopy, involving variable stiffness and slim colonoscopes and propofol sedation, bowel preparation remains the only drawback for the patient, and capsule endoscopy is still far from clinical application for mass screening [14].

Colon VCE: Costs

For mass screening, the ideal tool should have three main advantages: high sensitivity and specificity, noninvasiveness, and low cost. Compared with FOBT, the early findings for colon capsule endoscopy indeed show much better clinical results, and it could also be considered to be noninvasive, even though impaction, because of anatomy or unrecognized disease, will be always a possible side effect. However, if we consider the actual cost of the device (about 510 euros), no healthcare system will be able to bear this financial burden. In France, for example, there are 10 million inhabitants between 50 and 75 years old to be taken into account for screening. Mass production and industrial competition might reduce the cost, as we have seen in the past for biopsy forceps or, to take another example, for digital cameras. We can reasonably expect the price to be halved, but this would still represent an enormous amount of money. The cost of the time-consuming data reading could also be reduced with more efficient software and an extensive use of nurses, but we would still be a long way away from the overall cost of FOBT (less than 10 euros) or flexible sigmoidoscopy (60 euros).

The Future of VCE Technology

The Immediate Future

Capsule technology has already been improved, thanks to the competition between Given Imaging and Olympus Medical Systems Image resolution, a crucial feature from the point of view of diagnosis, is the main advantage of the Olympus video capsule. In response, Given Imaging has released a new capsule with improved resolution and a wider angle of view. Similarly, regarding length of battery life, the latest product from both companies provides for 8 h of digestive tract examination. More efficient software is another way of improving clinical benefit, by reducing reading time and applying some tools for automatic detection of abnormal images. Although at present the use of the "redness signal" has proved disappointing overall, other tools have been developed. Mathematical algorithms in the latest Olympus Medical Systems software allow a global view of 500 to 2000 still pictures in overview mode, and this could be practically useful in capsule colonoscopy. Both Olympus Medical Systems and Given have also developed a skip mode for moving pictures, and further automation software can be expected soon.

Capsule Procedures: Nurses or Physicians?

As we might expect the number of capsule procedures to increase on a large scale; we should consider that most of the time-consuming examination could be carried out by nurses. Not only might nurses monitor the patient, especially during the prolonged colon capsule examination, but they could also be involved in reading data. With the use of a clear protocol, and after initial training, nurses could select all abnormal pictures for the final overall diagnosis by the physician.

Overall Cost and Benefits

Even if technologies are improved, the overall cost of the device will be unacceptable for the time being. In France, the nasogastroscopy cost for complete esogastroduodenal examination is 96 euros compared with 510 euros for the capsule. For colonic screening, the difference in cost compared with FOBT or sigmoidoscopy is even greater. The reluctance of most healthcare providers to pay for small-bowel capsule endoscopy is linked to numerous overoptimistic clinical reports, the drawback of media pressure, and leaking of multicenter randomized trials. We are a very long way from routine clinical use of the capsule for the esophagus and colon.

Technological Visions

VCE will, of course, be improved. We are already seeing the importance of more advanced software, but the next developments should be with the device itself. We now envisage a capsule whose movement can be controlled. The engineers at Olympus Medical Systems have recently demonstrated possible magnetic control of the capsule, and we may be sure that Given Imaging engineers are working on some similar concept. If developed, this tool would allow large-bowel examination from the anus, but also more careful examination of the esophagus and stomach. The future development of the capsule will also involve biopsy or release of drugs for local treatment of digestive tract tumors. The capsule will have a clear clinical benefit for our patients when, in routine clinical practice, we can remotely control the capsule and use it to treat patients. At present, however, this possibility is still in the realm of science fiction.

Conclusion

VCE is definitely the gold standard for small-bowel examination, but we are still at an early stage with regard to the esophagus and colon. Nowadays medical devices, as are drugs, must be evaluated in four steps: the esophageal application of the capsule is at stage 2, where early clinical trials and assessments of potential benefit are conducted, and the colon capsule is at stage 1, where feasibility is evaluated. Overoptimistic "hyped-up" reporting and mass media coverage have, in fact, the most negative effect on the development of a clinically useful device. Competition between manufacturers should be based only on the technology and science. "Patient friendliness" is a marketing concept, as patient tolerance is well assessed by an already published scale. Nonmedical media coverage is an enormous mistake as the interests of potential shareholders are totally opposed to those of patient benefits and healthcare budgets. On the other hand, we dream, with Israeli and Japanese engineers, of a more advanced device, because we have seen the enormous clinical benefits for our patients as conventional endoscopy improved step by step over the past 40 years (from the fiberoptic scope to the video endoscope, high-definition endoscope, and NBI). This is why we can conclude that the future is bright for the video capsule.

References

1. Fleischer D (1994) 2020 Vision. Gastrointest Endosc 40:109–111
2. Rösch T, Eickhoff A, Fritscher-Ravens A, et al (2007) The new scopes: broadening the colonoscopy marketplace. Digestion 76:42–50
3. Cotton PB, Barkun A, Ginsberg G, et al (2006) Diagnostic endoscopy: 2020 vision. Gastrointest Endosc 64:395–398
4. Eisen GM (2006) Capsule endoscopy indications. ASGE Clinical Update 14:1
5. Eliakim R, Sharma VK, Yassin K, et al (2005) A prospective study of the diagnostic accuracy of PillCam ESO esophageal capsule endoscopy versus conventional upper endoscopy in patients with chronic gastroesophageal reflux diseases. J Clin Gastroenterol 39:572–578
6. Ramirez FC, Shaukat MS, Young MA, et al (2005) Feasibility and safety of string, wireless capsule endoscopy in the diagnosis of Barrett's esophagus. Gastrointest Endosc 61:741–745
7. Eisen GM, Eliakim R, Zaman A, et al (2006) The accuracy of PillCam ESO capsule endoscopy versus conventional upper endoscopy for the diagnosis of esophageal varices: a prospective three-center pilot study. Endoscopy 38:31–35

8. Lapalus MG, Dumortier J, Fumex F, et al (2006) Esophageal capsule endoscopy versus esophagogastroduodenoscopy for evaluating portal hypertension: a prospective comparative study of performance and tolerance. Endoscopy 38:36–41
9. Lin OS, Schembre DB, Mergener K, et al (2007) Blinded comparison of esophageal capsule endoscopy versus conventional endoscopy for a diagnosis of Barrett's esophagus in patients with chronic gastroesophageal reflux. Gastrointest Endosc 65:577–583
10. Sharma P, Wani S, Rastogi A, et al (2008) The diagnostic accuracy of esophageal capsule endoscopy in patients with gastroesophageal reflux disease and Barrett's esophagus: a blinded, prospective Study. Am J Gastroenterol 103:525–532
11. Gerson L, Lin OS (2007) Cost-benefit analysis of capsule endoscopy compared with standard upper endoscopy for the detection of Barrett's esophagus. Clin Gastroenterol Hepatol 5:319–325
12. Eliakim R, Fireman Z, Gralnek IM, et al (2006) Evaluation of the PillCam colon capsule in the detection of colonic pathology: results of the first multicenter, prospective, comparative study. Endoscopy 38:963–970
13. Schoofs N, Deviere J, Van Gossum A (2006) PillCam colon capsule endoscopy compared with colonoscopy for colorectal tumor diagnosis: a prospective pilot study. Endoscopy 38:971–977
14. Fireman Z, Kopelman Y (2007) The colon: the latest terrain for capsule endoscopy. Dig Liver Dis 39:895–899

Oropharynx and Hypopharynx

Endoscopic Diagnosis and Treatment of Superficial Cancer in the Oropharynx and Hypopharynx

MANABU MUTO

Summary. Although early detection of oropharyngeal and hypopharyngeal cancer has been rather difficult, narrow-band imaging (NBI) technology makes it possible. NBI is an innovative optical technology that can clearly visualize the microvascular structure of the organ surface when it is combined with magnifying endoscopy. This breakthrough opened a brand-new door of endoscopic diagnosis, not only of head and neck cancer but also of other gastrointestinal tract cancer. This new diagnostic strategy is based on microvascular morphological changes in the organ surface. Superficial squamous cell carcinoma of the oropharynx and hypopharynx shows typical characteristics. A well-demarcated brownish area and scattered irregular foci of microvascular proliferation projecting to the dysplastic squamous epithelium are the typical endoscopic features of the lesions. The number of detections of superficial cancer has increased over the past few years. For these superficial cancers, endoscopic treatment, generally accepted as a standard treatment for early cancer in the gastrointestinal field, is applied as a minimally invasive treatment. The endoscopic mucosal resection (EMR) cap method, endoscopic subepithelial dissection method, or endoscopic laryngopharyngeal surgery is performed under general anesthesia. Collaboration with otorhinolaryngologists and anesthesiologists is very important to successfully perform EMR in this region. This field also has problems directly linked to quality of life, such as swallowing and utterance. The establishment of early detection and of less invasive treatment is anticipated to provide great benefit to the patients.

Key words. Superficial cancer, Head and neck cancer, Narrow band imaging, Early diagnosis, Minimally invasive treatment

Introduction

One decade ago, although the pharyngeal space is the entrance to any endoscopic examination of the upper gastrointestinal (GI) tract, who could have anticipated that a GI endoscopist could find an early cancer in this region? At that time, no GI

Department of Gastroenterology and Hepatology, Kyoto University Graduate School of Medicine, 54 Kawaharacho, Shogoin, Sakyo, Kyoto 606-8577, Japan

endoscopist knew the endoscopic characteristics of superficial cancer in the pharynx, especially in the oropharyngeal and hypopharyngeal mucosal sites, because most of the cancer in this region had been diagnosed at an advanced stage with a large tumor. In addition, cancer in the oropharynx and hypopharynx has been considered to be the field of the ENT (ear-nose-throat) doctors.

Narrow-band imaging (NBI), which is one of the biggest technological breakthroughs in the GI endoscopic field, makes it possible to detect an early cancer in this region [1–3]. Thus, the number of superficial cancer in the oropharyngeal and hypopharyngeal mucosal sites detected by GI endoscopists has increased during the past few years. Here, we review the Japanese experience of endoscopic diagnosis and endoscopic treatment for superficial cancer in the oropharynx and hypopharynx.

"Early Cancer" or "Superficial Cancer" in the Oropharynx and Hypopharynx

The definition of "early cancer" or "superficial cancer" in the head and neck region has not been determined. In a way, early cancer means superficial cancer that shows good prognosis. However, the long-term prognosis and even the natural history of superficial pharyngeal cancer are unknown. In addition, in cases of GI tract cancer, invasion depth in the wall is one of the factors for the definition of early cancer because invasion depth is closely associated with lymph node metastasis. However, there is no classification of the invasion depth of cancer in the oropharyngeal and hypopharyngeal wall in the Japanese Criteria of Head and Neck Cancer (in Japanese) [4] and the TNM classification (sixth edition) by the International Union Against Cancer (UICC) [5]. Therefore, it is difficult to evaluate the risk for lymphatic metastasis on the basis of invasion depth in the wall in head and neck region.

To date, only "carcinoma in situ" [or "high grade intraepithelial neoplasia" by the World Health Organization (WHO) classification] reflects histological invasion depth. However, according to the statistics from 29 institutes nationwide in 2001 by the Japan Society of Head and Neck Cancer [6], carcinoma in situ was found in only 1 of 218 hypopharyngeal cases and none of 162 oropharyngeal cases. This finding indicates that it is markedly difficult to detect carcinoma in situ in the oropharynx and hypopharynx. In other words, there has been little clinical and pathological information about carcinoma in situ in the oropharynx and hypopharynx. It should be also noted that the definition of carcinoma in situ differs between Japan and Western countries, and it is also defined as high-grade dysplasia according to the Vienna Classification [7].

It is apparent that the superficial type of neoplasia has been increasingly identified during clinical practice. Therefore, we should immediately determine the terminology of these lesions. We herein prefer to use the term superficial cancer for slightly elevated, flat, or slightly depressed lesions, because their prognosis and risk of lymph node metastasis are uncertain.

Diagnosis of "Superficial Cancer" in the Oropharynx and Hypopharynx

We first reported that NBI observation with magnified endoscopy allowed detection of carcinoma in situ in the oropharynx and hypopharynx [1]. The detection rate and diagnostic accuracy of superficial cancer by NBI are quite high compared to conventional white light observation [8]. In the ENT field, ENT fiber combined with NBI can detect a superficial cancer [9].

Why is NBI useful to detect superficial cancer in the oropharynx and hypopharynx? NBI combined with magnifying endoscopy can clearly visualize minute vascular structures on the organ surface [10,11]. It has been known that abnormal changes in shape and irregular dilatation and meandering of minute vessels are observed even at the early phase of carcinogenesis, such as carcinoma in situ in the squamous epithelium (Fig. 1). Then, we can see endoscopically these changes as a hallmark, microvascular proliferation pattern (Figs. 1, 2) [1–3,9]. Inoue et al. reported that changes

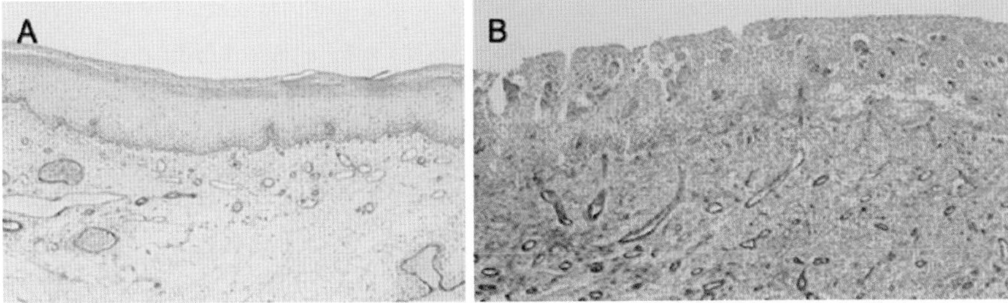

Fig. 1. Normal squamous cell epithelium (**A**) and squamous cell carcinoma in situ (**B**) in the pharynx. Abnormal changes in shape and irregular dilatation and meandering of minute vessels are observed in carcinoma in situ and the subepithelial layer (**B**). These changes are represented less in normal epithelium (**A**)

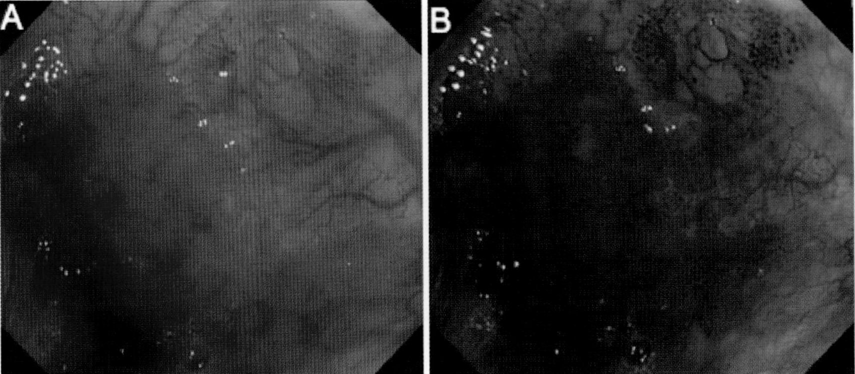

Fig. 2. Carcinoma in situ of right pyriform sinus of the hypopharynx. It is difficult to recognize the lesion by conventional white light observation (**A**), but a well-demarcated brownish area can be easily recognized by narrow-band imaging (NBI) (**B**).

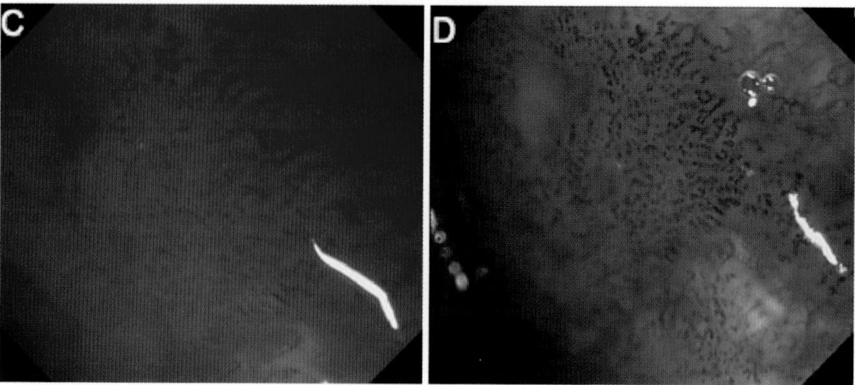

Fig. 2. The irregular microvascular pattern is difficult to identify by white light observation even under high magnification (**C**), whereas NBI clearly visualized the irregular microvascular pattern (**D**)

in the intraepithelial papillary capillary loop (IPCL) were a useful indicator for early squamous cell carcinoma in the esophagus [12]. Similar changes were observed in the oropharynx and hypopharynx. In addition, distinct boundaries were formed between the tumor lesion and normal epithelium and they were recognized as "brownish areas" by NBI observation (see Fig. 2) [1–3,9]. To date, superficial oropharyngeal and hypopharyngeal cancer has also been detected by careful observation, but advancement of GI endoscopy systems such as NBI has dramatically improved detection of superficial cancer in the oropharynx and hypopharynx.

Indication of Endoscopic Treatment

Radiotherapy or surgical resection has been a standard treatment for head and neck cancer for a long time. However, these modalities are apparently invasive for superficial cancer. Endoscopic mucosal resection (EMR) is an ideal treatment because EMR is considerably less invasive than surgical resection and can preserve these organs and functions.

EMR is theoretically indicated only for the lesions with no or extremely low risk for lymphatic metastasis. In the GI tract including the esophagus, stomach, and colon, the absolute indications have been determined based on detailed analysis using a large number of surgically resected cases, and EMR for superficial cancer is now generally accepted. On the other hand, the risk for lymphatic metastasis of superficial pharyngeal cancer has been unclear because of lack of information. What lesions we should treat by the EMR method?

In general, carcinoma in situ is recognized as a neoplasia without risk of metastasis. Therefore, when we consider the absolute indication of EMR for superficial cancer in the oropharyngeal and hypopharyngeal mucosal sites, it should be limited to lesions such as carcinoma in situ because of the lack of risk of metastasis.

There is another possibility of EMR for superficial cancer in the oropharynx and hypopharynx. If EMR can remove a superficial but slightly invasive cancer completely, this method could be a comparable method of local resection with external incision of the neck. This method provides great benefit of minimal invasiveness to the patients because it causes no skin injury.

To extend the indications, further accumulation of such cases is needed, which would clarify the maximum invasion depth under the squamous epithelium without the risk of metastasis. Early cancer would also be eventually defined.

EMR of Oropharyngeal and Hypopharyngeal Superficial Cancer

When EMR is carried out for suspected carcinoma in situ in the oropharynx and hypopharynx, it is necessary to confirm there is no lymphatic or distant metastasis by computed tomography (CT) or magnetic resonance imaging (MRI), with the possibility of subepithelial invasion being taken into account. The relationship between degrees of subepithelial invasion and frequency of lymphatic metastasis remains to be clarified, as already mentioned. However, because carcinoma in situ in the oropharynx and hypopharynx with minute subepithelial invasion is also found in some cases of neck lymphatic metastasis with an unidentified primary lesion, caution should be employed for such cases. Moreover, because oropharyngeal and hypopharyngeal carcinoma in situ has rarely been detected to date, no treatment guidelines are currently present.

T1 cancer according to the Japanese Criteria for Head and Neck Cancer and TNM classification by the UICC is defined as a lesion 2 cm or smaller, irrespective of invasion depth, and in cases of no lymphatic or distant metastasis, standard treatment is radiation therapy alone. However, in cases of radiation therapy, because saliva secretion is greatly decreased by the injury to the salivary glands, and serious problems for daily life, such as dryness in the oral cavity and taste abnormality, are induced, such treatment should be avoided if possible.

On the other hand, when the lesion size is small and surgical resection is possible, there are two methods: by an oral approach and by an external incision. In cases of oropharynx, satisfactory resection may be possible by an oral approach, but in cases of hypopharynx, an external incision is necessary, and it is expected that endoscopic approaches would reduce the burden for patients in view of invasiveness and cosmetic aspects.

It should be noted that general anesthesia is required because of the risk of aspiration into the airway when EMR is performed for oropharyngeal and hypopharyngeal carcinoma in situ. In addition, the fact that EMR for oropharyngeal and hypopharyngeal carcinoma in situ is currently an explorative treatment has to be fully explained to the patients and their family for informed consent. In this situation, EMR should be indicated when the following conditions are satisfied.

1. Carcinoma in situ or carcinoma with minute subepithelial invasion is diagnosed.
2. The size is within two or three subregions.
3. Clinically, there is no lymphatic or distant metastasis.

When subepithelial invasion and vascular infiltration are found after resection, degrees of risk for metastasis are currently unidentified. In cases of head and neck cancer, there is no concept of preventive lymphadenectomy, in contrast to GI cancer, and subepithelial invasion and vascular infiltration do not always indicate the requirement of therapy such as lymphadenectomy and radiation therapy. Therefore, currently such cases should be carefully followed up and, when lymphatic metastasis is found, surgical lymphadenectomy and radiation therapy (or chemoradiation therapy) need to be considered.

When the lesion for EMR is found to be unexpectedly large and surgical resection is more appropriate, it is better to change therapy from EMR to standard treatments, i.e., radiation therapy and surgical resection.

EMR Methods

EMR Cap Method

EMR using the cap method (EMRC) was previously reported [13]. EMRC is performed mostly by the aspiration method with a soft hood (Fig. 3). This method is technically easy, but there is a limitation of the size of resection in one session. Thus, EMRC should be indicated for small lesions less than 10 mm in which en bloc and complete resection could be expected.

Endoscopic Subepithelial Dissection Method

The endoscopic subepithelial dissection method (ESD) is based on the endoscopic submucosal dissection method for the stomach [14]. If the lesion is larger than 10 mm, the ESD method should be indicated because this method is useful to obtain a large specimen en bloc (Fig. 4).

Endoscopic Laryngopharyngeal Surgery

Endoscopic laryngopharyngeal surgery (ELPS) was first reported by Sato et al. [15]. This method is quite useful to maintain a wide working space in the pharynx (Fig. 5). It makes the procedure easier, and a larger specimen can be easily obtained.

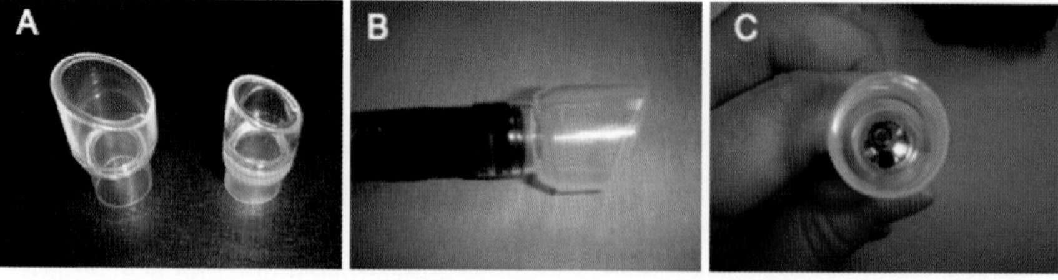

Fig. 3. Endoscopic mucosal resection (EMR) using a soft plastic hood (**A**, *left*) and a hard type hood (**A**, *right*). **B** Soft hood attached to tip of endoscope. **C** En face view

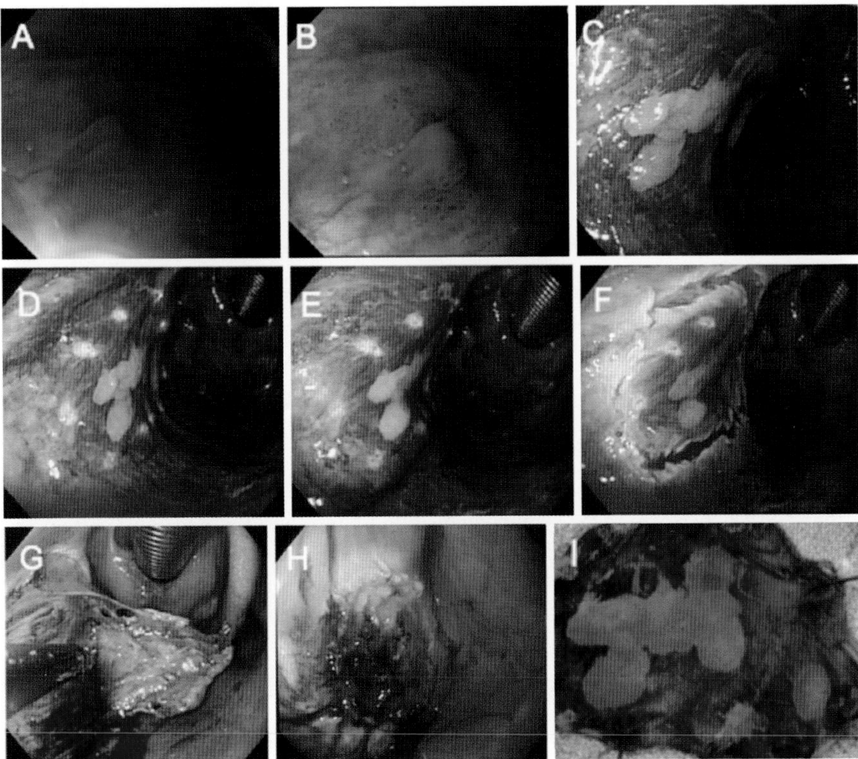

FIG. 4. Endoscopic subepithelial dissection (ESD) method. **A** A slightly reddish-colored lesion could be detected in the oropharynx; however, the margin is difficult to identify by conventional white light. **B** NBI revealed a slightly brownish area and scattered tiny brownish dots in the lesion. **C** The lesion is evidently recognizable as a nonstained lesion by iodine glycerine solution. **D** The incision line is indicated with several coagulating spots being marked along 5–10 mm outside the definite margin of the target lesion using a needle knife. **E** To make blunt dissection of the subepithelial layer, a saline solution containing diluted epinephrine (0.02 mg/ml) is injected into the subepithelial layer just outside the marking spots. **F** Circumferential incision of the mucosa is performed with a needle knife. **G** Subepithelial dissection is performed under the condition of lifting up the lesion toward the direction of the traction power of grasping forceps inserted directly per os. **H** Mucosal defect after ESD. **I** Ex vivo Lugol staining revealed that the resected specimen contained a cancerous lesion

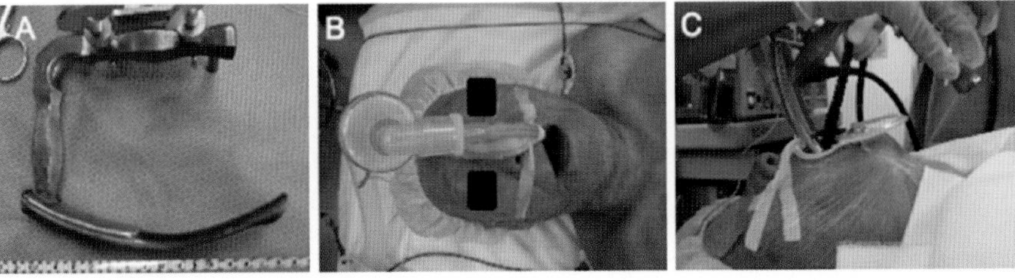

FIG. 5. Endoscopic laryngopharyngeal surgery. **A** A curved type rigid laryngoscope originally developed by Dr. Y. Sato, Kasawaki Hospital, Japan. **B** Transoral intubation and fixation at the angle of the mouth on the opposite side of the lesion. **C** Careful insertion of curved type rigid laryngoscope.

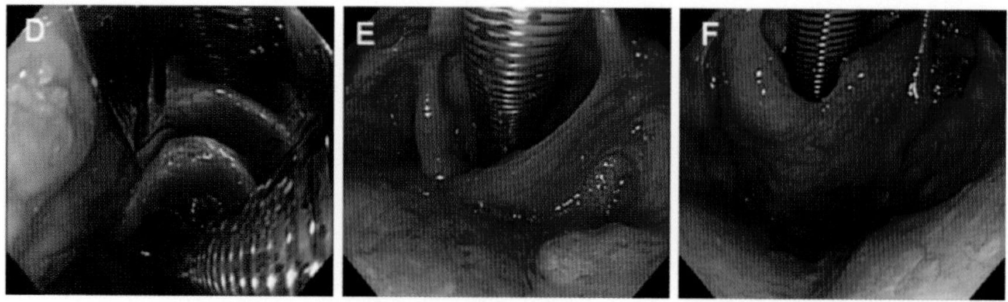

Fig. 5. **D** The tip of laryngoscope is gently inserted into the vallecula. **E** Pharyngeal space is usually narrowed. **F** After lifting up the whole larynx, the working space becomes wider

EMR Procedure

When EMR is performed for oropharyngeal and hypopharyngeal lesions, close communication between otorhinolaryngologists and anesthesiologists is indispensable. Unless it is secured, EMR of oropharyngeal and hypopharyngeal lesions should not be performed for reasons of consideration for the safety of the patient.

Examinations and Preparation before EMR

Given the requirement of general anesthesia, electrocardiography and evaluation of respiratory function are necessary. In addition, it is necessary to confirm the presence or absence of infection according to the standard of the institute. As the preparation on the day before treatment, a restriction on eating after supper and intake of a laxative are routinely done.

Day of EMR

On the day of EMR, a glycerin enema is given in consideration of incontinence during anesthesia. In addition, necessary drip infusion is done to secure the intravenous route, and nutrition is given because no intake is allowed on the day of EMR.

EMR Under General Anesthesia

Because general anesthesia is a common procedure, reference of other textbooks is recommended.

1. The supine position is recommended. The reasons are that (1) it reduces influx of iodine into the larynx and inflammation of the pharyngeal mucosa, and (2) surgical fields of the oropharynx and hypopharynx are easy to secure when the larynx is lifted with a laryngoscope (personal communication with Drs. Yasushi Sato and Yasushi Omori, Kawasaki Municipal Kawasaki Hospital, Kanagawa, Japan). Details of the laryngoscope are described later.

2. An oral approach is selected for tracheal intubation, and the tracheal tube is fixed at the angle of the mouth on the opposite side of the lesion. Fixation of a tracheal tube on the same side of the lesion narrows the surgical space in the pharynx.

3. Next, a laryngoscope is inserted and the whole larynx is lifted. As a laryngoscope is a rigid scope and compression by the device may break the teeth, it is recommended to construct a mouthpiece in advance. In addition, it is desirable to ask an experienced otorhinolaryngologist to place a laryngoscope to avoid potential injury to the larynx and pharynx.

4. Staining with iodine solution is currently the best method to identify the lesion as commonly accepted. Therefore, although the extent of the lesion is evaluated correctly by staining with iodine solution, presence or absence of multiple lesions should also be explored by spraying iodine solution over the whole oropharynx and hypopharynx.

5. As the iodine solution may overflow from the angle of the mouth and cause skin staining, it is recommended to put Opsite tapes on both angles of the mouth.

6. It is desirable to use iodine solution at half the concentration used for staining the esophagus to reduce chemical inflammation (about 1%).

7. It is necessary to pay attention to prevent influx of iodine solution into the larynx.

8. EMR for oropharyngeal and hypopharyngeal lesions is performed by appropriate methods [12]. It is sometimes difficult to employ the aspiration method for the lesion in the right pyriform recess and posterior parts of the annulus in the hypopharynx because of their anatomy. In addition, because the posterior wall of the hypopharynx is thin in the subepithelial layer, the aspiration method is hard to apply. For such lesions, the subepithelial dissection method should be considered.

9. After resection, presence or absence of pharyngeal edema is checked, and sodium thiosulfate (Detoxol, a neutralizer for iodine glycerin solution) is sprayed before the end of the procedure.

Management After EMR

Oral intake is prohibited even after full awakening on the day of EMR. On the next day after EMR, the degree of chemical inflammation and pharyngeal edema by iodide is examined by endoscopy, and water intake is begun. Because it is easier to swallow meals at certain solidity levels than fluid meals, porridge at intermediate solidity and chopped food are begun on day 2 after EMR. If possible, it is recommended to confirm no aspiration occurs at the meal. Meals are gradually changed to more solid meals, and patients are discharged about 1 week later. In about 1 week, chemical inflammation adjacent to the lesion by iodine solution is alleviated and only the resected area remains as an ulcer. Although healing depends on the size of resection, the ulcer becomes a scar in about 1 month. Therefore, during the follow-up period, endoscopy is performed about 1 month later to confirm scarring of the ulcer and presence or absence of remnants of the lesion, and endoscopy is repeated to detect metachronous multiple cancers 3 months later, 6 months later, and then every 6 months.

Conclusion

Oropharyngeal and hypopharyngeal carcinoma in situ, which used to be undetected, has been found by GI endoscopy rather than laryngoscopy as a consequence of the advances in diagnostic capability. Thus, EMR, established for gastrointestinal early cancer, has been applied for such lesions. However, this field is new with a short history, and a number of matters remain to be clarified. It is necessary to accumulate a large number of cases and elucidate long-term outcomes for establishment of appropriate treatment guidelines. On the other hand, this field also has problems directly linked to QOL (quality of life), such as swallowing and utterance. The establishment of early detection and of less invasive treatment is anticipated to provide great benefits to patients.

References

1. Muto M, Nakane M, Katada C, et al (2004) Squamous cell carcinoma in situ in oropharyngeal and hypopharyngeal mucosal sites. Cancer (Phila) 101:1375–1381
2. Muto M, Katada C, Sano Y, et al (2005) Narrowband imaging: a new diagnostic approach to visualize angiogenesis in the superficial neoplasm. Clin Gastroenterol Hepatol 3:S16–S20
3. Muto M, Ugumori T, Sano Y, et al (2005) Narrow band imaging combined with magnified endoscopy for the cancer at the head and neck region. Dig Endosc 17:S23–S24
4. Japan Society for Head and Neck Cancer (2001) General rules for clinical studies on head and neck cancer, 3rd edn. Kanehara Shoten, Tokyo
5. International Union Against Cancer (UICC) (2002) TNM classification of malignant tumors, 6th edn. Wiley-Liss, New York
6. Japan Society for Head and Neck Cancer Registry Committee (2005) Report of head and neck cancer registry of Japan: clinical statistics and registered patients, 2001. Jpn J Head Neck Cancer 31:60–80
7. Schlember RJ, Riddell RH, Kato Y, et al (2000) The Vienna classification of gastrointestinal epithelial neoplasia. Gut 47:251–255
8. Muto M, Saito Y, Ohmori T, et al (2007) Multicenter prospective randomized controlled study on the detection and diagnosis of superficial squamous cell carcinoma by back-to-back endoscopic examination of narrowband imaging and white light observation. Gastrointest Endosc 65:AB110
9. Watanabe A, Tsujie H, Taniguchi M, et al (2006) Laryngoscopic detection of pharyngeal carcinoma in situ with narrowband imaging. Laryngoscope 116:605–654
10. Gono K, Yamazaki K, Doguchi N, et al (2003) Endoscopic observation of tissue by narrow band illumination. Opt Rev 10:1–5
11. Gono K, Obi T, Yamaguchi M, et al (2004) Appearance of enhanced tissue feature in narrow-band endoscopic imaging. J Biomed Opt 9:568–577
12. Inoue H, Honda T, Nagai K, et al (1997) Ultra-high magnification endoscopic observation of carcinoma in situ of the oesophagus. Dig Endosc 9:16–18
13. Inoue H, Takeshita K, Hori H, et al (1993) Endoscopic mucosal resection with a cap-fitted panendoscope for esophagus, stomach and colon mucosal lesions. Gastrointest Endosc 39:58–62
14. Muto M, Miyamoto S, Hosokawa A, et al (2005) Endoscopic mucosal resection in the stomach using the insulated-tip needle-knife. Endoscopy 37:178–182
15. Sato Y, Omori T, Tagawa M (2006) Treatment of superficial carcinoma in the hypopharynx. Nippon Jibiinkoka Gakkai Kaiho 109:581–586 (in Japanese with English abstract)

Esophagus

Diagnosis of Esophageal and Gastric Carcinoma Using Transnasal Ultrathin Esophagogastroduodenoscopy

TAKASHI KAWAI[1], TETSUYA YAMAGISHI[1], and FUMINORI MORIYASU[2]

Summary. In Japan, rapid spread in the use of transnasal ultrathin esophagogastroduodenoscopy (UT-EGD) is reported. Problems have been identified with the new technique, however, including poor endoscopic imaging quality. In this study, we investigated detection rates for esophageal and gastric cancers using transnasal UT-EGD, and compared endoscopic imaging quality between UT-EGD and conventional EGD (C-EGD). The subjects were 959 patients who underwent transnasal UT-EGD. We investigated the detection rates for esophageal cancer, gastric cancer and gastric adenoma. We compared endoscopic image between UT-EGD and C-EGD. We detected 2 cases of esophageal cancer, 13 of gastric cancer and 5 of gastric adenoma. The detection rate for esophageal and gastric cancer was 1.56% (15/959). The border between an abnormal area and the surrounding mucosa was less distinct on the UT-EGD image than on the C-EGD image in 5 cases, and similar clarity was seen in 2 cases. In this study the esophageal-gastric cancer detection rate was high at 1.56%. Although we found no difference in the ability to distinguish abnormalities between UT-EGD and C-EGD, it is possible that problems with determining the extent or depth of invasion of lesions may arise compared with C-EGD image.

Key words. Transnasal esophagogastroduodenoscopy (TN-EGD), Ultrathin esophagogastroduodenoscopy (UT-EGD), Gastric cancer, Esophageal cancer

Introduction

In recent years, ultrathin esophagogastroduodenoscopy (UT-EGD) using the transnasal approach has attracted considerable attention. With this method, an ultrathin endoscope 5–6 mm in diameter is inserted through the nose. Garcia et al. compared sedated transoral conventional esophagogastroduodenoscopy (C-EGD) with unsedated transnasal UT-EGD in a randomized trial, and found no significant difference between groups in either patient satisfaction with the procedure or willingness

[1]Endoscopy Center, Tokyo Medical University Hospital, 6-7-1 Nishi-Shinjuku, Shinjuku-ku, Tokyo 160-0023, Japan
[2]Fourth Department of Internal Medicine, Tokyo Medical University, Tokyo, Japan

to undergo repeat EGD using the same method [1]. Studies comparing transnasal UT-EGD with unsedated transoral C-EGD also reported good patient tolerance [2,3]. Japanese studies of the benefits of transnasal UT-EGD in terms of patient satisfaction and its effects on cardiopulmonary function found significantly less discomfort during insertion of the endoscope, or trouble breathing or nausea during the procedure, in comparison with transoral C-EGD. The double product (heart rate × systolic blood pressure × 10^{-2}), known to correlate well with myocardial oxygen consumption, rose significantly at the time the endoscope was introduced into the esophagus with transoral C-EGD, whereas little or no change was seen during transnasal UT-EGD procedures, indicating the safety of the latter technique [4,5].

In Japan, a rapid spread in the use of transnasal UT-EGD is reported. Problems have been identified with the new technique, however, including poor endoscopic imaging quality and inferior rinsing function of lens (washing the endoscope charge-coupled device with water). In this study, we investigated detection rates for esophageal and gastric cancers using transnasal UT-EGD and compared imaging quality between ultrathin and conventional endoscopes.

Subjects and Methods

The subjects were 959 patients who underwent transnasal UT-EGD between January 2005 and September 2007. Their average age was 57.0 ± 15.6 years, with a male : female ratio of 1.32 : 1. The patients were stratified with three steps. In Step 1, we investigated the detection rates for esophageal cancer, gastric cancer and gastric adenoma. In Step 2, of the subjects, 78 patients with a history of cardiac disease or cerebral infarction were taking low-dose aspirin at the time of their procedure. All subjects underwent transnasal UT-EGD without ceasing their low-dose aspirin, and we investigated the rates of successful transnasal insertion, and epistaxis or other hemorrhage. We also investigated the detection rates for esophageal cancer, gastric cancer, and gastric adenoma. We surveyed each subject concerning how many times they had undergone EGD. In Step 3, the patients were 7 subjects who underwent transoral C-EGD within 2 months of detection of esophageal cancer, gastric cancer, or gastric adenoma by transnasal UT-EGD. They comprised 1 with esophageal cancer, 4 with gastric cancer, and 2 with gastric adenoma. We compared endoscopic findings of the degree of atrophy (Kimura/Takemoto classification [6]), the mucosal properties of the lesion and surrounding mucosa, and the border between the lesion and its surrounds, between transnasal UT-EGD and transoral C-EGD images.

The transnasal UT-EGD used were the GIF-N260 and GIF-XP260N of Olympus Medical Systems, Tokyo, Japan, and the EG470N, EG530N and EG530N2 of Fujinon-Toshiba ES Systems CO. LTD, Tokyo, Japan. The C-EGD used were the GIF-XQ240 and GIF-Q260 (Olympus Medical Systems).

Results

In Step 1, we detected 2 cases of esophageal cancer, 13 of gastric cancer, and 5 of gastric adenoma. The detection rate for esophageal and gastric cancer was 1.56% (15/959). The type for the cases of esophageal cancer was 0-IIa in 1 case and 0-IIb in the other. The type for the cases of gastric cancer was 0-Ia in 1 case, 0-IIa in 2 cases, 0-IIa + IIc in 1 case, 0-IIc in 8 cases, and type 2 in 1 case. Case 1 was a 57-year-old woman with a type 0-IIc gastric carcinoma on the greater curvature of the middle gastric body. The histological findings were of signet-ring cell carcinoma (Fig. 1). Case 2 was a 77-year-old man with a type 0-IIa esophageal carcinoma in the mid-esophagus. The histological findings were of squamous cell carcinoma (Fig. 2).

In Step 2, subjects had undergone EGD only 1.08 ± 0.26 times on average. The rate of successful transnasal endoscopic insertion was 96.2% (75/78), with the middle turbinate route used in 73.3% and the inferior turbinate route in 26.7%. The incidence of epistaxis was 2.6% (2/75), one case each for both routes. The detection rate for esophageal and gastric cancer was 6.4% (5/78), with one case of esophageal cancer, four of gastric cancer, and two of gastric adenoma. The type for the one case of esophageal cancer was 0-IIa, and the type for the cases of gastric cancer was one case each of 0-I, 0-IIa, 0-IIc, and type 2.

In Step 3, no difference was found in the degree of endoscopically observed mucosal atrophy using the Kimura/Takemoto classification between transnasal UT-EGD and C-EGD. Pale discoloration of atrophic areas of gastric mucosa could be seen more clearly in transnasal UT-EGD images than with C-EGD. Case 3 was a 67-year-old man. In the left-hand picture (UT-EGD image), we can see pale discoloration of an atrophic area of gastric mucosa on the lesser curvature of the gastric body more strongly than

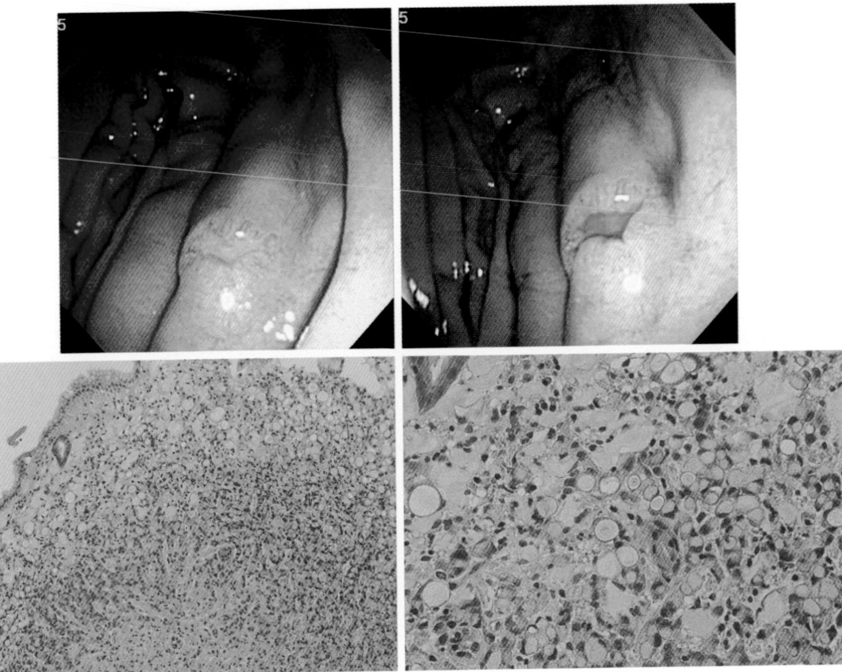

Fig. 1. Case 1 was a 57-year-old woman with a type 0-IIc gastric carcinoma on the greater curvature of the middle gastric body. The histological findings were of signet-ring cell carcinoma

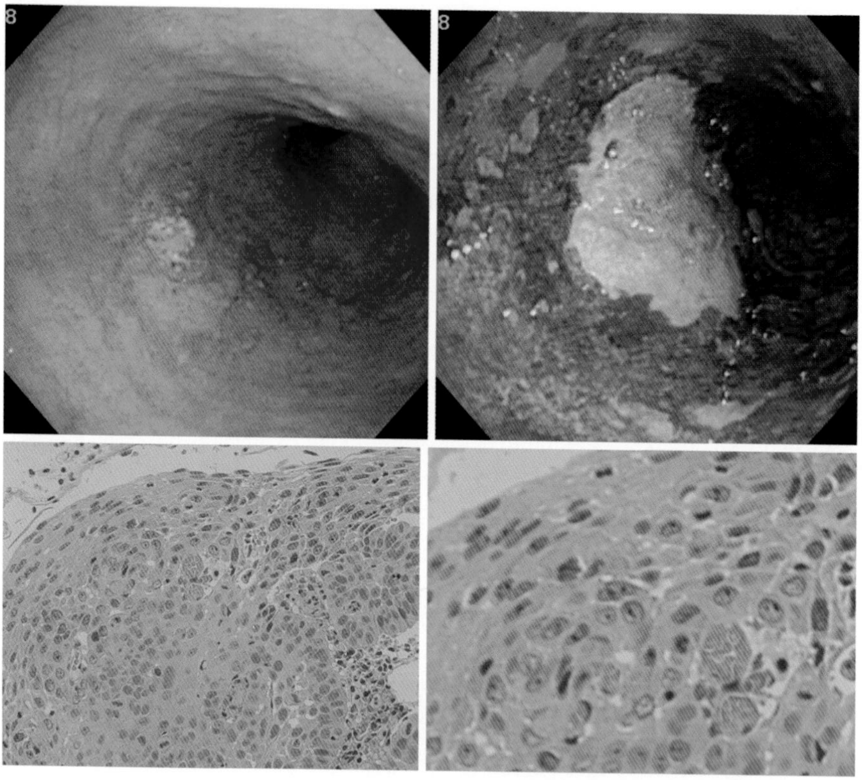

Fig. 2. Case 2 was a 77-year-old man with a type 0-IIa esophageal carcinoma in the mid-esophagus. The histological findings were of squamous cell carcinoma

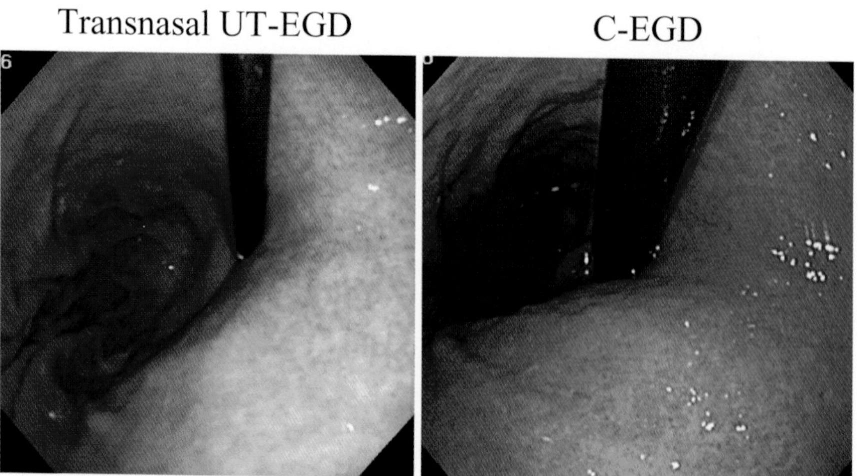

Fig. 3. Case 3 was a 67-year-old man. Pale discoloration of the area of gastric mucosal atrophy from the gastric body lesser curvature is more pronounced in the ultrathin esophagogastroduodenoscopy (UT-EGD) image on the *left* than in the conventional esophagogastroduodenoscopy (C-EGD) image on the *right*

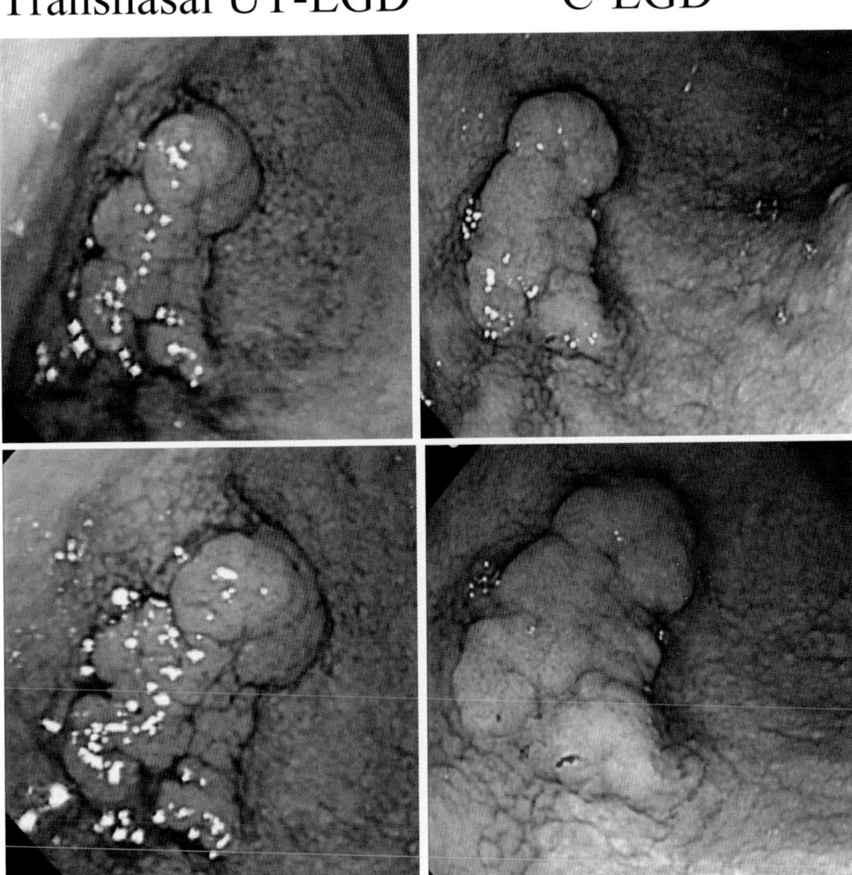

Fig. 4. Case 4 was a 52-year-old man with a well-differentiated type 0-IIa gastric carcinoma on the anterior wall of the greater curvature of the gastric angle. Rough granularity of the mucosal surface is more pronounced in the UT-EGD image on the *left* than in the C-EGD image on the *right*

in the right-hand picture (C-EGD image). Rough granularity of the mucosa in the target area is more pronounced in the UT-EGD than the C-EGD image (Fig. 3). The border between an abnormal area and the surrounding mucosa was less distinct on the UT-EGD image than on the C-EGD image in five cases, and similar clarity was seen in two cases. Case 4 was a 52-year-old man with a well-differentiated type 0-IIa gastric carcinoma on the anterior wall of the greater curvature of the gastric angle. Rough granularity of the mucosal surface is more pronounced in the left-hand picture (UT-EGD image) than in the right-hand picture (C-EGD image) (Fig. 4). Case 5 was a 63-year-old man with well-differentiated type 0-IIc gastric carcinoma on the greater curvature of the gastric antrum. Rough granularity of the mucosal surface is increased,

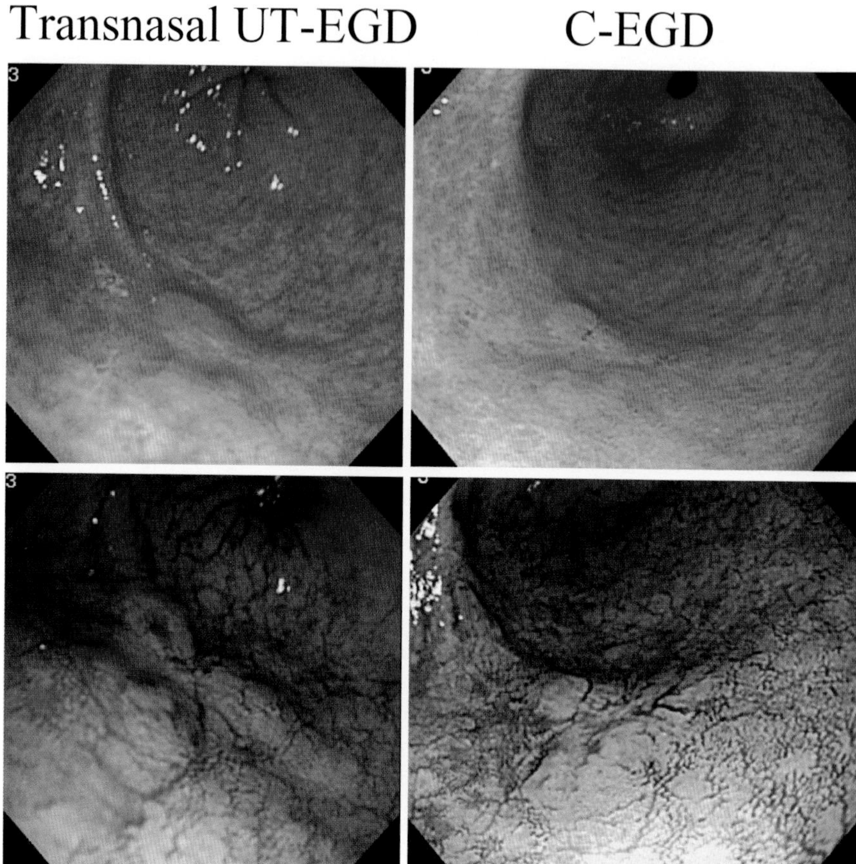

Fig. 5. Case 5 was a 63-year-old man with well-differentiated type 0-IIc gastric carcinoma on the gastric antrum greater curvature. Rough granularity of the mucosal surface is increased, and the border with the surrounding mucosa less clear, in the UT-EGD image on the *left* than in the C-EGD image on the *right*

and the boundary with the surrounding mucosa less clear, in the left-hand picture (UT-EGD image) than in the right-hand picture (C-EGD image) (Fig. 5).

Discussion

Although a number of studies have reported reduced patient discomfort with ultra-thin transnasal endoscopy, few have addressed diagnostic accuracy with this method. Saeian et al. compared the diagnostic accuracy of unsedated UT-EGD and sedated C-EGD for esophageal varices in 15 patients with hepatic cirrhosis. They found that UT-EGD was able to accurately diagnose esophageal varices and was a safe, low-cost method [7]. In another study, the same group reported that transnasal endoscopy accurately detects Barrett's metaplasia and dysplasia, including pathohistological findings, equally as well as conventional transoral endoscopy [8]. There have been few reports concerning diagnosis of gastric cancer using transnasal endoscopy, however. Despite concerns that imaging quality for transnasal UT-EGD is inferior in comparison with C-EGD, in this study the esophageal-gastric cancer detection rate was high, at 1.5%. In general, reported outpatient annual detection rates for gastric cancer, including this institution, are of the order of 0.5%–1.0%. When we restricted the subject population to patients on low-dose aspirin therapy in Step 2, the detection rate rose to 6.4%. One reason for the high detection rates for esophageal and gastric cancers may be explained by the low number of endoscopies previously undergone by this group. Transnasal UT-EGD can occupy an important position as a technique that can identify disease in patients who have until now been too afraid to undergo endoscopy.

Olympus Medical Systems have already announced that imaging quality obtained with ultrathin endoscopes is inferior to that provided by conventional diameter endoscopes. There have been no reports, however, of any observed differences in imaging quality in actual clinical use. In our comparison of images obtained with UT-EGD and C-EGD, we found differences in how the mucosal properties were perceived. Using UT-EGD, lesions took on a rough granular appearance, and the boundary with the surrounding mucosa was indistinct in several cases. Although we found no difference in the ability to distinguish abnormalities between UT-EGD and C-EGD, it is possible that problems with determining the extent or depth of invasion of lesions may arise with the former technique. Further studies are required to investigate whether UT-EGD can detect small flat (type IIb) lesions.

Although imaging quality with UT-EGD is inferior to that provided by C-EGD, at present it provides high detection rates for esophageal and gastric cancers, and is also a promising endoscopic technique for the future.

References

1. Garcia RT, Cello JP, Nguyen MH, et al (2003) Unsedated ultrathin EGD is well accepted compared with conventional sedated: a multicenter randomized trial. Gastroenterology 125:1606–1612
2. Bikner B, Fritz N, Schatke W, et al (2003) A prospective randomized comparison of unsedated ultrathin versus standard esophagogastroduodenoscopy in routine outpatient gastroenterology practice: does it work better through the nose. Endoscopy 35:647–651
3. Press C, Charton JP, Schumacher B, et al (2003) A randomized trial of unsedated transnasal small-caliber esophagogastroduodenoscopy (EGD) versus peroral small-caliber EGD versus conventional EGD. Endoscopy 35:641–645
4. Kawai T, Miyazaki I, Yagi K, et al (2007) Comparison of the effects on cardiopulmonary function of ultrathin transnasal versus normal diameter transoral esophagogastroduodenoscopy in Japan. Hepatogastroenterology 54:766–772
5. Yagi J, Adachi K, Arima N, et al (2005) A prospective randomized comparative study on the safety and tolerability of transnasal esophagogastroduodenoscopy. Endoscopy 37:1226–1231

6. Kimura K (1972) Chronological transition of the fundic-pyloric border determined by stepwise biopsy of the lesser and greater curvatures of the stomach. Gastroenterology 63:584–592
7. Saeian K, Staff D, Knox J, et al (2002) Unsedated transnasal endoscopy: a new technique for accurately detecting and grading esophageal varices in cirrhotic patients. Am J Gastroenterol 97:2246–2249
8. Saeian K, Staff D, Vasilopoulos S, et al (2002) Unsedated transnasal endoscopy accurately detects Barrett's metaplasia and dysplasia. Gastrointest Endosc 56:472–478

Magnifying Endoscopic Findings with Narrow-Band Imaging System in the Esophagus

Mototsugu Kato[1], Yuichi Shimizu[1], and Masahiro Asaka[2]

Summary. New techniques such as magnifying endoscopy and narrow-band imaging (NBI) are being accepted for diagnosis in esophageal fields. Especially, magnifying endoscopic examination with the NBI system is used to examine suspicious areas of mucosa not visible during conventional endoscopic examination. These endoscopic techniques are also used for diagnosis for nonmalignant disease. Because NBI accurately identifies the microvascular architecture of the surface mucosa, it clearly detects dyspepsia and carcinoma as a brownish area. Conventional endoscopy with NBI is useful for screening examinations in esophagus and pharynx. The advantage of the NBI system is that dye is not required. The main advantage of magnifying endoscopy with NBI is the improved visualization of intrapapillary capillary loops (IPCL). Morphological change and irregular arrangement of IPCLs are associated with inflammation and neoplasia of the esophagus. The characteristic changes of magnified appearance in squamous cell carcinoma are dilation, weaving, and variation in size and shape of IPCL. Magnifying endoscopic observation with NBI of IPCLs in esophageal epithelium is useful for diagnosis of nonerosive reflux disease, which cannot be visualized with conventional endoscopy. The patterns of IPCL in inflammatory mucosa are simply dilation and elongation with regular arrangement. Assessment of the IPCL pattern using magnifying endoscopy with NBI is important for diagnosis of esophageal squamous neoplasia and esophageal inflammatory disease.

Key words. Magnifying endoscopy, NBI, Esophageal cancer, dysplasia, nonerosive reflux disease (NERD)

Introduction

Although the incidence of esophageal adenocarcinoma has increased dramatically in Western countries during the past two decades, esophageal squamous cell carcinoma has been continuously dominant in Asian countries, including Japan. Endoscopic

[1]Division of Endoscopy, Hokkaido University Hospital, North 14, West 5, Kita-ku, Sapporo, Hokkaido 060-8648, Japan

[2]Department of Gastroenterology, Hokkaido University Graduate School of Medicine, Sapporo, Japan

resection is often used to treat early esophageal carcinoma because of its minimal invasiveness and satisfactory outcome. The early stage of squamous cell carcinoma with invasion to the lamina propria mucosa is indicated for endoscopic resection because such tumors are known to have a low risk of lymph node metastasis. Therefore, detection in the early stage of esophageal cancer is necessary to avoid invasive surgery and the combination treatment of chemotherapy and radiation. Some techniques such as chromoendoscopy, magnifying endoscopy, and narrow-band imaging (NBI) are used to examine suspicious areas of mucosa not visible during conventional endoscopic examination. The development of these techniques has led to detection of increasing numbers of early-stage esophageal squamous cell carcinomas. These endoscopic techniques are also used for diagnosis for nonmalignant disease.

Combination of Magnifying Endoscopy and Narrow-Band Imaging System

Advanced endoscopic techniques, such as magnifying endoscopy, NBI, and autofluorescence imaging (AFI), have recently been developed through image processing and digital technology to improve the accuracy of diagnosis of gastrointestinal disease. Compared with conventional endoscopy, magnifying endoscopy can visualize the microstructure and microvascularity of gastrointestinal surface mucosa [1]. The microsurface structure of the mucosa, the so-called pit pattern, includes the normal structure as well as abnormal structure changed through inflammation and carcinogenesis. Microvascular architecture includes normal vascular system and tumor microvessels related to tumor angiogenesis. Assessment of differences in microsurface structure and microvascular architecture provides useful information to diagnose histological findings. Magnifying colonoscopies with dye spraying are often used for histological diagnosis and invasive diagnosis of colorectal tumor according to pit pattern classification. As it seems that magnified observation did not have an impact in routine endoscopic examination of the upper gastrointestinal tract, magnifying endoscopy has not been widely used in clinical practice for the upper gastrointestinal tract. However, some important studies using magnifying endoscopy in the upper gastrointestinal tract were recently published in the clinical field of esophageal cancer, Barrett's epithelium, gastric cancer, gastritis, and gastroesophageal reflux disease (GERD). On the other hand, the NBI system has been introduced into gastrointestinal endoscopy at the same time. NBI consists of interference filters for illumination of the target in narrow red, blue, and green bands of the spectrum [2]. NBI is based on the phenomenon that depth of light penetration depends on wavelength. The precise mechanism of NBI technique is described in other chapters. NBI highlights the contrast imaging of structure and vascularity of surface mucosa without the need for dye. NBI is combined with magnifying endoscopy to clearly observe morphological change of microvessels in surface mucosa of the gastrointestinal tract [3]. Magnifying endoscopies with NBI system are now available in the world. Magnifying endoscopic examination with the NBI system has been accepted for diagnosis in esophageal and gastric fields.

Detection of Superficial Esophageal Lesions Using the NBI System

Detection of squamous cell carcinoma in an earlier stage in the esophagus benefits patients. Iodine staining during endoscopic examination enhances detection of early squamous cell carcinoma of the esophagus. The mechanism of iodine staining of the squamous epithelium is based on a chemical reaction between glycogen produced in squamous cell epithelium and iodine. Glycogen interacting with iodine turns brown. As areas with lesser amounts of glycogen interact little with iodine, squamous neoplasia and esophagitis show up as unstained areas. Therefore, chromoendoscopy with iodine is clinically useful for detecting squamous epithelial dysplasia or squamous cell carcinoma. However, iodine solution sprayed over the whole esophagus often causes allergic reaction, irritation, and uncomfortable symptoms such as chest pain and heartburn. NBI is also useful for the detection of squamous epithelial dysplasia and squamous cell carcinoma [4]. Because NBI accurately identifies the microvascular architecture of surface mucosa, it clearly delineates the margin of dyspepsia and carcinoma as a brownish area (Fig. 1). The color change of dyspepsia and carcinoma

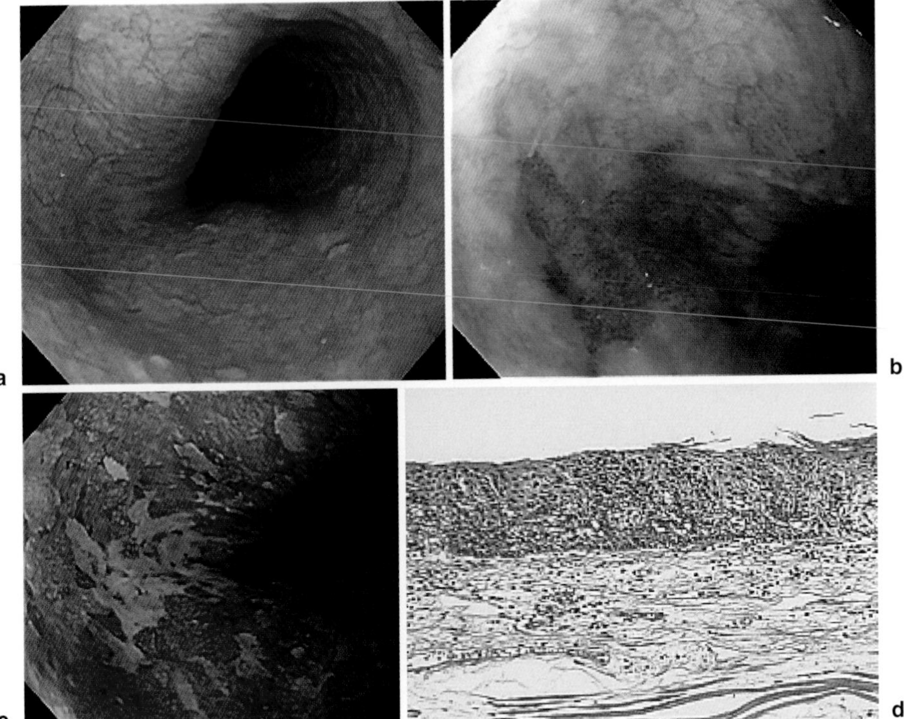

Fig. 1. **a** A superficial esophageal lesion was difficult to detect by conventional endoscopy. **b** Conventional endoscopy with narrow-band imaging (NBI) system enhanced detection of the superficial esophageal lesion as a *brownish area*. **c** Chromoendoscopy with iodine detected the superficial esophageal lesion as an *unstained area*. **d** Histological examination of the resected specimen revealed squamous cell carcinoma in situ

lesions to brown is based on irregular foci of microvascular proliferation. As the density of microvascularity increases, the brown stain in NBI becomes darker. Monma et al. reported that conventional endoscopy with NBI is useful for detecting early squamous cell carcinoma of esophagus without iodine staining [5]. The advantage of the NBI system is that dye is not required. Screening with NBI for dyspepsia or carcinoma in pharynx and larynx is far more useful because iodine is not used. Patients with squamous cell carcinoma of the esophagus were often associated with background mucosa showing many minute noncancerous unstained areas (so-called scattered type) [6]. These patients have a high risk of metachronous multiple esophageal carcinomas. In the case of the scattered type, the usefulness of the NBI system has not been clarified.

Diagnosis of Squamous Cell Carcinoma Using Magnifying Endoscopy with the Narrow-Band Imaging System

The combination of the NBI technique and magnification imaging increases the ability to diagnose the malignant potential of esophageal lesions. The main advantage of magnifying endoscopy with NBI is the improved visualization of intrapapillary capillary loops (IPCL). IPCLs are observed beneath the basement membrane of the epithelium in the normal esophageal squamous epithelium (Fig. 2). In the imaging of conventional endoscopy, IPCLs are usually shown as dot-like structures with regular intervals of about 100 μm in esophageal mucosa. Under magnified imaging, normal IPCL are hairpin shaped and small in diameter. Morphological change and irregular arrangement of IPCLs are associated with inflammation and neoplasia of esophagus. The characteristic changes of magnified appearance in squamous cell carcinoma are dilation, weaving, and variation in size and shape of IPCL.

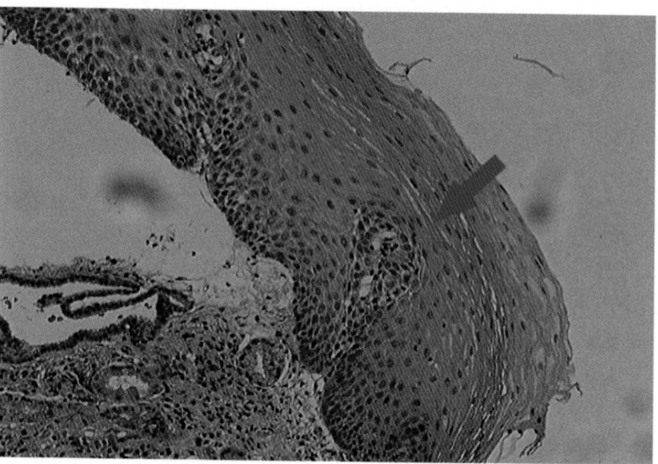

Fig. 2. Intraepithelial capillary loop (IPCL) in normal squamous epithelium (*arrow*)

Inoue et al. classified the IPCL pattern as follows [7]. Type I is positively stained with iodine, while IPCL do not differ from the normal pattern. Type II is positively stained with iodine, IPCL have one or two of four characteristic changes, and elongation and/or dilation is commonly seen. Type III is negatively stained with iodine, while IPCL have no changes or minimal changes. Type IV is negatively stained with iodine, and IPCL have three of four characteristic changes described in type V. Type V is negatively stained with iodine, and IPCL have all four characteristic changes such as dilation, tortuous weaving, caliber changes, and different shapes in each IPCL, indicating carcinoma in situ. Cancer infiltration depth is estimated by the degree of destruction of the IPCL and the range of affected vessels. In general, there is a change in the IPCL, which are gradually destroyed by cancer infiltration. The original IPCL shape remains basically unchanged in mucosal cancer. In submucosal cancer, the IPCL is totally destroyed, and novel tumor vessels appear. Kumagai et al. reported that the accuracy rate of diagnosis regarding the depth of superficial esophageal cancers was 83.1% according to the Inoue classification of magnified IPCL imaging [8].

Arima et al. reported their classification of microvascular patterns using magnifying endoscopy [9]. Type 1 was characterized by thin, linear capillaries in subepithelial papillae, similar to the normal mucosa. Type 2 was characterized by distended, dilated vessels in subepithelial papillae. The structure of capillaries was preserved, and their arrangement was relatively regular. Type 3 was characterized by destruction of vessels in subepithelial papillae, spiral vessels of irregular caliber, and crushed vessels with red spots. Type 4 was characterized by irregular multilayered, irregularly branched, reticular vessels. Type 1 vessels are commonly seen in normal mucosa. Most type 2 vessels are usually found in lesions with inflammatory changes, but can be associated with atypia. Type 3 vessels are characteristically seen in severe dysplasia and m1 or m2 cancers. The size of avascular areas (AVA) surrounded by distended type 4 vessels is related to the depth of tumor invasion. Reticular vessels are commonly seen in poorly differentiated cancers. When type 3 and type 4 vessels are considered the diagnostic criteria for severe dysplasia and cancers, the rate of differential diagnosis is 99.0% [9]. Therefore, magnifying endoscopy with NBI is able to evaluate the depth of squamous cell carcinoma by observation of difference in IPCLs (Fig. 3). Also, observation of IPCL change was useful for diagnosing the horizontal extent of cancer. Minute changes in IPCL such as dilation and elongation were reported to be suggestive of inflammatory changes in the esophagus.

Possibility of Diagnosis for Nonerosive Reflux Disease

Magnifying endoscopic observation with NBI of capillary vessels in esophageal epithelium is useful for diagnosis of nonerosive reflux disease (NERD), which cannot be visualized with conventional endoscopy. Gastroesophageal reflux disease (GERD) is associated with acidity. The mechanisms that contribute to the development of GERD include frequent and transient relaxation of the lower esophageal sphincter, impaired esophageal clearance of regurgitated gastric acid, presence of hiatus hernia, and delayed gastric emptying. Symptoms of heartburn and regurgitation are the most important for diagnosis of GERD in the clinical setting. Because endoscopic

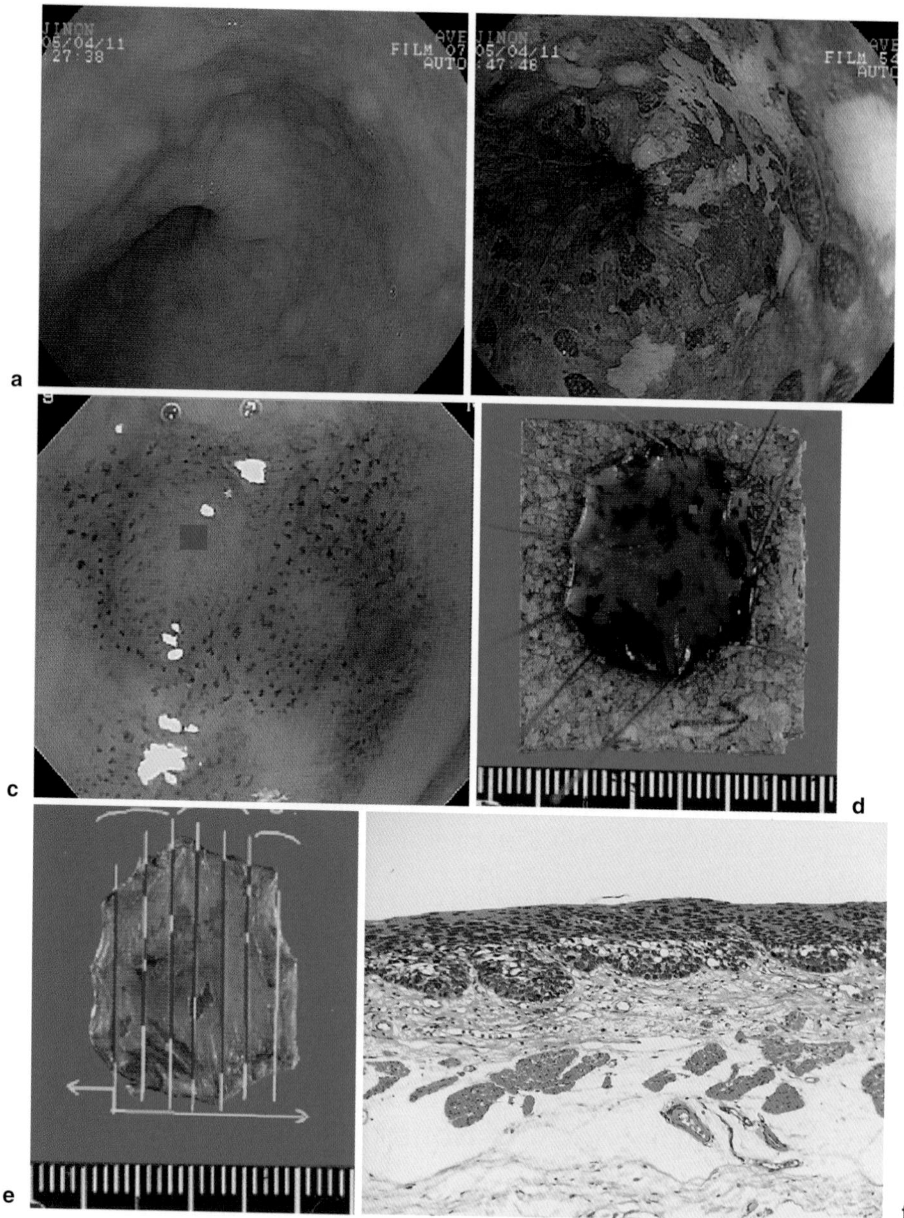

FIG. 3. **a** One superficial flat lesion, maximum 6 mm in diameter, was detected in the middle portion of the esophagus. **b** Iodine dyeing revealed it clearly as an *unstained area*. **c** Magnifying endoscopy with the NBI system showed morphological change and irregular arrangement of IPCL. **d** Endoscopic submucosal dissection was performed to remove the 19 × 11 mm specimen without complications. **e** Mapping of the resected specimen showed an area of squamous cell carcinoma in situ. The tumor size was 6 mm in maximum diameter without lymphatic and venous invasion. Cut ends of the resected specimen were both carcinoma negative. **f** Histological examination of the resected specimen revealed squamous cell carcinoma in situ

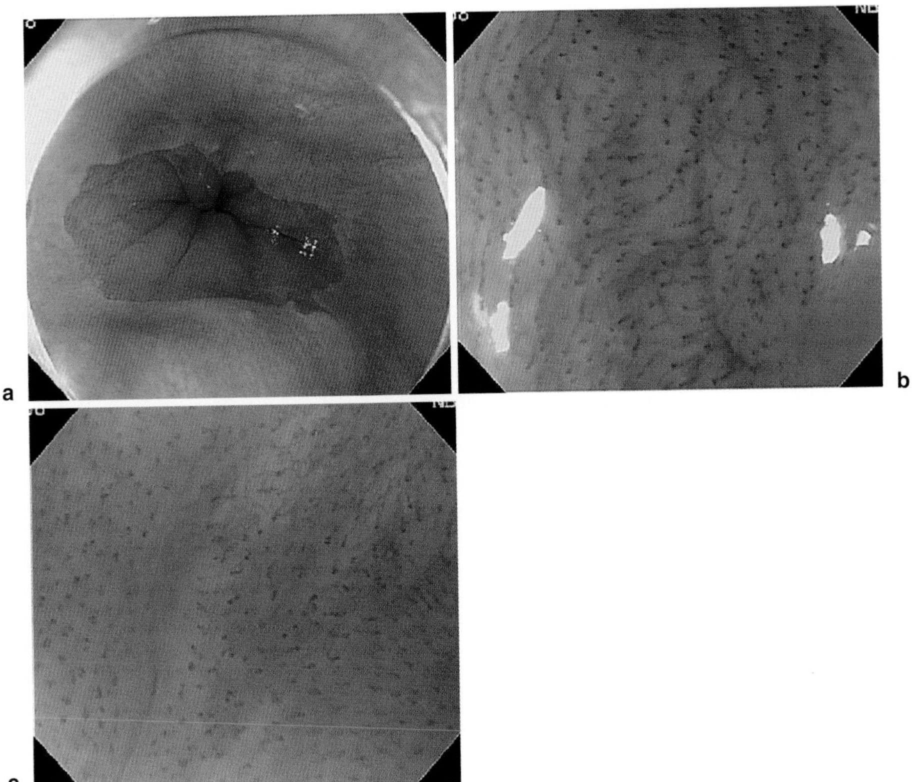

FIG. 4. **a** Magnifying endoscopy without the NBI system did not identify morphological changes of IPCL in patients with nonerosive reflux disease. **b, c** Magnifying endoscopy with the NBI system shows simple dilation and elongation of IPCLs at the lower site of esophagus in patients with nonerosive reflux disease.

examination is also widely used for diagnosis of GERD, GERD is classified according to the severity of esophageal mucosal breaks in the Los Angeles classification. However, about half of GERD patients reveal no abnormality under conventional endoscopy. GERD with negative endoscopic findings is called NERD. Diagnosis of NERD tends to be limited by the resolution of conventional endoscopy. In other words, there is the possibility to overlook minute mucosal changes.

Kato et al. reported magnified endoscopic observation of IPCL just above the mucosa of the esophagogastric junction in patients with reflux symptoms in whom no erosion was detected by conventional endoscopy [10]. Dilation and elongation of IPCL are detected significantly more often in NERD compared with controls (Fig. 4). NBI with magnifying endoscopy improved the accuracy of magnifying endoscopy for assessment of IPCLs. Thickness of the basal cell layer and/or length of papillae indicate histological changes of GERD. There are significant differences between dilated and regular IPCL in term of thickness of basal cell layer and length of papillae.

Conclusion

The morphology of IPCL is affected by inflammation and neoplasia. Magnifying endoscopic observation with NBI for IPCL is useful for diagnosis of esophageal squamous neoplasia and esophageal inflammatory disease. The assessment of IPCL pattern could benefit diagnosis of not only squamous cell carcinoma but also NERD. The patterns of IPCL in inflammatory mucosa are simply dilation and elongation with regular arrangement. The characteristic pattern of IPCL in malignant mucosa is disappearance of regularity such as irregular arrangement, irregular alignment, different size, different shape, and irregular dilation.

References

1. Kato M, Shimizu Y, Nakagawa S, et al (2005) Usefulness of magnifying endoscopy in upper gastrointestinal tract: history and recent studies. Dig Endosc 17:S5–S10
2. Kuznetsov K, Lambert R, Rey JF (2006) Narrow-band imaging: potential and limitations. Endoscopy 38:76–81
3. Lambert R, Kuznetsov K, Rey JF (2007) Narrow-band imaging in digestive endoscopy. Sci World J 7:449–465
4. Muto M, Sano Y, Fujii S, et al (2006) Endoscopic diagnosis of intraepithelial squamous neoplasia in head and neck and esophageal mucosal sites. Dig Endosc 18:S2–S5
5. Monma K, Yoshida M, Funada N, et al (2006) Endoscopic detection of early esophageal cancer by the narrow band imaging system. Stomach Intest (Tokyo) 41:151–164
6. Shimizu Y, Tsukagoshi H, Fujita M, et al (2001) Endoscopic screening for early esophageal cancer by iodine staining in patients with other current or prior primary cancers. Gastrointest Endosc 53:1–5
7. Inoue H (2001) Magnification endoscopy in the esophagus and stomach. Dig Endosc 13:S40–S41
8. Kumagai Y, Inoue H, Kawano T (2004) Magnifying endoscopic observation of superficial esophageal carcinoma. Dig Endosc 16:277–281
9. Arima M (2005) Evaluation of microvascular patterns of superficial esophageal cancers by magnifying endoscopy. *Esophagus* 2:191–197
10. Kato M, Yamamoto J, Shimizu Y, et al (2006) Magnifying endoscopic findings of nonerosive reflux disease. Dig Endosc 18(suppl):S33–S35

Current Perspective on Endocytoscopic Diagnosis in the Esophagus Based on the Multicenter Study at the Endoscopic Forum Japan

Mitsuhiro Fujishiro

Summary. Owing to the emergence of endocytoscopy, real-time in vivo observation of living cells in the gastrointestinal tract becomes possible through a flexible endoscope. However, we have no evidence concerning the impact of endocytoscopy on clinical practice so far. Consequently, we conducted a pilot multicenter study of endocytoscopy at the Endoscopy Forum Japan (EFJ) 2006 as the first step. The study revealed that the endocytoscopic image and horizontal conventional histological image were quite similar for normal and cancerous squamous cells in the esophagus when clear endocytoscopic images were obtained. The study also showed some limitations of endocytoscopy. The greatest problem is how to obtain consistent reproductions of endocytoscopic images of sufficient quality. After overcoming this limitation, adequate knowledge of endocytoscopic images of dysplasia and inflammatory changes, among others, as well as normal and cancerous images may become another problem to be solved. The study itself did not reveal the usefulness of endocytoscopy in clinical practice; however, the future direction of EFJ and further advancement in diagnostic endoscopy, including endocytoscopy under the aegis of EFJ, may result from this multicenter study.

Key words. Endocytoscopy, Optical biopsy, Magnifying endoscopy, Esophagus, Automatic diagnosis

Introduction

Contact endoscopy was first described by Hamou [1] as microhysteroscopy used to examine the surface of the genital tract at high magnification in 1979. Thereafter, the application has been extended to otolaryngology [2] and for the gastrointestinal tract, colorectal lesions became the first targets of ultrahigh-magnification endoscopy in 1982 [3]. In those days, however, the techniques were still in an experimental stage

Department of Gastroenterology, Graduate School of Medicine, The University of Tokyo, 7-3-1 Hongo, Bunkyo-ku, Tokyo 113-8655, Japan

and further improvements were needed to apply the techniques to clinical practice. In recent years, real-time histological analysis at endoscopy, known as "optical biopsy," has developed owing to remarkable advances in endoscopic technologies; and several methods, including laser coherent microscopy, optical computed tomography, and endocytoscopy, are promising for potential clinical use. Natural images can be obtained by using endocytoscopy alone, because this system uses white light and is quite similar to an optical microscope, which provides a great advantage over other systems when applying histopathological knowledge to the interpretation of the images [4]. A study performed at a leading hospital shows the potential of an endocytoscopic histological classification of epithelial atypia in the esophagus with an overall accuracy of 82% regarding the differentiation between malignancy and nonmalignancy [5]. This result means that endocytoscopy may replace endoscopic biopsy to some extent. To validate the obtained results, we conducted the following study in cooperation with the experts participating in the Endoscopy Forum Japan (EFJ) 2006.

The Study Design and Results of the Multicenter Study

An earlier study was conducted in an in vivo setting. When considering the technique applied to clinical practice, the data obtained in an in vivo setting are essential. However, we had not really known what the obtained images represent and whether they are consistent with histology. So, to evaluate quality and characteristics of the obtained images more precisely, our pilot study was planned to be performed in an ex vivo setting. Furthermore, because our first goal was to reach a consensus about endocytoscopic images of cancerous and noncancerous squamous cells in the esophagus, targeted tissues for observation were 27 endoscopically or surgically resected human esophagi obtained between May 2006 and July 2006 at the participating institutions for coexisting esophageal squamous cell carcinomas.

The tissues were stained by 1% iodine solution before formalin fixation within 1 h after excision to identify cancerous (unstained) and noncancerous (stained) areas. After targeting the points of observation (one cancerous point and one noncancerous point per esophagus), 10% sodium thiosulfate solution (Detoxol; Banyu Pharmaceutical, Tokyo, Japan) was scattered on the tissues to neutralize the staining and washed with physiological saline. Subsequently, after 60 s soaking in 1% methylene blue solution, the tissues were observed by using endocytoscopy. The details of the study design have been described previously [6].

Among 54 areas of observation (27 cancerous and 27 normal areas), evaluable pairs of an endocytoscopic image and a horizontal histological picture were obtained only at 12 cancerous areas and 14 normal areas. Twenty-eight areas (15 cancerous and 13 normal areas) were excluded from further analysis because clear endocytoscopic images were not obtained for 19 areas (11 cancerous and 8 normal areas) and clear images of horizontal histological sections of the mucosal surface could not be obtained for 9 areas (4 cancerous and 5 normal areas).

The sets of images were categorized as "similar," "dissimilar," and "indefinable" by unanimous agreement of all the panels at a technology session entitled "Clinical impact of the endocytoscopy system in the upper gastrointestinal tract" of the Endos-

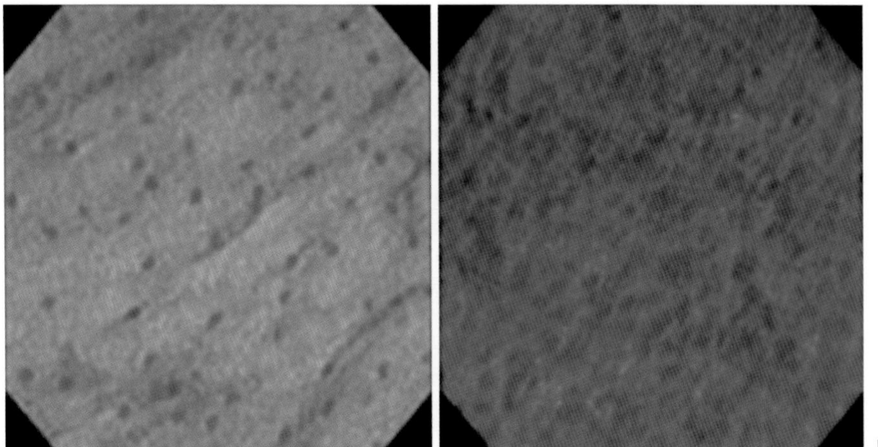

FIG. 1. Endocytoscopic image of noncancerous and cancerous squamous cells in the esophagus. **a** Noncancerous image. **b** Cancerous image. 1% methylene blue, ×450 on 14-inch monitor

copy Forum Japan 2006 according to the following factors: (1) pattern of the cellular arrangement and density; (2) size and shape of the cells; (3) size and shape of the nuclei; and (4) nuclear-to-cytoplasmic ratio.

The comparison revealed that all endocytoscopic images were quite similar to the corresponding horizontal histological pictures without exception, and all the sets were categorized as "similar." The pattern of the cellular arrangement and density (structural atypia), and size and shape of the nuclei (nuclear atypia) were morphologically identical between endocytoscopy and histology. However, comparisons of size and shape of cells and nuclear : cytoplasmic ratios were difficult because identification of cytoplasm in endocytoscopic images was not possible, likely because of poor staining of the cytoplasm. Endocytoscopic images obtained at cancerous areas showed increased cellular density with completely irregular arrangements and uneven sizes and shapes of nuclei, whereas those obtained at normal areas showed regular cellular arrangements and even regular sizes and shapes of nuclei (Fig. 1). Mean total numbers of the nuclei per endocytoscopic image calculated by image analyzing software (Image-Pro; Nippon Roper, Tokyo, Japan) were 129 ± 14.8 at normal areas and 550 ± 66.5 at cancerous areas, with a significant difference between the groups ($P < 0.0001$). The detailed results of this multicenter study were published in the journal *Gastrointestinal Endoscopy* as an original article [7].

Limitations and Problems

The first criticism of this study may be the ex vivo setting. We have to push forward to the next step, which is an in vivo setting, to evaluate the usefulness of endocytoscopy in clinical practice. However, even though this study was conducted in an ex vivo setting, 19 images of endocytoscopy (35%) were insufficient to evaluate in detail in terms of image quality. This evidence suggests that the appropriate preconditioning is necessary for endocytoscopic observation. We consider some of the limitations of this study to be Lugol staining immediately before observation and the lack of use of a mucolytic agent before methylene blue staining. So far, chromoendoscopy using iodine is considered to be the standard process to detect the existence of esophageal squamous cell carcinoma, especially in superficial macroscopic types with minute morphological changes, and is often unavoidable. Technical advancements in virtual chromoendoscopy without iodine staining, such as narrow-band imaging techniques, may give us other alternatives. We did not consider the latter when making the protocol because intensive washing by physiological saline was considered to be sufficient to dislodge any remaining mucus on the ex vivo specimens.

Another reason for differences in the results between a previous study conducted by Inoue et al. [5] and this study may be the scopes used for testing—an integrated type in the former study and a probe type in the latter. Succeeding recent studies in Western countries revealed fairly low accuracy (54%) in the esophagus [8] and a lack of sufficient image quality, especially in Barrett's esophagus [9], using a probe type of endocytoscope, similar to that found in this study. The difference between the two scopes lies not only in how they access a lesion but also how they obtain endocytoscopic images: the former adapts a reconstruction of the processed image from the sequential illumination of the three primary colors (red, blue, and green); in contrast, the latter adapts a way to record the real image which has been reached without a filter. When the former system is employed, we can easily change the light applied and the color to make the reconstructed image appropriate. Thus, the possibilities of endocytoscopy may increase and nonstaining endocytoscopy may become the norm in the near future.

When endocytoscopic images with sufficient quality were obtained, this study also revealed that it was quite easy to differentiate between normal and cancerous squamous cells when endoscopists had some knowledge of the histopathology. Thus, we could delineate three groups: definite cancer, which should be treated; definite normal, which can be followed without treatment; and, indefinite lesion, which should be investigated by endoscopic biopsy. Greater knowledge and expertise in the use of endocytoscopic images for endocytoscopic diagnosis of dysplasia with different grades, inflammatory changes, or diseases other than cancer, we can reduce the number of endoscopic biopsies.

Future Direction for Endocytoscopy

Real-time in vivo observation of living cells may bring us a new diagnostic approach that omits biopsy before treatment. This may be realized in endocytoscopic diagnosis, which saves on costs and time needed for the many processes before microscopic examination and lessens the burden of pathologists' work. Furthermore, a biopsy may cause fibrosis under the lesion, as well as creating a potential risk of postprocedural bleeding. The former must be taken into account as a major risk when the lesion is the target for endoscopic resection because the fibrosis may make it impossible to lift the lesion, even after submucosal fluid injection, which interferes with safe endoscopic resection. The latter concern always disturbs us when endoscopy is performed for patients with thrombocytopenia or coagulopathy and those who are taking anti-coagulant or antiplatelet medicine.

I believe the idea to observe living cells in real time is not wrong. However, we have to overcome several hurdles before endocytoscopic diagnosis becomes standard in daily practice, as already mentioned. When the present impact and possibilities of endocytoscopy are considered, there are two possible future directions: to obtain clear images that mimic completely those of hematoxylin and eosin (H&E) staining, and the partial substitution of histopathology, which discriminates among normal, cancerous, and indefinable images, as automatic diagnosis. The latter direction may already be applicable in clinical practice, because the nuclear number in cancerous images obtained by endocytoscopy was about four times higher than that of a normal sample. This suggests the possibility of making a correct automatic diagnosis of cancerous tissue only through detection of the total nuclear (dark staining) area per image [10]. What remains for us to do is to create an algorithm and computer software to make an automatic diagnosis. Although the percentage of indefinable cases that need endoscopic biopsy may be high at present, technical refinement may decrease this rate soon.

In summary, we have attempted to reach consensus among experts of different institutions in a multicenter study using the novel diagnostic modality of endocytoscopy. Although endocytoscopy has some limitations to be considered before application in daily practice, I believe we are moving toward establishing a new direction for EFJ, as well as a new diagnostic field of gastrointestinal endoscopy.

Acknowledgments. The author thanks Dr. Manabe Muto (Division of Digestive Endoscopy and Gastrointestinal Oncology, National Cancer Center Hospital East, Kashiwa, Japan), Dr. Kaiyo Takubo (Department of Clinical Pathology, Tokyo Metropolitan Institute of Gerontology, Tokyo, Japan), Dr. Yoshitaka Sato (Digestive Disease Center, Showa University Northern Yokohama Hospital, Yokohama, Japan), Dr. Mitsuru Kaise (Department of Endoscopy, The Jikei University School of Medicine, Tokyo, Japan), Dr. Yasumasa Niwa (Department of Gastroenterology, Nagoya University, Aichi, Japan), Dr. Mototsugu Kato (Division of Endoscopy, Hokkaido University School of Medicine, Sapporo, Japan), who made possible the conception, design, and data collection of the multicenter study described in this chapter. The author also thanks Mr. Sakae Takehana and Mr. Nobuyuki Doguchi of Olympus Medical Systems, Tokyo, Japan, for their pertinent comments on the technical aspects of the endocytoscopy system.

References

1. Hamou JE (1980) Microhysteroscopy: a new technique in endoscopy and its applications. Acta Endosc 10:415–422
2. Andrea M, Dias O, Santos A (1995) Contact endoscopy during microlaryngeal surgery: a new technique for endoscopic examination of the larynx. Ann Otol Rhinol Laryngol 104:333–339
3. Tada M, Nishimura S, Watanabe Y, et al (1982) A new method for the ultramagnifying observation of the colon mucosa. Kyoto Pref Univ Med 91:349–354

4. Kumagai Y, Iida M, Yamazaki S (2006) Magnifying endoscopic observation of the upper gastrointestinal tract. Dig Endosc 18:165–172
5. Inoue H, Sasajima K, Kaga M, et al (2006) Endoscopic in vivo evaluation of tissue atypia in the esophagus using a newly designed integrated endocytoscope: a pilot trial. Endoscopy 38:891–895
6. Muto M, Fujishiro M, Sato Y, et al (2007) Multicenter study design of the ex vivo evaluation of endocytoscopy in esophageal squamous cell carcinoma. Dig Endosc 19: S153–S155
7. Fujishiro M, Takubo K, Sato Y, et al (2007) Potential and present limitation of endocytoscopy in diagnosis of esophageal squamous cell carcinoma: a multi-center ex vivo pilot study. Gastrointest Endosc 66:551–555
8. Eberl T, Jechart G, Probst A, et al (2007) Can an endocytoscope system (ECS) predict histology in neoplastic lesions? Endoscopy 39:497–501
9. Pohl H, Koch M, Khalifa A, et al (2007) Evaluation of endocytoscopy in the surveillance of patients with Barrett's esophagus. Endoscopy 39:492–496
10. Kodashima S, Fujishiro M, Takubo K, et al (2007) Ex vivo pilot study using computed analysis of endocytoscopic images to differentiate normal and malignant squamous cell epithelia in the esophagus. Dig Liver Dis 39:762–766

Endoscopic Ultrasound-Guided Fine-Needle Aspiration Biopsy (EUS-FNA) for Mediastinal Abnormalities via the Esophagus

Atsushi Irisawa[1], Takuto Hikichi[2], and Hiromasa Ohira[1]

Summary. When suspicious mediastinal abnormalities, such as enlarged lymph nodes, are viewed radiographically, these patients are often sent for diagnostic procedures to obtain a tissue diagnosis. Endoscopic ultrasound-guided fine-needle aspiration biopsy (EUS-FNA) for mediastinal abnormalities is a safe, sensitive, minimally invasive method for pathological evaluation of the abnormalities, definitive diagnosis, and identification of the staging of malignancies. Moreover, it has marked advantages for patient management. Actually, EUS-FNA is a complementary modality in the diagnosis and staging of malignant lesions (not only gastrointestinal cancer but also cancers derived from nondigestive organs) in the posterior mediastinum.

Key words. EUS-FNA, Mediastinum, Lymph node, Cancer staging

Introduction

Endoscopic ultrasound (EUS) has great advantages over computed tomography (CT) and other imaging modalities because it allows assessment of the echo structure in lesions <1 cm diameter [1] and provides an opportunity to obtain material from abnormal lesions via the gastrointestinal wall for tissue confirmation using endoscopic ultrasound-guided fine-needle aspiration biopsy (EUS-FNA). The indication of EUS-FNA includes many different fields; it is recognized as a new imaging modality that is useful for diagnosis of mediastinal lesions, especially for evaluation of mediastinal nodal staging of gastrointestinal/pancreatobiliary [2,3] and lung cancer [4], and mediastinal adenopathy of unknown causes [5,6]. Originally, lymph node echofeatures of EUS were used to predict malignant involvement only in periesophageal and periintestinal lymph nodes in patients with esophageal cancer [7]. Although echofeatures are helpful, lymph node sampling provides cytological diagnosis that impacts patient management through definitive diagnosis, prognosis stratification, preopera-

[1]Department of Internal Medicine 2, Fukushima Medical University School of Medicine, 1 Hikarigaoka, Fukushima City, Fukushima 960-1295, Japan
[2]Department of Endoscopy, Fukushima Medical University Hospital, 1 Hikarigaoka, Fukushima City, Fukushima 960-1295, Japan

tive planning, and selection of chemotherapy and radiation therapy. This chapter reviews the practical aspects and recent developments in EUS-FNA of mediastinal abnormalities.

Anatomy of the Mediastinum on Curved Linear EUS

General View

In Japan, not many endosonographers perform EUS-FNA for mediastinal lesions. One factor hindering the use of mediastinal EUS-FNA is the difficulty in understanding the EUS anatomy of the mediastinum with curved linear array EUS. It is important to understand the EUS anatomy of the mediastinum to perform EUS-FNA with safety and certainty.

Most structures that are visible by EUS in the mediastinum are anterior to the esophagus, which necessitates consideration of mediastinal anatomy from a posterior perspective. In performing curved linear array EUS, it is desirable to imagine the structure of blood vessels in the mediastinum. From this point of view, the procedure of curved linear array EUS for the mediastinum is divided into eight steps in terms of landmarks as follows: liver (hepatic vein), abdominal aorta (including diaphragmatic crus), inferior vena cava, azygos vein, heart (especially right atrium, left ventricle, ascending aorta, and pulmonary artery), trachea, aortopulmonary window, and aortic arch. The EUS-FNA standardization committee in Japan [8] recommended the EUS procedure for mediastinum as described herein. The scope is rotated to observe 360° around the esophagus when the landmark is identified.

Procedure of Observation Using Curved Linear Array EUS

The eight procedural steps for the mediastinum using curved linear array EUS are the following.

Step 1: The left lobe of the liver is visible on the screen when the scope is inserted into the stomach with the controls free. Now rotate the scope clockwise to visualize the hepatic vein and the inferior vena cava (IVC) (Fig. 1).

Step 2: After identification of the liver, rotate the scope clockwise to observe the abdominal aorta. While observing the aorta, withdraw the scope slightly while rotating it counterclockwise, until a long triangular hypoechoic structure is visible in front of the aorta. This is the diaphragmatic crus, which is an important landmark for defining the boundary between the abdominal cavity and the mediastinum (Fig. 2). After evaluating this region, withdraw the scope while viewing the aorta to observe the surroundings of the thoracic aorta.

Step 3: After identification of the IVC again, withdraw the scope to observe the right atrium.

Step 4: Rotate the scope clockwise to observe the entire surroundings of the esophagus. Then withdraw the scope slightly until the azygos vein, which is viewed as a

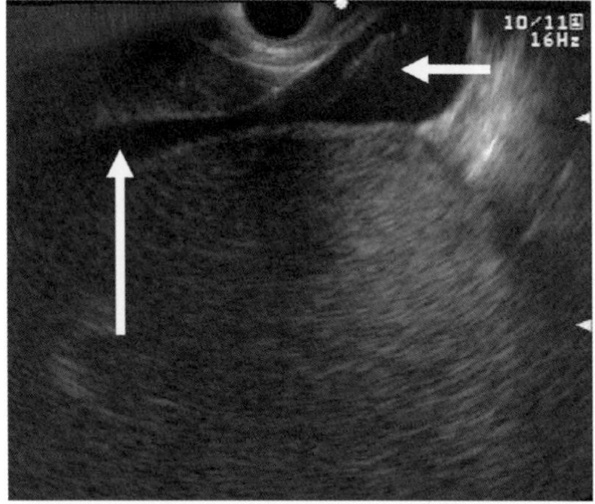

Fig. 1. Endoscopic ultrasound (EUS) shows the hepatic vein (*long arrow*) and inferior vena cava (*short arrow*)

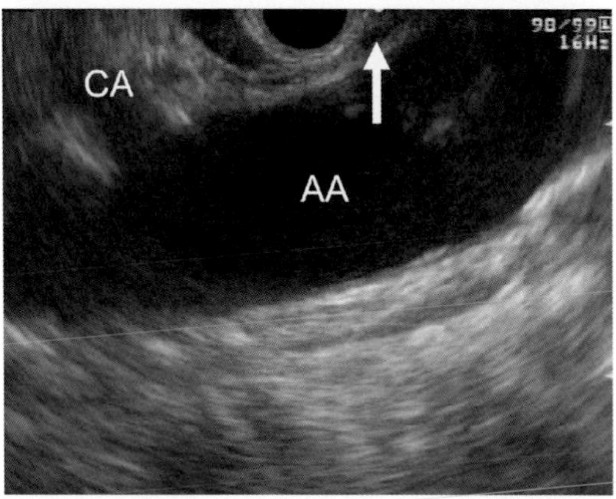

Fig. 2. EUS shows the abdominal aorta (*AA*), celiac artery (*CA*), and diaphragmatic crus (*arrow*)

thin and longitudinal echolucency close to the wall of the esophagus, is identified. Rotate the scope further clockwise to observe the descending aorta also. The descending aorta is a home base of the mediastinum (Fig. 3).

Step 5: Rotate the scope counterclockwise to return to the position described in Step 3, then withdraw the scope while rotating it further counterclockwise to visualize the left atrium, left ventricle, aortic valve, ascending aorta, and right pulmonary artery (Fig. 4).

Step 6: While watching the right pulmonary artery, withdraw the scope while rotating it slightly counterclockwise to view the trachea, which is identified as multiple-echo lines (Fig. 5). The multiple-echo line end is the tracheal bifurcation into the left and right main bronchi. This is an important view for localizing subcarinal lymph nodes for FNA.

Step 7: Visualize the right pulmonary artery again (Step 5), and withdraw the scope while rotating it counterclockwise; the arch of the aorta comes into view as a large

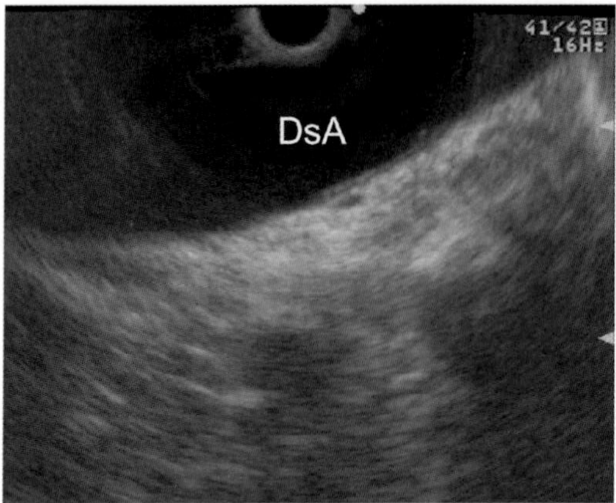

Fig. 3. EUS shows the descending aorta (*DsA*) in mediastinum

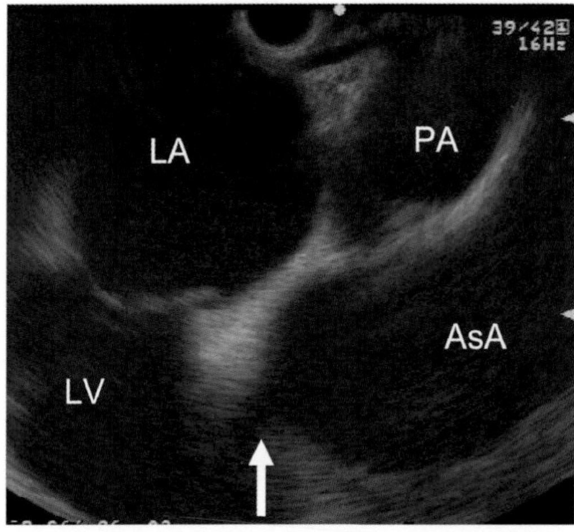

Fig. 4. EUS shows the left atrium (*LA*), left ventricle (*LV*), aortic valve (short arrow), ascending aorta (*AsA*), and right pulmonary artery (*PA*)

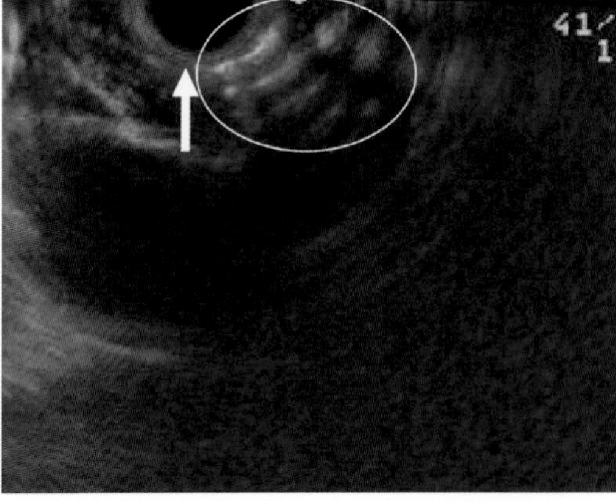

Fig. 5. EUS shows the trachea, which is identified as multiple-echo lines (*circled*). The multiple-echo line end is the tracheal bifurcation into the left and right main bronchi (*arrow*)

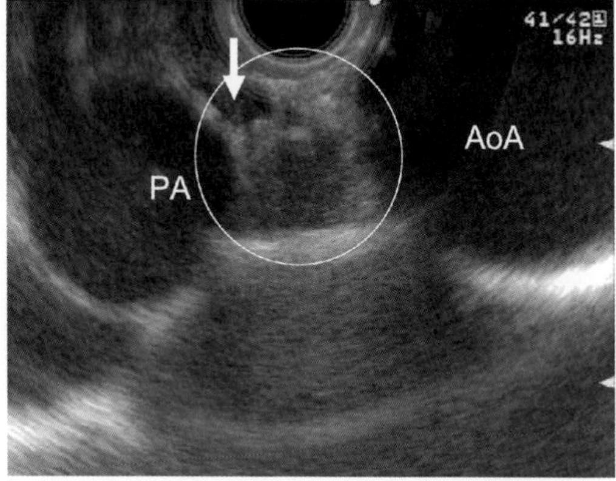

Fig. 6. EUS shows the two blood vessels [aortic arch (*AoA*) and right pulmonary artery (PA)], and the region between these blood vessels is the aortopulmonary window (AP window) (*circled*). A swollen lymph node is seen (*arrow*)

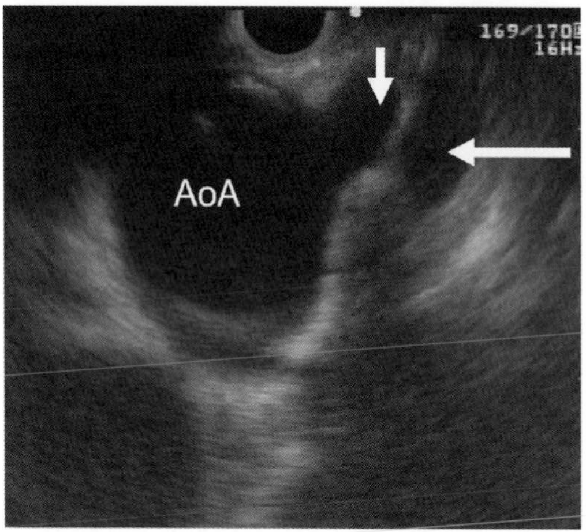

Fig. 7. EUS shows the left subclavian artery (*short arrow*) and left common carotid artery (*long arrow*)

circular structure adjacent to the esophagus on the right side of the image. The region between the two blood vessels is the aortopulmonary window (AP window) (Fig. 6). This area is important for FNA of mediastinal lymph nodes.

Step 8: While observing the aortic arch, withdraw the scope while rotating it counterclockwise to visualize the left subclavian artery and left common carotid artery (Fig. 7). Rotating the scope further counterclockwise at this level makes it possible to observe the brachiocephalic artery.

Procedure of EUS-FNA for Mediastinal Lesion

The procedure of EUS-FNA for mediastinal lesions is fundamentally the same as for other organs. It is desirable that all patients undergo standard upper endoscopy before the EUS-FNA. Before the procedure, sedative drugs are used to provide moderate conscious sedation while the examination is performed in the left lateral decubitus

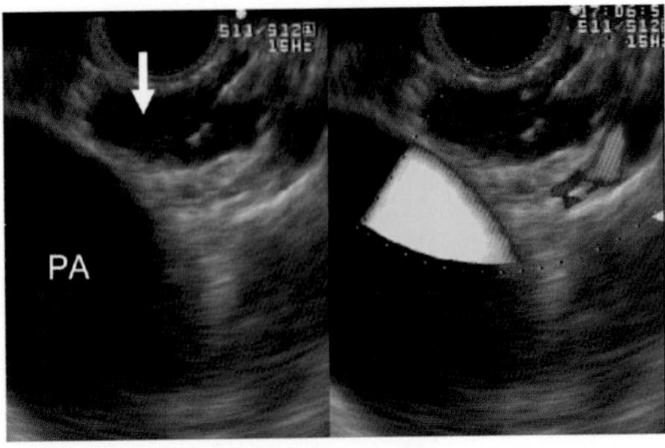

Fig. 8. Endoscopic ultrasound-guided fine-needle aspiration biopsy (EUS-FNA) for mediastinal enlarged lymph nodes (*arrow*) at AP window

position. Then, EUS-FNA is performed using an echoendoscope with an electronic multielement curved linear array ultrasound transducer and a 19-gauge or 22-gauge needle. Because a strongly angled operation of the scope is unnecessary for EUS-FNA for the mediastinum, a 19-gauge needle is easily useful, in contrast to other organs. When the lesion is identified using EUS, the needle is advanced through the wall of the esophagus into the target lesion or lesions, and material is aspirated using a 10- or 20-ml syringe (Fig. 8). No suction need be used, thereby avoiding contamination when only blood is aspirated using the procedure described above. Usually, two to four passes into the target are needed. Attendance of a cytopathologist on site at the time of the procedure is helpful for the certainty and safety of EUS-FNA, to determine if sufficient cellular material is obtained during each FNA, and to avoid unnecessary passes of the aspiration needle in cases of adequate samples. Prophylactic antibiotics before the procedure are used at the discretion of the endoscopist.

Usefulness of EUS-FNA for Mediastinal Abnormalities

The major indications of EUS-FNA for mediastinal lymph nodes are the staging of gastrointestinal and lung cancer and definitive diagnosis of enlarged lymph nodes of unknown cause. Serna et al. [9] demonstrated the usefulness of EUS-FNA in a comparative study between EUS-FNA and mediastinoscopy for diagnosis of mediastinal malignancy. They concluded that mediastinoscopy and EUS-FNA target different areas of the mediastinum and might be complementary for evaluation of mediastinal malignancy. To date, several good results in EUS-FNA for mediastinal lymph nodes have been reported. Larsen et al. [10] showed that EUS-FNA had a sensitivity of 92%, specificity of 100%, positive predictive value (PPV) of 100%, negative predictive value (NPV) of 80%, and an accuracy of 94% for cancer of the mediastinum in 79 patients having a mediastinal lesion in whom the final diagnosis was verified. In addition, Hernandez et al. [11] reported that the diagnostic accuracy of EUS-FNA was 84%; nevertheless, the most frequent indication in 59 patients with mediastinal lymphadenopathy was failed diagnosis by bronchoscopy (54%). Many studies have shown no major complications from EUS-FNA for mediastinal lesion.

EUS-FNA for Mediastinal Lymph Nodes for Cancer Staging

Recently, EUS-FNA for lung mass (including cancer staging and its diagnosis) has come to be performed often. Eloubeidi et al. [12] demonstrated that EUS-FNA has a higher predictive value than either the ^{18}F-fluorodeoxyglucose positron emission tomography (FDG-PET) scan or computed tomography (CT) scan for posterior mediastinal lymph nodes for staging of patients with non-small cell lung cancer (NSCLC). Moreover, Annema et al. [4] reported that, from the perspective of surgical procedures for lung cancer, EUS-FNA prevented 70% of scheduled surgical procedures because of the demonstration of lymph node metastases in NSCLC (52%), tumor invasion (T4) (4%), tumor invasion and lymph node metastases (5%), small cell lung cancer (8%), or benign diagnoses (1%); moreover, its sensitivity, specificity, and accuracy for EUS in mediastinal analysis were 91%, 100%, and 93%, respectively. On the basis of these reports, Hernandez et al. [13] performed a retrospective review of an established prospective database of all patients undergoing EUS-FNA of a primary lung neoplasm adjacent to the esophagus during January 2001–August 2005 in one tertiary care center. They concluded that EUS-FNA is a safe, cost-effective, and accurate initial diagnostic modality for the diagnosis of lung lesions adjacent to the esophagus or invading the mediastinum.

Several reports have described mediastinal FNA for staging of gastrointestinal/pancreatobiliary cancer. Hahn and Faigel [3] demonstrated that 11 of 66 patients who have advanced pancreatobiliary cancer had enlarged mediastinal lymph node on EUS, and that 4 of 9 patients who had undergone EUS-FNA had adenocarcinoma cells (M1 on TNM classification) in the aspirate from the mediastinal lymph node. In these patients, additional surgical aggression was avoided. In others, the usefulness of mediastinal FNA for metastasis of renal cancer, breast cancer, and malignancies in the head and neck was also demonstrated as a case report. These reports underscore the importance of observation of mediastinum to evaluate cancer staging in patients with advanced carcinoma in the abdominal cavity, pancreatobiliary and gastric/colonic cancer, and in nondigestive organs. Although several reports have described mediastinal EUS-FNA for staging of esophageal cancer [2], it is controversial whether EUS-FNA is required in Japan. Therefore, its review is omitted from this chapter.

EUS-FNA for Mediastinal Lymph Nodes of Unknown Origin

Several reports among the literature have described diagnosis of mediastinal lymph nodes of unknown origin. Catalano et al. [5] reported the usefulness of EUS-FNA in 26 patients with mediastinal masses of unknown origin. They showed that EUS-FNA was successful in directing subsequent workup in 77% (20 of 26) and therapy in 73% (19 of 26), and concluded that the emergence of transesophageal EUS-FNA of the mediastinum provides the ability to alter subsequent workup and therapy, obviating the need for more invasive diagnostic studies such as thoracotomy. For benign disease, Fritscher-Ravens et al. [6] reported diagnosis of sarcoidosis using EUS-FNA, and determined that the respective specificity and sensitivity of EUS-FNA were 94% and 100%. Moreover, these studies established the role of EUS-FNA in patients presenting with idiopathic mediastinal masses in most cases, particularly for those with malignant disease.

EUS-FNA for Mediastinal Abnormalities Excluding Lymph Nodes

As for abnormalities in the mediastinum aside from enlarged lymph nodes, cysts are a representative example. Most are benign; they represent a substantial fraction of the space-occupying lesions endosonographers encounter in the mediastinum. Congenital foregut cysts are the most common mediastinal cysts and probably arise as a result of aberrant development of the primitive foregut. Foregut cysts are categorized based on their anomalous embryonic origin into bronchogenic and neuroenteric cysts. Bronchogenic cysts represent 50%–60% of all mediastinal cysts, whereas enterogenous cysts, which include esophageal duplication and neuroenteric cysts, constitute, respectively, 5%–10% and 2%–5%. Few reports describe EUS-FNA for mediastinal cystic lesion. Although it is controversial whether EUS-FNA is necessary to diagnose mediastinal cystic lesion, Wildi et al. [14] indicated the role of EUS-FNA for mediastinal cyst from their case series: when a lesion is clearly anechoic (i.e., cystic), FNA should generally be avoided because of the risk of infection; conversely, when a lesion is hypoechoic, a solid tumor cannot be reliably distinguished from a mucin-filled cyst and FNA should be considered.

Conclusion

EUS-FNA for mediastinal abnormalities is a safe, sensitive, minimally invasive method for pathological evaluation, definite diagnosis and staging of malignancies. Moreover, it has a marked impact on patient management. However, when transesophageal EUS-FNA is considered the best option for a patient with mediastinal abnormalities, then it should be performed by a physician who is properly trained in this technique.

References

1. Vilman P (1996) Endoscopic ultrasonography guided fine needle aspiration biopsy of lymph nodes. Gastrointest Endosc 43:S24–S29
2. Vazquez-Sequeiros E, Norton ID, Clain JE, et al (2001) Impact of EUS-guided fine-needle aspiration on lymph node staging in patients with esophageal carcinoma. Gastrointest Endosc 53:751–757
3. Hahn M, Faigel DO (2001) Frequency of mediastinal lymph node metastases in patients undergoing EUS evaluation of pancreaticobiliary masses. Gastrointest Endosc 54:331–335
4. Annema JT, Versteegh MI, Veseliç M, et al (2005) Endoscopic ultrasound-guided fine-needle aspiration in the diagnosis and staging of lung cancer and its impact on surgical staging. J Clin Oncol 23:8357–8361

5. Catalano MF, Rosenblatt ML, Chak A, et al (2002) Endoscopic ultrasound-guided fine needle aspiration in the diagnosis of mediastinal masses of unknown origin. Am J Gastroenterol 97:2559–2565
6. Fritscher-Ravens A, Sriram PVJ, Topalidis T, et al (2000) Diagnosing sarcoidosis using endosonography-guided fine-needle aspiration. *Chest* 118:928–935
7. Catalano MF, Sivak MV Jr, Rice T, et al (1994) Endosonographic features predictive of lymph node metastases. Gastrointest Endosc 40:442–446
8. EUS-FNA Standardization Committee (2007) Standard imaging technique for ultrasound-guided fine needle aspiration using curved linear array echoendoscope. Dig Endosc 19:S180–S205
9. Serna DL, Aryan HE, Chang KJ, et al (1998) An early comparison between endoscopic ultrasound-guided fine-needle aspiration and mediastinoscopy for diagnosis of mediastinal malignancy. Am Surg 64:1014–1018
10. Larsen SS, Krasnik M, Vilmann P, et al (2002) Endoscopic ultrasound guided biopsy of mediastinal lesions has a major impact on patient management. Thorax 57:98–103
11. Hernandez LV, Mishra G, George S, et al (2004) A descriptive analysis of EUS-FNA for mediastinal lymphadenopathy: an emphasis on clinical impact and false negative results. Am J Gastroenterol 99:249–54
12. Eloubeidi MA, Cerfolio RJ, Chen VK, et al (2005) Endoscopic ultrasound-guided fine needle aspiration of mediastinal lymph node in patients with suspected lung cancer after positron emission tomography and computed tomography scans. Ann Thorac Surg 79:263–268
13. Hernandez A, Kahaleh M, Olazagasti J, et al (2007) EUS-FNA as the initial diagnostic modality in centrally located primary lung cancers. J Clin Gastroenterol 41:657–660
14. Wildi SM, Hoda RS, Fickling W, et al (2003) Diagnosis of benign cysts of the mediastinum: the role and risks of EUS and FNA. Gastrointest Endosc 58:362–368

Endoscopic Submucosal Dissection for Esophageal Cancer

Tsuneo Oyama

Summary. According to Japan Esophageal Society guidelines for the treatment of esophageal cancer, the absolute indication for endoscopic mucosal resection (EMR) is defined as m1–m2 esophageal cancer, while the relative indication is defined as m3–sm1 esophageal cancer. The incidence of lymph node metastasis of esophageal cancer relates closely to the depth of invasion, vascular invasion, and tissue type. En bloc resection is essential for investigating these parameters.

The rate of en bloc resection of esophageal EMR was as low as 23%–57% because the resected area was limited to 15.1–23.9 mm. On the other hand, in our experience that of endoscopic submucosal dissection (ESD) was 95% and the perforation rate was 0%. Piecemeal resection may not permit an adequate histopathological examination and may cause a high local recurrence rate.

In this chapter, we describe the basic procedure and treatment results of ESD in the esophagus. Bleeding and perforation are the major complications, and the use of a hook knife with a spray coagulation current is useful to cut the small vessels without bleeding. When a large vessel or an artery is found, precoagulation with hemostatic forceps is useful to prevent bleeding. The most important points to prevent perforation are to observe the submucosal layer well before submucosal dissection, and to know how to use a hook knife.

Key words. ESD, EMR, Esophageal cancer, Squamous cell carcinoma

Squamous Cell Carcinoma

Esophageal endoscopic submucosal dissection (ESD) is indicated for cancer with no or minimal risk of lymph node metastasis. When the lesions are classified according to the depth of invasion as intraepithelial carcinoma (m1), restricted within the proper mucosal layer (m2), adjacent to or invading the muscularis mucosa (m3), invading the submucosal layer to 200 micrometer or less (sm1), or more (sm2), then the incidence of lymph node metastasis was reported to be 0%, 0%–5.6%, 8%–18%, 11%–53%, and 30%–54%, respectively [1–3]. Therefore, under the 2002 Japan Esopha-

Department of Gastroenterology, Saku Central Hospital, 197 Usuda, Saku, Nagano 384-0301, Japan

geal Society guidelines for the treatment of esophageal cancer, the absolute indication for endoscopic mucosal resection (EMR) is defined as m1–m2 esophageal cancer as well as two-thirds or less extension of the circumference, while the relative indication is defined as m3–sm1 esophageal cancer as well as three-quarters or more mucosal defect after EMR [4].

Oyama et al. [3] reported that an analysis of 749 patients with m3–sm1 cancer revealed that the incidence of lymph node metastasis of m3 cancer was 9.3% and that of sm1 was 19.3%, that risk factors for lymph node metastasis represented a longitudinal extension of 50 mm or more, poorly differentiated carcinoma, and positive vascular invasion, and that the incidence of lymph node metastasis was 4.6% in the absence of these risk factors.

Barrett's Esophageal Cancer

There are limited superficial cases among patients with Barrett's esophageal cancer, which is more prevalent in Western countries. Therefore, the incidence of lymph node metastasis of the disease has not been reported. Bollschweiler et al. [5] reported that an analysis of pT1 esophageal adenocarcinomas in 36 patients revealed that the incidence of lymph node metastasis of mucosal cancer was 0%, while the incidence of sm1, sm2, and sm3, as well as all types of submucosal invasive cancer, was 22%, 0%, 78%, and 41%, respectively. To date, there have been no reports that superficial Barrett's esophageal cancer within the mucosa showed positive lymph node metastasis. Therefore, Barrett's esophageal cancer restricted within the mucosa and high-grade dysplasia can be considered as indications for endoscopic treatment.

Preoperative Examination

Endoscopy, endosonography, and computed tomography (CT) should all be carried out to examine the depth of invasion, the presence of lymph node metastasis, and metastasis to other organs.

Since squamous cell carcinoma does not stain with iodine staining, the range of lateral advancement can easily be determined. Sometimes, however, the range of lateral advancement of Barrett's esophageal adenocarcinoma may be difficult to determine. Therefore, the lateral margin is found by using chromoendoscopy with indigo carmine spray, or magnifying endoscopy with narrow-band imaging (NBI), as well as biopsy of the peripheral tissue.

Endoscopic Mucosal Resection (EMR)

A flat lesion is deformed into a polyp-like shape which can be snared using aspiration or with a grasper in EMR procedures. EMR is a simple technique, but the rate of en bloc resection is as low as 23%–57% because the resected area per resection is limited to 15.1–23.9 mm [6,7]. Therefore, the local recurrence rate was reported to be as high as 7.8%–20% [8,9]. In addition, more fractionated resections tended to lead to a higher local recurrence rate [9].

Endoscopic Submucosal Dissection (ESD) [10,11]

As stated above, en bloc resection is essential in order to fully investigate the risk factors of lymph node metastasis. ESD was developed for precise and large en bloc resections.

Marking

The thickness of the esophageal wall can vary depending on the air content; it may become as thin as about 2–3 mm when the wall is extended. A hook knife (KD-620LR, Olympus Medical Systems, Tokyo, Japan) is attached to the mucosa with the knife stored in the sheath and a moment of forced coagulation (60 W) (ICC200 or VIO300D, Erbe, Tübingen, Germany) can safely provide a mark (Figs. 1–3).

Submucosal Injection

Since the proper muscular layer of the esophageal wall is thinner than that of the gastric wall, and is always in motion according to the heart beats, sufficient space should be secured between the mucosa and the proper muscular layer by submucosal injection. Therefore, it is best to use solutions with a higher viscosity than that of physiological saline, such as 10% glycerol (Glyceol; Chugai Pharmaceutical, Tokyo, Japan), or 2–4-fold diluted sodium hyaluronate (Artz 1%, Kaken Pharmaceutical,

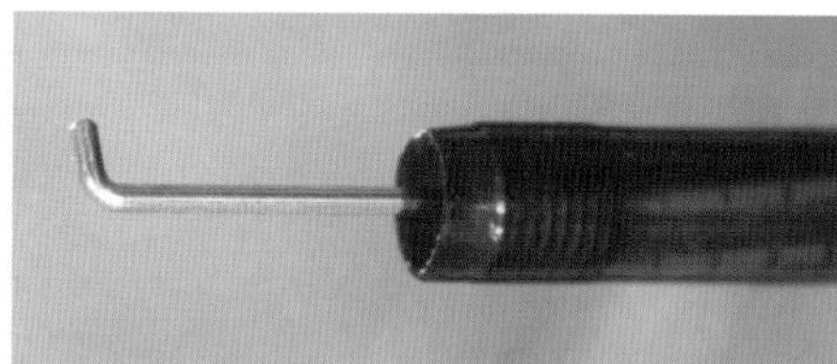

Fig. 1. A hook knife. The tip of the needle knife is angled to the right. The knife can be turned in any direction by rotation of the handle

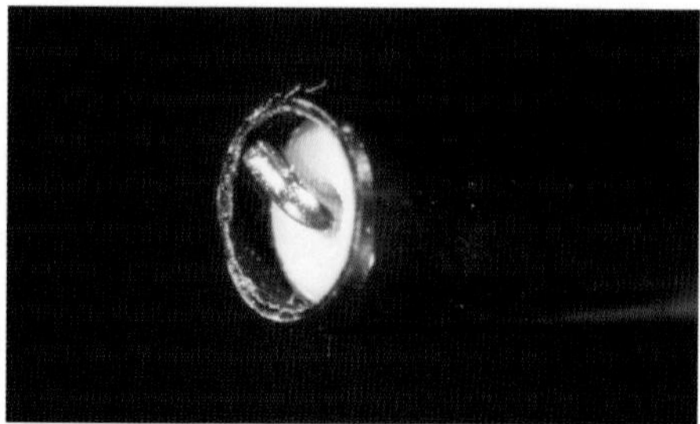

Fig. 2. The tip of the knife can be retracted into the top of the sheath

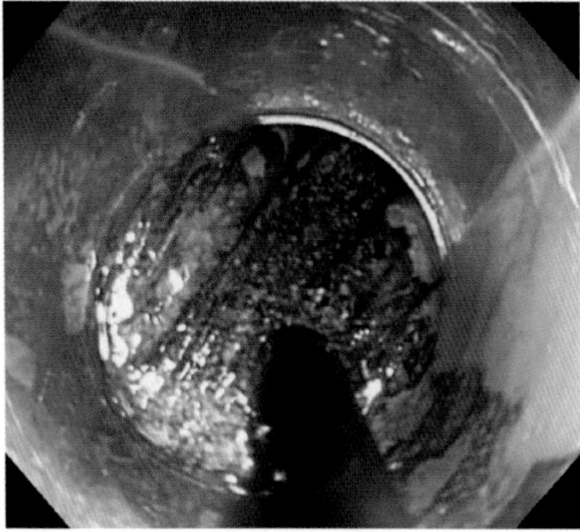

Fig. 3. A mark can be safely placed when the tip of the knife is retracted into the sheath and brought into contact with the mucosa for a moment of forced coagulation (60 W)

Tokyo, Japan; Suvenyl 1%, Chugai Pharmaceutical). To prevent bleeding, epinephrine should be added at 5 μg/ml into the local administration solution.

Mucosal Incision

A dry cut mode (effect 5, 60 W) is suitable for mucosal incisions because it can prevent bleeding. When a hook knife is used, perforation can be prevented by inserting the hook part into the submucosal layer and hooking the mucosa to the esophageal lumen for cutting (Figs. 4 and 5). A deep incision may damage the vessels, leading to bleeding. It is important to make a shallow incision in the mucosa initially, and to incise the submucosal layer more deeply under observation.

Then the mucosa on the oral side is incised in a similar manner. After the submucosal layer on the oral side is well visualized, a lateral mucosal incision is made. The direction of the hook knife has to be turned toward the esophageal lumen, and then inserted into the submucosal layer by sliding the knife backward. The mucosa is then elevated to the lumen and an electric incision is performed (Figs. 6 and 7). In general, the IT knife (KD-610L, Olympus Medical Systems) is not used for esophageal ESD owing to a high risk of perforation, but it may occasionally be useful for a mucosal incision from the anal side to the oral side. The optimal device should be selected and used according to the site and conditions.

Submucosal Dissection

For submucosal dissection, an electrosurgical mode with a high hemostatic capability, such as spray coagulation and a dry cut, should be selected because it enables us to control bleeding easily. To perform the submucosal dissection safely, a sufficient bulge should be maintained in the submucosal layer. Then the fibers of the submucosal tissue are hooked with a knife directed toward a safer space, followed by repeated brief energization. The knife can be used safely in the direction from the closed to the open space after the incised part is opened by the transparent hood. A local injection

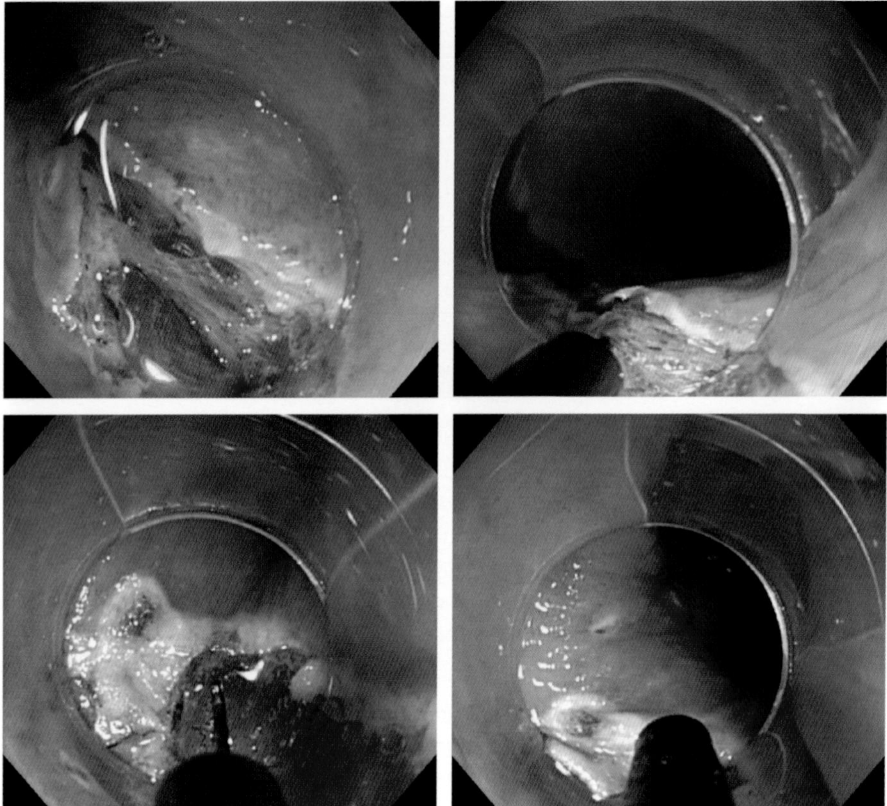

Fig. 4–7. The hook knife must be turned toward the esophageal lumen and inserted into the submucosal layer, which slides over the back of the knife. The mucosa is then elevated to the lumen and can be cut safely. A hook knife is also useful for mucosal incisions

is added after a circumferential incision, followed by a tunnel-shaped dissection of the center of the lesion and then the fibers on both sides are dissected. A tunnel-shaped dissection of the central part allows counter traction using a transparent hood, providing more efficient dissection (Figs. 8–10).

In patients with Barrett's esophageal cancer, the submucosal layer may be accompanied by severe fibrosis due to scarring after reflux esophagitis or esophageal ulcers. In this case, a submucosal topical injection of highly viscous sodium hyaluronate may be useful. If the lesion will not bulge sufficiently, then the operator should forgo endoscopic dissection and choose another treatment.

Hemostasis Using a Knife [11]

When bleeding occurs during mucosal incision or dissection, the area should be flushed using a water-jet system as soon as possible to find the origin of the bleeding.

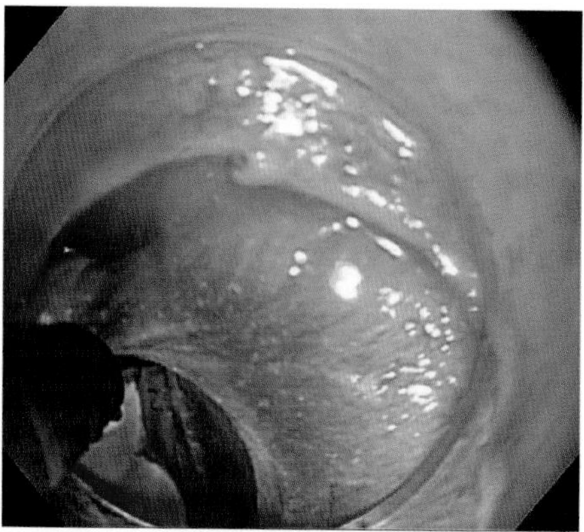

Fig. 8. The submucosal fibers are hooked with the knife

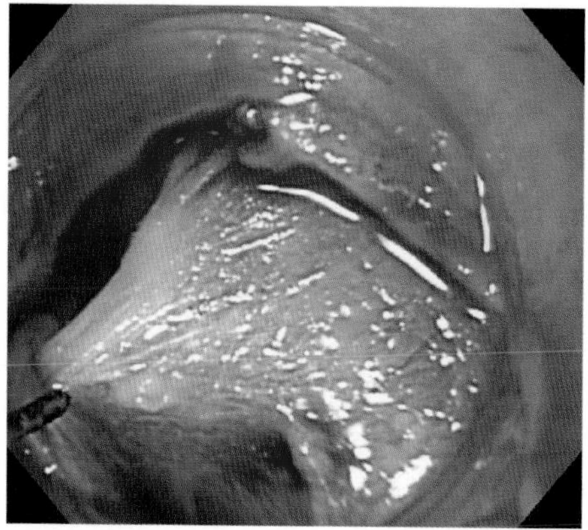

Fig. 9. The fibers are pulled into the transparent hood and are then cut in dry cut mode

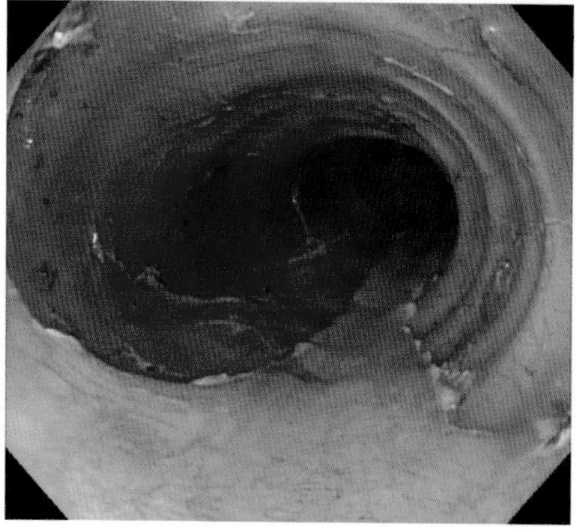

Fig. 10. Endoscopy revealed a huge ESD ulcer. There was no perforation or bleeding

For an oozing bleed, a knife tip is brought close to the origin and an electrical discharge is carried out with a spray mode to obtain hemostasis (effect 2 and 60 W with a hook knife). Since prolonged electrification may cause perforation, it should be performed for a brief moment only. Electrification by pushing the tip into the lesion may also cause perforation, and therefore it is important to maintain an optimal distance using a transparent hood.

Hemostatic Procedures Using Hemostatic Forceps

Hemostatic forceps are useful in cases of more active or spurting bleeding. After flushing with a water-jet to find the origin of the bleeding, the origin is grasped accurately with the hemostatic forceps. After that, reflushing with a water-jet may enable us to determine whether the origin has been grasped accurately. Then the forceps are elevated a little, and soft coagulation is performed with the forceps kept away from the proper muscular layer, followed by electrification for a moment with effect 5 and 40 W to obtain hemostasis.

Prevention of Bleeding

Bleeding may worsen the visual field, leading to a higher risk of accidents. Inadvertent coagulation of the blood may create an impaired field of vision. Incision and dissection while preventing bleeding are more desirable than hastily attempting hemostasis after bleeding starts. Regular transparent hoods are available for full observation of the submucosal layer. If small vessels with a diameter of 0.5 mm are observed, bleeding can be prevented through a careful incision using spray coagulation (effect 2 and 60 W with a hook knife). If vessels with a larger diameter are observed, bleeding can be prevented through precoagulation, which consists of grasping such vessels with hemostatic forceps, soft coagulation, and electrification for a short time with effect 5 and 40 W followed by an incision (Figs. 11–13).

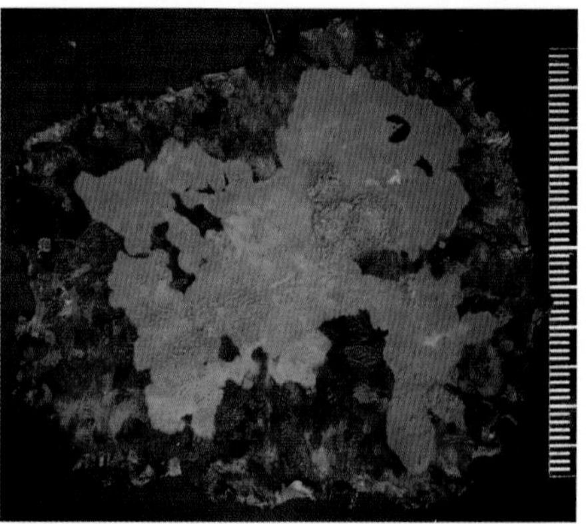

FIG. 11. The resected specimen clearly showing an iodine-demarcated unstained lesion. The cancer was 60×52 mm in area. The pathological diagnosis was a squamous cell carcinoma, the invasion depth was m2, and the lateral and vertical margins were negative

Table 1. Endoscopic evaluation of tissue atypia (EA).

I. Endoscopic structual atypia (ESA)
  a. evaluation of structural atypia (pit pattern classification)
  b. evaluation of vascular pattern (IPCL type classification)
II. Endoscopic cytological atypia (ECA)
  (ECA classification)

summarize and introduce our concept of EA as it is described in Table 1. Recent advancement of image enhancing technology, particularly NBI [2], made magnified images further recognizable. In 1990th present author reported the usefulness of vascular changes in the esophageal cancer [3,4].

In 2003, ultra-high magnification endoscopy has been developed to observe cell level structure in vivo [5–7]. Cellular-level image is interpreted with ECA (ndocytoscopic evaluation of tissue atypia) classification [8].

Those efforts are remarkably useful to detect early-stage GI cancer and to confirm superficially extending area of the neoplastic lesion during ESD.

On the other hand in the field of therapeutic endoscopy ESD was established recently [9]. The present authors developed a triangle-tip knife intending easy dissection even for un-skilled hands [10]. Development of ESD brought us a less-invasive endoscopic treatment with organ preservation.

Magnifying Endoscopy in the Esophagus (IPCL Pattern Classification)

Magnification of Normal Esophageal Mucosa

Superficial capillary pattern of the normal squamous mucosa of the esophagus was described in figure 1 [3]. In the normal mucosa IPCL, which rises perpendicular from the branching vessel, is barely recognizable with normal observation. By using the magnifying endoscope such as GIF-Q160Z, 180Z (Olympus) and GIF-Q240Z, H260Z (Olympus) which has magnification capability up to 80 times, the IPCL of the normal mucosa is identified as red dots. NBI makes capillary vessel recognizable much better. Branching vessel located at the deeper layer is observed as green, and IPCL involved in epithelium is observed as brown loops (brown dots).

Magnifying Endoscopic Diagnosis of IPCL Pattern Irregularity in the Esophageal Squamous Cell Carcinoma

In carcinoma of the esophageal squamous epithelium, four characteristic changes of IPCL pattern are detected in the non-iodine stained area. Those factors are dilatation,

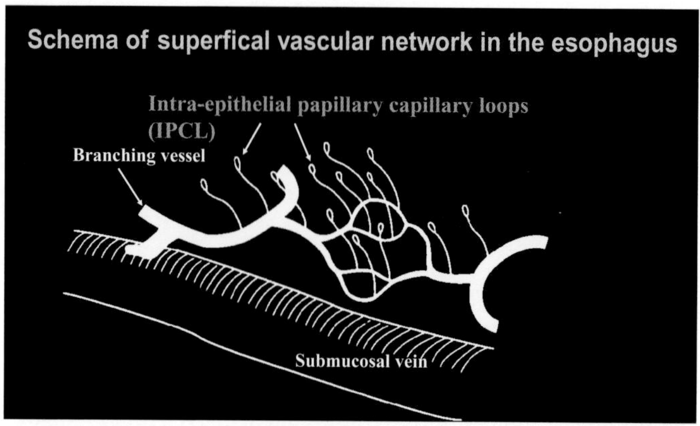

Fig. 1. Schematic drawing of magnifying endoscopic findings for superficial blood vessels in the squamous esophagus

Superficial blood vessels in the esophageal mucosa consist of branching vessels which extend to the horizontal plane and exist immediately above the lamina muscularis mucosae. IPCL rises from a branching vessel perpendicularly. The blood vessel, which can be observed under regular non-magnifying endoscopy is the branching vessel. When esophageal squmaous mucosa is magnified up to around 100 times through a magnifying endoscopy, looping vessels (IPCL) are observed. IPCL is demonstrated brown dots under NBI enhanced observation.

meandering, caliber change and uneven form in each IPCL (Figure 2) [4]. Changes in the IPCL progress gradually from normal mucosa, reactive changes, dysplasia, finally to cancer. Stratified squamous epithelium in the pharynx and esophagus has no pit pattern likely to be observed in glandular epithelium in stomach and colon. Magnifying endoscopy allows an observation of micro-vascular structure in the squamous epithelium. In the squamous epithelium, intra-papillary capillary loop (IPCL) is observed by magnifying endoscopy. IPCL demonstrates characteristic changes in its figure according to the tissue atypia and is directly related to the tissue characterization of a minute lesion [4].

Actual diagnosis consisted of two steps. First step is to detect a lesion as brownish area or as non-iodine stained lesion. Next step is to observe suspected area with high magnification and then evaluate IPCL pattern.

It is categorized from Type I (normal mucosa) to Type V (carcinoma). Type II is often equivalent to re-generative tissue or inflammation, Type III is a border line lesion which is often related to low-grade intraepithelial neoplasia, Type IV and V is equivalent to high-grade intraepithelial neoplasia, and TypeV-1 is characteristically reflecting carcinoma in situ (Figure 3). We consider that this reflects the structural irregularity of the tissue. However, under newly developed NBI processing, IPCL change is more easily to observe because NBI creates a noticeable contrast of vascular system from background tissue. It is significant that endoscopic diagnosis of flat mucosal lesion is possible by classifying the IPCL pattern in magnified image. It is endoscopically decided that IPCL Type III needs not to

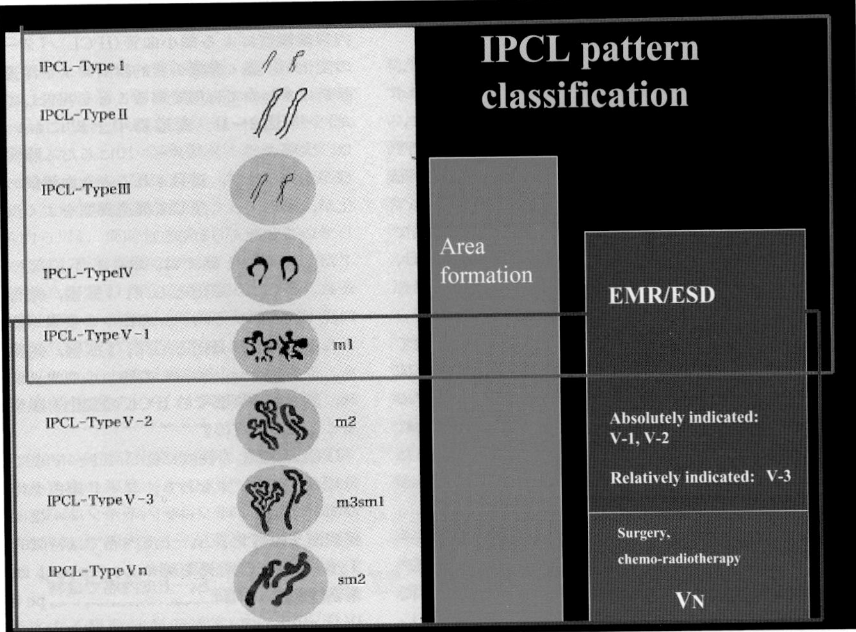

Fig. 2. IPCL pattern classification

IPCL pattern classification includes two sets of diagnostic criteria.

IPCL pattern classification from IPCL Type I to IPCL Type V-1 demonstrates the tissue characterization for flat lesion (square with red line). IPCL pattern classification from IPCL type V-1 to IPCL type VN reflects cancer infiltration depth (square with blue line).

IPCL Type III corresponds to border line lesion which potentially includes esophagitis, low-grade intraepithelial neoplasia. IPCL type III should be considered for a further follow-up study. In IPCL type IV, high-grade intraepithelial neoplasia or carcinoma in situ appears, and then further treatment with EMR/ESD should be considered. EMR/ESD should be also considered for IPCL type V-1 and type V-2 as they are definite m1 or m2 lesion with no risk of lymph node metastasis. To IPCL type V-3 lesion which corresponds to m3 lesion, diagnostic EMR/ESD should be applied as a complete biopsy to decide treatment strategy. Furthermore, IPCL type VN corresponds to a new tumor vessel, which is the cancer often associated with sm2 invasion with significantly increasing risk of lymph node metastasis, and the surgical treatment or chemoradiotherapy should be recommended.

be treated with periodical survey. IPCL Type IV and V need to be treated with EMR/ESD.

Invasion-Depth Diagnosis Standards for Superficial Carcinoma (Based on the Changes in IPCL)

In non-magnified endoscopic diagnosis, concavity of the lesion and/or the degree of the uplift and change in the shape by air feeding are major criteria used to determine the depth diagnosis. Diagnosis of sm massive invasive cancer is actually sufficient

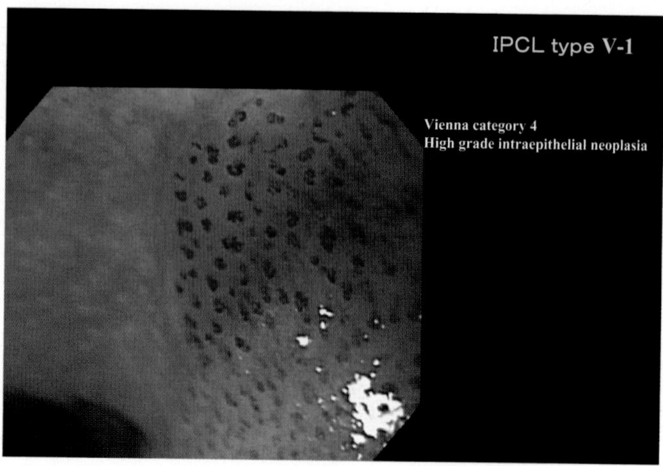

FIG. 3. NBI magnifying image of SCC in situ in the esophagus. IPCL type V-1.
NBI enhances vascular system and then recognition of IPCL becomes better.
In m1 lesion IPCL demonstrates typical changes that include four characteristic factors; dilatation, meandering, changes in caliber, unevenness in each IPCL.

enough only by non-magnified observation, magnifying endoscopic findings are considered as an additional information to non-magnified endoscopic diagnosis. Destructive change of IPCL with appearance of tumor vessels is a characteristic feature to the submucosally invasive tumor. The IPCL pattern classification of a superficial vessel is based on serial changes to the IPCL in squamous epithelium. In m1 lesion IPCL demonstrates typical changes that include four characteristic factors; dilatation, meandering, changes in caliber, unevenness in each IPCL. When it advances to m2, and m3, destructive changes of IPCL advance gradually. Therefore, changes that occur from IPCL Type II to IPCL Type V-2 take place within the mucosal layer keeping original IPCL structure partly. That resulted changes to the IPCL exists within a vertical plane. These changes are further extended and new tumor vessels appear in the submucosal cancer (Figure 2). The IPCL pattern VN (new tumor vessels) is characteristic to sm deep invasion (sm invasion depth is 200 micro and more). In contrast, irregularly arranged IPCL in m3/sm1 involves the advance destruction of the original IPCL and run on horizontal plane.

IPCL type V-1 and V-2 which often corresponds to m1/m2 lesion in histology, a changed IPCL still runs perpendicular. In IPCL type V-3 and VN which closely relates to sm cancer in histology, IPCL runs horizontal direction.

The Diagnostic difference between IPCL Type V-3 and VN is based upon the caliber of the new tumor vessels, and the histological depth where it appears. Tumor vessel which appears in IPCL type VN is around 10 times larger than irregular vessel which appears in IPCL type V-3.

We performed upper GI endoscopy using magnifying endoscopy for 648 consecutive cases. Among them 250 cases received NBI magnifying endoscopy. The correct diagnosis ratio was 78%. All inconsistencies except one were in one category only.

One case of m1 lesion was over-estimation of submucosal invasive cancer during magnifying endoscopic survey. By reviewing the videotape, magnifying observation of previous biopsy scar looked like the finding of sm massive invasive cancer.

NBI enhancement technology enables to observe capillary vessel with high contrast to background mucosa. According to the grade of changes in IPCL pattern, treatment strategy for flat epithelial lesion can be estimated.

The Route to Detect 1-mm Cancerous Lesion

Recently, even the super-minute 1mm neoplasia can be detected by utilizing NBI image enhancement. We have observed isolated 22 lesions out of 17 cases in the esophagus. When the mucosa is observed under white-light endoscopic observation, first attention needs to be paid to reddening area. A novel developed NBI allows us to detect this type of lesion as brown spot much easier. We suspect cancer when we find the following four conditions while performing magnifying endoscopic observation of a reddening spot white light or a brown spot in NBI enhanced image:

(1) area formation,
(2) loss of visibility of branching vessels in the lesion,
(3) marginal elevation of surrounding mucosa,
(4) change in vascular pattern with IPCL Type IV and V-1

Whenever all above 4 factors being recognized, we strongly suspect carcinoma in situ (Category IV of the Vienna classification).

In Vivo Observation of Living Cancer Cell Using Endocytoscopy

The most recent innovation of endoscopic imaging is visualization of the cellular level [5–7]. Cell nucleus can be observed by endocytoscopy. During endocytoscopic observation esophageal mucosa is stained with 0.5% methylene blue. To interprete endocytoscopic findings practically the ECA classification (endocytoscopic evaluation of tissue atypia) was newly introduced [8] (Figure 4). Endocytoscopic findings were graded from I to V by ECA classification. In the definite malignant lesion, cell nuclei were seen as enlarged and irregularly arranged (ECA-V). Overall accuracy of endocytoscopy in differentiating between non-malignant (Category I-III in Vienna classification) and malignant pathology (Category IV, V) was 82% in the squamous esophagus.

Furthermore, CM (crystal violet and methylene blue) double staining technique which is expected to be similar to Hematoxylin & eosin staining was developed by the present authors. By utilizing this double staining technique in vivo ECA classification became to be applied to gastric lesions.

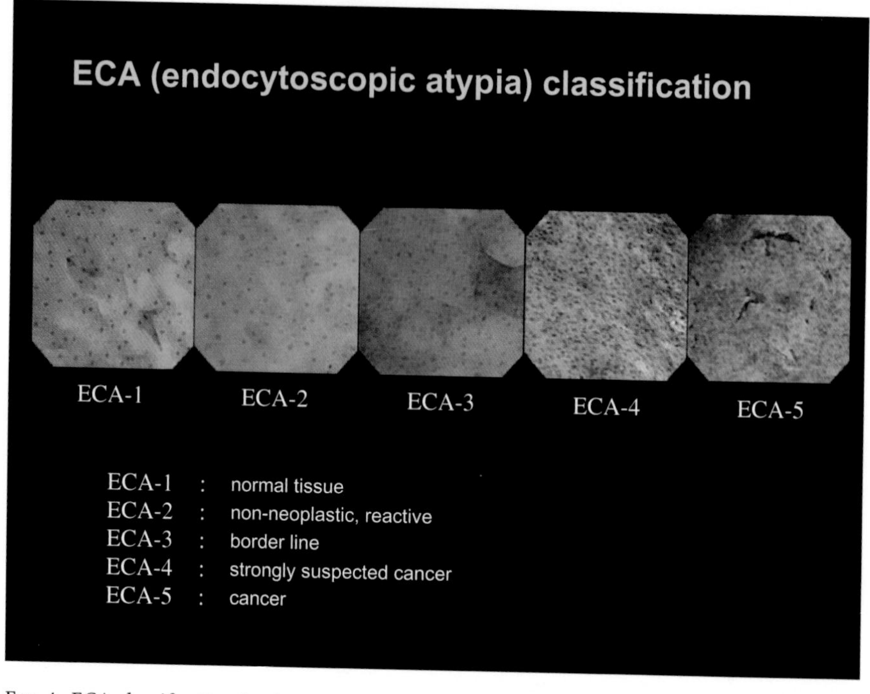

Fig. 4. ECA classification (endocytoscopic classification of tissue atypia).

Endocytoscopic images were classified into five categories as endocytoscopic atypism (ECA)

ECA-1. Large cytoplasm-rich cells with rhomboidal shape are regularly arranged. Small nuclei are located at the centre of them. This image corresponds to healthy squamous epithelium in the esophagus.

ECA-2. Cell margin often becomes round. Different-size small nuclei are observed in the esophagus. The image often reflects inflammatory or reactive changes.

ECA-3. Cell becomes smaller in size, but nuclei are still compact in the esophagus. The image often observed in border-line lesions.

ECA-4. Number of cell increases with increased nucleus/cytoplasm ratio (NC ratio) in the esophagus. This image strongly suggests malignant lesion.

ECA-5. Various size cells are irregularly arranged with high NC ratio in the esophagus. The image is recognized endoscopically as definite malignant lesion.

EMR/ESD as a Minimally Invasive Endoscopic Treatment

As methods to improve the prognosis of esophageal and gastric cancer, we are conducting the following two strategies; detection of early stage cancer and treating it by EMR/ESD (endoscopic mucosal resection/endoscopic submucosal dissection)]. In other words, our goal is to detect early-stage carcinoma during the endoscopic screening. If you have an ability to detect a 1mm neoplasia, then you would hardly overlook the 5 mm or 10 mm neoplasia. The other strategy is to conduct minimally invasive treatments according to clinical stage of carcinoma. Once the lesion is detected, accurate diagnosis for the clinical stage is mandatory to decide the strategies to each case. A minimally invasive treatment which is expected to be most effective to cure is conducted according its clinical stage. Intra-mucosal neoplasia has extremely low risk of lymph node metastasis, and therefore EMR/ESD is applied to such lesions.

EMR (Cap Technique)

In 1993 cap technique was reported by the present author [11]. It enables a quick resection of the mucosal lesion. Now it applies to a less than 1 cm lesion. Endoscopic mucosal resection (EMR) or endoscopic submucosal dissection (ESD) is an endoscopic treatment which provides a specimen for histopathological analysis. Generally, mucosal cancer without lymph node metastasis is the best candidate for these procedures. So far, the author and colleague experienced EMR in total more than 400 cases in all gastrointestinal lesions mainly by the EMRC procedure.

ESD Using "Triangle"-Tip Electrocautery Knife (TT Knife)

In the late 1990s, Hosokawa K and Ono H et al. advocated the IT Knife technique [9]. This technique enabled to perform mucosal resection in *en bloc* fashion even for a superficially widely spreading lesion. One-piece specimen regardless the size of the lesion contributes well to create accurate map of superficial tumor extension and invasion depth. Later, this technique was named ESD (endoscopic submucosal dissection) which is discriminated from conventional EMR. Ono H is the first doctor who demonstrated that ESD was technically feasible and it can be generally applied in clinical setting. Subsequently, other devices including Hook knife and Flex knife have been developed. Meanwhile, Yamamoto H et al have made it possible to keep the mucosal layer raised from the muscle layer surface for a longer period using sodium hyaluronate, which enables whole ESD procedure much technically easier and safer.

Less than 1 cm lesions receive EMR by using a cap device (EMR-C). Not-less-than-1 cm lesions receive ESD using TT knife. From October 2003 to February 2007, more than 250 cases received ESD in our hospital. General anesthesia with intra-tracheal intubation was applied to 78 consective cases of ESD. If the procedure is estimated to take more than 2 hours for treatment, the ESD was actually performed under general anesthesia.

A Newly Designed "Triangle"-Tip Knife for ESD

TT knife is a monopolar electrocautery knife, which allows pass electrical current even at the tip triangle plate [10] (Figure 5). Triangle shape of the distal plate enables to hook the tissue in any direction without adjusting the direction of the device. Hook knife which has also been commercially available can be applied to target mucosa as long as controlling direction of the hook appropriately by the assistant. In order to free operators from having to pay attention to controlling the orientation of the hook tip, the authors designed a knife with a triangular shape. A triangle shape of the tip allows the knife to hook the target mucosa into any direction regardless of the direc-

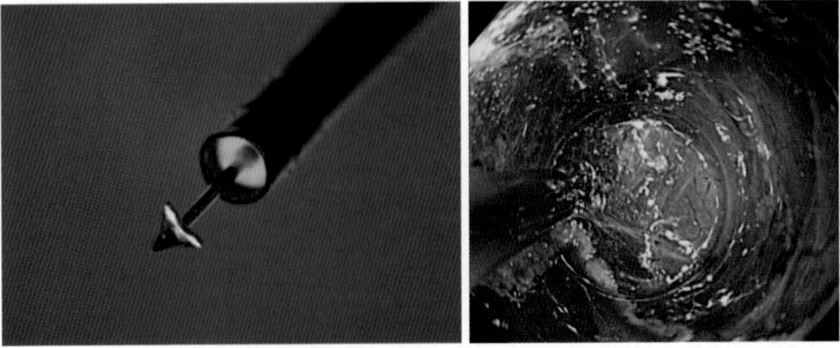

Fig. 5. "Triangle"-tip knife.
Electrocautery knife. Triangle tip allows us to catch target mucosa up into any direction without controlling the axis of the device.

tion in which TT knife advances in. A single device of TT Knife is used in all processes of ESD from marking to submucosal dissection. Only coagulating forceps is additionally used particularly in hemostasis for bleeding or in coagulation for exposed vessel.

ESD procedure consists of two parts; circumferential resection and submucosal dissection. In the phase of circumferential resection, marginal cutting is carried out using the TT Knife after confirming surface lifting of the target mucosa with local injection. The output of energy source is in the Endo-Cut mode, Effect 3 with 120 W (ICC200, ERBE) or in the Swift Coagulation mode, Effect 4 with 40 W (Vaio, ERBE). When the triangular plate is lightly touched onto the mucosal surface with intermittent current supply, the triangle plate by itself is easily cutting into the submucosal layer as an initial cutting of the mucosa. After triangle plate is inserted into submucosal layer, target mucosa is lifted up by TT Knife into the lumen of GI tract slightly applying a certain tension onto the mucosa itself. The TT Knife can be advanced in any directions in which the endoscope shaft is swung. Incision is advanced along the peripheral edge of the lesion until circumferencial cut is completed. A technical key to continue a safe marginal cutting is to lift up a target mucosa toward the lumen of GI tract by hooking it with TT knife plate. Repeated application of this manipulation enables to complete a cirmumferential marginal cutting.

The second phase of ESD is dissection of the submucosal plane. Local injection of sodium hyaluronate is recommended during dissection of the submucosal layer. This solution keeps the mucosa raised up for a longer period than saline or glyceol alone so as to make submucosal dissection much easier. By submucosal injection of hyaluronic acid submucosal layer will be swollen and be recognized as a blue band with color of indigo carmine. In contrast, the surface of muscle layer is observed as whitish plane at the bottom of blue-band submucosal layer. When the cap on the endoscopy tip is positioned to the submucosal layer, stretched submucosal fibers are easily dissected by the tip of triangle tip knife with electrocautery. Submucoal dissection is continued until the complete resection will be achieved. Dissection will be carried out with the forced coagulation mode at 60 W (ICC, ERBE) or swift coagulation mode at 40 W (Vaio, ERBE).

Significance of en bloc *Resection for Superficial Neoplasia*

The most crucial decision for the patient is whether to proceed surgical treatment in order to resect lymph nodes. Deep submucosal invasion, infiltration pattern and vessel permeation of cancer cell on the ESD specimen are the crucial factors to proceed surgical intervention. Once cancer invades into deep submucosl layer the lesion has 10–50% risk of lymph node metastasis that is expected to be curatively treated by laparoscopic surgery. For precise histological evaluation of the target lesion, en bloc resection is considered to be essential. In a piecemeal resection, precise evaluation of the lateral margin of the lesion and even the infiltration depth of cancer becomes impossible.

Selection of Method; "TT Knife ESD" or "Cap-EMR"?

"Cap" procedure is, in principle, based upon a snare polypectomy, so that the procedure time is short but the size of resected specimen is limited. "Triangle"- tip knife enables en bloc resection even for a large superficially spread lesion, but it takes relatively longer operating time. For a small lesion it is not necessary to use a triangle tip knife, and EMR with cap (a large oblique hard cap with a rim, Olympus) is easily applied and then quickly resected. In the esophagus less than 2 cm lesion can be easily resected in en bloc fashion by EMR using a cap device. Even in the stomach less than 1 cm lesion can be resected in en bloc fashion. A size of the resected specimen by cap is affected with the thickness of the mucosa.

References

1. Kudo S, Kashida H, Tamura T, et al (2000) Colonoscopic diagnosis and management of nonpolypoid early colorectal cancer. World J Surg 24:1081–1090
2. Sano Y, Saito Y, Fu KI et al (2005) Efficacy of magnifying chromoendoscopy for the differential diagnosis of colorectal lesions. Dig Endosc 17:105–116
3. Inoue H, Honda T, Yoshida T et al (1996) Ultra-high magnification endoscopy of the normal esophageal mucosa. Dig Endosc 8:13–138
4. Inoue H, Honda T, Nagai K et al (1997) Ultra-high magnification endoscopic observation of carcinoma in situ of the esophagus. Dig Endosc 9:16–18
5. Kumagai Y, Monma K, Kawada K (2004) Magnifying chromoendoscopy of the esophagus: in-vivo pathological diagnosis using an endocytoscopy system. Endoscopy 36:590–594
6. Inoue H, Kazawa T, Sato Y, et al (2004) In vivo observation of living cancer cells in the esophagus, stomach, and colon using catheter-type contact endoscope, "Endo-Cytoscopy system". Gastrointest Endoscopy Clin N Am 14:589–594
7. Inoue H, Kudo S, Shiokawa A (2005) Technology insight: laser-scanning confocal microscopy and endocytoscopy for cellular observation of the gastrointestinal tract. Nature Clinical Practice Gastroenterology & Hepatology 2:31–37
8. Inoue H, Sasajima K, Kaga M, et al (2006) Endoscopic in vivo evaluation of tissue atypia in the esophagus using a newly designed integrated endocytoscope: a pilot trial. Endoscopy 38:891–895
9. Ono H, Kondo H, Gotoda T et al (2001) Endoscopic mucosal resection for treatment of early gastric cancer. Gut 48:225–229

10. Inoue H, Sato Y, Kazawa T (2004) Technique of endoscopic submucosal dissection using a newly developed triangle-tip Knife. Stomach and Intestine 39:73–75
11. Inoue H, Takeshita K, Hori H et al (1993) Endoscopic mucosal resection with a cap-fitted panendoscope for esophagus, stomach, and colon mucosal lesions. Gastrointest Endosc 58–62

Barrett's Esophagus

Endoscopic Diagnosis of Barrett's Esophagus and Esophageal Adenocarcinomas

Kazuyoshi Yagi, Atsuo Nakamura, and Atsuo Sekine

Summary. The use of methylene blue and acetic acid in magnifying endoscopic diagnosis of intestinal metaplasia in Barrett's esophagus has been reported previously. Recently, the use of acetic acid or narrow-band imaging (NBI) has been described in magnifying endoscopic diagnosis of intramucosal adenocarcinomas arising from Barrett's esophagus. Diagnosis by NBI is based on the examination of microvascular patterns. The characteristic microvascular patterns of intramucosal adenocarcinomas in Barrett's esophagus are the mesh pattern and the loop pattern. The former appears on the lesion with dense round pits and the latter tend to appear on the lesion with elongated cancerous crypts. Acetic acid is used in the two methods of magnifying endoscopic diagnosis of adenocarcinoma: enhanced-magnification endoscopy and dynamic chemical magnifying endoscopy. In the former, the structure of the mucosal surface is observed after enhancement of the surface color with acetic acid to a clear white. In the latter, the difference between cancerous and noncancerous lesions is observed on the basis of the difference in duration of the whitening. These magnified views are very clear and facilitate the accurate diagnosis of cancerous lesions that are difficult to diagnose by conventional endoscopy. Because they help delineate the extent of cancerous lesions, these new methods of diagnosis support curative surgery of adenocarcinoma in Barrett's esophagus by endoscopic submucosal dissection.

Key words. Barrett's esophagus, Esophageal adenocarcinoma, Magnifying endoscopy, Acetic acid, Dynamic chemical endoscopy

Introduction

The incidence of esophageal adenocarcinoma originating from Barrett's esophagus has been steadily increasing in Western countries. Barrett's esophagus is defined as replacement of the normal esophageal squamous epithelium by columnar epithelium containing intestinal metaplasia. The epithelial cells in Barrett's esophagus are

Department of Internal Medicine, Niigata Prefectural Yoshida Hospital, Tsubame, Niigata 959-0242, Japan

heterogeneous and resemble those of the gastric fundus, gastric cardia, or intestine. The process of transformation of these cell clusters to resemble intestinal epithelium is known as specialized intestinal metaplasia (SIM). SIM is similar in appearance to the incomplete intestinal metaplasia that is seen in the stomach. SIM is recognized as the precursor of esophagus adenocarcinoma [1]. However, because of the poor endoscopic characteristics of SMI, biopsy is the only validated procedure for diagnosis of SIM in Western countries.

Endoscopic resection, such as endoscopic mucosal resection (EMR) and endoscopic submucosal dissection (ESD), has been reported as an alternative treatment for esophageal adenocarcinoma [2,3]. However it is difficult to endoscopically diagnose mucosal adenocarcinomas arising from Barrett's esophagus the same as their precursors. To ensure complete endoscopic removal of the diseased mucosa, accurate endoscopic diagnosis of SIM and early-stage Barrett's adenocarcinoma should be achieved. Recently, the use of magnifying endoscopy with acetic acid infiltration or narrow-band imaging (NBI) has received worldwide attention [3–5] because these novel imaging technologies may allow precise diagnosis of the existence and extent of esophageal adenocarcinomas. Here, we describe the mucosal pattern of Barrett's esophagus and the magnifying endoscopic appearance of adenocarcinoma when various methods are used. Our subjects were nine patients with early-stage adenocarcinoma arising from Barrett's esophagus.

Techniques of Enhanced-Magnification Endoscopy and Magnifying Endoscopy with Narrow-Band Imaging (NBI)

Acetic acid-enhanced magnification endoscopy was first reported by Guelrud et al. [4]. Instillation of acetic acid gives the columnar mucosa a whitened appearance and the structure of the mucosa can then be observed clearly by magnifying endoscopy. Thus, 10 ml 1.5% (v/v) acetic acid was sprinkled at low pressure onto the esophageal mucosa by means of a syringe attached to the accessory channel of the endoscope.

NBI is a video endoscopic imaging technique for enhanced display of mucosal microstructure and capillaries of the superficial mucosal layer obtained when using a narrow-band filter [wavelength ranges of the new RGB (red-green-blue) filters: 485–515 nm for red (R), 430–460 nm for green (G), and 400–430 nm for blue (B)], which wavelengths are different from conventional filters, to the RGB of a plane sequential endoscope, and by changing the spectral feature of the observation light relative to that of the narrow-band filters [6].

Magnified Views of Barrett's Esophagus by Enhanced Magnifying Endoscopy

We previously observed 53 patients with columnar-lined esophagus by this method and defined four patterns; 110 biopsy specimens of each pattern were obtained [3]. The four types are type I, small round pits of uniform size and shape ("corpus" type);

TABLE 1. Correlation of acetic acid-enhanced magnifying endoscopic views with histopathological findings.

	Histological classification (*n*, %)			
Endoscopic classification	Fundic type	Cardiac type	Intestinal metaplasia	Total
Type I	11 (100%)	0	0	11
Type II	2 (4%)	45 (82%)	8 (15%)	55
Type IIIa	0	10 (29%)	24 (71%)	34
Type IIIb	0	1 (10%)	9 (90%)	10
Total	13	56	41	110

Source: Data reproduced from [3]

type II, slit-reticular pattern with horizontally elongated mucosal pits ("cardiac type"); type IIIa, gyrus pattern; and type IIIb, villous pattern [3]. The correlations between the magnified pattern and histological type of mucosa are shown in Table 1. Type IIIa and IIIb are thought to be magnified views of intestinal metaplasia. Goda et al., using NBI, reported the characteristic magnified patterns of intestinal metaplasia as cerebriform, fine mucosal, and with ivy- or DNA-like capillaries [5].

Regardless of the method chosen, it is very important for the diagnosis of Barrett's adenocarcinoma that we have a clear understanding of the patterns of nonneoplastic epithelium, including intestinal metaplasia, under magnification.

Diagnosis of Adenocarcinoma in Barrett's Esophagus

We diagnosed nine patients with early-stage esophageal adenocarcinoma arising from Barrett's esophagus (Table 2). Five patients had mucosal adenocarcinomas. Four of them were treated with ESD and one by surgery. Three patients had submucosal invasion; one was treated by EMR (the grade of submucosal invasion was found to be sm1), one by surgery, and one by surgery after EMR because sm2 invasion was

TABLE 2. Data from Niigata Prefectural Yoshida Hospital of nine cases of esophageal adenocarcinoma arising from Barrett's esophagus(BE).

Case	Sex	Type of BE	Endoscopic classification	Depth	Microvascular pattern	Response to acetic acid	Therapy
1	M	SSBE	IIb	sm2	Irregular	Not tested	EMR + surgery
2	M	SSBE	IIb	m	Unclear	Not tested	Surgery
3	M	SSBE	IIa + IIc + III	sm2	Irregular	Not tested	Surgery
4	M	SSBE	IIa + IIb	sm1	Irregular mesh	Not tested	EMR
5	M	LSBE	IIa + IIb	m	Loop pattern	Minute grain-like pattern	ESD
6	F	SSBE	IIc	m	Unclear	Minute grain-like pattern	ESD
7	F	SSBE	IIa	m (?)	Mesh pattern	Early disappearance of whitening (dynamic chemical endoscopy)	No therapy

Table 2. *Continued.*

Case	Sex	Type of BE	Endoscopic classification	Depth	Microvascular pattern	Response to acetic acid	Therapy
8	M	SSBE	Ia + IIb	m	Mesh pattern	Early disappearance of whitening (dynamic chemical endoscopy)	ESD
9	M	SSBE	IIa	m	Mesh pattern	Early disappearance of whitening (dynamic chemical endoscopy)	ESD

SSBE, short segment Barrett's esophagus; LSBE, long segment Barrett's esophagus; sm, submucosal; m, mucosal; EMR, endomucosal resection; ESD, endoscopic submucosal dissection

recognized in the histological specimen. One patient had other severe disease and elected not to undergo treatment.

Five adenocarcinomatous lesions had characteristic microvascular patterns, and five were imaged clearly after instillation of acetic acid. The endoscopic and magnifying endoscopic views are shown.

Microvascular Pattern of Adenocarcinoma

The microvascular patterns of adenocarcinoma are divided into two types. One is the mesh type, in which each cancerous crypt is surrounded by an interconnecting mesh network of microvessels that expands horizontally around the crypt. The second type is the loop type, in which there are loop-like microvessels with abnormal density, size, or form; these often have a thick dot-like or stick-like appearance. The loops do not appear to be connected and are distributed vertically around the cancerous crypts. Two of the cases that had mesh patterns are described next.

Case 7. The conventional endoscopic findings are shown in Fig. 1A. The slightly elevated lesion is visible above a squamous epithelial island. The area surrounded by the yellow box in Fig. 1A was observed by GIF 240Z with magnification; the mesh pattern is apparent (Fig. 1B). The size and shape of each network was irregular. The mesh pattern was highlighted by magnifying endoscopy using NBI (Fig. 1C). This area with the mesh pattern was classed as a differentiated adenocarcinoma on histopathological examination.

Case 8. The conventional endoscopic view of this case is shown in Fig. 2A. Figure 2B is a magnified view of the box in Fig. 2A. This magnified view shows the mesh pattern of the microvessels and indicated differentiated adenocarcinoma. This lesion was resected by ESD; a magnified view of the resected specimen after acetic acid sprinkling is given in Fig. 2C, which covers the same area shown in Fig. 2B. Small, round pits and mesh-like microvessels surrounding the pits are seen. This structure is the basic mesh pattern seen with magnifying endoscopy.

The case that had a loop pattern is described next.

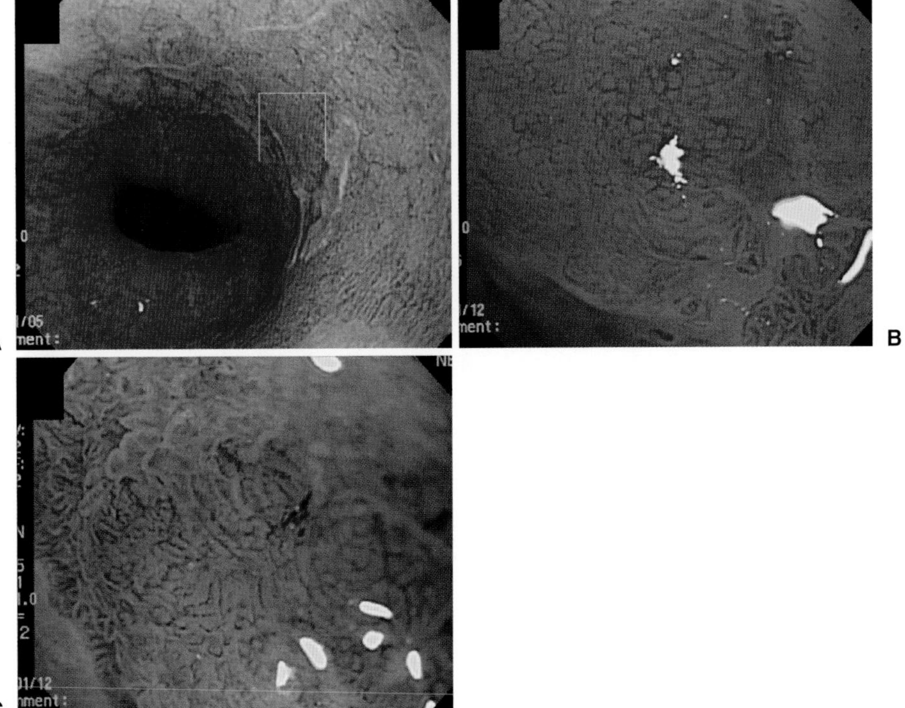

FIG. 1. **A** Conventional endoscopic view of lesion in Case 7. **B** Magnifying endoscopic view of the area delineated by the *yellow box* in **A**. A mesh pattern is visible. **C** The area in **B** as it appears on magnifying endoscopy with narrow-band imaging (NBI)

Case 5. The conventional endoscopic appearance is shown in Fig. 3A. Figure 3B is a magnified view of the box in Fig. 3A. A granular pattern of irregular size is seen, along with loop-like microvessels that are irregular in size and form. These microvessels form a pattern of loops vertically distributed in a network of microvessels surrounding each cancerous crypt.

The finding of both the aforementioned characteristic microvascular patterns together (mesh and loop) by magnifying endoscopy would strongly suggest that the lesion is a differentiated adenocarcinoma.

Use of Acetic Acid to Diagnose Adenocarcinoma

Acetic acid is used in two ways in the diagnosis of adenocarcinoma. One way is to enhance the appearance of the mucosal structure by whitening it [3]. The other is in dynamic chemical endoscopy, in which the acetic acid-induced whitening disappears from the cancerous area earlier than from the noncancerous area [7].

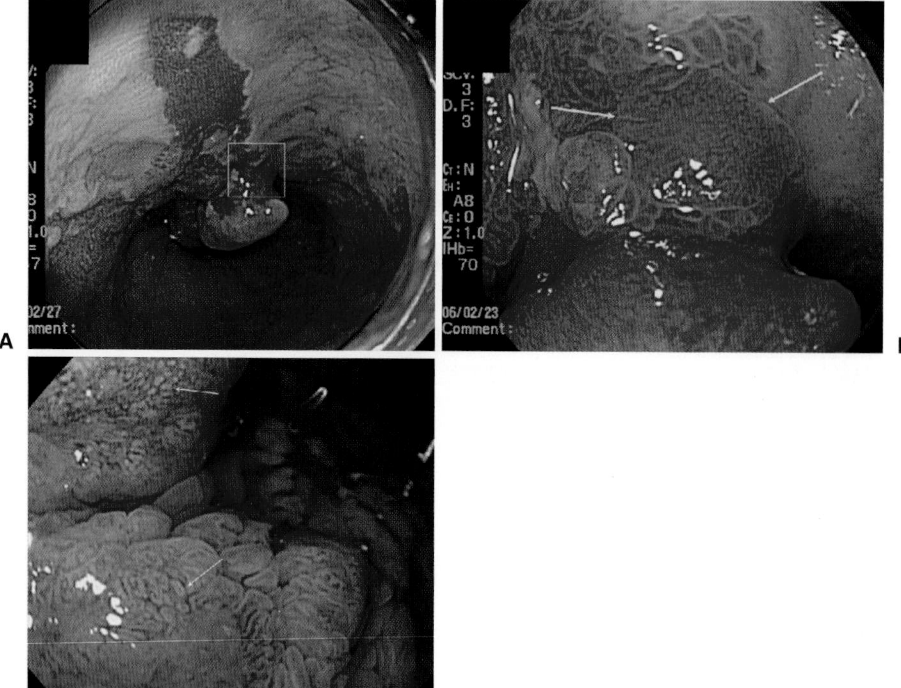

FIG. 2. **A** Conventional endoscopic view of lesion in Case 8. **B** Magnifying endoscopic view of *box* of **A**. A mesh pattern is visible (*yellow arrows*). **C** Magnifying endoscopic view of resected specimen after acetic acid sprinkling. Small round pits (indicating cancerous tissue) and mesh-like microvessels surrounding the pits are visible

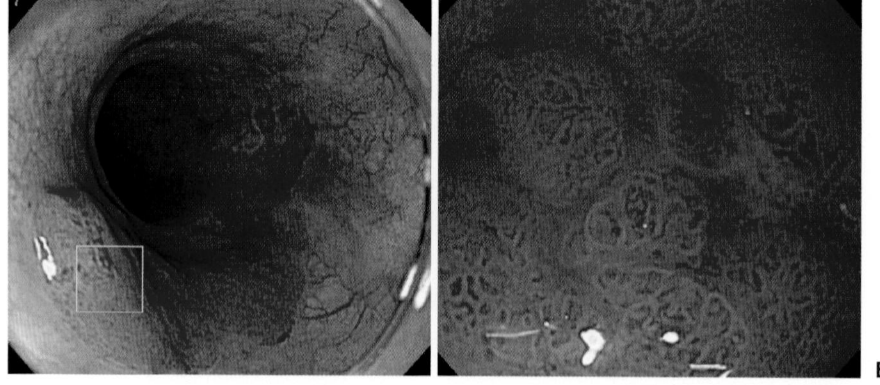

FIG. 3. **A** Conventional endoscopic view of a lesion in Case 5. **B** Magnifying endoscopic view of the *boxed area* in **A**. A granular pattern irregular in size with loop-like microvessels is visible

Use of Acetic Acid to Enhance Magnifying Endoscopy

The presence of an irregular tissue structure indicates a diagnosis of differentiated adenocarcinomas [3].

Case 5. Figure 4A is a conventional endoscopic view in this patient. A fine mucosal pattern can be seen, but the cancerous extent cannot be determined. Figure 4B is a magnified view of box 1 in Fig. 4A after the instillation of acetic acid. A regular pit pattern is apparent, indicating noncancerous mucosa. Histopathological examination of a biopsy specimen from this area revealed intestinal metaplasia. Figure 4C is a magnified view of box 2 in Fig. 4A after the instillation of acetic acid. A minute grain-like pattern can be seen on the left side (yellow arrows). This pattern is indicative of cancerous mucosa. The area surrounding the minute grain-like pattern has a regular pit pattern similar to that in Fig. 4B. This lesion was also resected by ESD, and the

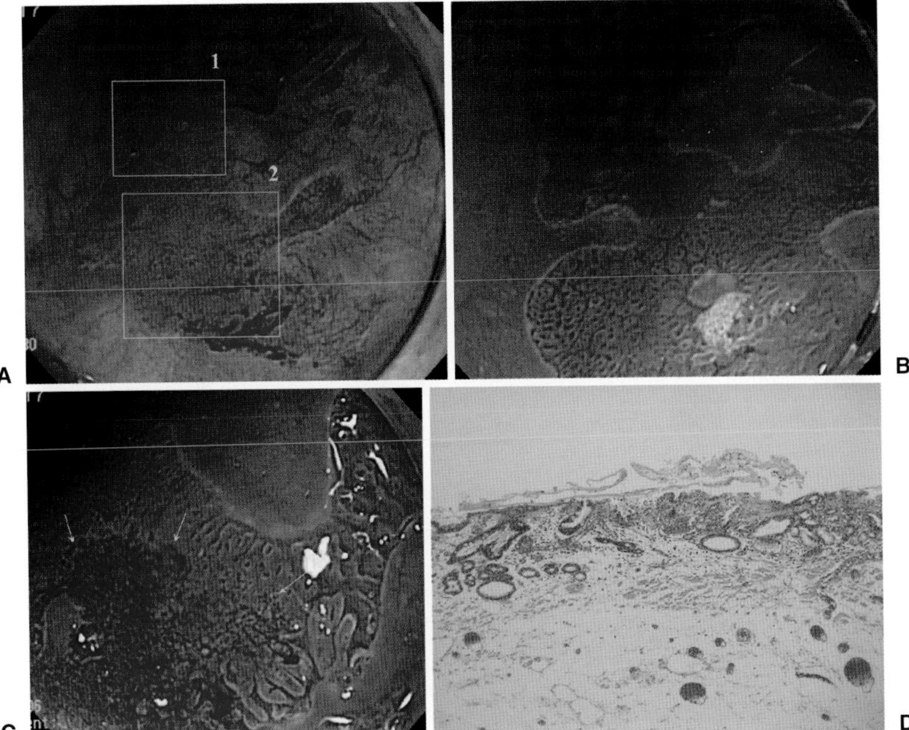

Fig. 4. **A** Conventional endoscopic view of lesion in Case 5. **B** Magnifying endoscopic view of the area in *box* 1 in **A** after instillation of acetic acid. Regular pits are visible. This was an area of intestinal metaplasia. (Reproduced from [3], with permission.) **C** Magnifying endoscopic view of the area in *box* 2 in **A** after instillation of acetic acid. A minute grain-like pattern is visible on the *left side* (*yellow arrows*). This was an area of well-differentiated adenocarcinoma. (Reproduced from [3] with permission.) **D** Histological findings of this area. At the *right* is cancerous tissue and at the *left* is intestinal metaplasia

histological finding is shown in Fig. 4D. On the right side of Fig. 4D is cancerous tissue, and on the left side is intestinal metaplasia.

Use of Acetic Acid in Dynamic Chemical Magnifying Endoscopy [7]

This magnifying endoscopic examination with acetic acid is different from other conventional endoscopic diagnoses based on the anatomic characteristics of the lesion, because this methodology utilizes the difference in chemical response to acetic acid between normal and cancerous mucosa. The mucosal color is whiter after acetic acid application and dynamically changes, with different rates of speed, depending on the histological characteristics of the lesion.

Case 7. The conventional endoscopic appearance of a lesion in this case is shown in Fig. 5A. After instillation of acetic acid, all the mucosa, including cancerous epithelium, shows an aceto-white reaction. Several seconds after acetic acid instillation, the aceto-whitening of the cancerous area began to disappear, but the noncancerous mucosa continued to show aceto-whitening (Fig. 5B). The extent of the cancer can be diagnosed by the area indicated by arrows in Fig. 5B.

Case 8. Figure 6A is a conventional endoscopic view of a lesion. Figure 6B is a magnified view of the boxed area in Fig. 6A; it shows a tubular pattern not typical of cancer. After instillation of acetic acid, the area in the box displays aceto-whitening (Fig. 6C), but the aceto-whitening began to disappear after several seconds (Fig. 6D,E; yellow arrows). This reaction indicated the presence of cancerous tissue. The histopathology of the area is shown in Fig. 6F: the cancerous crypts have weak structural atypia and the stroma surrounding the cancerous crypts is rich. This histological feature gave the tissue the tubular pattern seen in the magnified view (Fig. 6B), making it difficult to categorize the tissue as cancerous with magnification alone. However, dynamic chemical endoscopy indicated this area to be cancerous because of the early disappearance of aceto-whitening.

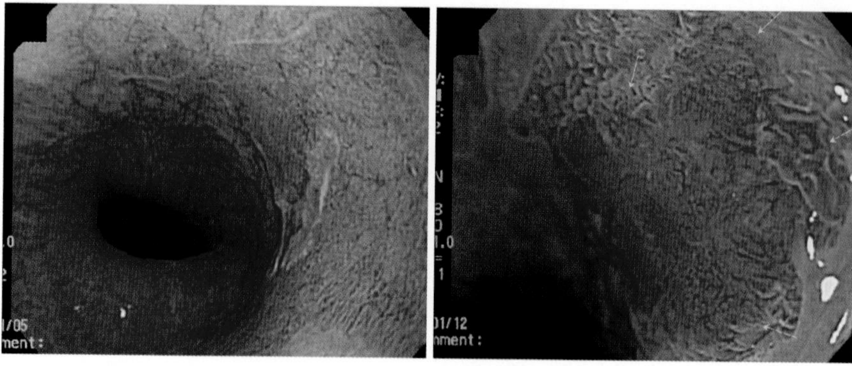

Fig. 5. **A** Conventional endoscopic view of lesion in Case 7. **B** Several seconds after the instillation of acetic acid, the aceto-whitening of the cancerous area has begun to disappear. The extent of the cancer is delineated by the area indicated by the *arrows*

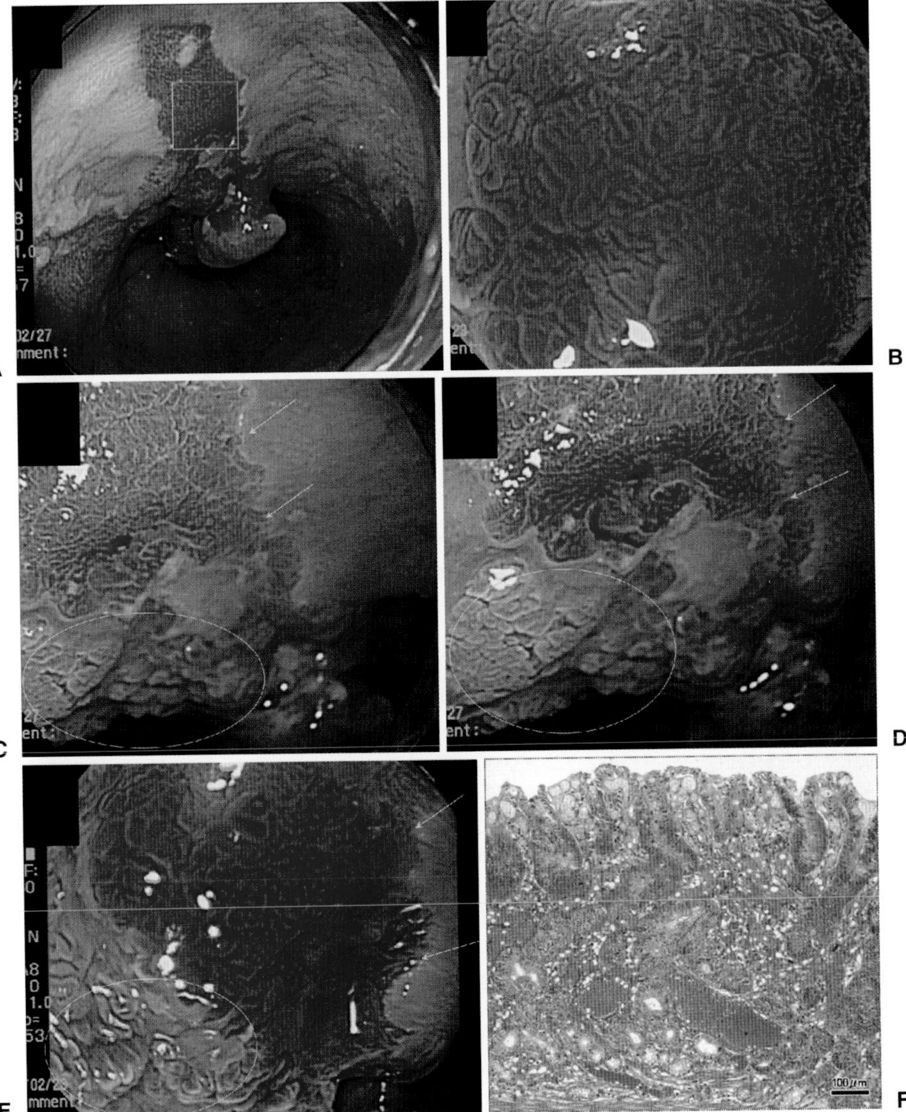

Fig. 6. **A** Conventional endoscopic view of a lesion in Case 8. **B** Magnifying endoscopic view of the *boxed area* in **A**. **C** Magnifying endoscopic view of the *boxed area* in **A** (*yellow arrows*) and of the *circled area* in Fig. 7 (*yellow oval*) after acetic acid sprinkling. **D** Magnifying endoscopic view of the *boxed area* in **A** and of the *circled area* in Fig. 7 10 s after acetic acid sprinkling. The aceto-whitening of the *yellow arrow area* began to disappear (*yellow arrows*), although aceto-whitening of the *circled area* was still present (*yellow oval*). **E** Magnifying endoscopic view of the *boxed area* in **A** and of the *circled area* in Fig. 7 20 s after acetic acid sprinkling. The aceto-whitening of the *yellow arrow area* had disappeared (*yellow arrows*), although aceto-whitening of the circled area was still present (*yellow oval*). **F** Histopathology of the *boxed area* in **A**. Cancerous crypts have weak structural atypia, and the stroma surrounding them is rich

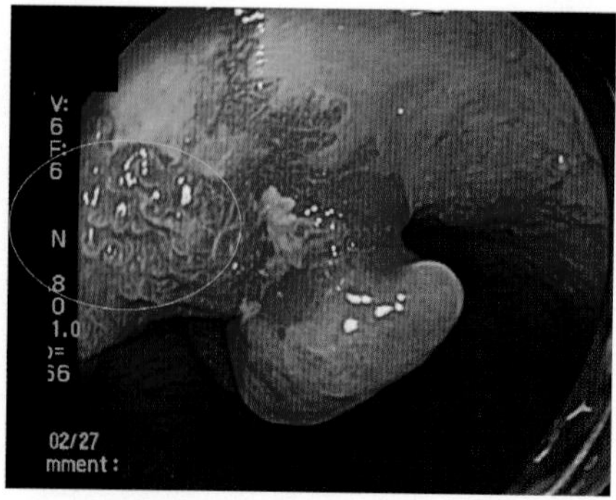

Fig. 7. Conventional endoscopic view of a lesion in Case 8. The *enclosed area* (*yellow oval*) has a granular pattern

Figure 7 is another conventional endoscopic view of the lesion in Case 8. The magnified view in the enclosed area shows a granular pattern. The microvascular pattern was not observed, and it was impossible to determine whether this lesion was cancerous. Dynamic chemical endoscopy was therefore done (Fig. 6C). After instillation of acetic acid, the circled area showed aceto-whitening and continue to show whitening (Fig. 6D,E). Because the aceto-whitening in this area continued for 1 min after instillation of acetic acid, the lesion here was classified as noncancerous. Intestinal metaplasia was ascertained by biopsy and histopathological examination.

Discussion

Magnifying endoscopic examination had been used for diagnosis of intestinal metaplasia of Barrett's esophagus [3–5,8,9]. Recently, it has also been used for the diagnosis of mucosal adenocarcinoma arising from Barrett's esophagus [2,3,5]. In particular, magnifying endoscopy has been reported to be of practical use for determining the extent of adenocarcinoma in Barrett's esophagus before endoscopic resection [2,3].

Diagnosis of Barrett's adenocarcinoma has been established by modifying magnifying endoscopic diagnosis of gastric mucosal cancer [7,10–12].

The views obtained by magnifying endoscopy under conventional light and magnifying endoscopy with NBI differ in that (1) magnifying endoscopy with NBI reveals almost all the fine microvessels surrounding the cancerous crypts, which often show a regular rather than an irregular microvascular pattern, whereas magnifying endoscopy with conventional light tends to emphasize the irregularity of the microvessels in cancerous tissue; and (2) different endoscopists show the same magnified views by magnifying endoscopy using NBI, whereas different endoscopists show different magnified views when they use magnifying endoscopy with conventional light. Point 1 can be regarded as a disadvantage of using NBI, but with knowledge of cancerous structure—the so-called pit pattern—it is easy to correctly identify the microvascular pattern by magnifying endoscopy using NBI [12]. In intramucosal noninvasive cancer, the microvessels of the cancerous tissue tend to form a pattern that imitates that of the feeding vessels surrounding the crypts. In invasive cancer, the microvessels of the cancerous tissue tend to have an interrupted pattern that does not resemble that of the feeding vessels. We previously classified microvascular patterns of noninvasive gastric intramucosal cancer into mesh and loop patterns [12]. The adenocarcinomas arising from Barrett's esophagus are thought to show the same types of microvascular pattern. The mesh pattern consists of horizontally connected microvessels (Figs. 1B,C, 2B), and with this pattern there tend to be round pits of cancerous tissue (Fig. 2C). The meshed microvessels are located inside the stroma surrounding the round pits of the cancerous crypts.

In the loop pattern, there were loop-like microvessels with abnormal density, size, or form; they often appeared as thick dot-like or stick-like microvessels (Fig. 3B). The loops did not appear to be connected, in contrast to the mesh pattern. This pattern appeared to form a network from bottom to top vertically, with the loops at the surface of the cancerous tissue. With this pattern there tended to be a tubular or granular structural, not round pits. Case 5 showed a loop pattern (Fig. 3B), and the granular structure was revealed by acetic acid sprinkling.

Guelrud et al. described a technique that they named enhanced-magnification endoscopy; it combines magnifying endoscopy with the instillation of acetic acid [4]. They classified Barrett's epithelium into four patterns: I, round pits with a characteristic pattern of circular dots arranged in a regular and orderly manner; II, reticular with circular or oval pits that are regular in shape and arrangement; III, villous with no pits present but a fine villiform appearance with regular shape and arrangement; and IV, ridge with no pits present but a thick villous convoluted shape with a cerebriform appearance with regular shape and arrangement [3]. Guelrud et al. found that the rate of detection of intestinal metaplasia in pattern III and pattern IV epithelium in patients with previously diagnosed Barrett's esophagus was 87% and 100%, respectively [4]. Endo et al. reported the same result using magnifying endoscopy with methylene blue [8]. Guelrud did not describe the magnified appearance of adenocarcinoma arising from Barrett's esophagus, but enhanced-magnification endoscopy with acetic acid application has been used by other endoscopists and is reported to be practical use in the diagnosis of adenocarcinomas [3]. Case 5 is a good example (Fig. 4B,C).

Dynamic chemical magnifying endoscopy is the same as enhanced-magnification endoscopy in that both techniques use acetic acid, but the mechanism of diagnosis differs. When we were studying the use of acetic acid-enhanced magnifying endoscopy in the diagnosis of gastric cancer and adenoma, we realized that the duration of acetic-whitening differed between gastric carcinoma and noncancerous gastric mucosa: aceto-whitening disappeared earlier in carcinoma than in the noncancerous mucosa [7]. Therefore, a clear contrast between the cancerous and noncancerous mucosa appears and is very useful in determining the extent of the cancerous lesion. Endoscopy using acetic acid is different from chromoendoscopy because no dyes are used and the chemical response of the mucosa to acetic acid produces the whitening changes. The change in the degree of whitening with time and the dependency of the duration of whitening on the histology led us to call this new technique dynamic chemical endoscopy [7].

Figure 5B (Case 7) shows typical dynamic chemical endoscopic views with good contrast. Figure 6C,D,E (Case 8) illustrates how the dynamic chemical mechanism can be used to determine whether a lesion is adenocarcinomatous.

In conclusion, the use of magnifying endoscopy with the addition of NBI or acetic acid is a progressive step in the diagnosis of adenocarcinoma arising from Barrett's esophagus.

References

1. Spechler SJ, Goyal RK (1996) The columnar-lined esophagus, intestinal metaplasia, and Norman Barrett. Gastroenterology 110:614–621
2. Yagi K, Nakamura A, Sekine A, et al (2002) Magnified view of adenocarcinoma in short segment Barrett's esophagus treated by endoscopic mucosal resection. Gastrointest Endosc 55:278–281
3. Yagi K, Nakamura A, Sekine A, et al (2006) Endoscopic diagnosis of mucosal adenocarcinomas and intestinal metaplasia of columnar-lined esophagus using enhanced-magnification endoscopy. Dig Endosc 18:S21–S26
4. Guelrud M, Herrera I, Essenfeld H, et al (2001) Enhanced magnification endoscopy: a new technique to identify specialized intestinal metaplasia in Barrett's esophagus. Gastrointest Endosc 53:559–565
5. Goda K, Tajiri H, Ikegami M, et al (2007) Usefulness of magnifying endoscopy with narrow band imaging for the detection of specialized intestinal metaplasia in columnar-lined esophagus and Barrett's adenocarcinoma. Gastrointest Endosc 65:36–46
6. Gono K, Yamazaki K, Doguchi N, et al (2003) Endoscopic observation of tissue by narrow band illumination. Opt Rev 10:211–215
7. Yagi K, Aruga Y, Nakamura A, et al (2005) The study of dynamic chemical magnifying endoscopy in gastric neoplasia. Gastrointest Endosc 62:963–969
8. Endo T, Awakawa T, Takahashi H, et al (2002) Classification of Barrett's epithelium by magnifying endoscopy. Gastrointest Endosc 55:641–647
9. Sharma P, Weston AP, Topalovski M, et al (2003) Magnification chromoendoscopy for the detection of intestinal metaplasia and dysplasia in Barrett's oesophagus. Gut 52:24–27
10. Yao K, Iwashita A, Yao T (2004) Early gastric cancer: proposal for a new diagnostic system based on microvascular architecture as visualized by magnified endoscopy. Dig Endosc 16:S110–S117
11. Nakayoshi T, Tajiri H, Matsuda K, et al (2004) Magnifying endoscopy combined with narrow band imaging system for early gastric cancer: correlation of vascular pattern with histology. Endoscopy 36:1080–1084
12. Yagi K, Nakamura A, Sekine A (2007) Comparative study of microvascular architecture and pit pattern in gastric differentiated adenocarcinomas. Gastrointest Endosc 65:AB354

Narrow-Band Imaging in the Diagnosis of Barrett's Esophagus

Christopher R. Lynch and Prateek Sharma

Summary. Barrett's esophagus (BE) is the premalignant lesion for the majority of patients with esophageal and gastroesophageal junction adenocarcinoma, a cancer rapidly rising in incidence in the United States and western Europe. Endoscopic diagnosis of BE and neoplasia arising from within a BE segment continues to be a challenge and is typically dependent on random biopsies. Because of the focal and patchy nature of intestinal metaplasia and neoplasia, novel endoscopic approaches aimed at improving current screening and surveillance strategies have been explored. Narrow-band imaging (NBI) with or without magnification endoscopy is a new endoscopic technique that changes the optical filters of the current sequential lighting video endoscopes to spectral narrow-band filters. Use of a higher intensity of blue light with narrow-band filters allows detailed imaging of mucosal and vascular surface patterns with a high degree of resolution. Studies to date have yielded promising results for NBI alone or in combination with other advanced endoscopic techniques in the detection and surveillance of patients with BE.

Key words. Barrett's esophagus, Narrow-band imaging, Dysplasia, Esophageal adenocarcinoma, Screening and surveillance

Introduction

Barrett's esophagus (BE) has generated a great deal of interest in the gastroenterological community. It occurs in approximately 10% to 15% of patients with chronic gastroesophageal reflux disease (GERD) and is defined as the presence of columnar epithelium in the distal esophagus that contains specialized intestinal metaplasia on histological examination [1]. This metaplastic conversion carries with it the potential risk of future dysplastic transformation to esophageal adenocarcinoma (EAC). BE incurs a 30- to 50-fold greater risk of development of EAC with an absolute risk that

Division of Gastroenterology and Hepatology, Veterans Affairs Medical Center and University of Kansas School of Medicine, 4801 East Linwood Boulevard, Kansas City, MO 64128-2295, USA

approaches 0.5% annually [2]. It is estimated that approximately 13,000 to 15,000 people in the United States alone are affected by esophageal cancer annually. Although survival rates have improved in some countries during recent years, EAC remains a highly lethal cancer, with a 5-year survival rate of 10% to 20% in most Western populations [3]. This poor survival is a reflection of the advanced stage often present at diagnosis. The emergence of endoscopic methods of treatment of high-grade dysplasia (HGD) and early EAC such as photodynamic therapy and endoscopic mucosal resection demands that endoscopists accurately identify BE and then recognize dysplasia before the development of invasive EAC.

Limitations of Diagnosis and Surveillance of Barrett's

Many experts advocate an initial screening upper endoscopy for selected patients with GERD (e.g., those with frequent or long-standing symptoms). Standard white light endoscopy without biopsies can detect columnar-like epithelium but cannot confirm specialized intestinal metaplasia or dysplasia. Although strong clinical evidence is lacking, BE patients are typically enrolled in surveillance programs with the goal of identifying those patients who might benefit from therapy. Current guidelines for surveillance suggest periodically obtaining target biopsies at sites of endoscopically visible mucosal abnormalities (e.g., ulcers, nodules) along with random four-quadrant biopsies every 2 cm along the entire BE length [4]. In addition to being time consuming and labor intensive, this approach is limited by sampling error. Biopsy specimens from short segments of columnar-appearing mucosa reveal intestinal metaplasia in only 40% to 60% of patients [5]. This patchy and focal nature of intestinal metaplasia was further highlighted by a study of 570 patients undergoing upper endoscopy; although BE was suspected in 146 patients, only 60 patients had histological confirmation of BE [6]. Furthermore, early neoplasia in BE is not visible to the naked eye at standard endoscopy, and random biopsies sample only a very small proportion of the at-risk epithelium. As with BE, the distribution of dysplasia and early EAC is patchy and focal; standard white light endoscopy with random biopsies may fail to detect these lesions as well.

As the number of patients with reflux symptoms continues to increase, upper endoscopy is diagnosing an ever-increasing number of patients with BE. As these patients enter surveillance programs, it is highly desirable that endoscopists be able to accurately identify those patients with HGD or EAC early in the disease process so that curative therapies may be undertaken. As many of these patients may undergo endoscopic therapy, these measures may help in alleviating the considerable morbidity and mortality associated with esophagectomy for EAC. These reasons in combination with the limitations of current surveillance strategies make the development of improved techniques in the diagnosis and surveillance of BE essential.

Several new endoscopic techniques, including chromoendoscopy, magnification endoscopy, autofluorescence endoscopy, light-scattering spectroscopy, and optical coherence tomography, have been implemented either alone or in conjunction to aid in the diagnosis of intestinal metaplasia and dysplasia within the BE segment. More recently, narrow-band imaging (NBI), a new endoscopic technique for improving visualization of mucosal surfaces and capillary patterns without the use of dyes, has been studied in the diagnosis of BE and dysplasia.

Narrow-Band Imaging

Narrow-band imaging is a novel endoscopic technique that has been developed to improve the quality of endoscopic images and to enhance the visualization of the microvasculature and mucosal pattern of the gastrointestinal tract. This technique allows precise evaluation of the epithelium from which neoplasia arises. Narrow-band imaging has been shown to be useful in the diagnosis of head and neck cancers, BE, and early gastric and colon cancer [7–10].

NBI Endoscopy System

The sequential lighting method in standard video endoscopes has a rotation disk with RGB (red, green, blue) optical filters in front of a white light source, typically a xenon lamp. Narrow-band imaging technology uses spectral narrow-band optical filters instead of the full spectrum of white light. The penetration depth of light is dependent on its wavelength; the shorter the wavelength, the more superficial the penetration. The light absorption and scattering properties of tissue are strongly wavelength dependent such that blue light, which has a shorter wavelength, typically reaches into shallow surfaces. Therefore, in the visible spectrum, blue light penetrates only superficial areas of tissue (mucosal imaging) whereas red light penetrates most deeply. Thus, the use of blue light with the help of special narrow-band filters (415 nm, 445 nm, 500 nm) enables visualization of the superficial tissue structures. The major chromophore in esophageal tissues in the visible wavelength range is hemoglobin, which has a maximum absorptive wavelength near 415 nm, enabling NBI to detect vascular structures and patterns more effectively than standard endoscopy. In addition, narrow-band light delivered onto tissue surfaces undergoes less scattering than conventional RGB broadband light, leading to the production of clearer images (Fig. 1a,b). Switching between the RGB filters (standard white light endoscopy) and NBI filters is achieved by pressing a button on the endoscope, thus allowing the endosco-

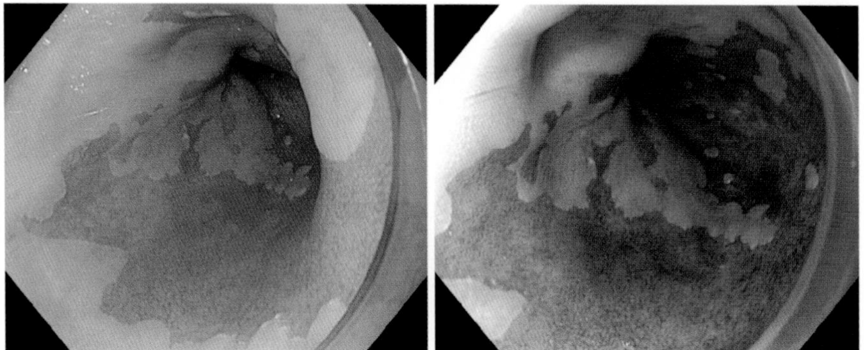

Fig. 1. Barrett's esophagus (BE). **a** Column of BE as seen with standard white light endoscopy. **b** The same column of BE as seen with narrow-band imaging (NBI)

pist to easily alternate between standard white light endoscopy and NBI at any time during the procedure. Usually a transparent cap is fitted on the distal end of the endoscope, allowing the mucosa in contact with the cap to be examined with minimal interference from esophageal motility. Biopsies can then be obtained from areas of interest.

NBI in Barrett's Esophagus

Several investigators have examined the role of NBI in the diagnosis and surveillance of BE patients. A number of classification systems for the mucosal and vascular patterns seen at NBI have been described. One such system characterizes the mucosal pattern as ridge/villous (Fig. 2a), circular (Fig. 2b), and irregular/distorted (Fig. 2c), and the vascular pattern as normal (Fig. 3a) and abnormal (Fig. 3b). Gono et al. reported improved endoscopic visualization of the pit pattern of BE mucosa compared with conventional endoscopy in 12 patients with known BE [11]. Hamamoto and colleagues similarly demonstrated that magnifying endoscopy with NBI was more useful than conventional magnifying endoscopy for the diagnosis of BE in a study of

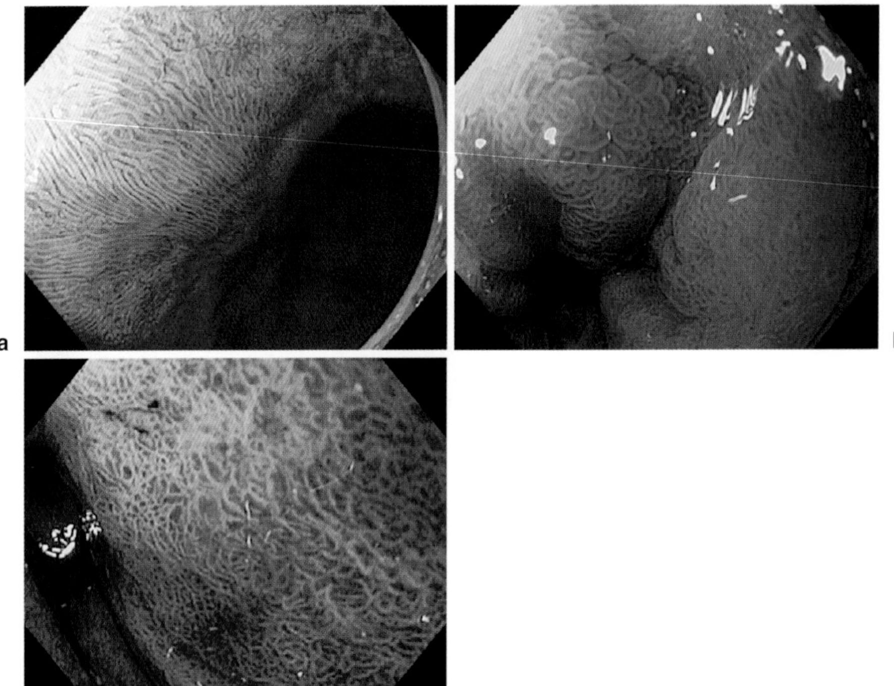

Fig. 2. NBI images of mucosal patterns. **a** Ridge/villous pattern illustrated by the presence of uniform longitudinally aligned ridges (*darker lines*) alternating with a villiform pattern (*lighter lines*). **b** Circular pattern illustrated by the presence of circular and/or oval areas arranged in a regular fashion. **c** Area with high-grade dysplasia (HGD), which appears distorted and irregular compared to the ridge/villous pattern

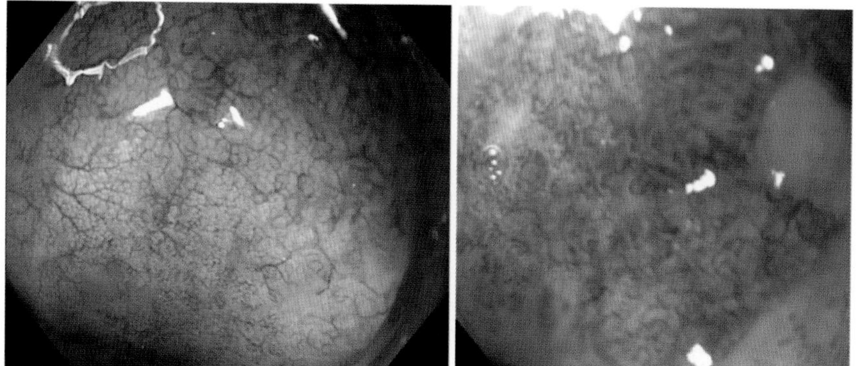

Fig. 3. NBI images of vascular patterns. **a** Normal pattern as illustrated by the fine capillary pattern showing normal size, shape, and distribution of small blood vessels. **b** Abnormal pattern, as illustrated by increased number, tortuosity, and corkscrew-type vessels

11 patients [8]. Kara et al. studied 28 patients with BE and 11 with HGD/EAC and showed that the presence of an irregular mucosal pattern or irregular vascular pattern was an independent predictor of HGD/EAC [12]. The authors emphasized that the "irregularity/non-uniformity" of a mucosal surface was more important than a specific mucosal pattern. The same investigators used NBI with magnifying endoscopy to image and biopsy areas in 63 BE patients to characterize the mucosal and vascular morphology in nondysplastic BE and HGD [13]. Nondysplastic BE was characterized by either villous/gyrus forming mucosal patterns with regular vascular patterns (80%) or flat mucosa with regular normal-appearing long branching vessels (20%). Irregular mucosal pattern, irregular vascular pattern, and the presence of abnormal blood vessels were the three abnormalities associated with HGD. In all areas with HGD ($n = 48$), at least one of these factors was present; 85% had two or more abnormalities. Furthermore, the frequency of these abnormalities showed a significant increase with increasing grades of dysplasia. The mucosal and vascular pattern seen by NBI had a sensitivity of 94%, a specificity of 76%, a positive predictive value of 64%, and a negative predictive value of 98% for detecting HGD. In another study, Sharma et al. assessed the potential of NBI with magnifying endoscopy for prediction of histology during screening and surveillance endoscopy in 51 patients [14]. In this study, images were graded according to mucosal pattern (ridge/villous, circular, and irregular/distorted) and vascular pattern (normal and abnormal) and correlated with histology in a prospective and blinded fashion. The sensitivity, specificity, and positive predictive values of the ridge/villous pattern for the diagnosis of intestinal metaplasia without HGD were 93.5%, 86.7%, and 94.7%, respectively. None of the biopsy samples from an area showing a ridge/villous pattern had HGD. The sensitivity, specificity, and positive predictive values of the irregular/distorted pattern for the presence of HGD were 100%, 98.7%, and 95.3%, respectively. None of the biopsy samples from an area of normal vascular pattern had HGD. However, in this study, NBI was unable to distinguish between areas of intestinal metaplasia and those of low-grade dysplasia (LGD). Goda and colleagues reported on 58 patients with BE, including 4 patients

with superficial EAC [15]. The authors divided the mucosal patterns seen at NBI into groups 1 to 5 ("spotty round or oval," "fine long straight branching," "digital to foliaceous villous," "cerebriform," and "irregular"); the capillary patterns were also divided into five categories (I–V). All EAC were detected with mucosal pattern 5 and capillary pattern V. Mucosal pattern 4 and capillary pattern IV significantly increased the possibility of specialized intestinal metaplasia. When the capillary pattern was used in combination with the mucosal pattern, the detection rate of BE was significantly higher. A number of additional studies published in abstract form have also reported promising results using NBI to assist with the diagnosis of BE and neoplasia using a variety of classifications of mucosal and vascular patterns.

These data suggest that NBI endoscopy may represent a significant improvement over standard white light endoscopy to detect intestinal metaplasia and to differentiate neoplastic and nondysplastic BE within a BE segment. A large multicenter study is currently underway to examine the diagnostic performance of NBI in a crossover study design comparing it to standard four-quadrant biopsies.

NBI in Combination with Other Endoscopic Techniques

A number of endoscopic imaging modalities have been studied in BE. Chromoendoscopy with and without magnification has been evaluated in the detection of intestinal metaplasia and neoplasia with mixed results. Kara and colleagues compared high-resolution endoscopy (HRE) with indigo carmine to HRE plus NBI for the detection of HGD or early EAC in 28 patients with BE [16]. The sensitivities of HRE + indigo carmine and HRE + NBI for the detection of HGD/early EAC were 93% and 86%, respectively. All patients with HGD/early EAC were identified by HRE alone; however, indigo carmine and NBI both detected additional nonneoplastic lesions that were not appreciated by HRE alone. This study suggests that NBI is at least as good as chromoendoscopy for imaging BE. Autofluorescence imaging (AFI) is based on the principle that excitation of tissues with light of a short wavelength gives rise to emission of light of a longer wavelength. This emission is caused by the excitation of a number of biological substances ("fluorophores"); submucosal collagen is the most important fluorophore in the gastrointestinal tract. In a proof-of-principle study, Kara et al. examined 20 BE patients with suspected or endoscopically treated HGD using HRE and AFI [17]. Suspicious areas were then reexamined using NBI with magnification before biopsy. AFI identified 47 suspicious lesions with 28 containing HGD (resulting in a false-positive rate of 40%). Subsequent evaluation with NBI showed that 14 of the 19 false-positive lesions had regular patterns on NBI, decreasing the false-positive rate to 10%.

Narrow-Band Imaging: Potential and Limitations

NBI endoscopy allows detailed inspection of mucosal and vascular patterns with a high level of resolution and contrast without the use of staining agents as are necessary in chromoendoscopy. The pitfalls with chromoendoscopy, such as difficulty achieving uniform coating of the mucosal surface with the staining agent, the need for additional equipment for dye spraying, and concealment of the superficial blood vessels by the dye, are avoided with NBI. No additional requirements for preparation and sedation of the patient are required, and NBI endoscopy is enabled easily by a manual switch on the handle of the endoscope. High-yield areas may be identified more readily, which may minimize the number of random nondiagnostic biopsies required, thus potentially reducing the time and cost of the procedure.

There are several limitations of NBI endoscopy in BE. The studies reported to date have been performed in high-risk patients at tertiary referral centers by experts in the field, thus limiting the generalizability of the results. No formal training in NBI endoscopy presently exists, thus adding another element of variability in interpretation of imaging. The lack of consensus in terminology describing mucosal and vascular patterns presents a similar obstacle to clinical practice. NBI alone may not be able to distinguish LGD from intestinal metaplasia [14]. There are no data on inter- and intraobserver variability of NBI findings; unacceptably high interobserver variability has been published in the magnification chromoendoscopy literature [18]. An international multicenter study of the utility and interobserver variability of a simplified mucosal and vascular classification system is currently underway.

Conclusions

NBI endoscopy represents a substantial improvement over standard white light endoscopy in the diagnosis of metaplasia, dysplasia, and even early cancer. The problems with current BE diagnostic and surveillance strategies highlight the need for developing novel methods of improving the efficacy of BE surveillance. Potential applications of NBI in BE patients include screening and surveillance, defining the extent of EAC, evaluation after ablation therapy, and defining the boundaries of neoplasia before endoscopic mucosal resection. Although preliminary studies of NBI in the diagnosis and surveillance of BE have been encouraging, large, multicenter, randomized controlled trials using validated and standardized terminologies and criteria are needed to evaluate the true potential of this imaging technology.

References

1. Spechler SJ (2002) Clinical practice: Barrett's esophagus. N Engl J Med 346:836–842
2. Sharma P, Falk GW, Weston AP, et al (2006) Dysplasia and cancer in a large multicenter cohort of patients with Barrett's esophagus. Clin Gastroenterol Hepatol 4:566–572
3. Eloubeidi MA, Mason AC, Desmond RA, et al (2003) Temporal trends (1973–1997) in survival of patients with esophageal adenocarcinoma in the United States: a glimmer of hope? Am J Gastroenterol 98:1627–1633
4. Sampliner RE (2002) Practice parameters committee of the ACG. Updated guidelines for the diagnosis, surveillance, and therapy of Barrett's esophagus. Am J Gastroenterol 97:1888–1895
5. Eloubeidi M, Homan R, Martz M, et al (1999) A cost analysis of outpatient care for patients with Barrett's esophagus in a managed care setting. Am J Gastroenterol 94:2033–2036
6. Eloubeidi M, Provenzale D (1999) Does this patient have Barrett's esophagus? The utility of predicting Barrett's esophagus at the index endoscopy. Am J Gastroenterol 94:937–943
7. Muto M, Nakane M, Katada C, et al (2004) Squamous cell carcinoma in situ at oropharyngeal and hypopharyngeal mucosal sites. Cancer (Phila) 101:1375–1381
8. Hamamoto Y, Endo T, Nosho K, et al (2004) Usefulness of narrow band imaging endoscopy for diagnosis of Barrett's esophagus. J Gastroenterol 39:14–20

9. Nakayoshi T, Tajiri H, Matsuda K, et al (2004) Magnifying endoscopy combined with narrow band imaging system for early gastric cancer: correlation of vascular pattern with histopathology. Endoscopy 36:1080–1084
10. Machida H, Sano Y, Hamamoto Y, et al (2004) Narrow band imaging in the diagnosis of colorectal mucosal lesions: a pilot study. Endoscopy 36:1094–1098
11. Gono K, Obi T, Yamaguchi M, et al (2004) Appearance of enhanced tissue features in narrow band endoscopic imaging. J Biomed Opt 9:568–577
12. Kara MA, Fockens P, Peters F, et al (2004) Narrow band imaging in Barrett's esophagus: what features are relevant for detection of high-grade dysplasia and early cancer? Gastroenterology 126:A50
13. Kara MA, Ennahachi M, Fockens P, et al (2006) Detection and classification of the mucosal and vascular patterns (mucosal morphology) in Barrett's esophagus by using narrow band imaging. Gastrointest Endosc 64:155–166
14. Sharma P, Bansal A, Mathur S, et al (2006) The utility of a novel narrow band imaging endoscopy system in patients with Barrett's esophagus. Gastrointest Endosc 64: 167–175
15. Goda K, Tajiri H, Ikegami M, et al (2007) Usefulness of magnifying endoscopy with narrow band imaging for the detection of specialized intestinal metaplasia in columnar-lined esophagus and Barrett's adenocarcinoma. Gastrointest Endosc 65: 36–46
16. Kara MA, Peters FP, Rosmolen WD, et al (2005) High-resolution endoscopy plus chromoendoscopy or narrow band imaging in Barrett's esophagus: a prospective randomized crossover study. Endoscopy 37:929–936
17. Kara MA, Peters FP, Fockens P, et al (2006) Endoscopic video autofluorescence imaging followed by narrow band imaging for detecting early neoplasia in Barrett's esophagus. Gastrointest Endosc 64:176–185
18. Meining A, Rosch T, Kiesslich R, et al (2004) Inter- and intra-observer variability of magnification chromoendoscopy for detecting specialized intestinal metaplasia at the gastroesophageal junction. Endoscopy 36:160–164

Magnifying Endoscopy in Combination with Narrow-Band Imaging and Acetic Acid Instillation in the Diagnosis of Barrett's Esophagus

Kyosuke Tanaka[1], Hideki Toyoda[1], and Edgar Jaramillo[2]

Summary. Barrett's esophagus (BE) is a condition of the distal esophagus involving columnar-lined epithelium (CLE) with intestinal metaplasia (IM). During conventional endoscopy, IM in CLE is not clearly identifiable. Here we describe a technique of magnifying endoscopy (ME) using narrow-band imaging (NBI) in combination with acetic acid instillation in the diagnosis of BE. Within 10–20 s after acetic acid instillation, the mucosal surfaces whiten and fine mucosal surface patterns become clearer with ME emphasized with NBI.

We classified CLE surface patterns into five types: type I, small round pits of uniform size and shape; type II, slit-like pits; type III, gyrus and villous pattern; type IV, irregular size and arrangement; type V, destructive pattern. A significant correlation between type III pattern and the presence of IM was observed (sensitivity 88.5%, specificity 90.2%, and overall accuracy 90.0%). Most adenocarcinomas expressed type IV or type V patterns. ME in combination with NBI and acetic acid instillation seems to be useful for identifying IM and early adenocarcinomas in CLE.

Key words. Barrett's esophagus, Endoscopy, Acetic acid, Narrow-band imaging, Neoplasms

Introduction and Background

Barrett's esophagus (BE) is a condition involving a columnar-lined esophagus (CLE) in which normal squamous mucosa is replaced by columnar epithelium. The columnar epithelium is heterogeneous, and is usually composed of fundic mucosa, cardiac mucosa, or a distinctive epithelial type known as specialized columnar epithelium. This specialized columnar epithelium, containing intestinal-type goblet cells, is the only type that carries an inherent risk of malignancy. For this reason, a diagnosis of

[1]Department of Endoscopic Medicine, Mie University Hospital, 2-174 Edobashi, Tsu, Mie 514-8507, Japan
[2]Department of Gastroenterology and Hepatology, Karolinska Universitetssjukhuset, Stockholm, Sweden

BE has been reserved for those patients where biopsy specimens of the distal esophagus demonstrate intestinal metaplasia (IM).

As IM in CLE is not identifiable with conventional endoscopy, several other endoscopic techniques have been used to obtain a diagnosis of BE. In chromoendoscopy, for example, Lugol's solution (an iodine-based absorptive dye) imparts a brown stain to glycogen-containing squamous epithelium, but does not stain CLE. Lugol staining accurately delimits the boundaries between squamous epithelium and CLE, but it does not provide definitive evidence of IM. A methylene blue solution (0.5%), which is absorbed by well-differentiated enterocytes, has also been proposed for the detection of IM and dysplasia in BE but results have been conflicting, with a number of articles reporting variable levels of sensitivity and specificity.

Enhanced magnifying endoscopy (EME) is a technique that combines magnifying endoscopy (ME) and the instillation of acetic acid [1]. The transient whitening of epithelial surfaces after contact with acetic acid is a consequence of an increase in surface opacity, and corresponds to a reversible alteration in the tertiary structure of some cellular proteins [2]. EME has been used not only to detect IM in BE [1,3], but also in the diagnosis of neoplasms of the stomach [4–6] and duodenum [7]. Narrow-band imaging (NBI; Olympus Medical Systems, Tokyo, Japan) is a new method of endoscopic imaging that is based on modifying the bandwidth of illuminating light via an optical filter. The diagnostic value of combining NBI with ME (NBI–ME) for the detection of BE has been described previously [8]. Recently, we observed CLE and gastric mucosa [9] using magnifying endoscopy combined with NBI and acetic acid instillation, and recorded a synergistic enhancement in image information with the use of these two techniques. Here we describe the application of magnifying endoscopy combined with NBI and acetic acid instillation for the study of BE.

Materials

Endoscopy System

High-resolution digital processors, such as the CV-260SL and CLV-260SL (Olympus Medical Systems), and endoscopes (GIF-Q240Z, GIF-H260Z; Olympus Medical Systems) with an optical zoom and an adjustable magnification in a continuous range up to ×80 were used. These systems also offer an NBI function. Images were viewed on a monitor (OEV 143, OEV 191, OEV191H; Olympus Medical Systems).

Adjustable Distal Cap Attachment

A short distal cap attachment (D-201-11 802, BK-162 for the GIF-Q240Z; Olympus Medical Systems) placed at the tip of the endoscope to maintain a fixed distance from the scope tip to the mucosal surface is useful but not essential. The distal attachment is also used to pool acetic acid or water between the endoscope tip and the mucosa at the time of acetic acid instillation.

Acetic Acid

Acetic acid (pKa 4.8) has the shortest carbon chain of any fatty acid. Glacial acetic acid diluted in water to a final concentration between 1% and 3% (pH 2.5–3.0) is used for in vivo applications. We found that the transient whitening of the mucosa is too weak with concentrations of acetic acid <1%, and that the acid maintains a pungent odor at concentrations ≥3%. For reasons of hygiene, a 15% stock solution of acetic is stored in a refrigerator. We often prepare 20 ml of 1.5% acetic acid by mixing 2 ml of 15% acetic acid with 18 ml water. Common vinegar, which generally contains 4%–6% acetic acid, can be diluted and used to achieve the same effect.

Endoscopic Procedure

Preparation for Endoscopy

The preparation for ME in combination with NBI and acetic acid instillation is similar to that for standard endoscopy. To dissolve the mucus layer of the esophagus and stomach, each patient ingests a solution containing 20 000 U pronase (Pronase MS; Kaken Pharmaceutical Products, Tokyo, Japan) and 1 g of $NaHCO_3$ in 50 ml water 10 min before the endoscopic procedure. Glucagon or an anticholinergic agent can be given to decrease gastrointestinal tract contractions and minimize the loss of reagents. We regularly prepare several 20-ml syringes filled with 1.5% acetic acid.

Magnifying Endoscopy in Combination with Narrow-Band Imaging and Acetic Acid Instillation

First, anatomical landmarks are identified by conventional endoscopy. The esophagogastric junction is defined by either the proximal margin of the gastric folds or the end of the palisade vessels. The squamo-columnar junction is defined by a sharp demarcation between squamous stratified epithelium and columnar lined mucosa.

After conventional observation, both standard ME and ME with NBI are performed to look for areas with IM and or neoplasia. Thereafter 10–20 cc of 1.5% acetic acid solution are sprinkled at low pressure onto the mucosa through the accessory channel of the endoscope using a 20-ml syringe. The minimal amount of acetic acid necessary to whiten the mucosa is applied, and excess acetic acid is removed by endoscope suction to prevent aspiration. Within 10 or 20 s after acetic acid instillation, the mucosal surfaces whiten and remain so for 3–5 min. The tip of the scope is positioned and fixed near the mucosal surface by the use of the distal cap attachment. Fine capillaries cannot be observed while the mucosal surface is whitened, but the fine pattern of the mucosal surface is clearly seen with ME. With the addition of NBI, the surface patterns are further emphasized and the observation time of the whitened mucosal surface is lengthened.

Figure 1 shows ME images of CLE. During conventional ME, the mucosal surface pattern was unclear (Fig. 1a). ME and NBI clarified both the capillary network and the mucosal surface pattern (Fig. 1b). ME after acetic acid instillation provided a more detailed mucosal surface pattern (Fig. 1c). ME with NBI after acetic acid instillation made the mucosal surface pattern appear even clearer and more vivid (Fig. 1d). The surface pattern in these images is type III (as described later), and further pathological examination of a biopsy specimen indicated IM.

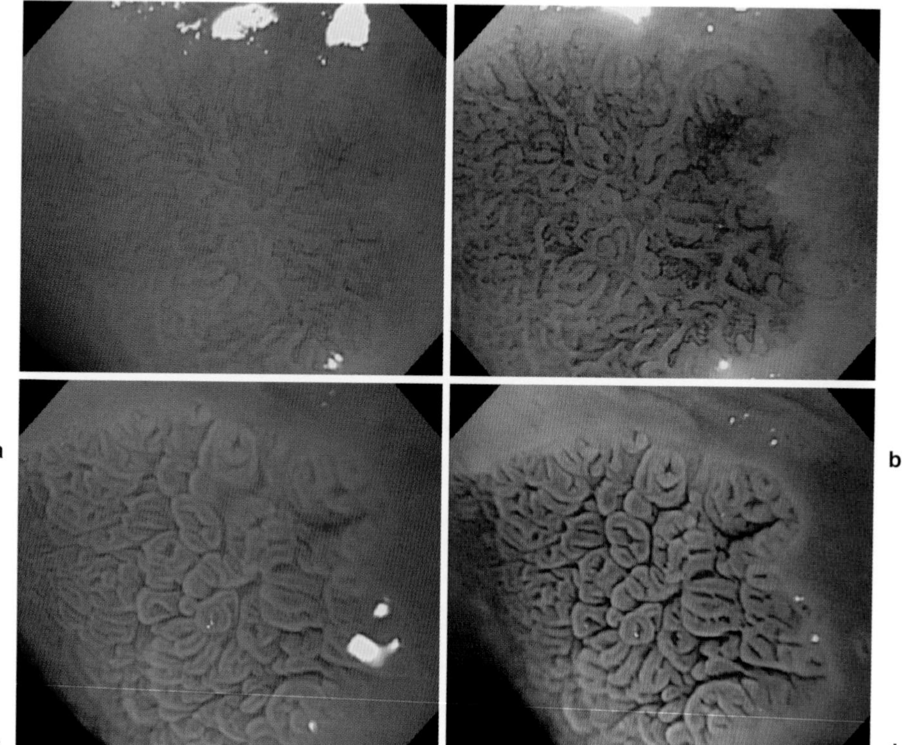

Fig. 1. Magnifying endoscopic images of a columnar-lined esophagus (CLE). **a** During conventional magnifying endoscopy (ME), the mucosal surface pattern is indistinct. **b** ME with narrow-band imaging (NBI) makes both the capillary network and the mucosal surface pattern appear clear. **c** Enhanced ME after acetic acid instillation provides a more detailed view of the mucosal surface pattern as a consequence of an increase in surface opacity. **d** ME with NBI after acetic acid instillation makes the mucosal surface pattern appear even clearer and more vivid

Figure 2 shows magnified endoscopic images of an early carcinoma in BE. Using conventional ME, the mucosal surface pattern is indistinct (Fig. 2a). ME with NBI showed irregular microvessels and an irregular mucosal surface pattern (Fig. 2b). After acetic acid instillation and with ME an irregular mucosal surface pattern is seen (Fig. 2c). ME in combination with NBI after acetic acid instillation provided a clearer view of the mucosal surface pattern (Fig. 2d). The surface pattern in these images was classified as type IV (as described later), and pathological examination of the resected specimen indicated a well-differentiated adenocarcinoma.

Surface Pattern Classification (Nonneoplastic Mucosa)

Guerlud et al. [1] described four different surface patterns in Barrett's mucosa: type I, round pits; type II, reticular (circular or oval pits); type III, villous (fine villiform appearance without visible pits); type IV, ridged (thick villi with a convoluted, cerebriform appearance without visible pits). In a nonprospective study, these authors

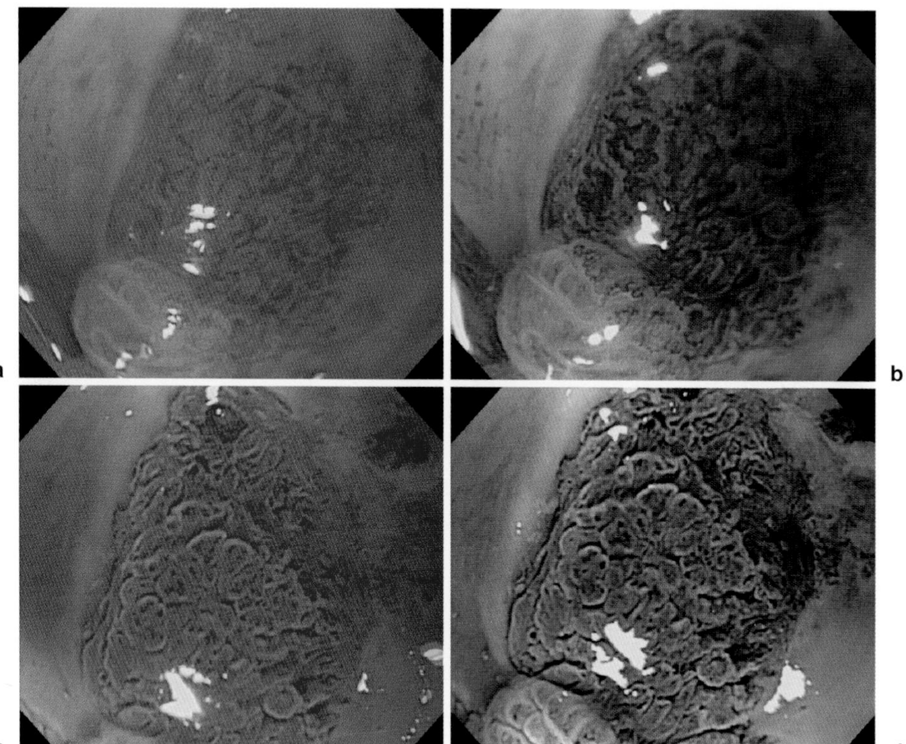

Fig. 2. Magnifying endoscopic images of an early carcinoma in Barrett's esophagus. **a** During ME the mucosal surface pattern is indistinct. **b** ME with NBI shows irregular microvessels and an irregular mucosal surface pattern. **c** Enhanced ME after acetic acid instillation shows an irregular mucosal surface pattern. **d** ME with NBI after acetic acid instillation provides a clearer view of the irregular mucosal surface pattern. The surface pattern in these images was classified as type IV, and pathological examination of the resected specimen indicated a well-differentiated adenocarcinoma

reported that in patients with previously diagnosed BE, the rates of detection of IM in mucosa with pattern III or pattern IV were 87% and 100%, respectively.

Based on these finding, we originally devised a classification of nonneoplastic mucosa surface patterns in CLE with three types: type I, small round pits of uniform size and shape (Fig. 3a); type II, slit-like pits (Fig. 3b); type III, gyrus and villous patterns (Fig. 3c,d) [3]. In a prospective study, we reported a significant correlation between pattern type III and the detection of IM (sensitivity 88.5%, specificity 90.2%, and overall accuracy 90.0%) [3].

Surface Pattern Classification (Adenocarcinoma)

The prevention of advanced cancer relies on the early recognition of carcinoma more than the detection of IM in CLE. Once early cancer is detected, different endoscopic methods (including endoscopic submucosal dissection) are available to treat early carcinoma in BE completely.

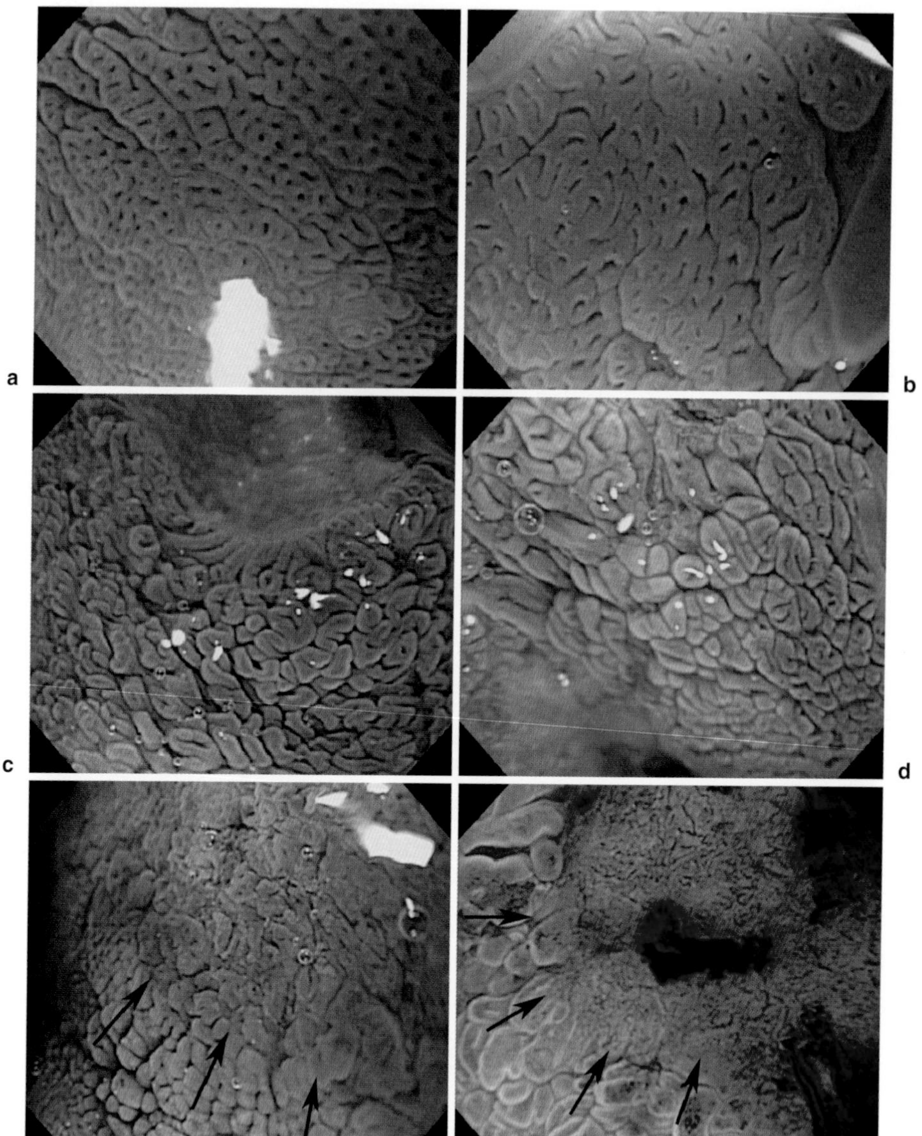

Fig. 3. Classification of CLE surface patterns. **a** Type I, small round pits of uniform size and shape. **b** Type II, slit-like pits. **c,d** Type III, gyrus and villous patterns. **e** Type IV, irregular arrangement and size (*arrows*). **f** Type V, destructive pattern (*arrows*)

Screening for Gastric Cancer in Japan

Takahiro Kozu[1], Hiroko Shoda[1], Yukio Muramatsu[1], and Daizo Saito[2]

Summary. Gastric endoscopy has not yet been recommended for organized or population-based cancer screening because at the moment, the sole criterion for evaluating the effectiveness of cancer screening is the reduction in the death rate, and not the mere detection of cancer. Nevertheless, compared with X-ray screening, which has normally been recommended, endoscopic screening is better at finding small lesions, at finding cancer at its earlier stages, making it more easily and economically treatable, and allows on-the-spot biopsies. Opportunistic, individually initiated screening by endoscopy is more and more in demand. Therefore, its excellent efficacy needs to be matched by improved toleration, improved safety, and improved manpower efficiency so that it can be standardized and utilized to its full diagnostic, therapeutic, and quality-of-life potential.

Key words. Gastric cancer, Screening, Endoscopy

Introduction

In Japan, cancer screening based on monitoring the death from cancer of elderly patients has been managed by the government since 1983, and radiological gastrography (X-ray) is recommended because of its effectiveness in decreasing the rate of death from gastric cancer.However, owing to remarkable progress in endoscopy technology in the past quarter of a century, endoscopy has become the most popular method of examination not only in clinical situations, but also for screening purposes. However, there are some problems which still have to be solved, such as toleration, safety, and manpower, before mass screening by endoscopy can ever be considered. The purpose of this chapter is to consider the present problems and solutions, and search for a standardization that will make mass utilization possible.

[1]National Cancer Center, Research Center for Cancer Prevention and Screening, Cancer Screening Division, 5-1-1 Tsukiji, Chuo-ku, Tokyo 104-0045, Japan
[2]National Cancer Center Hospital, Endoscopy Division, Tokyo, Japan

Assessment of Effectiveness

In Japan, the most common methods of screening for gastric cancer are radiological gastrography (X-ray), pepsinogen assay, *Helicobacter pylori* antibody count, and endoscopy. An evaluation by a study group from the Ministry of Welfare, in a report entitled "Gastric Cancer Guidelines Based on the Evaluation of Effectiveness" stated that the X-ray is an effective screening method owing to its cohort study result, but that the pepsinogen assay was doubtful, and a *Helicobacter pylori* antibody count was not effective. The guidelines also reported that "screening endoscopy is not recommended for population-based screening" because there is no evidence that it decreases the cancer death rate, but that it may be used for opportunistic screening, and is available with informed consent when sought by an individual (Table 1).

Screening by Endoscopy

Advantages

A nationwide research study (including only institutions which have more than 500 cases per year) into screening endoscopy for gastric cancer reported that 287 gastric cancers were detected out of 93 909, that the detection rate was 0.31%, and that the rate of early gastric cancer cases was 67.9% (195 cases). On the other hand, the detection rate by X-ray screening was 0.094% and its ratio of early cancer was 68.4%. The ratio of early cancer was the same, but when the overall cancer detection rate was found to be 0.14% in subsequent tests, the detection rate by endoscopy was shown to be 3–4 times that by X-ray, which proves that endoscopy is very precise [1] (Table 2).

Table 1. Summary of present "recommendations" for gastric cancer screening.

	Population-based Screening	Opportunistic Screening
X-ray	Recommended	Recommended
PG	Not recommended	As decided by individual
HP	Not recommended	As decided by individual
GF	Not recommended	As decided by individual

PG, Pepsinogen; HP, Helicobacter pylori antibody; GF, gastroscopy

Table 2. Result of screening by endoscope.

Number of receivers	93,909
M	50,876 (54.2%)
F	43,033 (45.8%)
Detected lesion and detection rate	
Gastric cancer	287 (0.31%)
(Early GC 195)	(0.21%)
Gastric ulcer	4,435 (4.72%)
Gastric polyp	7,627 (8.12%)

*Detection rate by X-ray screening: 0.094% (GC)

High Precision in Diagnosis

An endoscopy examination used to be the second test to check the details of a lesion after X-ray detection and to make a final diagnosis, but based on nationwide endoscopy screening research, endoscopy is now known to be the most precise method of checking the gastrointestinal tract.

Biopsy

When abnormal findings are detected, a histological diagnosis from a biopsy specimen is helpful whenever it is difficult to make a diagnosis from endoscopic findings.

Subjective Organs

Not only the stomach, but also the esophagus and duodenum, can easily be observed by panendoscopy.

Selection of Subjects

Of course the subjects screened should be in the high-risk age group, but as there is no possibility of exposure to radiation, younger subjects are not contraindicated. Even subjects who have paralysis, difficulty in hearing, or any other physical handicap can be examined easily because they do not have to change position during the examination.

Problems

Toleration

The level of technique varies widely depending on the examiner, even with a thin scope or sedation. The trend for transnasal endoscopy has shown that the most difficult part is insertion into the esophagus from the throat. Even when the examination has been completed very smoothly with deep sedation, over-inflation can cause abdominal fullness or nausea afterwards. Therefore examiners have to have a good technique so that the patient is comfortable even after the examination is finished.

Complications

An endoscopy examination has a few risks, such as shock from the preparation medicine, perforation, or infection. Research by the Japan Gastroenterological Endoscopy Society (1998–2002) reported that the complication rate was 0.12% (997/826 313) with panendoscopy. The death rate was 0.0076% (63/826 313), and 19 cases died from the observation examination only (without biopsy or therapeutic endoscopy). The complication rate due to preparation was 0.0059% (754/12 844 551), and the death rate was 0.00011% (14/12 844 551). The frequency was highest in cases with anti-bowel-movement medicine or sedation [2] (Table 3).

TABLE. 3. Complications of Endoscopie examinations for recently 5 years.

Whole (including ERCP, CS)	Pan-endoscope
Total No.: 12,844,551	Total No.: 8,263,813
Complicaitons: 4,412 (0.032%)	Complicaiton: 997 (0.012%)
By preparation	Death: 63 (0.00076%)
Complicaitons: 754	Observation: 19
Death: 14	Biopsy: 1
Local anesthesia: 1	Stop bleeding: 10
Mixed: 6	Polypectomy, EMR: 4
Sedation only: 2	Varices therapy: 16
Analgesic drug: 2	PEG: 8
others: 3	Others: 5

Japan Gastroenterological Endoscopy Society (1998–2002)

Infection

Infections thought to be related to the use of endoscopy are reported to be hepatitis B virus (HBV) (1 case), hepatitis C virus (HCV) (1 case), *H. pylori* (2 cases), blood poisoning (1 case), and one other, but it is nearly impossible to confirm direct cause and effect. Medical accidents totaled 144 cases, and glutalaldehyde-dependent eye and skin diseases, as well as asthma, are rather common. HBV infections totaled 3 cases, and HCV infections totaled 8 cases [2].

Omissions

Yoshida et al. [3] have presumed that when there is an outbreak within 3 years of an endoscopic examination it will be a false negative, and have retrospectively found a rate of 25.6% (62 cases out of 242). It has also been reported that the majority of those cases (58 lesions = 83.9%) were unnoticed during the endoscopy, while 10 lesions (14.7%) were unnoticed in a biopsy. Hosokawa et al. [4] examined stomach cancer detection performance retrospectively for 3 years, and reported finding 18.3% of false-negative examinations (150/820). In order to decrease the number of false-negative examinations, it is suggested that both examination technique and observation accuracy need to be increased by means of further practice and also by a more positive use of biopsies.

Manpower

An endoscope examination needs at least 5 min for adequate observation, image taking, and evaluation. The examination time is not very different from that needed for a radiographic examination, but the preliminary questionnaire, the set-up, and the post-examination rest all require specialized staff. If the skill of all examiners is considered to be equal, the processing capacity is proportional to the number of examining physicians, but compared with radiologists, the number of endoscopists, especially those engaged in screening, is clearly much smaller, and the present situation is thought likely to continue. In short, it is impossible to increase the number of

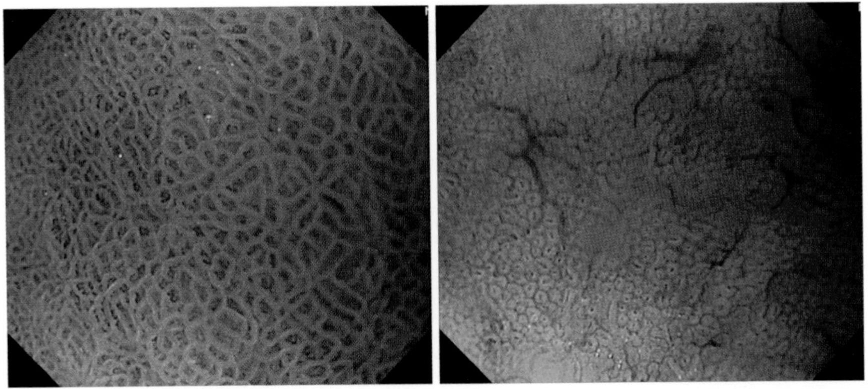

Fig. 1. Magnification endoscopy (ME) findings with narrow-band imaging (NBI) of the normal gastric mucosa. **A** Gastric antrum: (1) microvascular (MV) architecture, a regular coil-shaped subepithelial capillary network (SECN) pattern with absence of a regular collecting venule (CV) pattern; (2) microsurface (MS) structure, a regular linear or reticular crypt-opening pattern. **B** Gastric body: (1) MV architecture, a regular honeycomb-like SECN pattern with presence of a regular CV pattern; (2) MS structure, a regular oval crypt-opening pattern. [From Yao K, Iwashita A, Matsui T, et al (2007) The process of endoscopy diagnosis and the endoscopic findings. Nihon Medical Center, Tokyo, pp 334–342, with permission of Nihon Medical Center Ltd.]

Gastric Body (Fig. 1B)

Basic microanatomical findings: (1) MV architecture: a regular honeycomb-like SECN pattern with presence of a regular CV pattern; and (2) MS structure: a regular oval crypt-opening pattern.

Description: A polygonal loop of a subepithelial capillary surrounds each gastric crypt opening, and these loops form a honeycomb-like network beneath the epithelium and converge onto a collecting venule [1–4]. With regard to the MS structure, the crypt opening demonstrates a round or oval shape. If there is no pathological change such as *Helicobacter pylori* gastritis in the mucosa, both the MV architecture and the MS structure consistently show a regular pattern in both shape and arrangement

Chronic Gastritis

As the ME findings of the gastric mucosa with chronic gastritis (Fig. 2) have not yet been fully investigated, a comprehensive classification has not been established. However, with regard to the gastric body mucosa with chronic *Helicobacter pylori*-associated gastritis, a systematic investigation had been carried out [5,6].

Gastric Body

The basic microanatomical findings and classification for chronic gastritis follow.

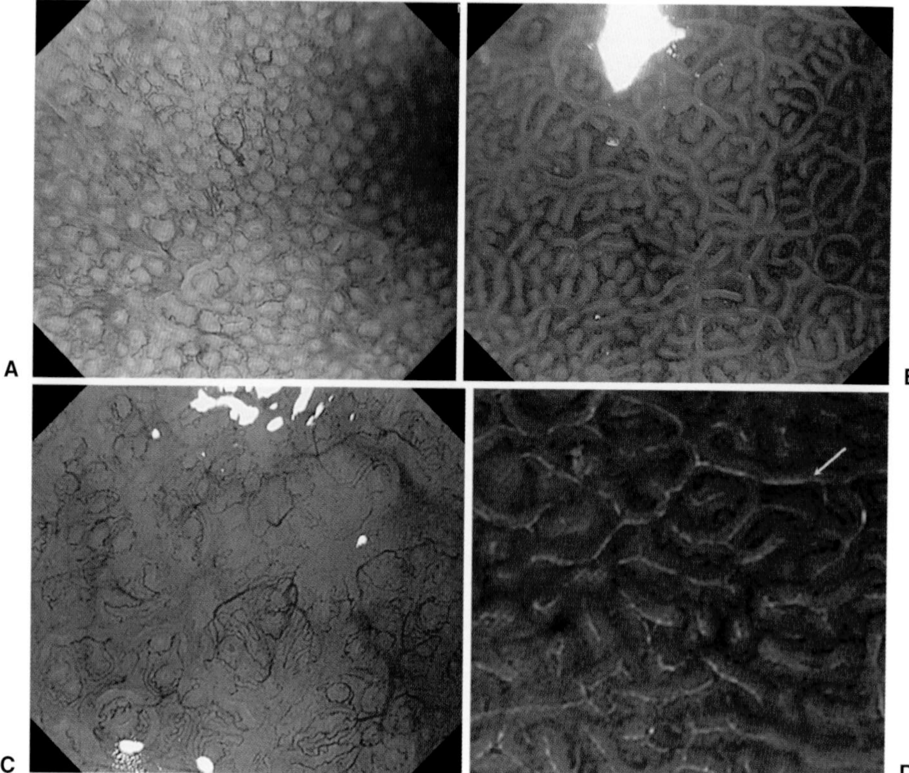

Fig. 2. ME findings with NBI of the gastric body mucosa with *Helicobacter pylori (HP)*-associated chronic gastritis and gastric atrophy. Type 1 is shown in Fig. 1B. **A** Type 2: (1) MV architecture, a regular honeycomb-like SECN pattern with absence of a regular CV pattern; (2) MS structure, a regular oval/tubular crypt-opening pattern. [From Yao K, Iwashita A, Matsui T, et al (2007) The process of endoscopy diagnosis and the endoscopic findings. Nihon Medical Center, Tokyo, pp 334–342, with permission of Nihon Medical Center Ltd.). **B** Type 3: (1) MV architecture, loss of a regular honeycomb-like SECN pattern with absence of a regular CV pattern; (2) MS structure, a regular but enlarged white oval/tubular crypt-opening pattern. (From Anagnostopoulos GK, Yao K, Kaye P, et al.,[5] with permission of Elsevier Inc.). **C** Type 4 (1) MV architecture, loss of a regular honeycomb-like SECN pattern with presence of a slightly irregular CV pattern (one of the CVs is indicated by an *arrow*); (2) MS structure, flat or non-structural type with absence of MS pattern. **D** Light blue crest (LBC): the edge of the epithelial surface with intestinal metaplasia is fringed with linear light-blue reflection of the light (one of the LBCs is indicated by an *arrow*)

Type 1 (Fig. 1B): (1) MV architecture: a regular, honeycomb-like SECN pattern with presence of a regular CV pattern; and (2) MS structure: a regular oval crypt-opening pattern.

Type 2 (Fig. 2A): (1) MV architecture: a regular, honeycomb-like SECN pattern with absence of a regular CV pattern; and (2) MS structure: a regular oval/tubular crypt-opening pattern.

Type 3 (Fig. 2B): (1) MV architecture: loss of a regular honeycomb-like SECN pattern with absence of a regular CV pattern; and (2) MS structure: a regular but enlarged white oval/tubular crypt-opening pattern.

Type 4 (Fig. 2C): (1) MV architecture: loss of a regular honeycomb-like SECN pattern with presence of a slightly irregular CV pattern; and (2) MS structure: flat or nonstructural type with absence of MS pattern.

Clinical relevance: Magnification endoscopy (ME) has also been reported to be useful for identifying *Helicobactor pylori (HP)*-associated gastritis and gastric atrophy (Fig. 2) [5]. The type 1 pattern is highly predictive for normal gastric mucosa with negative findings for *HP* infection; the type 2 or 3 pattern is predictive for the *HP*-infected stomach, and the type 4 pattern is predictive for gastric atrophy. This classification was made through modification of the original findings of both Yagi and Nakagawa [5].

Light-Blue Crest

Uedo et al. reported an interesting concept and new application of NBI with magnifying endoscopy for the diagnosis of gastric intestinal metaplasia (Fig. 2D) [6]. They indicated that a distinctive finding called light-blue crest (LBC) was a good indicator of histological intestinal metaplasia, which is a risk factor for the development of differentiated (intestinal) type gastric cancer. The LBC was defined as a fine, blue-white line on the crests of the epithelial surface or gyri as visualized by magnification endoscopy with NBI.

Early Gastric Cancer

For basic microanatomical findings and VS classification for early gastric cancer, see Fig. 3 [1,2,7,8].

(1) Microvascular architecture (V)
  1. Regular microvascular pattern (RMVP): microvessels appear regular in shape and arrangement.
  2. Irregular microvascular pattern (IMVP): microvessels appear irregular in shape and arrangement (tortuous or irregularly branched microvessels of various sizes with abnormal caliber).

(2) Microsurface structure (S)
  1. Regular microsurface pattern (RMSP): linear/reticular/tubular/papillary type; presence of a clear regular linear, reticular, tubular or papillary pattern
  2. Irregular microsurface pattern (IMSP): significant irregularity of the linear/reticular/tubular/papillary pattern.
  3. Absent microsurface pattern (AMSP): flat or nonstructural type with absence of MS pattern.

(3) Presence or absence of a demarcation line.

Description: we were the first to demonstrate characteristic ME findings of early gastric cancer based on the MV architecture as visualized by the ME with WLI [1,7], and then, after developing ME with the NBI technique, we reported additional findings based on the MS structure as visualized by ME with NBI [2,8]. With reference to

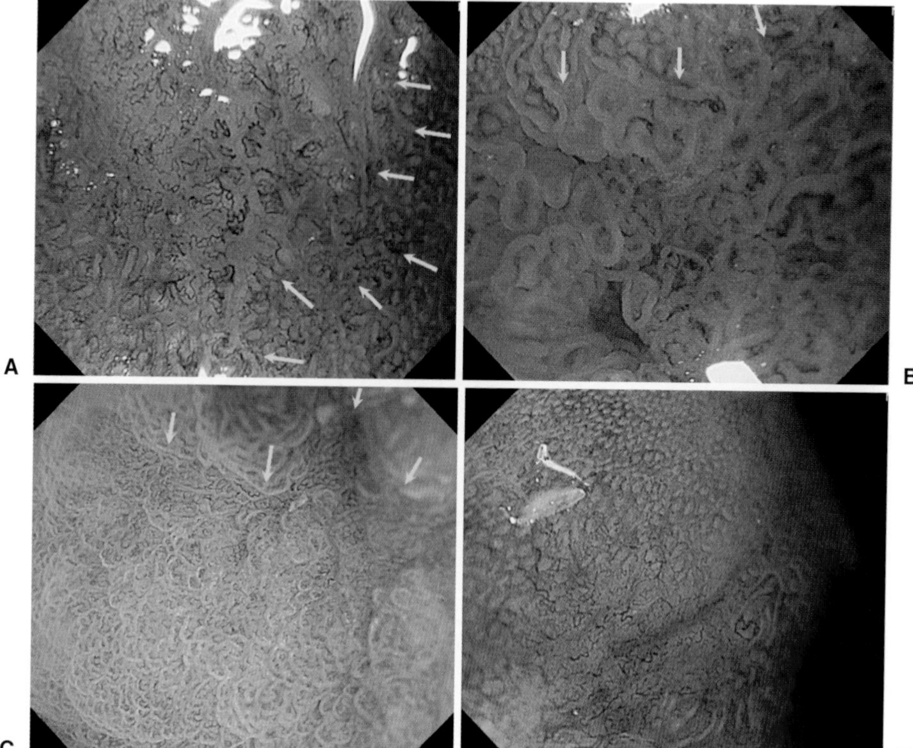

FIG. 3. Representative ME findings with NBI of early gastric cancer according to VS classification system. **A** Differentiated carcinoma: (1) MV architecture, presence of an irregular microvascular pattern (IMVP); (2) MS structure, irregular microsurface pattern (IMSP), significant irregularity of the reticular/tubular pattern; (3) demarcation line (*arrows*), present between cancerous and noncancerous mucosa. [From Yao K, Nakamura M, Nagahama T, et al (2007) How to determine the horizontal margin of early gastric cancer by using a novel magnification endoscopic technique. Stomach and Intestine (Tokyo) 42:735–745, with permission of Igaku-Shoin Ltd.). **B** Differentiated carcinoma: (1) MV architecture, presence of an irregular microvascular pattern (IMVP); (2) MS structure, irregular microsurface pattern (IMSP), significant irregularity of the papillary pattern; (3) demarcation line (*arrows*), present. **C** Differentiated carcinoma: (1) MV architecture, presence of an irregular microvascular pattern (IMVP) with a demarcation line; (2) MS structure, irregular microsurface pattern (IMSP), significant irregularity of the reticular/tubular pattern; (3) demarcation line (*arrows*), present. **D** Undifferentiated carcinoma: (1) MV architecture, loss of regular microvascular pattern (RMVP); (2) MS structure; loss of regular microsurface pattern (RMSP) plus absence of microsurface pattern (AMSP); (3) demarcation line, absent. [From Yao K, Iwashita A, Matsui T, et al (2007) The process of endoscopy diagnosis and the endoscopic findings. Nihon Medical Center, Tokyo, pp 334–342, with permission of Nihon Medical Center Ltd.)

TABLE 1. VS classification system for making a correct diagnosis between cancerous and noncancerous pathology in the stomach.

	Noncarcinoma	Carcinoma
Microvascular (MV) architecture	RMVP	IMVP
Microsurface (MS) structure	RMSP	IMSP

V, microvascular architecture; S, microsurface structure;
RMVP, regular microvascular pattern; IMVP, irregular microvascular pattern; RMSP, regular microsurface pattern; IMSP, irregular microsurface pattern

the foregoing basic microanatomical findings, the noncancerous background mucosa (Fig. 2) consistently shows RMVP plus either RMSP or AMSP; however, the ME with NBI findings characteristic for early gastric cancer differ depending upon the histological type, that is, differentiated or undifferentiated type. With regard to the ME with NBI findings of differentiated carcinoma, in the cancerous mucosa, both the RMVP and the RMSP had disappeared; instead, RMVP plus either AMSP or IMSP is present. Furthermore, a demarcation line can be detected between the cancerous and noncancerous mucosa. On the other hand, in the ME findings of undifferentiated carcinoma, the cancerous mucosa only shows loss of RMVP plus either loss of RMSP or AMSP.

Accordingly, because the ME findings characteristic for differentiated carcinoma seem to be specific for malignant tissue, the following clinical application is possible.

1. Differential diagnosis between focal gastritis and small flat gastric cancer [9,10].
2. Determining the margin of the early gastric cancer for curative endoscopic resection [9,11].

Proposal for a New Diagnostic System of Early Gastric Cancer Produced by ME and NBI in the Stomach

In accordance with the basic principles for the new diagnostic system produced by ME and NBI, we herein propose VS classification system for making a correct diagnosis between cancerous and noncancerous pathology in the stomach, as shown in Table 1. The criterion for making a diagnosis of cancerous pathology is the presence of either an IMVP or an IMSP, whereas the criterion for the diagnosis of noncancerous pathology is the absence of both an IMVP and an IMSP. This classification system can be commonly used in both high-grade dysplasia/early cancer in Barrett's esophagus and early gastric cancer, because adenocarcinoma arises commonly from chronically inflamed columnar epithelium in Barrett's esophagus and the stomach [8,12].

In conclusion, the most important advantage of magnification endoscopy with NBI is that it can visualize both the MV architecture and the MS structure without the need to introduce any artificial materials (such as dye or acetic acid) into the human body. Magnification endoscopy with NBI is a promising method to be utilized as the standard endoscopy technique because it is quick, safe, and accurate for making a precise diagnosis of gastrointestinal pathology.

Acknowledgments. We thank Miss Katherine Miller (Royal English Language Centre, Fukuoka, Japan) for correcting the English used in this manuscript. This work was supported in part by a Grant-in-Aid from the Ministry of Health, Labor and Welfare of Japan.

References

1. Yao K, Oishi T (2001) Microgastroscopic findings of mucosal microvascular architecture as visualized by magnifying endoscopy. Dig Endosc 13:S27–S33
2. Yao K, Nagahama T, Hirai F, et al (2007) Clinical application of magnification endoscopy with NBI in the stomach and the duodenum. Comprehensive atlas of high-resolution endoscopy and narrow-band imaging. Blackwell, Boston, pp 83–103
3. Yao K, Iwashita A (2006) Clinical application of zoom endoscopy for the stomach (in Japanese with English abstract). Gastroenterol Endosc 48:1091–1101
4. Yao K (2004) Gastric microvascular architecture as visualized by magnifying endoscopy: body mucosa and antral mucosa without pathological change demonstrate two different patterns of microvascular architecture. Gastrointest Endosc 59: 596–597
5. Anagnostopoulos GK, Yao K, Kaye P, et al (2007) High-resolution magnification endoscopy can reliably identify normal gastric mucosa, *Helicobacter pylori*-associated gastritis, and gastric atrophy. Endoscopy 39:1–6
6. Uedo N, Ishihara R, Iishi H, et al (2006) A new method of diagnosing gastric intestinal metaplasia: narrow-band imaging with magnifying endoscopy. Endoscopy 38: 819–824
7. Yao K, Oishi T, Matsui T, et al (2002) Novel magnified endoscopic findings of microvascular architecture in intramucosal gastric cancer. Gastrointest Endosc 56:279–284
8. Yao K, Takaki Y, Matsui T, et al (2008) Clinical application of magnification endoscopy and narrow band imaging in the upper gastrointestinal tract: new imaging techniques for detecting and characterizing GI neoplasia. Gastrointest Endosc Clin N Am (in press)
9. Yao K, Iwashita A, Kikuchi Y, et al (2005) Novel zoom endoscopy technique for visualizing the microvascular architecture in gastric mucosa. Clin Gastroenterol Hepatol 3: S23–S26
10. Yao K, Iwashita A, Tanabe H, et al (2007) Novel zoom endoscopy technique for diagnosis of small flat gastric cancer, a prospective, blind study. Clin Gastroenterol Hepatol 5:869–878
11. Yao K, Yao T, Iwashita A (2002) Determining the horizontal extent of early gastric carcinoma: two modern techniques based on differences in the mucosal microvascular architecture and density between carcinoma and non-carcinomatous mucosa. Dig Endosc 14:S83–S87
12. Anagnostopoulos GK, Yao K, Kaye P, et al (2007) Novel endoscopic observation in Barrett's oesophagus using high resolution magnification endoscopy and narrow band imaging. Aliment Pharmacol Ther 26:501–507

Diagnosis of Gastric Cancer by Magnifying Endoscopy with Narrow-Band Imaging: Impact and Clinical Feasibility of Narrow-Band Imaging for Accomplishing Endoscopic Pathology

Mitsuru Kaise

Summary. Although early and precise endoscopic diagnosis of gastric cancer is crucial for reducing its high mortality rates, the diagnosis is difficult because of the broad and heterogeneous appearances of neoplastic mucosa and inflamed gastric mucosa. Narrow-band imaging yields very clear endoscopic images of fine mucosal structures (FMS) and microvessels and has advanced magnifying endoscopic diagnosis into a new stage, endoscopic pathology. Significant microvascular findings related to superficial depressed gastric cancer (0IIc) are dilation, abrupt caliber alteration, and heterogeneity in shape and tortuousness, and those of FMS are complete or partial disappearance. The histopathology of gastric cancer is predictable according to microvascular patterns; fine network pattern and corkscrew pattern correspond to well- and poorly differentiated adenocarcinomas, respectively. Although we have to fully utilize these endoscopic findings for accomplishing endoscopic pathology, the relative importance of the two microstructures differs according to the macroscopic appearance of gastric cancers. In superficial elevated gastric cancer (0IIa), FMS findings such as heterogeneity in shape have greater meaning than microvascular findings because of the frequent absense of irregular microvessels. In superficial flat gastric cancer (0IIb), irregular microvessels enclosed in a villous or papillary microstructure named intrastructural irregular vessel (ISIV) is specific, and the relative importance of FMS is lower.

Key words. Gastric cancer, Magnifying endoscopy, Narrow-band imaging (NBI), Endoscopic pathology

The Impact of Narrow-Band Imaging on Magnifying Endoscopic Diagnosis for Gastric Cancer

Although magnifying endoscopic diagnosis for gastric disorders including gastric cancer has been attempted in past decades [1], the diagnostic approach did not

---

Department of Endoscopy, The Jikei University School of Medicine, 3-25-8 Nishishinbashi, Minato-ku, Tokyo 105-8641, Japan

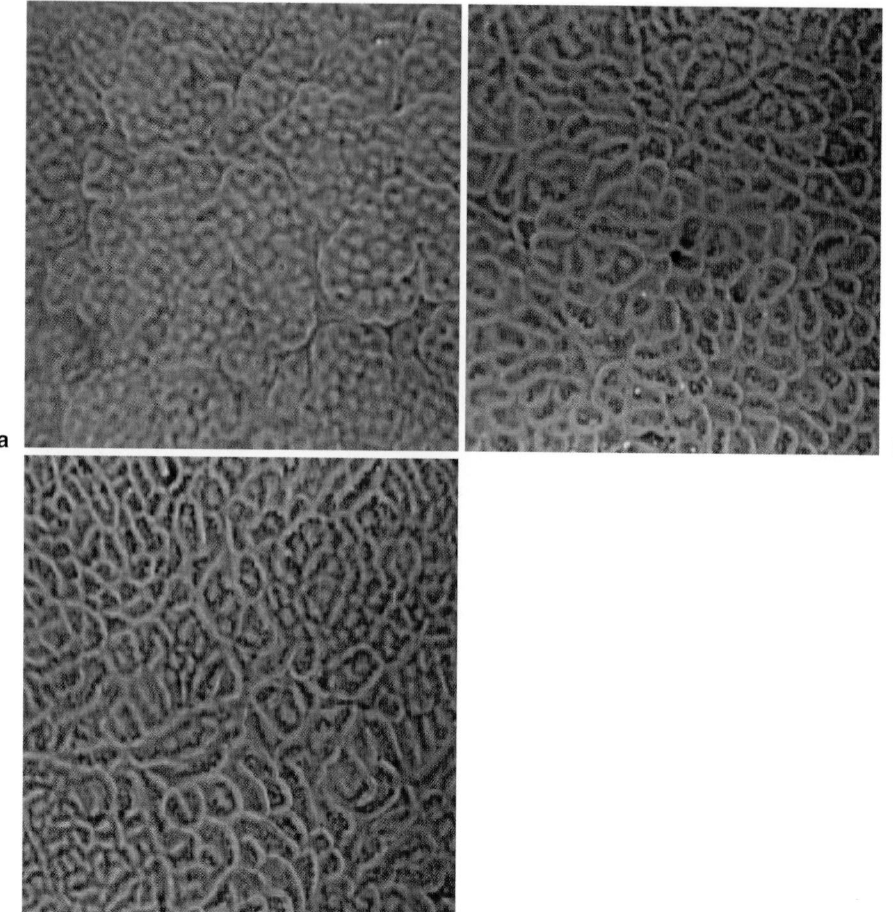

Fig. 1. Normal mucosal images obtained by magnifying endoscopy with narrow-band imaging (NBI). **a** On the mucosal surface of the gastric fundic gland are microvessels surrounding the gland pits, which show a honeycomb pattern. **b** On the mucosal surface of the gastric pyloric gland, microvessels are included in papillary or tubular pits. **c** On the mucosal surface of glands of the intermediate zone, microvessels surround the tubular type pit and stripe pit

succeed well because of the complicated microstructures of the gastric mucosa and gastric neoplasia. Three different proper gastric glands (Fig. 1) show diverse appearances of mucosal microstructures with modification by atrophy, chronic inflammation, and metaplasia (Fig. 2). The histopathological spectrum of gastric cancer is broad (Fig. 3). In a number of cases, pathological appearances are not homogeneous in one cancerous lesion, and a histologically mixed type often exists.

The development of magnifying video-endoscopy combined with narrow-band imaging (NBI) has changed this situation and opened a new era. NBI yields very clear

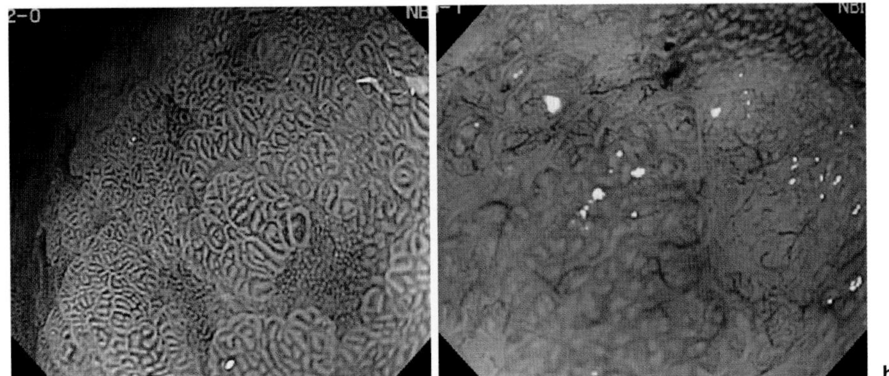

FIG. 2. Modifications of gastric microstructures by atrophy, chronic inflammation, and metaplasia. **a** *Helicobacter pylori*-infected pyloric mucosa lined with a small round, tubular, or gyrus-like pattern of fine mucosal structure, which is different from normal pyloric mucosa (**b**). **b** Atrophic gastric mucosa: fine mucosal structures disappear and stretched microvessels appear

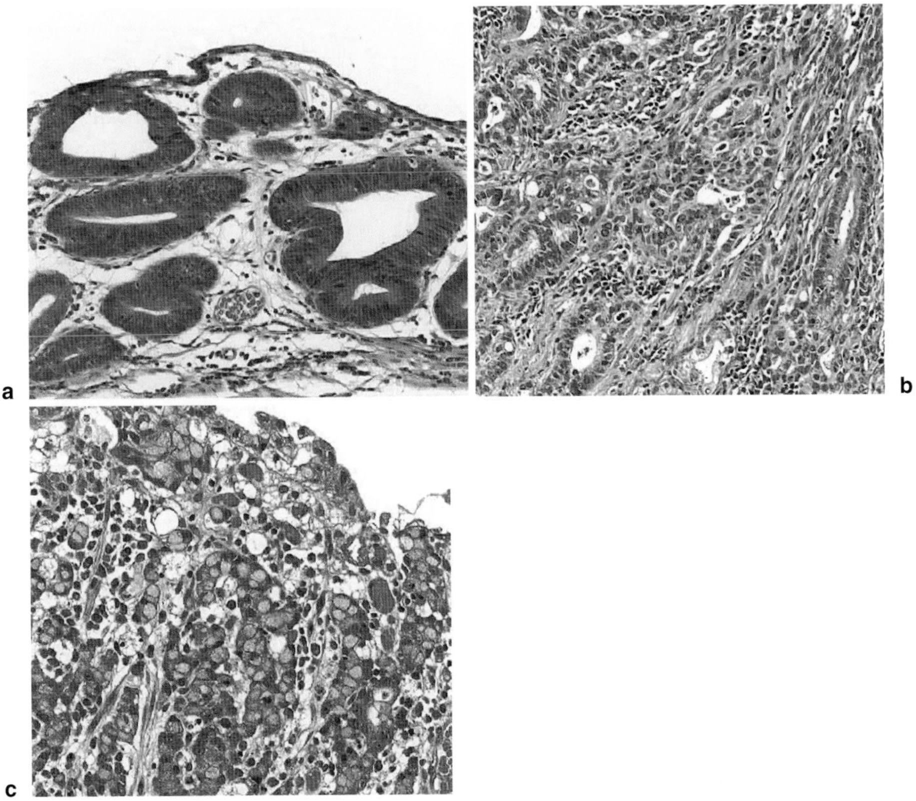

FIG. 3. Histopathological classification of gastric cancer. Gastric cancer shows a broad spectrum of histopathology, which is one of the reasons gastric microstructural findings are complicated. **a** Well-differentiated tubular adenocarcinoma; **b** moderately differentiated adenocarcinoma; **c** poorly differentiated adenocarcinoma

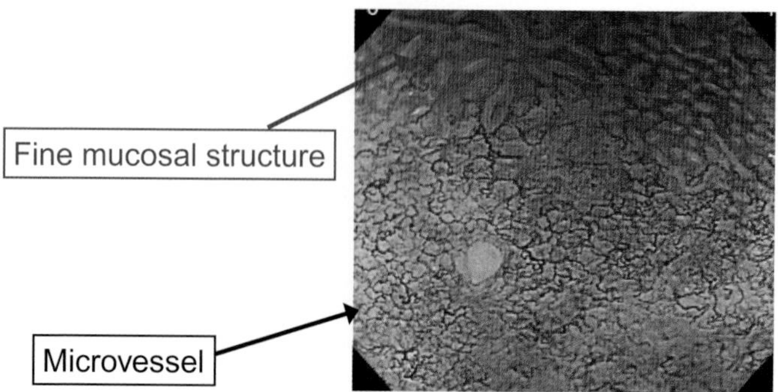

FIG. 4. A representative image of early gastric cancer obtained by magnifying endoscopy with NBI. NBI yields very clear images of fine mucosal structure (FMS) as well as microvessels of the gastric mucosa, which has advanced magnifying endoscopic diagnosis into a new stage, endoscopic pathology

images of fine mucosal structure (FMS) as well as microvessels of the gastric mucosa (Fig. 4), which has advanced magnifying endoscopic diagnosis into a new stage, endoscopic pathology.

Strategy for Diagnosing Gastric Cancer by Magnifying Endoscopy with NBI

The strategy for magnifying endoscopic diagnosis of gastrointestinal cancers is organ specific (Fig. 5). Because the esophagus lined with squamous epithelia does not show any FMS, magnifying endoscopic diagnosis for squamous esophageal cancer solely depends on the findings of microvessels called the intrapapillary capillary loop (IPCL), which is very specific for squamous epithelium. In contrast, magnifying endoscopic diagnosis for colon cancer can be achieved on the findings of FMS, the so-called pit patterns. For magnifying endoscopic diagnosis of gastric cancer, we have to fully utilize the findings of FMS as well as microvessels to overcome the diagnostic difficulties. Therefore, NBI is essential for magnifying endoscopic diagnosis of gastric cancer.

Another critical point in the strategy for magnifying endoscopic diagnosis of gastric cancer is the "macroscopic appearance-specific" approach. Gastric cancers show broad spectra in both microscopic and macroscopic appearance. Superficial gastric cancers are classified into three subtypes based on macroscopic appearance: superficial elevated type (0IIa), superficial depressed type (0IIc), and superficial flat type (0IIb). Although magnifying endoscopic diagnosis of gastric cancer depends on the findings of FMS as well as microvessels, the relative importance of the two microstructures differs according to the macroscopic subtypes of gastric cancers (Fig. 6).

Colon neoplasia:
diagnosable with fine mucosal structure

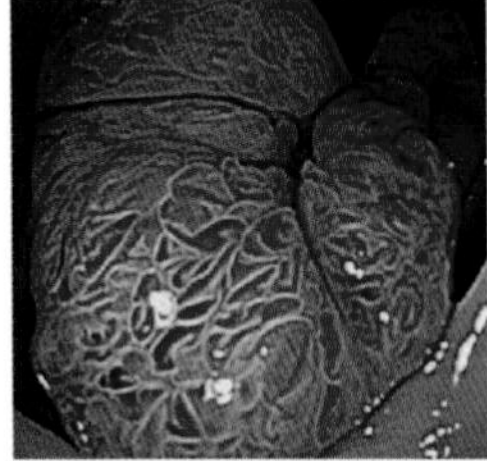

Esophageal neoplasia (squamous cell CA):
diagnosable with microvessel

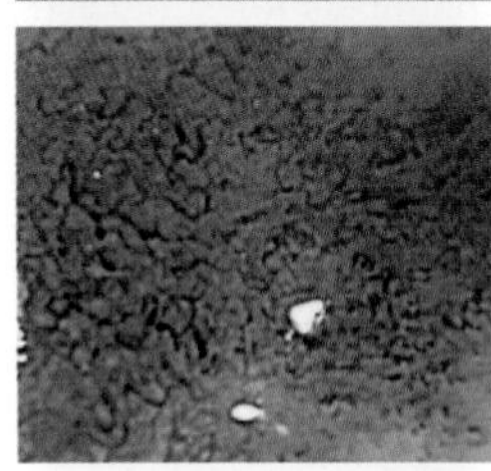

Gastric neoplasia:
diagnosable with fine mucosal structure+ microvessel

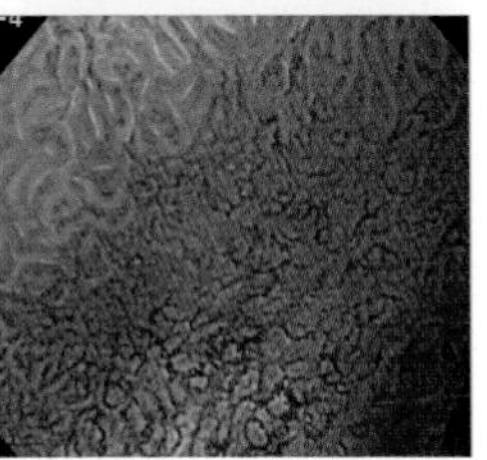

Fig. 5. Organ-specific differences in strategy of magnifying endoscopic diagnosis with NBI. Relative weights of fine mucosal structure and microvessel findings in magnifying endoscopic diagnosis are very different between esophagogastro-intestinal tracts in an organ-specific manner

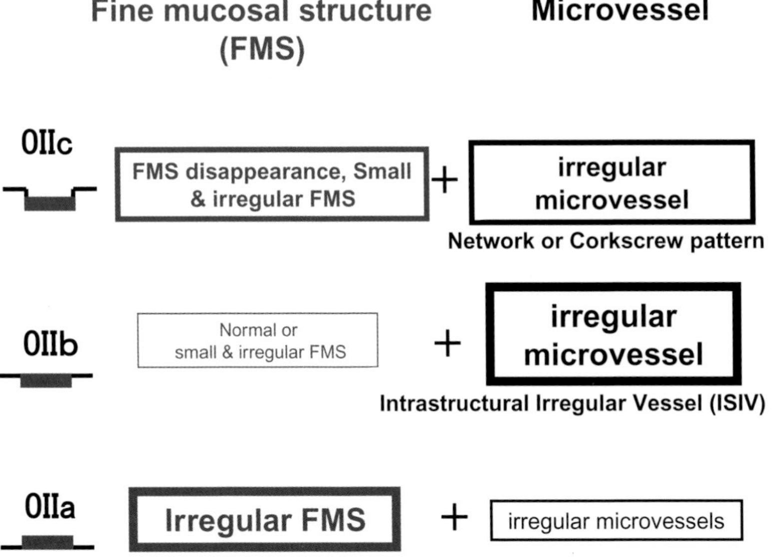

Fig. 6. "Macroscopic appearance-specific" approach in magnifying endoscopic diagnosis for superficial gastric cancer. The relative importance of findings of fine mucosal structure and microvessels in magnifying endoscopic diagnosis with NBI is very different between superficial depressed, flat, and elevated gastric cancers

Diagnosis of Superficial Depressed Gastric Cancer (0IIc) by Magnifying Endoscopy with NBI

Diagnostic Criterion for Superficial Depressed Gastric Cancer (0IIc)

We have conducted a study to clarify a universal criterion of magnifying endoscopic diagnosis for superficial depressed gastric cancer. Static images of depressed lesions (0IIc cancers and benign depressions mimicking cancer) obtained by magnifying endoscopy with NBI were displayed to pleural endoscopists without any clinical information, who scored the existence or absence of findings of microvessels and FMS shown in Table 1. Microstructural findings significantly related to gastric cancer were as follows: dilation, abrupt caliber alteration, heterogeneity in shape and tortuousness of microvessels, and complete or partial disappearance of FMS. Statistical analysis showed that the triad of FMS disappearance, dilation, and heterogeneity in shape of microvessels is a tentative minimal criterion of superficial depressed gastric carcinoma by magnifying endoscopy with NBI.

Prediction of Gastric Cancer Histology by Magnifying Endoscopy with NBI

We have done a study to elucidate the correlation between the magnified endoscopic images obtained with NBI and the histological findings, especially with regard to the microvascular pattern [2]. Two hundred twenty-five cases of superficial depressed gastric carcinoma (152 well-differentiated adenocarcinomas and 75 poorly differenti-

TABLE 1. Irregular findings of microstructure detected by magnifying endoscopy with NBI.

(1) Findings of microvessel
**Dilation
**Heterogeneity in shape
**Abrupt caliber alteration
**Tortuousness
x Denseness
x Regionality
(2) Findings of fine mucosal structure (FMS)
**Complete disappearance
**Partial Disappearance
x Heterogeneity in shape
x Micrification

**indicates those related with gastric cancer
x indicates those not related with gastric cancer
▒ indicates minimal criterion.

ated adenocarcinomas) were enrolled in the study. Findings of microvessels were classified into two patterns: fine network pattern and corkscrew pattern (Fig. 7). The fine network pattern appears as a mesh, and abundant microvessels are well connected with one another. In contrast, the corkscrew pattern has isolated and tortuous microvessels, which appear like a corkscrew. The mixed type with network and corkscrew pattern was classified into one of the types according to the dominant finding. A fine network pattern was recognized in 68.4% of well-differentiated adenocarcinomas (intestinal type). The corkscrew pattern was observed in 85.3% of poorly differentiated adenocarcinoma (diffuse type). Therefore, we can predict gastric cancer histology according to vascular patterns demonstrated by magnifying endoscopy with NBI.

The evidence indicates that magnifying endoscopy with NBI could achieve endoscopic pathology in superficial depressed gastric cancer based upon both FMS and microvessel findings (Figs. 8, 9).

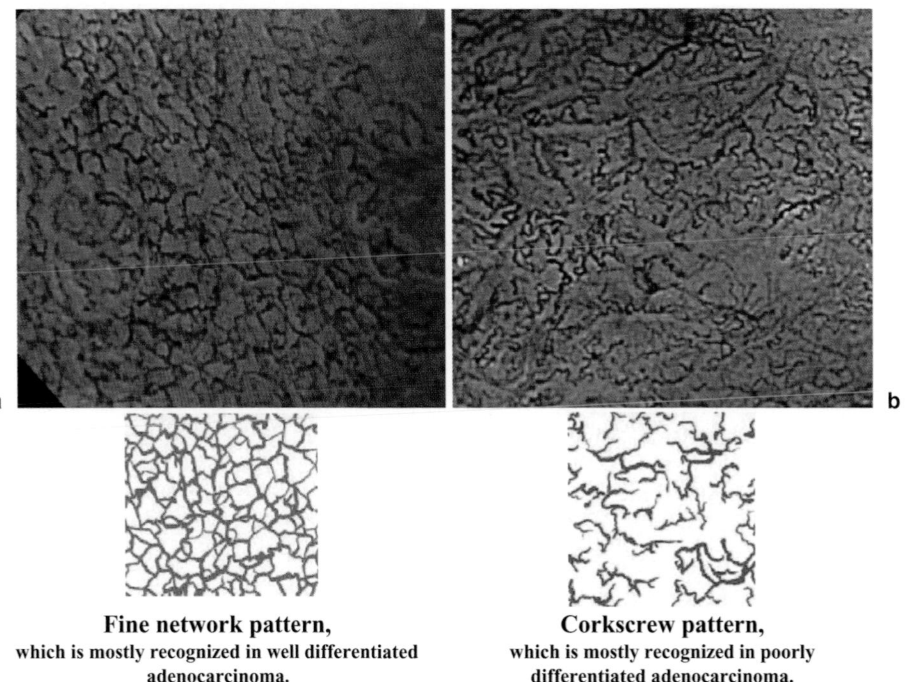

FIG. 7. Classification of irregular microvessels observed in superficial depressed gastric cancer. Irregular microvessels observed in superficial depressed gastric cancer can be classified into (**a**) fine network pattern and (**b**) corkscrew pattern. The fine network pattern appears as a mesh, and abundant microvessels are well connected with one another. In contrast, the corkscrew pattern is composed of tortuous microvessels, which are isolated or are branched but not much connected with one another. The fine network pattern is well recognized in well-differentiated adenocarcinoma, whereas the corkscrew pattern is recognized in poorly differentiated adenocarcinoma

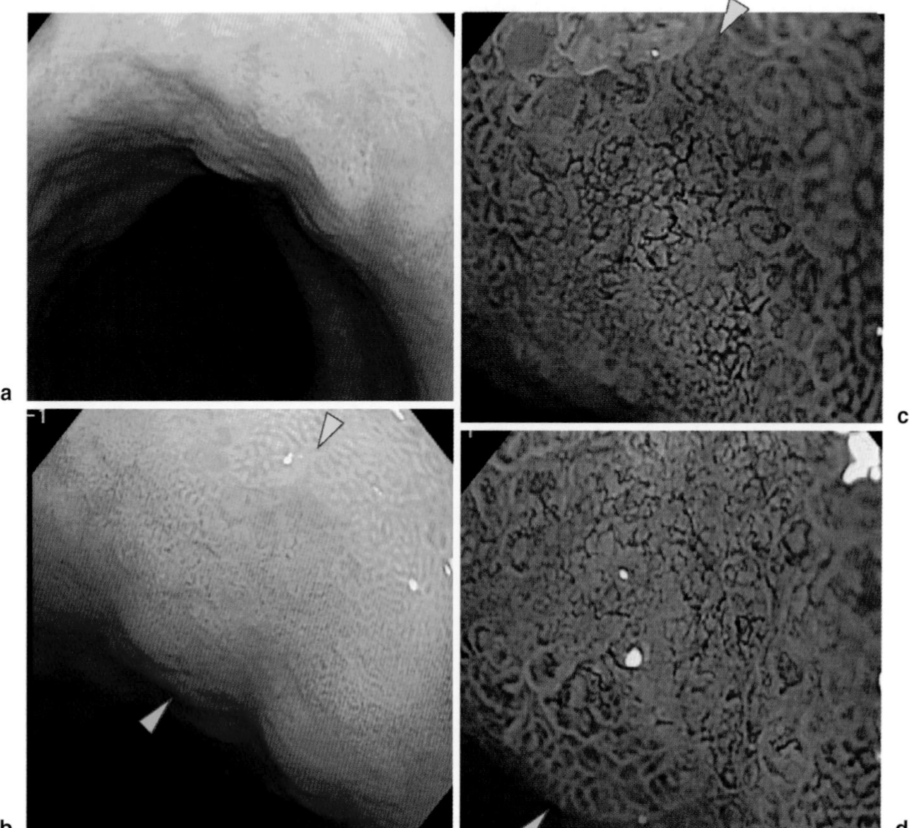

Fig. 8. Representative endoscopic images of superficial depressed gastric cancer (type 0IIc) composed of well-differentiated adenocarcinoma. Conventional endoscopy (**a**) and white light magnifying endoscopy (**b**) show the presence of a depressed lesion on the lesser curvature of the gastric corpus. It is difficult to recognize that the gastric depressed lesion is cancerous by white light endoscopy. Magnifying endoscopy with NBI demonstrates the depressed lesion to have no fine mucosal structure (FMS), but irregular microvessels of fine network pattern, indicating that it is a well-differentiated adenocarcinoma (**c**, **d**). The two portions are indicated by the arrowheads in Fig. 8b. Corresponds to the portions are indicated by the arrowheads in Fig. 8c and Fig. 8d, respectively.

Diagnosis of Superficial Elevated Gastric Cancer by Magnifying Endoscopy with NBI

The diagnostic approach established in superficial depressed neoplasias cannot be simply applied to superficial elevated cancer (0IIa) because the irregular microvasculature is frequently invisible. An elevated lesion shown in Fig. 10 looks like gastric

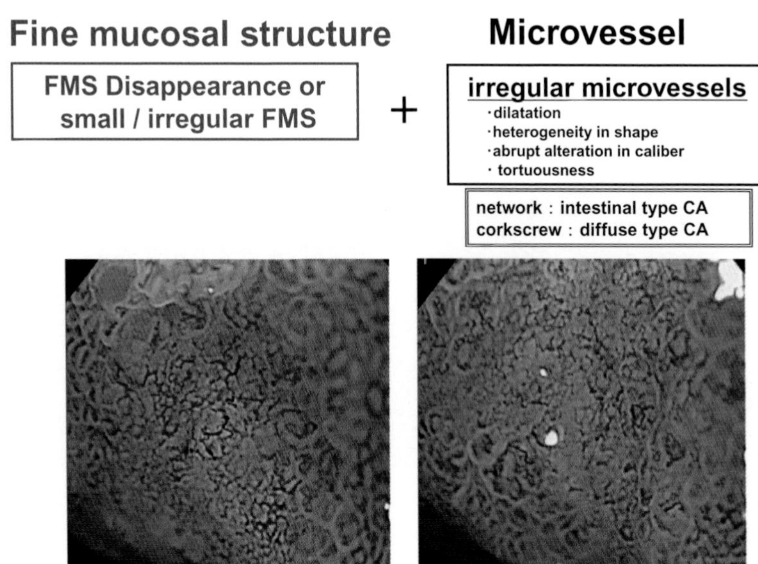

Fig. 9. Diagnostic rationale for superficial depressed cancer by magnifying endoscopy with NBI. For magnifying endoscopic diagnosis of superficial depressed gastric cancer, we have to fully utilize findings of fine mucosal structure (FMS) as well as microvessels to overcome diagnostic difficulties

adenoma by white light endoscopy (Fig. 10a,b) because its surface is white and smooth without irregularity. However, magnifying endoscopy with NBI demonstrates heterogeneity of FMS (Fig. 10c–e), suggesting that the lesion is cancerous but not adenomatous. Histopathology of the sample resected by ESD showed that it was superficial elevated gastric cancer composed of well-differentiated adenocarcinoma. In this case we could not recognize the irregular microvessels at all, meaning that the relative importance of FMS and microvessels in superficial elevated cancer differs from that in a depressed lesion, and FMS findings have greater meaning than irregular microvessels in 0IIa (Fig. 11).

Diagnosis of Superficial Flat Gastric Cancer by Magnifying Endoscopy with NBI

Superficial flat gastric cancer (0IIb) is hard to detect by endoscopy, but there are clues for its diagnosis by magnifying endoscopy with NBI. A 0IIb cancer shown in Fig. 12 displays a discolored area in the lesser curvature of the antrum. White light endoscopy could not demonstrate any information to diagnose the lesion as neoplastic. Magnifying endoscopy with NBI demonstrated that the lesion had relatively regular villous or papillary FMS, but irregular microvessels existed in the FMS

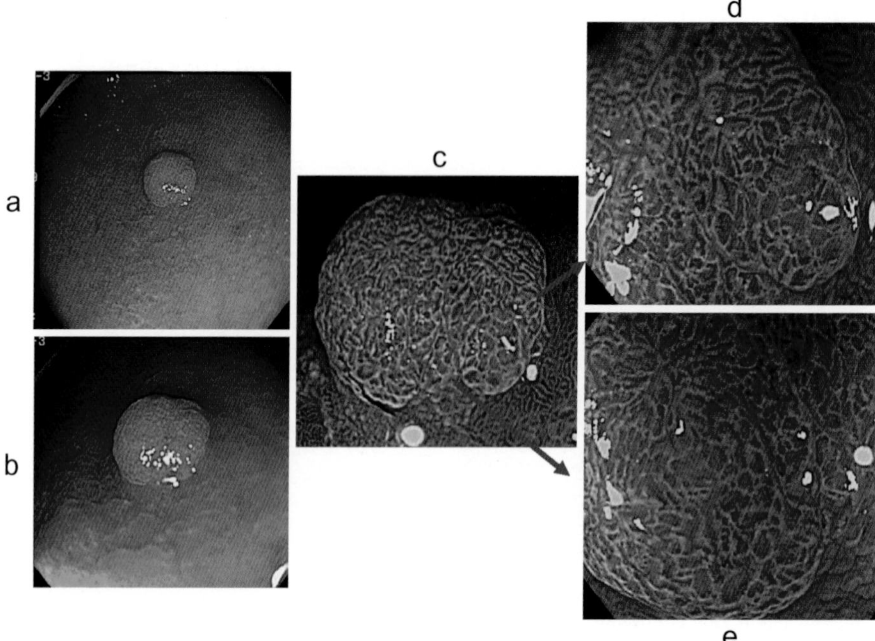

Fig. 10. Representative endoscopic images of superficial elevated gastric cancer (type 0IIa) composed of well-differentiated adenocarcinoma. Conventional endoscopy (**a**, **b**) shows a discolored elevated lesion on the gastric corpus. It is difficult to judge whether the lesion is gastric adenoma or gastric cancer. Magnifying endoscopy with NBI (**c**, **d**, **e**) shows heterogeneity of fine mucosal structures (FMS), suggesting that the lesion is cancerous. However, we could not recognize irregular microvessels on the surface of the lesion, which are almost always recognized in depressed gastric cancers, meaning that FMS findings have greater meaning than irregular microvessels in 0IIa cancer

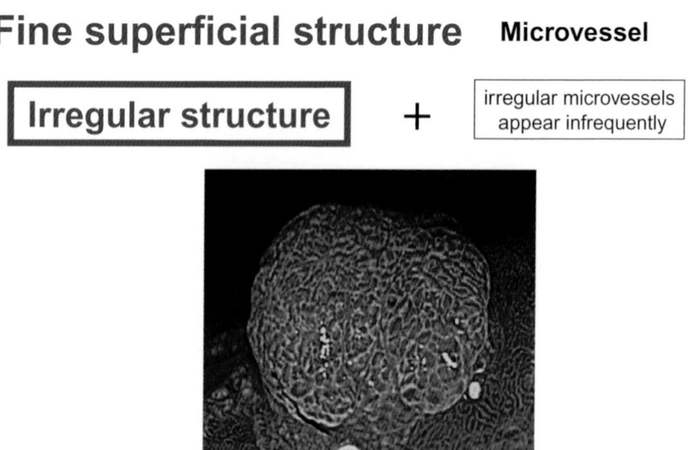

Fig. 11. Diagnostic rationale for superficial elevated cancer (type 0IIa) by magnifying endoscopy with NBI. FMS findings have relatively greater meaning than irregular microvessels in 0IIa cancer

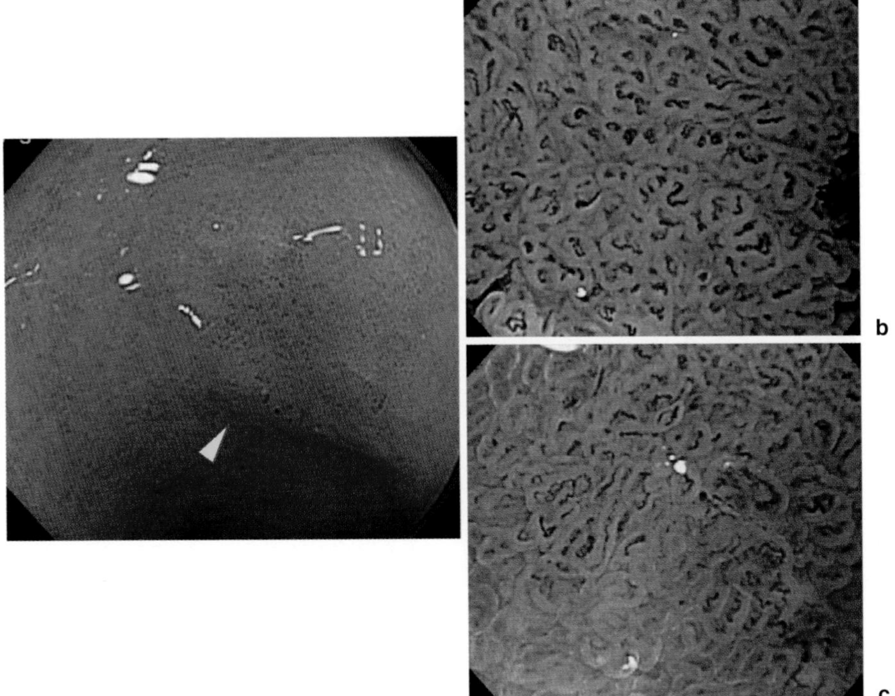

FIG. 12. Representative endoscopic images of superficial flat gastric cancer (type 0IIb) composed of well-differentiated adenocarcinoma. 0IIb cancer displays a discolored area in the lesser curvature of the antrum. White light endoscopy (**a**) could not display any definitive information to diagnose the lesion as neoplastic. Magnifying endoscopy with NBI demonstrated that the center of the lesion had villous or papillary shapes of fine mucosal structures that enclose irregular microvessels with dilation, heterogeneous shape, tortuousness, and abrupt caliber alteration (**b**). The existence of irregular microvessels indicates that the lesion is cancerous. The margin of the lesion can be clearly recognized by the existence of irregular microvessels in FMS at the rim of the lesion indicated by the *yellow arrowhead* in **a** (**c**)

(Fig. 12b). In the rim of the lesion, features of microvessels between the lesion and surrounding mucosa are distinct (Fig. 12c). Histopathology of the sample resected by ESD showed that it was superficial flat gastric cancer composed of well-differentiated adenocarcinoma.

We tentatively named the irregular microvessels as intrastructural irregular vessels (ISIV) (Fig. 13), which is different from irregular microvessels as shown in superficial depressed cancer in regard to the relationship of FMS. ISIV is found in villous or papillary FMS. In contrast, irregular microvessels found in superficial depressed cancer exist in areas where FMS disappear or are unclear. Although intrastructural microvessels are demonstrated in nonneoplastic gastric mucosa, those microvessels do not have characteristics of irregularity, that is, dilation,

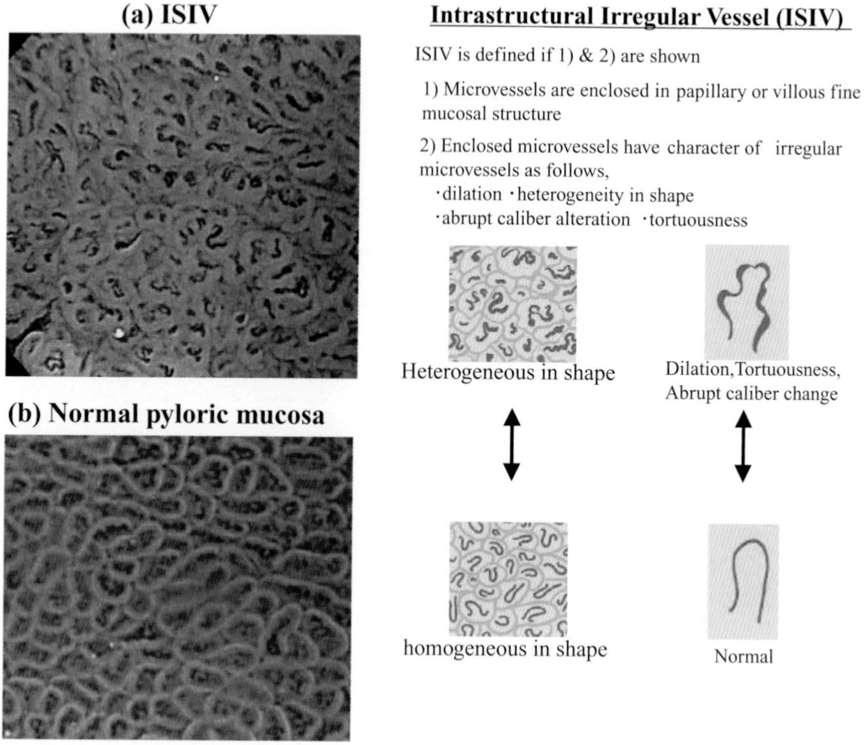

(a) ISIV

(b) Normal pyloric mucosa

Intrastructural Irregular Vessel (ISIV)

ISIV is defined if 1) & 2) are shown

1) Microvessels are enclosed in papillary or villous fine mucosal structure

2) Enclosed microvessels have character of irregular microvessels as follows,

·dilation ·heterogeneity in shape

·abrupt caliber alteration ·tortuousness

Heterogeneous in shape

Dilation,Tortuousness, Abrupt caliber change

homogeneous in shape

Normal

Fig. 13. An intrastructural irregular vessel (ISIV) is defined if microvessels enclosed in papillary or villous FMS have characteristics of irregular microvessels: dilation, heterogeneity in shape, abrupt caliber alteration, and tortuousness (**a**). Normal pyloric mucosa demonstrates microvessels enclosed papillary FMS, which mimic ISIV. However, those microvessels do not have characters of irregularity and are homogeneous in shape (**b**)

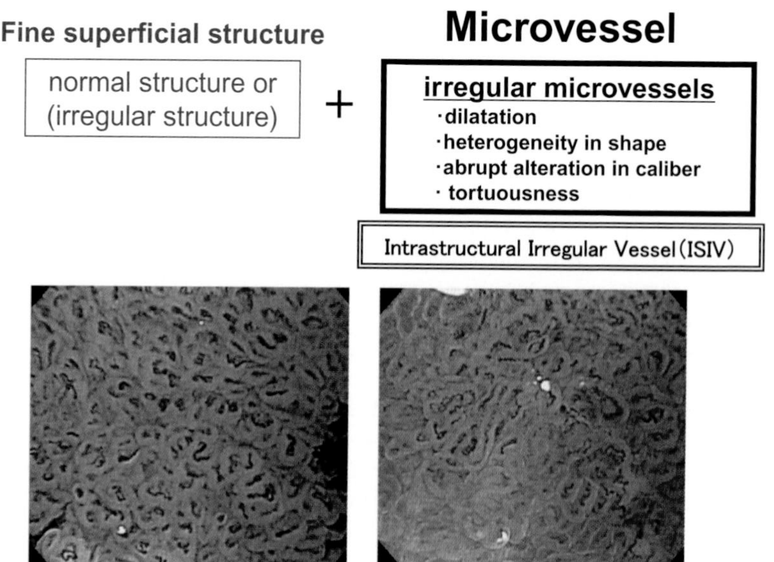

Fig. 14. Diagnostic rationale for superficial flat cancer (type 0IIb) by magnifying endoscopy with NBI. Findings of microvessels such as ISIV have relatively greater meaning than those of FMS in superficial flat gastric cancer

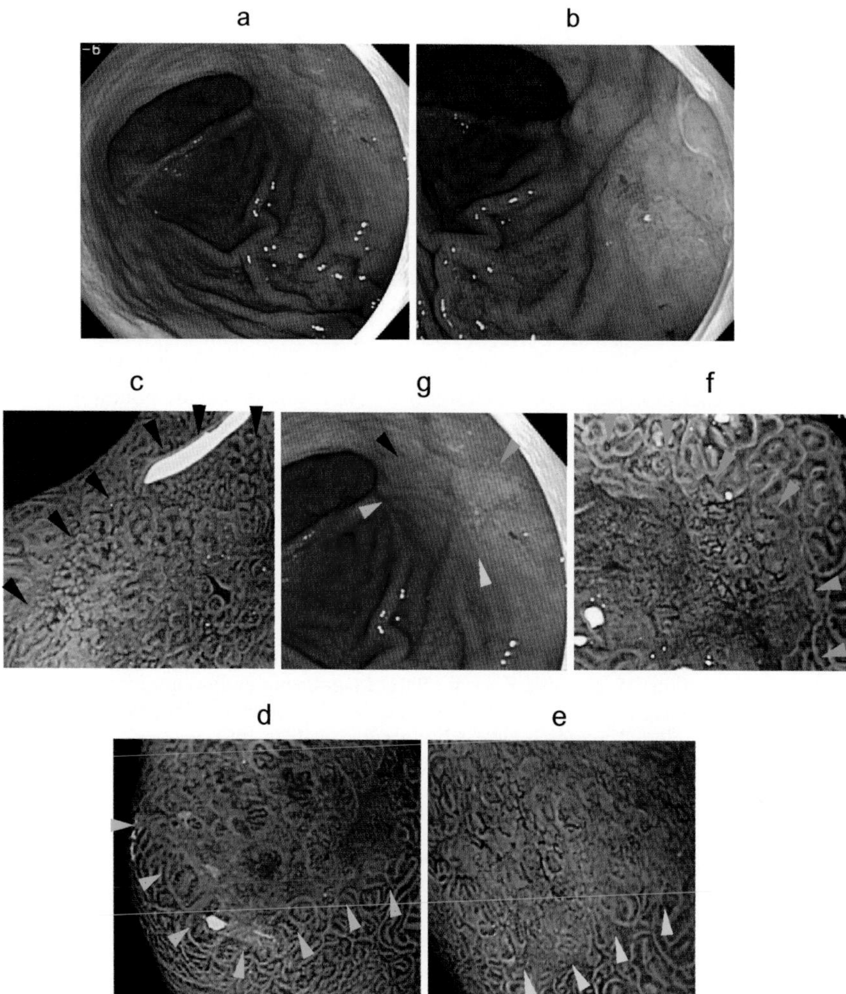

Fig. 15. A superficial gastric cancer with indefinite information on cancerous existence and margin by white light endoscopy. High-resolution white light endoscopy shows indefinite information on cancerous existence and margin (**a**, **b**). Magnifying endoscopy with NBI (**c**–**f**) conveyed clear images of irregular microstructures that demonstrate the margin of lateral cancerous extent very well. *Arrowheads* in **c**–**f** indicate the cancerous margins, whose positions correspond with *arrowheads* of the same color in **g**

abrupt caliber alteration, heterogeneity in shape, or tortuousness. We, therefore, can distinguish those found in nonneoplastic mucosa from ISIV. The diagnostic rationale for superficial flat cancer by magnifying endoscopy with NBI is shown in Fig. 14.

Application of Magnifying Endoscopy with NBI on Gastric ESD

Diagnosis of the lateral extent of cancerous infiltration is indispensable for endoscopic or surgical resection of gastric carcinoma. As around 20% of superficial gastric carcinomas do not give a clear borderline on conventional white light endoscopy, accurate endoscopic diagnosis plays a crucial role for a radical cure, especially in endoscopic resection. Endoscopic submucosal dissection (ESD), a recently developed superb method that enables an en bloc resection for large lesions, can achieve a more radical cure in combination with precise endoscopic diagnosis of the cancerous extent. Therefore, we usually perform ESD in combination with magnifying endoscopy with NBI, which can allow endoscopic and real-time pathology [3]. Figure 15a,b shows high-resolution endoscopic pictures of a gastric cancer that are not informative as to cancerous existence and extent on white light endoscopy. Magnifying endoscopy with NBI (Fig. 15c–f) conveyed clear images of irregular microstructures that demonstrate the margin of lateral cancerous extent very well, and ESD could be curatively carried out based on the findings of magnifying endoscopy with NBI.

References

1. Sakaki N, Iida Y, Okazaki Y, et al (1978) Magnifying endoscopic observation of the gastric mucosa, particularly in patients with atrophic gastritis. Endoscopy 10:269–274
2. Nakayoshi T, Tajiri H, Matsuda K, et al (2004) Magnifying endoscopy combined with narrow band imaging system for early gastric cancer: correlation of vascular pattern with histopathology (including video). Endoscopy 36:1080–1084
3. Sumiyama K, Kaise M, Nakayoshi T, et al (2004) Combined use of a magnifying endoscope with a narrow band imaging system and a multibending endoscope for en bloc EMR of early stage gastric cancer. Gastrointest Endosc 60:79–84

Autofluorescence Imaging Video-Endoscopy System for Diagnosis of Superficial Gastric Neoplasia

NORIYA UEDO, RYU ISHIHARA, and HIROYASU IISHI

Summary. An autofluorescence imaging video-endoscopy system (AFI) produces real-time pseudocolor images from computed detection of autofluorescence emitted by endogenous fluorophores in the mucosa. In the AFI images of the gastric body, the fundic mucosa appears purple, whereas atrophic mucosa appear bright green. Gastric tumors appear purple or green in the AFI images according to their morphology, i.e., elevated or depressed, respectively. Therefore, the color patterns of gastric tumors are classified into four types: purple tumors in a green background, purple tumors in a purple background, green tumors in a green background, and green tumors in a purple background. Purple tumors in a green background and green tumors in a purple background are readily distinguished by their color. In contrast, purple tumors in a purple background are difficult to define by color. Green tumors in a green background appear similar in color to the surrounding mucosa, but the tumor extension can be determined by their purple rim. Diagnostic accuracy of AFI for tumor extension was better (68%) than that by white light endoscopy (36%), but was not as good as chromoendoscopy (91%). The low accuracy rate was mainly caused by interference of an ulceration or scar, while the AFI diagnosed flat tumor extension more accurately than did white light images. Because the AFI could visualize flat or isochromatic tumor extension compared with white light endoscopy, it detected more multiple neoplasia in patients who underwent endoscopic treatment.

Key words. Autofluorescence endoscopy, Early gastric cancer, Atrophic gastritis, Chromoendoscopy, Endoscopic mucosal resection

Introduction

The incidence of gastric cancer has consistently decreased, but it remains the second most common cause of death from malignant disease worldwide, and the highest incidence in the world is in Japan. Early detection and early treatment have been considered to be an effective strategy for reduction of mortality from gastric cancers; thus, many efforts have been undertaken in this regard, such as encouraging mass screening and developing endoscopic diagnostic procedures.

Department of Gastrointestinal Oncology, Osaka Medical Center for Cancer and Cardiovascular Diseases, 3-3 Nakamichi 1-chome, Higashinari-ku, Osaka 537-8511, Japan

Chromoendoscopy is currently an essential procedure for detection and staging of gastric cancers in Japan. However, as it is somewhat complicated and time consuming, its routine use is limited. Therefore, the development of an effective and facile diagnostic method of endoscopy has been anticipated. In this chapter, we introduce one of the new diagnostic imaging technologies that uses a combination of autofluorescence and reflection imaging: the autofluorescence imaging video-endoscopy system (AFI; Olympus Medical Systems, Tokyo, Japan) and demonstrate its possible utility for the diagnosis of gastric neoplasia.

Principle of Autofluorescence Video-Endoscopy

When a short wavelength excitation light irradiates a substance called a fluorophore, that substance emits a longer wavelength light, that is, fluorescence. In the digestive tract, endogenous fluorophores, such as collagen, nicotinamide, adenine dinucleotide, flavin, and porphyrins, exist in both mucosa and submucosa; therefore, they emit a natural tissue fluorescence called autofluorescence when the excitation light illuminates the mucosa. An autofluorescence video-endoscopy system produces real-time pseudo-color images from detection of the autofluorescence. In the development and evaluation of fluorescence-based diagnostic technologies, either autofluorescence or fluorescence caused by an exogenously administered fluorescent drug such as 5-aminolevulinic acid is used. Because the autofluorescence video-endoscopy system only utilizes natural tissue fluorescence from an endogenous fluorophore, it does not require any drug administration or dye spraying, which may cause adverse patient effects.

Detection of abnormal lesions by autofluorescence video-endoscopy depends on changes in the concentration or depth distribution of endogenous fluorophores, changes in the tissue microarchitecture, or both, including altered mucosal thickness or blood (hemoglobin) concentration, which affect the fluorescence intensity or spec-

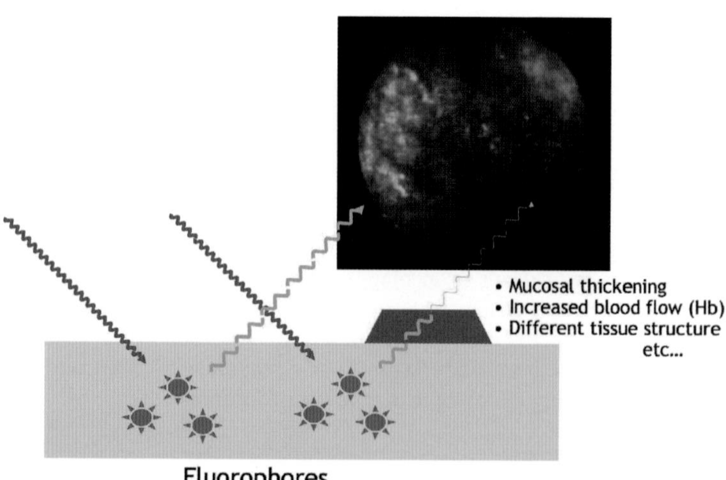

Fig. 1. Principle of autofluorescence endoscopy and possible mechanisms of color change

trum. Autofluorescence is basically reduced at the tumors compared with the normal mucosa [1]; possible mechanisms are shown in Fig. 1. The differences in the fluorescence features, mainly determined by the intensity, are represented as color differences in the autofluorescence video-endoscopy images.

Instruments of the New Autofluorescence Imaging System

Because earlier autofluorescence imaging systems used a fiberoptic endoscope and a heavy image-intensifying camera unit attached to the eyepiece, they failed to provide sufficient image quality and maneuverability. Thus, they were not suitable for general clinical use in this video-endoscopy era. The AFI system uses a dedicated video-endoscope (XGIF-Q240FY, XGIF-Q240FZ; Olympus Medical Systems), in which are incorporated two charge-coupled devices (CCDs) for the autofluorescence and white light modes. Thus, the appearance and maneuverability of the endoscope are the same as that of a conventional video-endoscope. Each mode is selected by pressing a small pushbutton on the control head for a few seconds. The AFI is the first imaging system that detects autofluorescence by a CCD incorporated in the video-endoscope.

In the autofluorescence mode, the excitation light for inducing autofluorescence (395–475 nm), and the narrowband green (G'-) light (550 nm) for recording reflection images, were illuminated sequentially from the light source through the rotation filter. An excitation light cut filter is incorporated with the CCD for the autofluorescence mode to permit only 490- to 625-nm wavelength light to intensify the CCD. When the G'-light is illuminated, reflection images are taken. The image possessor artificially colors the autofluorescence images to green, and the green reflection image to red and blue, and composite images are displayed on the video screen (Fig. 2).

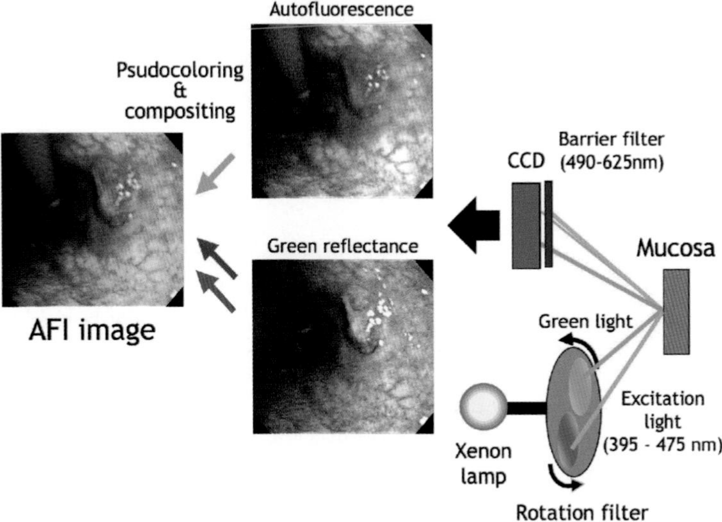

Fig. 2. Diagram of the autofluorescence imaging (AFI) system

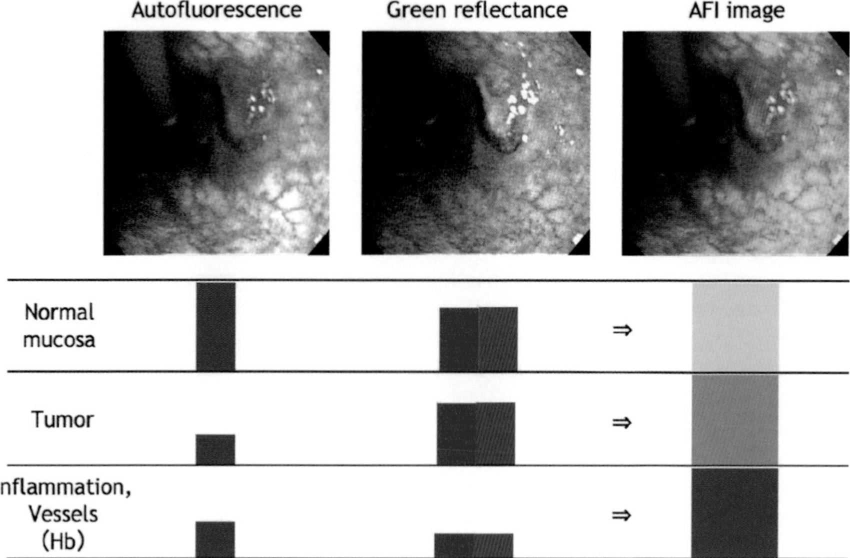

Fig. 3. Pseudo-color of the AFI system

The wavelengths of G'-light are determined by absorption features of hemoglobin. Normal mucosa emits bright autofluorescence, and thus the composite color appears bright green. Because a tumor absorbs autofluorescence well, it looks magenta, which is the complementary color of green. As hemoglobin absorbs both autofluorescence and G'-light (550 nm), areas containing more hemoglobin are displayed as dark green in the AFI image (Fig. 3).

In the white light mode, the light source provides red, green, and blue wavelength light sequentially by a rotation filter. As the CCD for the white light mode is the same as that equipped in EVIS GIF-Q240, diagnosis could be made with information from autofluorescence observation in addition to the high-resolution white light video images.

Diagnosis of Atrophic Gastritis

It is widely accepted that gastric cancers evolve through a multistep process starting with superficial gastritis, followed by atrophy with intestinal metaplasia (IM), dysplasia, and finally carcinoma. Thus, the identification of precursor status and follow-up of patients in whom these events occur could lead to diagnosis of gastric cancer at an early stage and to improved patient survival. We have demonstrated that the extent of atrophic gastritis observed by the endoscopic Congo red test was significantly related to the risk of development of gastric cancer by a long-term follow-up study [2].

Basically, the color of the digestive tract mucosa looks bright green in the AFI images [3,4]. However, that of the gastric mucosa is different because of the presence of the fundic gland, which characterizes the unique gastric function, acid secretion.

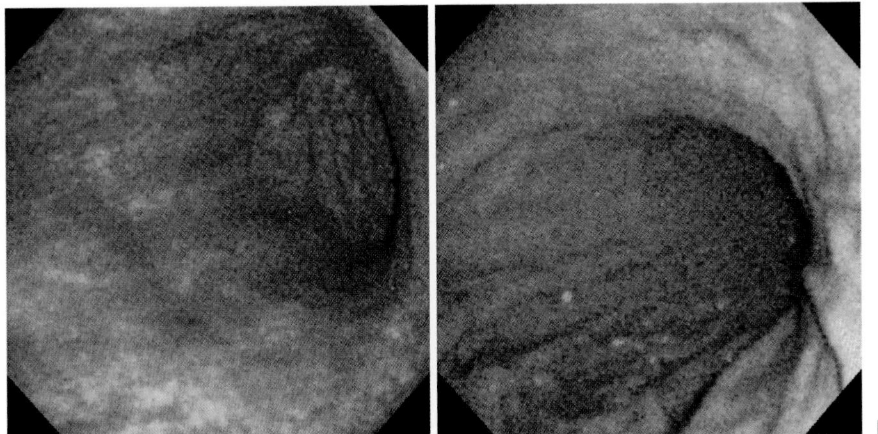

Fig. 4. In a *Helicobacter pylori*-negative patient, the gastric body mucosa looks *purple* (**a**), whereas in patients with extensive mucosal atrophy, it looks *green*, similar to the mucosa in the other digestive tract organs (**b**)

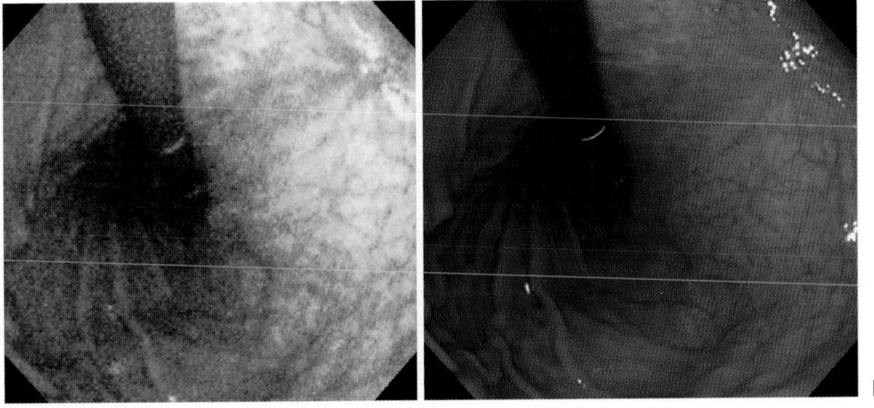

Fig. 5. In patients with atrophic gastritis, green mucosa in the gastric body (**a**) represents the extension of atrophic mucosa: pale mucosa with visible vascular pattern (**b**)

In patients who do not have atrophic gastritis, the gastric body mucosa appears purple (Fig. 4a), whereas it looks bright green in patients with extensive mucosal atrophy (Fig. 4b). Histological grading of biopsy specimens taken from the purple and green mucosa according to the visual analogue scale of the updated Sydney system indicated that green mucosa in the gastric body had significantly more atrophy and intestinal metaplasia scores compared to purple mucosa (Table 1). In the AFI images, therefore, the extent of the green mucosa in the gastric body represents the extent of atrophic gastritis with intestinal metaplasia (Fig. 5). The difference in the mucosal color could be explained by the thickness or vascular density of the fundic mucosa.

TABLE 1. Gastritis scores of body mucosa in accordance with AFI color.

	Color of the gastric body		
	Purple (n = 36)	Green (n = 26)	P value
Activity	0.9 ± 0.7	0.9 ± 0.8	0.624
Inflammation	2.1 ± 0.8	1.9 ± 0.5	0.975
Atrophy	1.6 ± 0.6	1.9 ± 0.8	0.030
Intestinal metaplasia	0.8 ± 1.2	2.0 ± 1.0	0.000

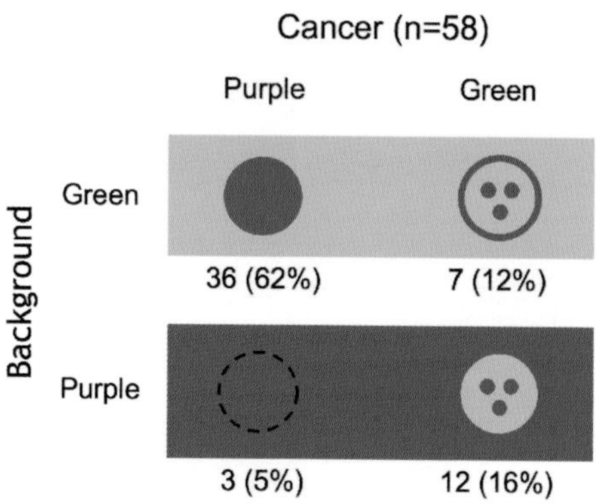

FIG. 6. Color patterns of early gastric cancers in the AFI images

Color Patterns of Superficial Gastric Neoplasia

Similar to the gastric mucosa, the color of gastric tumors varies from purple to green in the AFI images. Therefore, the color patterns of gastric tumors are classified into four types according to the colors of tumors and background mucosa: purple tumors in green background, purple tumors in purple background, green tumors in green background, and green tumors in purple background (Fig. 6). Green tumors in purple background (Fig. 7) and purple tumors in green background (Fig. 8) are readily distinguished by their color. In contrast, purple tumors in a purple background are difficult to define by the color, although their prevalence is low. For green tumors in a green background, the tumors appear similar in color to the surrounding mucosa, but they are rimmed by purple color, and there are sometimes purple nodules representing regenerative mucosa in the tumor (Fig. 9).

Investigating the association between tumor color and clinicopathological factors including morphology, histology, location, size, and background color in the AFI images, only morphological type (elevated to depressed: odds ratio of 16.4) and background color (green to purple: odds ratio of 3.4) were independent contributors to the tumor color [5]. Accordingly, elevated tumors basically look purple, whereas most of the depressed tumors look green. Recognition of those color patterns assists in interpreting the AFI findings of gastric neoplasia.

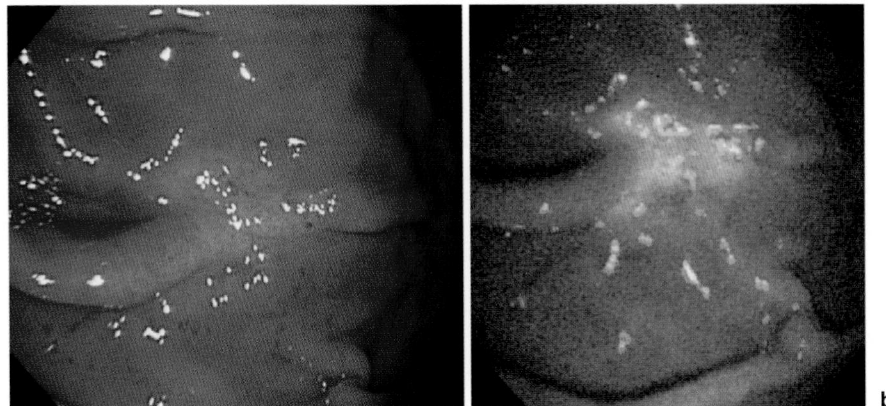

FIG. 7. A depressed type tumor in the fundic mucosa (**a**) looks *green* in purple background

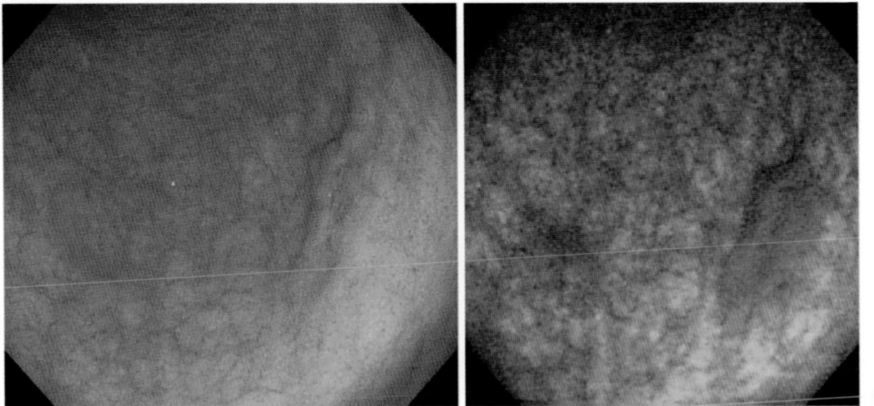

FIG. 8. Elevated type tumors in the atrophic mucosa (**a**) look *purple* in green background

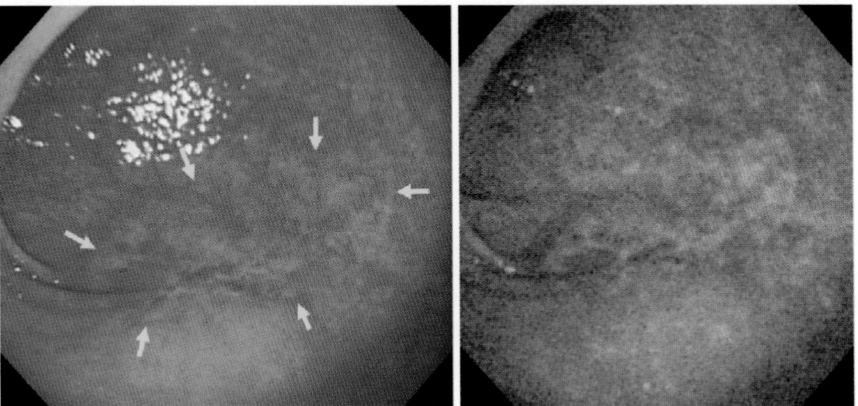

FIG. 9. A depressed type tumor in the atrophic mucosa (*yellow arrows* in **a**) appears similar in color to the green background. The tumor is rimmed by purple color, and *purple nodules* sometimes exist inside (**b**)

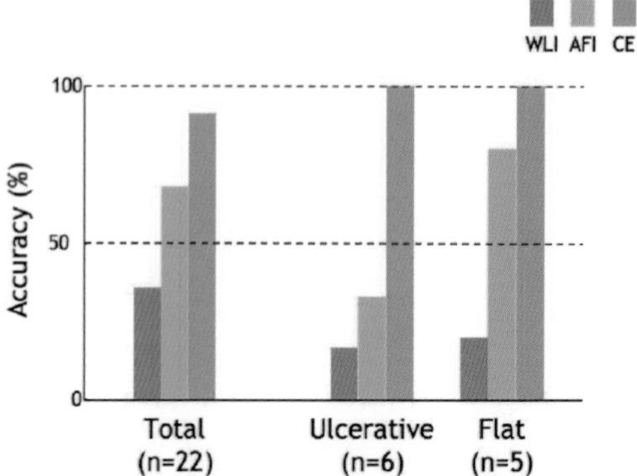

Fig. 10. Diagnostic accuracy for tumor extension. *WLI*, white light image (*red bars*); *AFI*, autofluorescence images (*green bars*); CE (*blue*), chromoendoscopy

Diagnosis of Tumor Extent

For diagnosis of tumor extent, we found that the diagnostic accuracy of AFI was better than that by white light endoscopy, but was not as same as that of chromoendoscopy [6]. In the subclass analysis, the low accuracy rate was mainly caused by interference with ulceration or scar, while AFI diagnosed flat tumor extension more accurately than white light images (Fig. 10).

Detection of Gastric Neoplasia by AFI

After endoscopic treatment of early gastric cancer, most of the gastric mucosa that may contain areas at high risk for developing gastric neoplasia, such as mucosa with atrophic gastritis and intestinal metaplasia, remain, in contrast to gastrectomy. Multiple cancers frequently develop in patients who underwent endoscopic resection of early gastric cancer: 3.8% in 5 years. Because AFI detected the flat tumor extension that was not evident in white light images, it could identify a small or flat malignancy or premalignant lesions that were undetectable by conventional white light endoscopy before they develop. On the basis of this hypothesis, we investigated the effectiveness of AFI on detecting multiple gastric neoplasia in 68 patients who underwent endoscopic mucosal resection for early gastric cancers. In that study, we compared the diagnostic ability of AFI and conventional white light images for multiple neoplasia other than the lesion, which was treated by endoscopic resection, in terms of chromoendoscopy with biopsy as a reference standard. AFI found seven early gastric cancers and one borderline lesion (median size, 5 mm) in seven patients, whereas white light observation found only one early gastric cancer in one patient (Table 2) [7].

TABLE 2. Diagnostic ability of autofluorescence imaging and white light imaging for multiple gastric neoplasia. (n = 68)

	Sensitivity	Specificity	PPV	NPV	Efficacy
AFI	1.00	0.79	0.36	1.00	0.82
[95% C.I.]	[1.00, 1.00]	[0.70, 0.89]	[0.16, 0.56]	[1.00, 1.00]	[0.76, 0.90]
WLI	0.13	0.94	0.20	0.90	0.86
[95% C.I.]	[0.00, 0.35]	[0.89, 0.99]	[0.00, 0.55]	[0.83, 0.97]	[0.77, 0.94]

AFI, autofluorescence imaging; WLI, white light imaging; PPV, positive predicting value; NPV, negative predicting value

Future Perspective

In this chapter, we described the diagnostic utility of AFI for diagnosis of gastric neoplasia in our experience. The AFI is the first autofluorescence endoscopy system incorporating CCD for autofluorescence observation, and it achieved the same maneuverability as conventional high-resolution video-endoscopy in general clinical use. Although there are currently several limitations in moderate resolution in images or low specificity [8,9] in some clinical settings, the technology has the potential to yield a new field in diagnosis of gastric neoplasia. Further evaluations for determining the optimum usage or settings and additional technological developments for improvement of specificity are required.

References

1. Mayinger B, Jordan M, Horbach T, et al (1993) Evaluation of in vivo endoscopic autofluorescence spectroscopy in gastric cancer. Gastrointest Endosc 59:191–198
2. Tatsuta M, Iishi H, Nakaizumi A, et al (1993) Fundal atrophic gastritis as a risk factor for gastric cancer. Int J Cancer 53:70–74
3. Kara MA, Peters FP, Ten Kate FJ, et al (2005) Endoscopic video autofluorescence imaging may improve the detection of early neoplasia in patients with Barrett's esophagus. Gastrointest Endosc 61:679–685
4. Uedo N, Iishi H, Ishinhara R, et al (2006) Novel autofluorescence video-endoscopy imaging system for diagnosis of cancers in the digestive tract Dig. Endosc 18:S131–S136
5. Kato M, Uedo N, Iishi H (2007) Analysis of color pattern of early gastric cancer by autofluorescence imaging videoendoscopy system. Gastrointest Endosc 65:AB356
6. Uedo N, Iishi H, Tatsuta M, et al (2005) A novel video endoscopy system by using autofluorescence and reflectance imaging for diagnosis of esophagogastric cancers. Gastrointest Endosc 62:521–528
7. Uedo N, Iishi H, Tekeuchi Y, et al (2005) Diagnosis of early gastric cancer using endoscopic screening with autofluorescence video-endoscopy. Endoscopy 37:A26
8. Uedo N, Higashino K, Ishihara R, et al (2007) Diagnosis of colonic adenomas by new autofluorescence imaging system: a pilot study. Dig Endosc 18:S131–S136
9. Kato M, Kaise M, Yonezawa J, et al (2007) Autofluorescence endoscopy versus conventional white light endoscopy for the detection of superficial gastric neoplasia: a prospective comparative study. Endoscopy 39:937–941

The Diagnosis of Gastric Cancer and Adenoma Using Endocytoscopy

Yasumasa Niwa and Hidemi Goto

Summary. Endocytoscopy is ultrahigh magnifying endoscopy based on contact light microscopy. Using this endoscopy, we could observe the nuclei and cytoplasm in living cells during ongoing endoscopy. For gastric adenoma and cancer, we could observe the abnormal arrangement of glands and the irregularity of the nuclei in the neoplasm. These endocytoscopic images directly contributed to the diagnosis of malignancy in the lesion because it allowed microscopic observation at the cellular level. Until now there have been some problems: unstable image acquisition because of the small, soft catheter; and the contrast agent, methylene blue, which has a detrimental effect when combined with strong white light. This system might be more useful and these drawbacks overcome if integrated with the usual magnifying endoscopy and ultrahigh magnifying endoscopy, and if a new contrast agent is developed, which could result in real optical biopsy during ongoing endoscopy.

Key words. Endocytoscopy, Ultrahigh magnifying endoscopy, Gastric cancer, Gastric adenoma, Optical biopsy

Introduction

In Japan we have investigated medical images with histological findings in the gastroenterological area. Morphological diagnosis, for example, X-ray and endoscopic images, has been advanced and has led to the highest level of the diagnosis of early gastric cancer in the world. Endoscopists especially always want to know the accurate histological diagnosis of gastrointestinal (GI) tract lesions immediately, and until now high vision endoscopy has been used for that clinical application. Moreover, magnifying endoscopy with or without narrow-band imaging (NBI) might satisfy some of the passion of endoscopists. This quality of endoscopic images has contributed to the diagnosis of malignant lesions and extent of neoplasms in the GI tract, but until now even with the use of such high-level endoscopy we cannot see the nucleus and cytoplasm in vivo. The final diagnosis as to whether the lesion is malignant or benign requires several days until the pathologist decides. Also, sometimes we may not obtain

Department of Gastroenterology, Nagoya Graduate School of Medicine, 65 Tsuruma-cho, Showa-ku, Nagoya 466-8550, Japan a biopsy from the GI tract mucosa because the patient is prescribed anticoagulant medicine or antiplatelet medicine for cardiovascular disease or cerebrovascular disease.

Recently, two types of ultrahigh magnification endoscopy have been developed, endocytoscopy and laser endoscopy. These endoscopies display at about 500 or 1000 fold magnification and show the cytoplasm in the living cell. Especially, endocytoscopy (ECS) is newly developed on the basis of light contact microscopy. This new endoscopy was collaboratively developed by Dr. Inoue and the Olympus Medical Systems Co., Tokyo, Japan. Its use was reported for superficial esophageal cancer by Kumagai and Inoue [1,2]. When pathologists diagnose the malignancy in the lesion, it is important to judge the arrangement and uniformity of the glands and the size, uniformity, and irregularity of nuclei. This most important point of this ultrahigh magnifying endoscopy is to observe the nucleus in the cell.

We used a prototype endocytoscopy system, which consisted of a soft-catheter-type endoscope with an outside diameter of 3.2 mm at the distal end (XEC-300-U; Olympus Medical Systems, Tokyo, Japan), a VISERA video system center (OTV-S7V; Olympus Medical Systems), and a high-brightness light source (CLH-SC; Olympus Medical Systems). When we apply this catheter type for clinical cases, we should select an endoscope with a larger working channel, such as the GIF-1T240 (Olympus Medical Systems). It has a magnification of 450× (on a 14-in. monitor) and provides a field of view covering a 300 × 300 μm area. An amount of 5 ml or less of 1% methylene blue is sprayed onto the surface mucosa of the stomach. The penetration depth of images is limited to 30 μm.

Case Presentation

The first case was early gastric cancer in a freshly resected stomach; this was superficial depressed gastric cancer (type IIc). The histology is moderately tubular adenocarcinoma. Ex vivo endocytoscopic images showed the cancer cells clearly. We could see the cytoplasm and nuclei in the freshly resected specimen in real time (Fig. 1a).

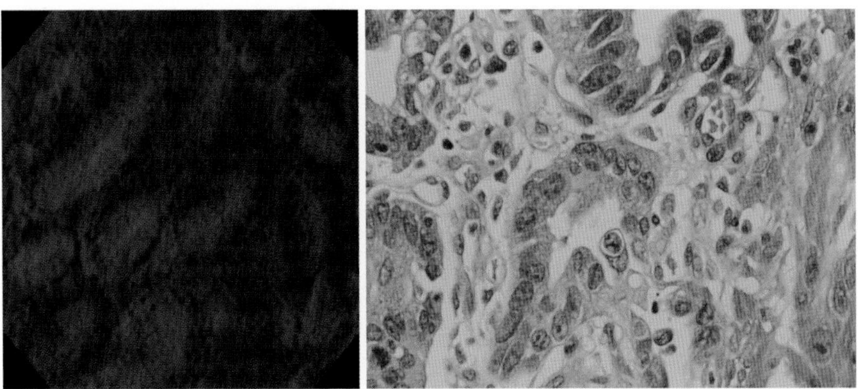

Fig. 1. **a** Endocytoscopic image of superficial depressed gastric cancer (type IIc) in freshly resected stomach. **b** Histological finding showed moderately differentiated tubular adenocarcinoma

The pathological picture agreed well with the endocytoscopic images (Fig. 1b). The freshly resected stomach presents a good condition for endocytoscopy because there is no new mucus being produced and covering the mucosa in the lesion. Fujishiro et al. reported the endocytoscopic diagnosis of esophageal cancer ex vivo, and they consistently obtained sufficient image quality of squamous cell carcinoma in a freshly resected specimen [3].

The following case was gastric adenoma, located on the lesser curvature at the lower gastric body (Fig. 2a). Endocytoscopic images were as follows: tubular glands were homogeneous in size; nuclei were fusiform and regularly arranged along the basement membrane; there was only a slight disorder of polarity; and cellular density was low (Fig. 2b).

The next case was superficial elevated gastric cancer (type IIa), located on the lesser curvature at the lower body. Endocytoscopic images were as follows: nuclei were arranged in the luminal side of the gland, and irregularly larger glands were observed (Fig. 3). This lesion was resected using endoscopic submucosal dissection (ESD). Histology showed well-differentiated adenocarcinoma, pT1(m), ly0, v0. Until now we could not distinguish differentiated tubular adenocarcinoma and gastric adenoma by endocytoscopic findings alone.

The last case was superficial type depressed gastric cancer (type IIc), located on the anterior portion at the upper body. Endocytoscopic images were as follows: there were marked deformities and enlargement of nuclei, and gastric gland structure was not recognized (Fig. 4). This histology was poorly differentiated tubular adenocarcinoma. Because of the patient's age and bronchial asthma, he underwent ESD therapy.

Endocytoscopic diagnosis depends on the abnormality of structures and cells. It is almost equivalent to the common histological diagnosis with hematoxylin and eosin (H&E) stain. There are many reports concerning the usefulness of endocytoscopy for the diagnosis of esophageal cancer. Kumagai et al. [1] reported the higher density of cells, the more irregular cell distribution, cell heterogeneity, and the higher irregularity of nuclei in esophageal cancer compared with that in the normal esophageal

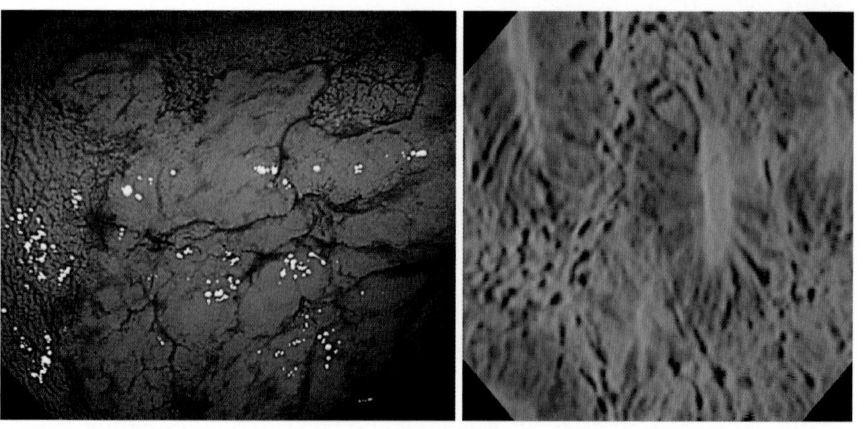

Fig. 2. **a** Endoscopic finding of gastric adenoma. **b** Endocytoscopic image of gastric adenoma in living cell

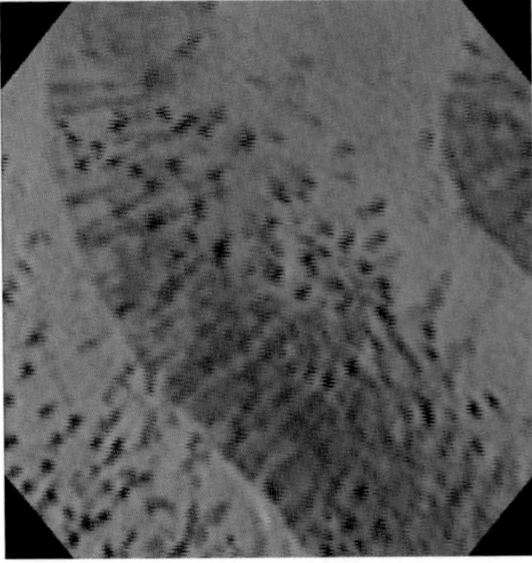

Fig. 3. Endocytoscopic image of superficial elevated gastric cancer (type IIa, well-differentiated tubular adenocarcinoma)

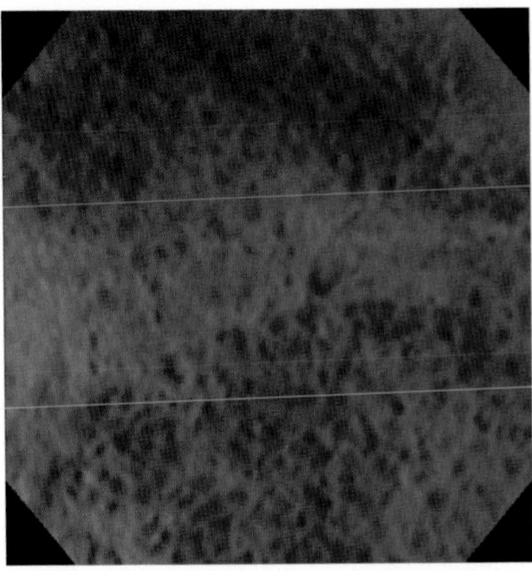

Fig. 4. Endocytoscopic image of superficial depressed gastric cancer (type IIc, poorly differentiated tubular adenocarcinoma)

mucosa. In general, it is common to diagnose the malignancy of columnar epithelium from the point of view of the arrangement of glands, the size and uniformity of glands, the size of nuclei, the ratio of nucleus to cytoplasm, and so on. However, we know it is easier and clearer to observe the esophageal mucosa than gastric mucosa using endocytoscopy because there is a smaller content of mucus in the esophagus than in the stomach. Mucus covering the lesion is one of the biggest factors that disturb the acquisition of high-quality endocytoscopic images. The catheter type of endocytoscopy has an advantage and a disadvantage. The advantage is that we can use conventional endoscopy and through the working channel obtain endocytoscopic images. The soft-catheter type of endocytoscopy also has limitations: the image is slightly smaller for the diagnosis of the structure of gastric glands, and we can see only one or two gastric glands in one frame. We must repeatedly move the endoscope to get new images to obtain an accurate diagnosis. Also, because of its instability, this type cannot regularly obtain high-quality endocytoscopic images. In the near future we will have integrated-type endoscopy combining the advantageous aspects of magnifying endoscopy and endocytoscopy. We might see endocytoscopic images that are larger than the present images. In the integrated type, we might be able to compare the usual magnifying endoscopy (80×) and ultrahigh magnifying endoscopy (400–500×).

Comparison Between ECS and Confocal Endomicroscopy

Confocal endomicroscopy is another super-magnifying endoscopy with which we can see the microstructure and the microvessels in the living cell after the injection of fluorescein sodium [4,5]. These images are digital images, which are clearer images. We compared the two super-magnification endoscopic methods in Table 1 [6]. Confocal endomicroscopy is still in the development stage because the acquisition of images is unstable, a higher quality of images is required, and the scopes used were still large and had need for a fluorescent agent, which has the potential to evoke allergy. The depth of observation was 0–30 μm for endocytoscopy and 0–250 μm for confocal endomicroscopy. On the other hand, endocytoscopy also has some problems to date. We must use methylene blue, which is reported to cause DNA damage in combination with the strong light used, for the endocytoscopic dye [7,8]. We need a safer and better contrast agent for endocytoscopy. Using endocytoscopy, we can see only the shallowest epithelium on the horizontal image. Because sometimes we contact and scrub the epithelium, we can see the shallowest epithelium come off.

Table 1. Ultra-high magnifying endoscopy.

	Endocytoscopy	Confocal endomicroscopy
magnification	Prototype I:450 (24Inc) Prototype II:1,100	500
method	Probe type or integrated endocytescopy Contact ultramagnifying endoscopy by optical image	Integrated type Administration of fluorescein. No intake into nucleus Intake into cytoplasm
Expression of nucleus	yes	Depend on contrast agent (Acriflavine can express nucleus.)
merits	Real time expression. The ratio of nucleus and cytoplasm was assessed.	Clear image. possibility of expression of target cell by the development of specific fluorescent material
demerits	Side effect of methylene blue	Allergy against fluorescent agent

Future

Knowing the histology in real time during ongoing endoscopy has led to the ability to give immediate judgment on the diagnosis of benign or malignant. Now we can observe the microsurface and microvascural structure of gastric lesion and diagnose the lateral margin of early gastric cancer clearly using magnifying endoscopy with NBI. If we have the integrated type of magnifying endoscopy and endocytoscopy, it will be very useful in deciding the margin of lesions for ESD. Ultrahigh magnifying endoscopy might bring us to a still higher level of endoscopic diagnosis.

References

1. Kumagai Y, Monma K, Kawada K (2004) Magnifying chromoendoscopy of the esophagus: in vivo pathological diagnosis using an endocytoscopy system. Endoscopy 36:590–594
2. Inoue H, Kazawa T, Satodate H, et al (2004) In vivo observation of living cancer cells in the esophagus, stomach, and colon using catheter type contact endoscope, "endocytoscopy system." Gastrointest Endosc Clin N Am 14:589–594
3. Fujishiro M, Takubo K, Sato Y, et al (2007) Potential and present limitation of endocytoscopy in the diagnosis of esophageal squamous-cell carcinoma: a multicenter ex vivo pilot study. Gastrointest Endosc 66:551–555
4. Kiesslich R, Burg J, Vieth M, et al (2004) Confocal laser endoscopy for diagnosing intraepithelial neoplasias and colorectal cancer in vivo. Gastroenterology 127:706–713
5. Kitabatake S, Niwa Y, Miyahara R, et al (2006) Confocal endomicroscopy for the diagnosis of gastric cancer in vivo. Endoscopy 38:1110–1114
6. Niwa Y, Miyahara R, Matsuura T, et al (2007) Endocytoscopy for esophageal cancer ex vivo. Dig Endosc 19:S166–S169
7. Olliver JR, Wind CP, Sahay P, et al (2003) Chromoendoscopy with methylene blue and associated DNA damage in Barrett's oesophagus. Lancet 362:373–374
8. Hardie LJ, Olliver JR, Wild CP, et al (2004) Chromoendoscopy with methylene blue and the risk of DNA damage. Gastroenterology 126:623 (author reply 623–624)

Endoscopic Ultrasonography Diagnosis for Depressed Type Early Gastric Cancer: Tissue Characterization in Cases Associated with Fibrosis

Junko Fujisaki

Summary. There is a limitation in the improvement of diagnostic accuracy in endoscopic ultrasonography (EUS) diagnosis because of the presence of scar in early gastric cancer. We evaluated EUS diagnosis of early gastric cancer with fibrosis applying measurement echo level. The 55 patients underwent EUS and were histologically confirmed to have early gastric cancer. All the cases underwent EUS and were diagnosed with fibrotis. We clipped an area of interest from the image and investigated the configuration of the margin of the clipped area. A histogram in the area of interest was measured on Photoshop. The overall diagnostic accuracy was 67% (37/55). Irregularity was identified in the marginal configuration of the third layer in 6/30 (20%) and in 11/25 (44%) of submucosal (SM) cancers. Difference in SM invasion and fibrosis by histogram showed the mean value of measurement of the area of interest by histogram was 90.7 for mucosal (M) cancer and 57.8 for SM cancer, showing a significant difference between M and SM cancer. The use of echo level can contribute to the tumor depth diagnosis in cases associated with scar. The combination of echo level and the configuration of the margin can increase the accuracy rate of early gastric cancer with fibrosis.

Key words. Early gastric cancer, EUS, Fibrosis, Tissue characterization, Echo level

Introduction

Since the establishment of fundamental knowledge about the walls and layers of the gastrointestinal tract by Aibe et al. [1], endoscopic ultrasonography (EUS) has been reported to be useful in the tumor depth diagnosis of early gastric cancer [2].

The diagnostic accuracy of EUS for early gastric cancer before endoscopic treatment has been reported to be more than 90%, demonstrating its usefulness. However, because of the presence of scar in gastric cancer, there is a limitation in the improvement of diagnostic accuracy, and different diagnostic criteria have been reported

Cancer Institute Hospital, 3-10-6 Ariake, Koto-ku, Tokyo 135-8550, Japan

[3–5]. Subsequently, the development of three-dimensional endoscopic ultrasonography (3D-EUS) has enabled us to obtain multiple images instantly once the lesion is scanned, even if we cannot choose an adequate image immediately, and to search for images at the deepest site after examination, thus contributing to improvement in the diagnosis of tumor depth [6,7].

Recently, a wide variety of therapies including endoscopic submucosal dissection (ESD) and laparoscopic treatment have been applied to cases associated with scar, necessitating an improvement in the accuracy of preoperative diagnosis of tumor depth. Efforts have been made to improve the diagnostic accuracy in cases with scar by focusing on the configuration of the EUS image. In this study, we focused on the difference in cell density in the invasive lesion and fibrosis layer as well as on the image configuration to investigate whether assessing the internal echo level may contribute to an improvement in diagnostic accuracy.

Materials and Methods

The study subjects included 55 patients in whom upper gastrointestinal endoscopy had revealed fold convergence macroscopically and diagnosis of early gastric cancer associated with ulcer scar had been made. The 55 patients underwent EUS and were histologically confirmed to have early gastric cancer, including 30 mucosal (M) cancers and 25 cancers with submucosal (SM) invasion. The diagnosis of tumor depth was according to the Japanese Classification of Gastric Carcinoma [8].

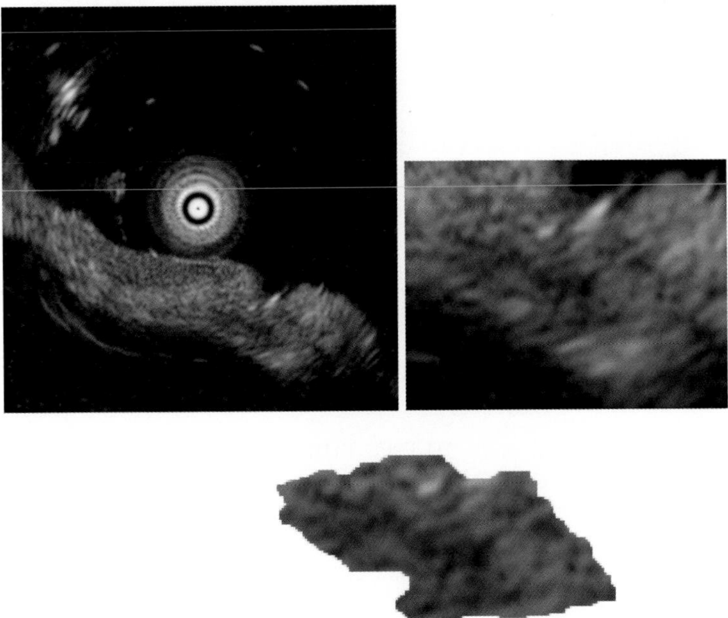

Fig. 1. An area of interest was clipped from the image, and the configuration of the margin of the clipped area was investigated

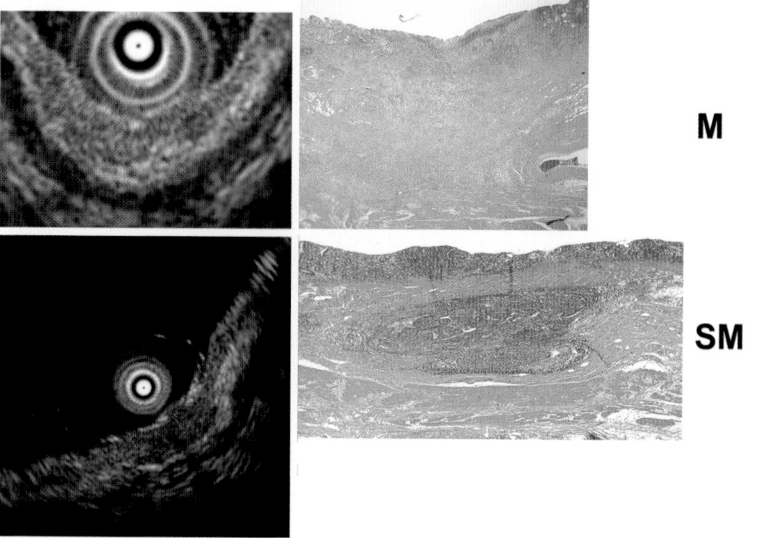

Fig. 2. The endoscopic ultrasonography (EUS) image was compared to the histology, focusing on the difference in the echo level between the area of cancer invasion and that of fibrosis. *M*, mucosal; *SM*, submucosal

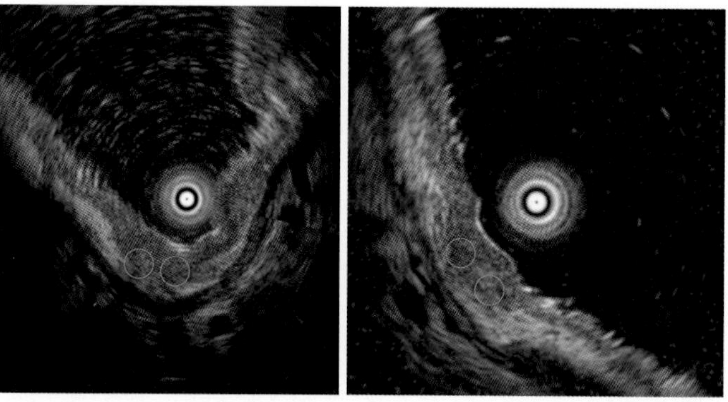

Fig. 3. Several areas of interest in the image of the third or deeper area were set

The instruments used were 3D-EUS, EUIP2, and EUIP2 viewer 12, 20 MHz (Olympus Medical Systems, Tokyo, Japan). EUS was carried out using a water-filling technique. An image was chosen from the 3-D images, and diagnostic accuracy of EUS was investigated. The diagnosis of tumor depth in cases with ulcer scar was based on the classification by Kida et al. [3]. We clipped an area of interest from the image and investigated the configuration of the margin of the clipped area (Fig. 1).

We compared the EUS image to histology and focused on the difference in the echo level between the area of cancer invasion and that of fibrosis (Fig. 2). We set several areas of interest in the image of the third or deeper layers (Fig. 3). A histogram in the

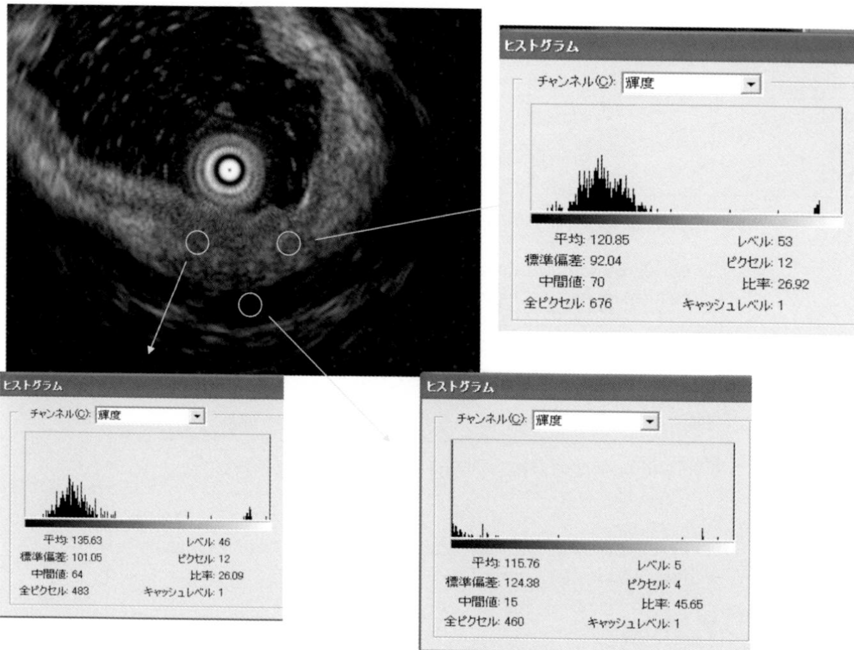

Fig. 4. Echo levels by the mean of the median values and by the difference in the median of the muscularis mucosa were compared

area of interest was measured on Photoshop. We compared echo levels by the mean of the median values and by the difference in the median of the muscularis propria layer (Fig. 4).

Results

Diagnostic Accuracy by EUS and Endoscopy

The overall diagnostic accuracy was 67% (37/55 cases). The diagnostic accuracy was 50% (15/30 cases) in M cancers and 80% (20/25) in SM cancers (Table 1). Furthermore, when SM cancers were divided into SM1 and SM2, the correct diagnosis was made in 15% (2/13) of cases for SM1 and 83% (10/12) of cases for SM2. When the accuracy was compared between endoscopic diagnosis and EUS diagnosis in 30 cases that were histologically diagnosed as M cancers, the proper diagnosis of M cancer was made by both EUS and endoscopy in 47% (14/30 cases). The diagnostic accuracy by EUS alone was 50% (15/30 cases). Overdiagnosis of M cancer as SM cancer was made by both EUS and endoscopy in 30% (9/30 cases) (Table 2). Thus, the presence of fibrosis in M cancers led to the overinterpretation as SM cancers and resulted in the overdiagnosis.

Among the 25 cases that were histologically diagnosed as SM cancers, the proper diagnosis of SM cancers was made in 28% (7/25) of cases by both endoscopy and EUS,

Table 1. EUS Diagnosis.

	EUS Diagnosis			
Pathological Diagnosis	M	SM1	SM2	Accuracy rate
M	15	7	8	15/30 (50)
SM1	3	2	8	2/13 (15)
SM2	2	0	10	10/12 (83)

Table 2. EUS and Endoscopically Diagnosis of depth especially intramucosal lesion. (n = 30)

	EUS	
Endoscopy	M (%)	SM (%)
M	14 (47)	6 (20)
SM	1 (3)	9 (30)

EUS and Endocopy Over diagnosis = 9 cases

Table 3. EUS and Endoscopically Diagnosis of depth especially submucosal lesion. (n = 25)

	EUS	
Endoscopy	M (%)	SM (%)
M	3 (12)	14 (56)
SM	1 (5)	7 (27)

Table 4. The Marginal Configration.

	Smooth	Irregularity of the margin	Case number (%)	
M	24	6	6/30 (20)	
SM1	7	6	6/13 (46)	11/25 (44)
SM2	7	5	5/12 (42)	

but in 84% (21/25) by EUS alone and 32% (8/25) by endoscopy alone, demonstrating the higher diagnostic accuracy in EUS (Table 3).

Marginal Configuration (Table 4)

Irregularity was identified in the marginal configuration of the third layer in 6/30 (20%) M cancers and in 11/25 (44%) SM cancers. Although marginal irregularity was infrequently found in M cancers, it was only seen in less than half of SM cancers.

Difference in SM Invasion and Fibrosis by Histogram (Table 5)

The mean value of measurements of the area of interest by histogram was 90.7 for M cancers and 57.8 for SM cancers, showing a significant difference between the M and SM cancers ($P < 0.01$).

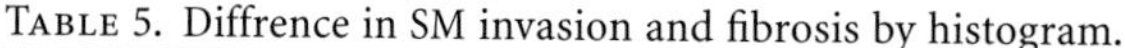
TABLE 5. Diffrence in SM invasion and fibrosis by histogram.

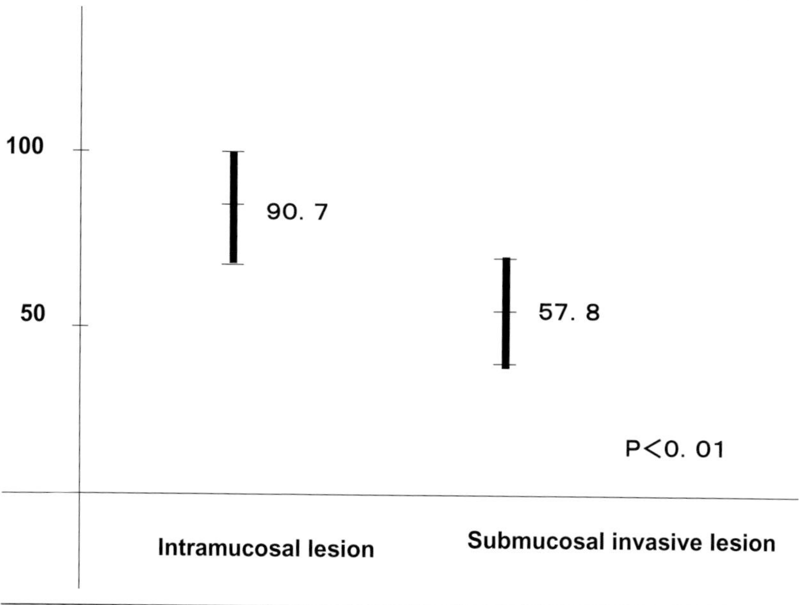

TABLE 6. Combination Diagnosis of Depth using Echo lebel and the marginal configuration.

	EUS			
Pathology	M	SM1	SM2	
M	20	6	4	20/30 (67)
SM1	2	2	9	2/13 (15)
SM2	1	0	11	11/12 (91)

Combination Diagnosis of Depth Using Echo Level and Marginal Configuration (Table 6)

Mean values of the histogram (upper, 90.7; lower, 57.8) were criteria of fibrosis and cancer invasion. Intramucosal cancer with fibrosis is progressing in accurate diagnosis using a combination of echo level and marginal configuration. Submucosal invasive lesion with fibrosis is progressing in accurate diagnosis also.

Case Presentation

EUS showed a depressed configuration, suggestive of a cancer with SM invasion, but subsequent histology revealed M cancer associated with ulcer fibrosis (Ul2) (Fig. 5).

The mean value of the histogram in the depressed lesion was 173 ± 23 and that in the muscularis propria layer was 23 ± 12, with a difference of 153 ± 11, showing a higher value than the mean in SM cancers. SM cancer was suspected by EUS image,

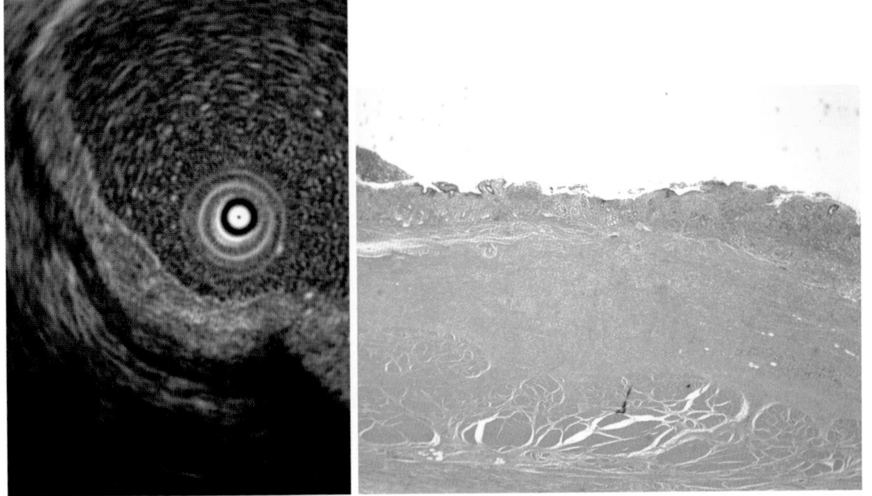

Fig. 5. **a** EUS showed a depressed configuration. **b** Histology revealed M cancer associated with ulcer fibrosis

but the mean value of the histogram suggested that the component was fibrosis alone.

Discussion

There have been many reports on tumor depth diagnosis of early gastric cancer. Although there have been satisfactory reports on the tumor depth diagnosis in determining the indication of EMR (endoscopic mucosal resection) or ESD (endoscopic submucosal dissection), the tumor depth diagnosis of early gastric cancer, in contrast to colon cancer, was influenced by the presence of scar. There is a limitation in the tumor depth diagnosis in cases associated with fibrosis, with a diagnostic accuracy limited to around 70% [3–5]. In addition, criteria for tumor depth diagnosis in cases associated with fibrosis slightly varies among reports [3–5]. In cases associated with fibrosis, it is not infrequent that determination of whether there is fibrosis alone or there is cancer invasion within fibrosis is difficult from the configuration alone.

Recently, UL (+) M cancer of less than 3 cm is regarded as a lesion of expanded indication for ESD by a treatment guideline for early gastric cancer [9]. In cases with UL (+), however, because it is difficult to dissect the fibrous part by ESD, an artifact on the resected specimen is strong and tumor depth diagnosis is difficult by histopathological examinations, requiring additional gastric resection in some cases. In addition, with the increasingly widespread application of ESD, this procedure can be performed as a conception of total biopsy; e.g., surgery is performed if SM (submucosal invasive lesion) is identified by histopathological examinations after ESD. As the technology of ESD advances, such a situation increasingly occurs, leading to lower levels of preoperative diagnosis and waste of medical funds. To improve the accuracy of tumor depth diagnosis for early gastric cancer, it is necessary to improve the diagnostic accuracy in UL (+). In the past, tumor depth diagnosis was made by changes

surgery. Proper staging can only be accomplished through histological analysis achieved by performing an endoscopic resection.

Indications for Endoscopic Resection of Early Gastric Cancer

Currently accepted indications for EMR of EGC include small intramucosal lesions of the differentiated type (Fig. 1) [6].

This guideline is based on the knowledge that larger-size lesions and undifferentiated type lesions are more likely to extend into the SM layer and thus have a higher risk of LN metastasis. In addition, en bloc resection of large lesions has oftentimes been too difficult technically until the more recent development of the ESD technique.

At present, the accepted indications for conventional EMR are (1) differentiated type elevated cancers ≤20 mm in diameter and (2) differentiated type small depressed lesions ≤10 mm without ulceration. All such lesions must be moderately or well-differentiated cancers confined to the mucosa and have no lymphatic or vascular involvement histologically.

Clinical observations have noted, however, that the present criteria for endoscopic resection may be too strict, leading to unnecessary surgery [3]. The currently accepted indications for endoscopic resection assumed conventional EMR as the primary treatment strategy. Recent advances in the ESD technique now make it possible, however, to resect larger intramucosal GC lesions and SM1 GC lesions, so expanded criteria have been proposed for endoscopic resection. The upper limit of the 95% confidence interval (CI) calculated from earlier studies, however, was too broad for clinical use because of small sample sizes.

Using a large database involving more than 5000 patients who underwent gastrectomy with meticulous R2 level LN dissection, Gotoda et al. [1] recently further defined the risk of LN metastasis in additional groups of EGC patients with increased certainty (Table 1). According to their intramucosal cancer findings, none of the 1230

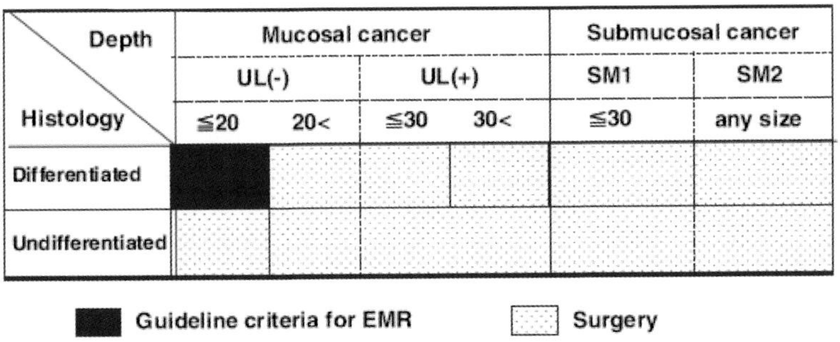

Depth	Mucosal cancer				Submucosal cancer	
	UL(-)		UL(+)		SM1	SM2
Histology	≤20	20<	≤30	30<	≤30	any size
Differentiated						
Undifferentiated						

Guideline criteria for EMR　　Surgery

Fig. 1. Current guideline criteria for endoscopic mucosal resection (EMR) of early gastric cancer (EGC)

Table 1. Early gastric cancer (EGC) with no risk of lymph node metastasis.

Criterion	Incidence (%)	95% CI
Intramucosal EGC Differentiated adenocarcinoma No lymphovascular invasion Irrespective of ulcer findings Tumor ≤30 mm in size	0/1230 (0%)	0%–0.3%
Intramucosal EGC Differentiated adenocarcinoma No lymphovascular invasion Without ulcer findings Irrespective of tumor size	0/929 (0%)	0%–0.4%
Undifferentiated intramucosal cancer No lymphovascular invasion Without ulcer findings Tumor ≤20 mm in size	0/141 (0%)	0%–2.6%
Minute submucosal penetration (SM1) Differentiated adenocarcinoma No lymphovascular invasion Tumor ≤30 mm in size	0/145 (0%)	0%–2.5%

differentiated lesions ≤30 mm in size was associated with LN metastasis regardless of ulceration (95% CI, 0%–0.3%). Similarly, none of the 929 differentiated lesions without ulceration was associated with LN metastasis regardless of lesion size (95% CI, 0%–0.4%).

As for SM invasive cancer, there was a significant correlation between tumors >30 mm in size and lymphatic-vascular involvement with an increased risk of LN metastasis. In addition, those cancers penetrating deep into the SM layer were the most likely to be associated with regional LN metastasis. The subgroup of 145 histologically differentiated lesions ≤30 mm in size with no lymphatic-vascular involvement and SM1 penetration as classified according to the Japanese Classification of Gastric Carcinoma, however, was entirely free of LN metastasis (95% CI, 0%–2.5%).

Last, none of the 141 undifferentiated histological lesions without ulceration ≤20 mm in size was associated with a positive LN finding (95% CI, 0%–2.6%). The mortality of patients who have undergone standard gastrectomy with LN dissection at our hospital is 0.2% to 0.5%. Considering surgical mortality and the 99% 5-year survival rate for mucosal cancer, considerable controversy exists concerning the appropriate treatment strategy for patients with mucosal cancer consisting of the undifferentiated histology type. A recent report based on a large series has shown that EGC with signet-ring cell carcinoma has a low rate of LN metastasis, suggesting that mucosal cancer with signet-ring cell carcinoma could also be a candidate for less-invasive surgery [7].

These groups of patients were shown to have a low risk or no risk of LN metastasis, which is significant when considering the risk of mortality from surgery. The results of this study have facilitated the development of an expanded list of candidates suitable for endoscopic resection primarily using the ESD technique [8] (Fig. 2), because

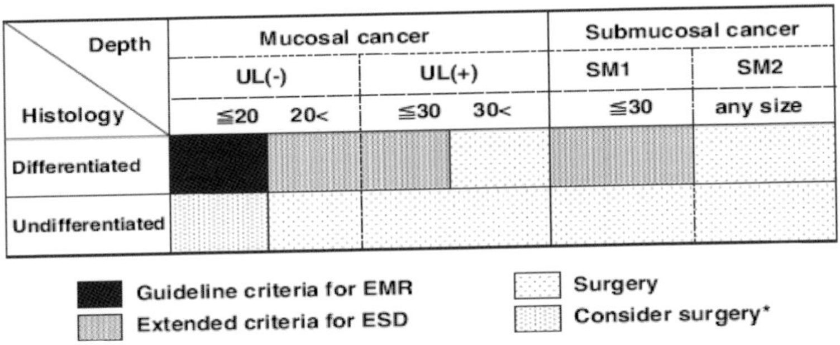

Depth / Histology	Mucosal cancer				Submucosal cancer	
	UL(-)		UL(+)		SM1	SM2
	≦20	20<	≦30	30<	≦30	any size
Differentiated						
Undifferentiated						

Guideline criteria for EMR
Extended criteria for ESD
Surgery
Consider surgery*

Fig. 2. Proposed expanded criteria for endoscopic mucosal resection (EMR) and endoscopic submucosal dissection (ESD) of early gastric cancer (EGC)

lesions covered by these proposed extended criteria for endoscopic resection would previously have been resected in a piecemeal fashion if treated by conventional EMR.

Importance of En Bloc Resection

EMR has been successfully practiced in Japan for the past two decades for the removal of small EGC. Outcomes involving EMR of larger intramucosal carcinomas of the stomach, however, have been less favorable. Piecemeal resections required during the removal of larger lesions can lead to a higher risk of local recurrence and make it more difficult for pathologists to render precise depth and margin assessments.

The minimal risk of LN involvement in large EGC coupled with the potential curative role of endoscopic therapy, however, has provided the impetus for the development of a new technique of endoscopic resection to overcome the limitations associated with piecemeal resections. ESD was specifically developed to allow en bloc resections of even larger lesions [9]. An en bloc resected specimen provides proper orientation, sectioning, and margin assessment, resulting in improved pathological examination. Accurate histopathology is critical because the criteria for a curative endoscopic resection are based on careful assessment of the serial sectioning of a pathological specimen. The ESD technique also allows en bloc resections to be performed through fibrotic SM tissue, which is commonly found during resections of ulcerated EGC.

Endoscopic Submucosal Dissection (ESD)

ESD for EGC has been explored since the early 1990s and is increasingly practiced throughout Japan. The popularity of the technique can be attributed to the technical ability to endoscopically remove large EGCs en bloc with less morbidity and mortality compared to the more invasive surgical alternatives.

ESD using a variety of specially created endoscopic knives has been developed for en bloc resection using a standard single-channel gastroscope (Fig. 3). This procedure has the major advantage of being able to achieve large and en bloc resections.

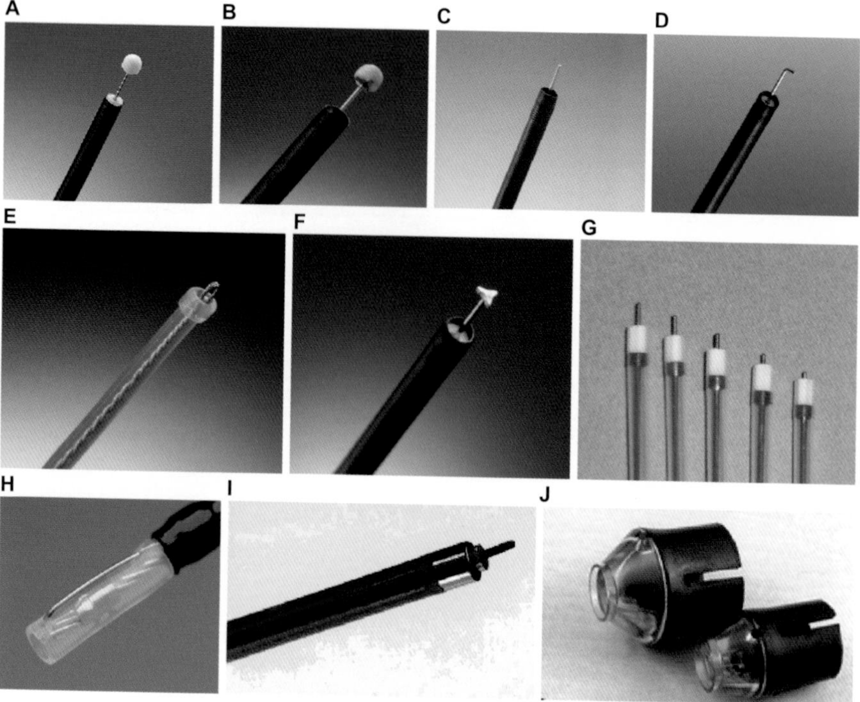

FIG. 3. Endoscopic devices for ESD. **A** Insulation-tipped surgical knife (IT knife) (KD-610L, Olympus Medical Systems). **B** Modified IT knife with three-pointed star blade (KD-611L, Olympus Medical Systems). **C** Needle knife (KD-1L-1, Olympus Medical Systems). **D** Hook knife (KD-620LR, Olympus Medical Systems). **E** Flex knife (KD-630L, Olympus Medical Systems). **F** Triangle-tipped knife (Olympus Medical Systems). **G** Flash knives with several needle lengths (Fujinon Toshiba ES Systems). **H** Mucosectom (DP-2518, Pentax). **I** Bipolar needle knife (B-knife; Xemex). **J** Small-caliber tip transparent (ST) hood (DH-15GR, 15CR; Fujinon Toshiba ES Systems)

ESD consists of three steps: first, injecting solution into the SM layer to separate the lesion from the muscle layer; next, predetermined circumferential cutting of the mucosa surrounding the lesion; and, finally, dissection of the SM connective tissue under the lesion.

Marking the periphery of the lesion (Fig. 4A–C) is performed using a standard needle knife (or hook knife, flex knife, triangle-tipped knife, or flash knife) with a forced 20 W coagulation current (ICC200; ERBE, Tubingen, Germany). After injection with diluted epinephrine (1 : 100 000) to raise the SM layer, a small initial incision (Fig. 4D) to insert the tip of an insulation-tipped surgical knife (IT knife) into the SM layer is made by a standard needle knife in the 80 W ENDO-CUT mode with effect 3 (ICC200, ERBE).

Circumferential mucosal cutting at the periphery of the marking dots (Fig. 4E–G) is then performed using the IT knife in 80 W ENDO-CUT mode. A ceramic ball at the tip of the IT knife prevents perforation of the muscle layer. After completion of the

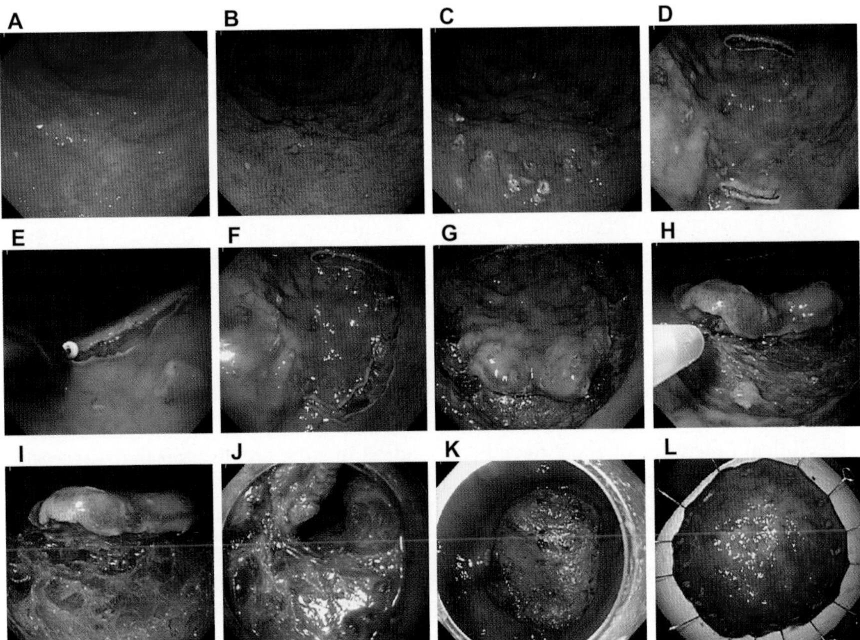

Fig. 4. ESD procedures. **A** Locally recurrent tumor on greater curvature of gastric antrum after piecemeal EMR. **B** Indigo carmine dye spray for determining tumor margin. **C** Markings made by needle knife with coagulation current. **D** Initial incision made using needle knife in ENDO-CUT mode after injection of diluted epinephrine. **E** Ceramic ball prevents perforation of muscle layer. **F** Mucosal cutting using IT knife in ENDO-CUT mode. **G** Circumferential mucosal cutting at periphery of marking dots. **H** Additional submucosal (SM) injection with diluted epinephrine after completing circumferential cutting. **I** Dissecting SM layer using IT knife in ENDO-CUT mode. **J** Attachment cap for stretching SM tissue. **K** Large ESD ulcer bed after complete en bloc resection without perforation. **L** Flattened periphery of ESD specimen using thin needles on plate

circumferential cutting, additional diluted epinephrine is injected into the SM layer (Fig. 4H).

The SM layer under the lesion is directly dissected (Fig. 4I) with the IT knife using a lateral movement. It is important to cut tangentially at the SM layer to avoid perforation. Indigo carmine dye previously injected into the SM layer helps to identify it. Additional diluted epinephrine can be injected into the SM at any time to raise and confirm the SM layer. An attachment cap (Olympus Medical Systems, Tokyo, Japan) is frequently used to provide traction for the resected specimen and help exfoliate the SM tissue (Fig. 4J). ESD can provide a large en bloc resection without size limitation (Fig. 4K). Finally, the resected specimen is retrieved using grasping forceps.

The ESD technique allows for the one-piece removal of ulcerated gastric lesions and the resection of recurrent EGC after an unsuccessful EMR. It was extremely difficult, if not impossible, to resect these lesions previously by conventional EMR techniques because SM fibrosis prevented adequate lifting of the mucosal lesion by SM injection.

Despite requiring additional technical skill and involving a longer procedure time, the ESD technique is now accepted as a standard treatment for EGC. In fact, the Japanese government recently approved insurance coverage for ESD treatment costs at twice the rate for conventional EMR, primarily because of its demonstrated effectiveness in the en bloc removal of large EGCs.

ESD is associated with significant drawbacks, however, including longer procedure times and a higher risk of complications. It also requires extensive training, so a standardized ESD training program is needed to ensure its successful dissemination in the future.

Clinical Outcomes of Endoscopic Resection for EGC

The clinical outcomes of EMR have been studied in such great detail that successful outcomes observed from these studies have allowed EMR to become the standard treatment for EGC in Japan. Kojima et al [10] reviewed the outcomes of EMR from 12 major Japanese institutions. The inject, lift and cut, EMR with a cap-fitted panendoscope (EMR-C), and EMR with ligatim (EMR-L) techniques were most commonly used and achieved en bloc resections in approximately three-quarters of all patients who underwent such techniques. The disease-specific survival rate was 99%, although not all studies reported long-term outcomes.

As previously indicated, however, standard EMR techniques are associated with a higher risk of recurrence, especially when resections are piecemeal or resection margins are not tumor free histologically. The risk of local recurrence after EMR varies from 2% to 35%. In some specialized centers in Japan, studies on the long-term outcomes of patients who have had endoscopic resections using the expanded criteria are currently under way. The incidence of metachronous multiple GC in patients who have undergone endoscopic resection on their first lesions also needs to be prospectively investigated to determine the appropriate interval for effective surveillance endoscopy.

Future Prospects

The endoscopic resection technique has been demonstrated to be safe, effective, and applicable to a wide range of clinical situations. Rapid technological progress in combination with the development of ESD has been responsible for advances in the endoscopic resection of not only EGC but also esophageal and colorectal cancers [11].

Although several endoscopic devices have been developed to make ESD easier and safer, this technique still requires a highly experienced endoscopist because the procedure is performed using a single gastroscope, thus requiring one-handed surgery. More recently, procedures involving countertraction of lesions such as percutaneous traction-assisted EMR (PTA-EMR), magnetic-anchor-guided (MAG) ESD, and sinker-assisted ESD have been described in various published reports.

To further extend the indications for treating EGC with less-invasive surgery, endoscopic resection combined with laparoscopic regional LN dissection should be given serious consideration. In addition, an endoscopic full-thickness resection technique is now being developed that should be available in the near future for the treatment of even deeper carcinomas without LN metastasis.

Conclusions

The major advantage of the ESD technique compared to standard EMR methods is that an en bloc resection with a tumor-free margin is possible even for large tumors and tumors with ulceration scarring. On the other hand, ESD has the following disadvantages: a longer procedure time, a higher complication rate for bleeding and perforation, and the requirement of a higher degree of technical skill. A suitable training program must be developed, therefore, before widespread dissemination of this technique will be feasible.

The development of the novel ESD technique and the recent detailed histopathological analysis of a large EGC series allow for the original EMR guideline criteria to be expanded so as to include ESD of EGC. The results so far have been highly encouraging, although long-term outcome data are still unavailable.

References

1. Gotoda T, Yanagisawa A, Sasako M, et al (2000) Incidence of lymph node metastasis from early gastric cancer: estimation with a large number of cases at two large centers. Gastric Cancer 3:219–325
2. Rembacken BJ, Gotoda T, Fujii T, et al (2001) Endoscopic mucosal resection. Endoscopy 33:709–718
3. Japanese Gastric Cancer Association (1998) Japanese classification of gastric carcinoma, 2nd English edition. Gastric Cancer 1:10–24
4. Sasako M, Kinoshita T, Maruyama K (1993) Prognosis of early gastric cancer (in Japanese with English abstract). Stomach Intest 28:139–146
5. Gotoda T, Sasako M, Ono H, et al (2001) An evaluation of the necessity of gastrectomy with lymph node dissection for patients with submucosal invasive gastric cancer. Br J Surg 88:444–449
6. Yamao T, Shirao K, Ono H, et al (1996) Risk factors for lymph node metastasis from intramucosal gastric carcinoma. Cancer (Phila) 77:602–606
7. Hyung WJ, Noh SH, Lee JH, et al (2002) Early gastric carcinoma with signet ring cell histology. Cancer (Phila) 94:78–83
8. Soetikno R, Kaltenbach T, Yeh R, et al (2005) Endoscopic mucosal resection for early cancers of the upper gastrointestinal tract. J Clin Oncol 23:4490–4498
9. Ono H, Kondo H, Gotoda T, et al (2001) Endoscopic mucosal resection for treatment of early gastric cancer. Gut 48:225–229
10. Kojima T, Parra-Blanco A, Takahashi H, et al (1998) Outcome of endoscopic mucosal resection for early gastric cancer: review of the Japanese literature. Gastrointest Endosc 48:550–554
11. Saito Y, Uraoka T, Matsuda T, et al (2007) Endoscopic treatment of large superficial colorectal tumors: a case series of 200 endoscopic submucosal dissections (with video). Gastrointest Endosc 66:966–973

Features of Therapeutic Devices for Gastric Endoscopic Submucosal Dissection and Basic Techniques

Naohisa Yahagi

Summary. Many endoscopic mucosal resection (EMR) techniques have been developed in Japan for the treatment of gastric mucosal lesions. They have become a popular practice not only in Japan but also in many Western countries. However, conventional EMR techniques have limitations in size and location. Piecemeal resection often becomes necessary in the case of large and difficult lesions. En bloc resection is desirable, because histological evaluations are essential to estimate the risk for lymph node metastasis, and prevention of local recurrence is also very important. To conduct reliable en bloc resection, endoscopic submucosal dissection (ESD) was developed using new electrosurgical knives specially designed for the ESD technique. The way of conducting an actual ESD procedure differs depending on the features of each knife. Operators should fully understand the features of these knives and select the appropriate one according to the situation and their skills. ESD is a wonderful technique that realizes en bloc resection of relatively large and difficult lesions that are impossible to treat by the conventional EMR technique.

Key words. Gastric ESD, IT knife, Hook knife, Flex knife, TT knife

Introduction

Many endoscopic mucosal resection (EMR) techniques have been developed in Japan for the treatment of gastric mucosal lesions. Among these techniques, strip biopsy [1] and aspiration mucosectomy using an attached hood on the tip of the endoscope [2,3] have become popular practices for their convenience. However, the specimens obtained by these techniques have limitations in size (approximately 10–20 mm, according to tumor location and operator skills), and piecemeal resection often becomes necessary in the case of larger tumors. En bloc resection is desirable, especially in larger tumors, because histological evaluations are essential to estimate the risk for lymph node metastasis. Moreover, it is also very important to prevent local

Department of Gastroenterology, Toranomon Hospital, 2-2-2 Toranomon, Minato-ku, Tokyo 105-8470, Japan recurrence, because a notably high recurrence rate after piecemeal resection has been reported [4]. There was a more reliable technique, endoscopic mucosal resection with hypertonic saline and epinephrine (ERHSE), done by incising the surrounding mucosa of the target lesion with a needle knife then resecting the lesion with a snare [5], but this technique still had limitations in size and location of the tumor, and it was rather difficult.

Endoscopic submucosal dissection (ESD) techniques using the diathermic needle knife [6], the insulated-tip diathermic knife (IT knife) [7], or the tip of a thin-type snare [8] have been introduced to overcome those disadvantages. However, different problems have emerged: safe control of the needle knife was difficult, precise control of the thin-type snare was troublesome, and the IT knife required unusual scope control for a successful procedure; also, higher complication rates for the IT knife, i.e., 22% of bleeding and 5% of perforation [9], were reported. Therefore, new instruments, including the hook knife, the flex knife, and the triangle tip (TT) knife, were developed to provide a much easier and safer ESD. The features of these devices and the settings of the standard ESD procedure are described in this chapter.

Materials for ESD Procedure

Endoscope

The maneuverability of the endoscope is the most important factor for successful ESD. The multibending scope (Fig. 1) (GIF-Q260-2TM, Olympus Medical Systems, Tokyo, Japan), which has a second bending channel at the proximal part of the conventional bending channel, is very useful for approaching difficult locations such as widely opened gastric angles, cardia, or fornix [10]. The water irrigation system integrated into therapeutic endoscopes (GIF Q260-2TM and GIF Q260-J; Olympus Medical Systems) is very useful to clarify the bleeding points during the procedure.

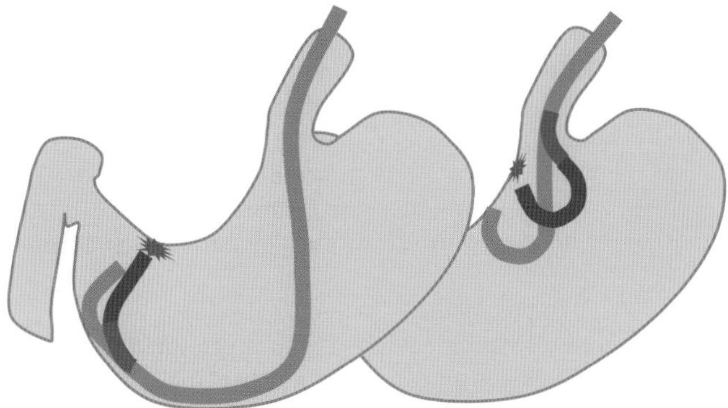

Fig. 1. The multibending scope has a second up-and-down channel at the proximal part of the conventional vending channel, which is very useful to approach a difficult location

Distal Attachment

It is strongly recommended to attach a transparent hood at the tip of the endoscope to conduct ESD safely. The edge of the hood can be used like a surgical forceps to open an incised wound to obtain better vision of the operating field, or to gently hold the tissue to help control the knife during incision and dissection.

Local Injection Solutions

Normal saline is the most popular injecting fluid for conventional EMR. However, the mucosal protrusion created with normal saline does not last long enough to provide sufficient time for submucosal dissection [11,12]. To create a long-lasting mucosal protrusion, several other fluids have been used for ESD. Among those, Glyceol® (Chugai Pharmaceutical, Tokyo, Japan; 10% glycerin, 5% fructose, 0.9% sodium chloride) is the most popular solution. For large and difficult cases, however, sodium hyaluronate is much better, because it can create a much higher protrusion and remains longer [11,12]. The clinical usefulness of a 0.4% sodium hyaluronate solution with an average molecular weight of 800000 kDa (Muco Up®; Johnson and Johnson, Tokyo, Japan; derivative type, rooster comb) was proved by a clinical study [13], and it was approved for endoscopic resection of gastric lesions in Japan. Usually, a small amount of epinephrine (0.001%) and an indigo carmine dye (0.004%) are mixed into the injection solution as they are useful for hemostasis and clear visualization of the submucosal layer.

Electrosurgical Knives

Several kinds of electrosurgical knives, specially designed for ESD, are commercially available in Japan (Fig. 2). Among them, the conventional needle knife, IT knife, hook knife, flex knife, and triangle tip (TT) knife are also obtainable in many Asian and European countries. The features of these widely available knives are briefly explained in this section.

a. Needle knife (KD-10Q-1; Olympus Medical Systems) (Fig. 2a)
   The needle knife has a fine tip and it allows a sharp incision, because the electric current is concentrated in its small contact area. It cuts most efficiently in any direction and is also available for dissection even in a severely scarred tissue. However, at the same time, it is a somewhat risky device, so that operators should control the knife very carefully to avoid perforation and severe bleeding throughout the procedure. To conduct safe ESD with this knife, it is advisable to attach a transparent hood and to use sodium hyaluronate as an injecting solution [6].
b. IT knife (KD-610L; Olympus Medical Systems) (Fig. 2b)
   The IT knife is a needle knife equipped with a ceramic ball at its point. This knife was originally developed to conduct a mucosal incision safely, as the point is insulated, preventing perforation. It is necessary to make a small mucosal incision using the other knife to insert the ceramic tip into the submucosa when the operator starts the procedure. It cuts very well in a longitudinal direction from the

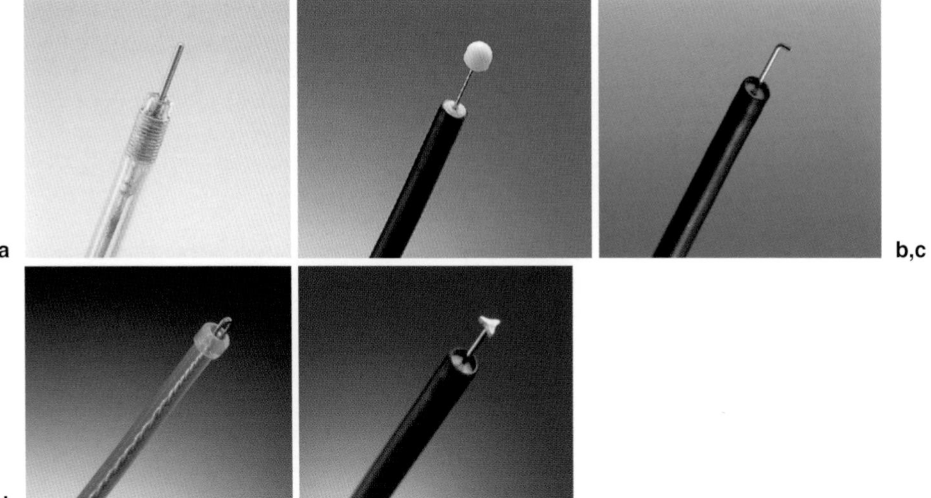

Fig. 2. Electrosurgical knives commercially available worldwide for endoscopic submucosal dissection (ESD). **a** A needle knife. **b** The insulated-tip diathermic (IT) knife. **c** The hook knife. **d** The flex knife. **e** The triangular tip (TT) knife. (Images provided by Olympus Medical Systems)

distal to proximal position, but it often requires much greater skill to cut in a lateral direction. The operation must control the endoscope, sometimes twisting it, as the ceramic tip disturbs lateral movement and the blade of this knife must contact the tissue on its side. Also, it sometimes becomes blind during submucosal dissection as a result of an unusual scope position. Although it is the most popular device for gastric ESD in Japan and provides a relatively fast procedure, it requires a longer learning curve.

c. Hook knife (KD-620LR; Olympus Medical Systems) (Fig. 2c)

The hook knife has a right-angled tip, 1 mm in size. The operator can hook and pull the tissue before cutting it. Therefore, it results in a very safe procedure, although only a limited amount of tissue can be cut at one time with this knife. Safety is further improved if operators use a transparent hood and pull the tissue into the hood before turning on the electricity. This knife has a rotating function so that operators can select any direction to hook. It is very useful, especially in difficult situations cased by severe fibrosis or poor maneuverability of the endoscope, because it can cut the tissue very precisely and safely by hooking the tissue [14].

d. Flex knife (KD-630L; Olympus Medical Systems (Fig. 2d)

The flex knife is the most maneuverable device owing to its soft and flexible nature [15]. The tip of the knife is rounded with a twined wire similar to a snare so as not to pierce the muscle layer with it. The length of the knife is adjustable according to the circumstances. The tip of the sheath is thickened, which can be used as a stopper, so that operators can control the depth of incision much easier. Because of this feature, a flex knife is less likely to cause perforation than a needle knife. It is very important to use a transparent hood to conduct a safe and smooth procedure. Although it is very handy and can be used for most ESD procedures, the operator should change to the other device in case of fibrosis because it is difficult to continue the procedure with this soft and flexible device.

e. TT knife (KD-640L; Olympus Medical Systems (Fig. 2e)

The TT knife is a needle knife equipped with a small triangle metallic tip at its point. Each projection of the triangle is 1 mm long, just the same length as the hook knife. The concept of this knife is very similar to the hook knife, i.e., hook and pull the tissue before cutting it, but it is not necessary to adjust the direction of the projection during the procedure. It can hook the tissue in any direction at any time so that the usage of this knife is very simple, just hooking the tissue from the proximal side to the distal side, although the incision line becomes relatively wider and rather zigzag in appearance. It is strongly recommended to use a transparent hood to maintain the safety zone.

High-Frequency Generators

The ICC 200 and ICC 350 (ERBE, Tubingen, Germany), which have an endocut mode and multiple coagulation modes, are very useful for the ESD technique. Rough standards of these generators for each knife are shown in Table 1.

A few years ago, a new HF generator, VIO 300D (ERBE, Tubingen, Germany), was introduced for ESD. It was regarded as a much more useful machine than previous models because it can reduce bleeding during the procedure with new high-frequency modes, dry cut, and swift coagulation. Rough standards of this generator for each knife are also shown in Table 1.

Other Devices

It is necessary to prepare some devices for hemostasis whenever we conduct ESD. The Coagrasper (Olympus Medical Systems) and hemostatic forceps (Pentax, Tokyo, Japan) are specific devices designed for hemostasis, which have a much smaller cup than hot biopsy forceps and can coagulate the bleeding vessels much precisely. The hot biopsy forceps is also applicable to this purpose, but it requires much higher output because of the relatively wider cup and it causes a stronger burning effect. In case of bleeding, it is very important for operators to pinch a bleeding vessel precisely, retract it, and coagulate with a minimal contact area. For this purpose, it is advisable to use special endoscopes that have a water irrigation system (Pentax, Olympus Medical Systems, and Fujinon Toshiba ES systems, Tokyo, Japan), as they are very useful to visualize the bleeding point.

It is important to prepare rotatable clip fixing devices (Olympus Medical Systems) ready to use at any time for perforation. The operators must close a perforated hole securely to avoid air leak and to prevent severe peritonitis.

TABLE 1. Rough standards of HF generators for each device

	ICC200			VIO300D				
	Mode	Output	Effect	Mode	Output	Effect	Duration	Interval
Needle Knife								
marking	Soft Coag	40 W		Soft Coag	80 W	5		
mucosal incision	Endo Cut	120 W	3	Endo Cut I		1	4	1
submucosal dissection	Forced Coag	25 W		Swift Coag	25 W	4		
IT Knife								
marking (using needle knife)	Forced Coag	20 W		Swift Coag	30 W	2 ~ 3		
pre-cut (using needle knife)	Endo Cut	80 W	3	Endo Cut I		2	3	3
	Auto Cut	80 W	3	Dry Cut	50 W	4		
mucosal incision	Endo Cut	80 W	3	Dry Cut	50 W	4		
				Endo Cut I		2	3	1
submucosal dissection	Endo Cut	80 W	3	Dry Cut	50 W	4		
	Forced Coag	50 W		Swift Coag	50 W	5		
				Endo Cut I		2	3	1
Hook Knife								
marking	Forced Coag	40 W		Forced Coag	40 W	2		
mucosal incision	Endo Cut	120 W	3	Dry Cut	60 W	3		
submucosal dissection	Forced Coag	60 W		Dry Cut	60 W	3		
Flex Knife								
marking	Soft Coag	50 W		Soft	50 W	5		
mucosal incision	Endo Cut	80 W	3	Dry Cut	40 W	4		
				Endo Cut Q		1	4	3
submucosal dissection	Forced Coag	40 W		Swift Coag	40 W	4		
TT Knife								
marking	Forced Coag	40 W		Forced Coag	40 W	2 ~ 3		
mucosal incision	Endo Cut	120 W	3	Swift Coag	60 W	3 ~ 4		
submucosal dissection	Forced Coag	40 W		Swift Coag	60 W	3 ~ 4		

General Strategy of Gastric ESD

To conduct ESD successfully, it is important to construct a strategy that includes the order of incisions and dissections of the mucosa and submucosa. Usually, mucosal incision should be made only for the area to be dissected, and then submucosal dissection should start immediately from the incised part, when we use a needle knife or the flex knife, because if operators perform circumferential mucosal incision and postpone submucosal dissection, the injected solution will easily drain from the incised wound, resulting in decrease of submucosal thickness. It becomes risky and difficult to complete the procedure in such a situation because these devices are usually used by pressing down on the target tissue.

On the other hand, circumferential incision is made before submucosal dissection when we use the IT knife, the hook knife, or the TT knife because the IT knife can dissect the submucosal tissue much faster by its long stroke while ensuring safety with the insulated tip. Also, the hook and the TT knife can dissect the submucosal tissues relatively more safely, retracting the tissue with their tips.

The operator should keep a sufficient submucosal fluid cushion throughout the procedure by an additional submucosal injection when necessary. It is also advisable to dissect the submucosa under direct vision, as far as possible, utilizing gravity and the transparent hood.

Gastric ESD is usually conducted under conscious sedation, using some sedatives and painkillers such as petidine chloride and diazepam. However, when the procedure time is estimated to be more than 2 h for a large or difficult lesion, it is better to conduct the procedure under general anesthesia.

Procedure of ESD

As described in the general strategy of gastric ESD, the way of conducting actual ESD procedures differs depending on the features of each device. The operators should fully understand the features of electrosurgical knives and select the one appropriate according to the situation and their skills.

In this section, a common ESD procedure using the flex knife is briefly described as one of the examples.

It is very important to adjust the knife length before using the flex knife: 0.5–1.0 mm long is enough for marking, and 1.5–2.0 mm long is enough for mucosal incision and submucosal dissection (Fig. 3.). The knife length must be checked just in front of the lens each time when it is inserted. The typical therapeutic process is as follows (Fig. 4).

1. Marking dots are made using the tip of the flex knife with the soft coagulation mode on the circumference of the target lesion (Fig. 4a).

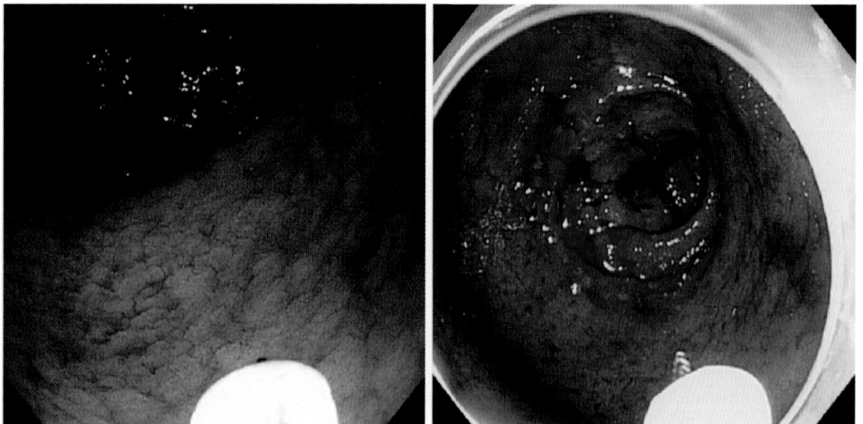

Fig. 3. The knife length of the flex knife is adjustable according to the situation: 0.5–1 mm is long enough for marking (**a**), and 1–2 mm is an appropriate length for mucosal incision and submucosal dissection (**b**)

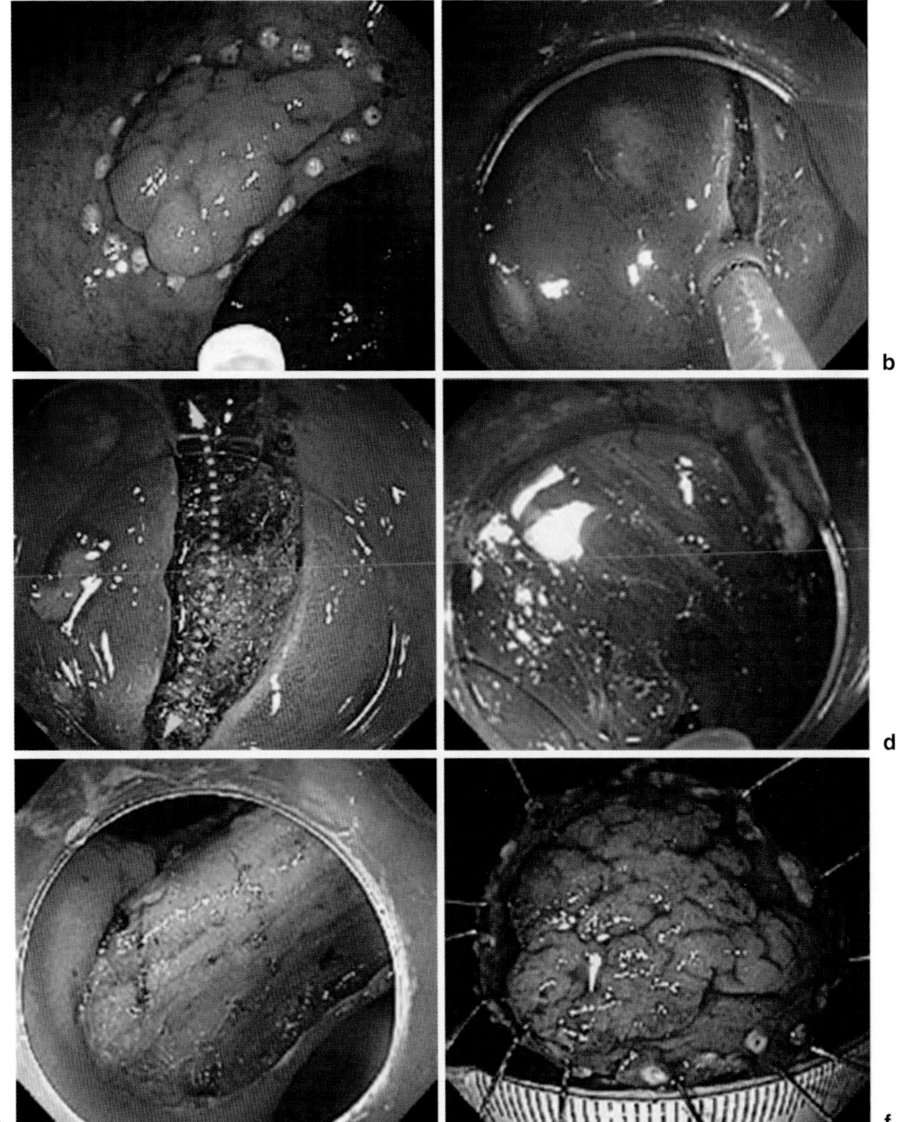

Fig. 4. Standard gastric ESD process. **a** Marking dots were placed a few millimeters outside the target lesion. **b** Mucosal incision is usually conducted in a very close position to control the knife precisely. A few centimeters is long enough for the initial mucosal incision. **c** Submucosal dissection should be begun immediately after the initial mucosal incision, tracing along the internal edge of the incised wound (*yellow dotted line*) with the knife. **d** A transparent hood is very useful for clear visualization of the operating field. The dissection line is usually set around one-third of the submucosa from the bottom. **e** Complete resection can be achieved even in the angulated position with this technique. **f** Precise histological evaluation is available with the completely resected specimen in an en bloc fashion

2. Glyceol® or Muco Up® with a small amount of indigo carmine and epinephrine is injected into the submucosal layer around the lesion to lift it up with a 23-gauge disposable injector needle.
3. Partial mucosal incision, slightly outside of the marking dots, is made by the flex knife with endocut mode or dry cut mode to separate the lesion from the surrounding normal mucosa (Fig. 4b). Usually, a few centimeters of mucosal incision is enough, each time, before submucosal dissection.
4. Submucosal dissection should progress immediately after each mucosal incision by tracing the internal side of the incision line with forced coagulation or swift coagulation mode (Fig. 4c). The operator should step on the foot pedal intermittently to control the direction and the extent of dissection.
5. It is important to utilize the transparent hood and gravity to obtain good visibility of the operative field during submucosal dissection (Fig. 4d). Also, the operator should maintain sufficient submucosal thickness of the target area with additional submucosal injection whenever necessary.
6. Repeat the foregoing steps of injection, mucosal incision, and submucosal dissection until the lesion is completely cut off from the gastric wall (Fig. 4e).
7. The resected specimen is retrieved and stretched on a cork or rubber board (Fig. 4f). After checking and documenting the marking dots and the direction of the specimen, the specimen is subjected to histopathological evaluation.

Conclusion

ESD is a new technique of endoscopic resection for superficial neoplasias of the gastrointestinal tract. It realizes en bloc resection of relatively large and difficult lesions that are impossible to treat by the conventional EMR technique. It is really a wonderful technique, but it requires a longer procedure time and involves relatively higher risk for complications. Therefore, the operator should acquire thorough knowledge, especially for new devices, and also should acquire sufficient skills to conduct safe and reliable ESD.

References

1. Tada M, Shimada M, Murakami F, et al (1984) Development of the strip-off biopsy (in Japanese with English abstract). Gastroenterol Endosc 26:833–839
2. Inoue H, Takeshita K, Hori H, et al (1993) Endoscopic mucosal resection with a cap-fitted panendoscope for esophagus, stomach, and colon mucosal lesions. Gastrointest Endosc 39:58–62
3. Torii A, Sakai M, Kajiyama T, et al (1995) Endoscopic aspiration mucosectomy as curative endoscopic surgery; analysis of 24 cases of early gastric cancer. Gastrointest Endosc 42:475–479
4. Hamada T, Kondo K, Itagaki Y, et al (1998) Possibility of complete resection by endoscopic mucosal resection using the piecemeal method (in Japanese with English abstract). Stomach Intest (Tokyo) 33:1609–1617
5. Hirao M, Masuda K, Asanuma T, et al (1988) Endoscopic resection of early gastric cancer and other tumors with local injection of hypertonic saline-epinephrine. Gastrointest Endosc 34:264–269

6. Yamamoto H, Koiwai H, Yube T, et al (1999) A successful single-step endoscopic resection of a 40 millimeter flat-elevated tumor in the rectum: endoscopic mucosal resection using sodium hyaluronate. Gastrointest Endosc 50:701–704
7. Ono H (2005) Endoscopic submucosal dissection for early gastric cancer. Chin J Dig Dis 6:119–121
8. Yahagi N, Fujishiro M, Kakushima N, et al (2004) Endoscopic submucosal dissection for early gastric cancer using the tip of an electrosurgical snare (thin type). Dig Endosc 16:34–38
9. Ookuwa M, Hosokawa K, Boku N, et al (2001) New endoscopic treatment for intramucosal tumors using an insulated-tip diathermic knife. Endoscopy 33:221–226
10. Yahagi N, Fujishiro M, Kakushima N, et al (2005) Clinical evaluation of the multi-bending scope in various endoscopic procedures of the upper GI tract. Dig Endosc 17: S94–S96
11. Yamamoto H, Yube T, Isoda N, et al (1999) A novel method of endoscopic mucosal resection using sodium hyaluronate. Gastrointest Endosc 50:251–256
12. Fujishiro M, Yahagi N, Kashimura K, et al (2004) Comparison of various submucosal injection solutions for maintaining mucosal elevation during endoscopic mucosal resection. Endoscopy 36:579–583
13. Yamamoto H, Yahagi N, Oyama T, et al (2008) Usefulness and safety of 0.4% sodium hyaluronate solution as a submucosal fluid "cushion" in endoscopic resection for gastric neoplasms: a prospective multicenter trial. Gastrointest Endosc 6:830–838
14. Oyama T, Kikuchi Y (2002) Aggressive endoscopic mucosal resection in the upper GI tract: hook knife method. Minim Invasive Ther Allied Technol 11:291–295
15. Yahagi N, Fujishiro M, Imagawa A, et al (2004) Endoscopic submucosal dissection for the reliable en bloc resection of colorectal mucosal tumors. Dig Endosc 16:S89–S92

Future Prospects of Endoscopic Submucosal Dissection from the Product Development Standpoint

Yasuo Miyano

Summary. Studies have been made into techniques for the minimally invasive treatment of early-stage mucosal lesions in the digestive tract. In the endoscopic field, various studies continue, primarily in Japan. One example is the development of endoscopic submucosal dissection (ESD), which has the potential to replace surgical operations. In particular, the endoscopic minimally invasive treatment of early-stage gastric mucosal lesions has steadily improved. It has emerged from its developmental phase and entered its practical phase. Olympus Medical Systems, Tokyo, Japan, has developed and marketed the IT knife, the IT knife 2, the flex knife, the hook knife, the triangle knife, and hemostatic forceps. This chapter describes how effective the ESD is by describing the features of the products listed above, and discusses the future of the therapy from the standpoint of an engineer.

Key words. ESD, IT knife, flex knife, Hook knife, Triangle knife

Introduction

In the 1990s, endoscopic mucosal resection (EMR) using the lifting and aspiration methods was a standard procedure to treat early-stage mucosal legions in the GI tract. The conventional EMR procedure has the disadvantage that it only allows piecemeal resection because of the technical limitations of the therapeutic devices. Therefore local recurrences sometimes occur. Although the endoscopic resection using hypertonic saline epinephrine (ERHSE) procedure can be used for resecting tissue en bloc, the devices used, in particular the diathermic knife, are cumbersome and require great skill by the physician.

To cope with this disadvantage, an improved technique, endoscopic submucosal dissection (ESD), has been developed. It is aimed at resecting a larger lesion with ease. In Japan, ESD has rapidly become widespread as a method of treatment for intramucosal tumors in the GI tract with the development of various therapeutic devices.

Therapeutic Products Development Department, Olympus Medical Systems Corp., 2951 Ishikawa-cho, Hachioji-shi, Tokyo 192-8507, Japan

Concepts and Design for Typical Therapeutic Devices

IT Knife and IT Knife 2

A doctor's concept for an IT knife was that a diathermic knife with an insulated tip at the distal end could prevent deep invasion of the tissue and facilitate an en bloc resection of a large area. With the insulated tip, the distal tip resists the flow of high-frequency current, thus allowing the electric current to pass only through the cutting knife. Therefore, when the knife is cutting the target tissue, the high-frequency current does not flow into tissue in contact with the IT tip. This mechanism is effective in preventing damage to the deep areas of tissue.

We have also developed a modified model, IT knife 2. This retains the basic performance of the IT knife and is much easier to use. For example, in the premodified type, it is difficult to cut tissue when the knife is perpendicular to the target tissue, or to make an incision in the lateral direction. Although endoscopists can get over such difficulties by controlling the angle of the endoscope, it requires great skill and technique.

After technical modifications, we have overcome these difficulties by providing three conductable fins at the joint between the distal tip and the nylon rod. Improvements have also been made to the shape of both the distal tip and the nylon tip (Figs. 1 and 2).

The key issues in designing and manufacturing these knives were the selection of the insulation material for the distal tip, and the adhesive strength between the IT tip and the knife. We have selected a biocompatible ceramic which has high insulation properties and heat-resistance. We had to overcome some difficulties of high-precision processing technology to make the distal ceramic tip only 2 mm in diameter. Another problem was how to connect the tip securely to a knife 0.4 mm in diameter. In IT knife 2, we had difficulties in modifying the method of connecting the distal tip because of its distinctive design.

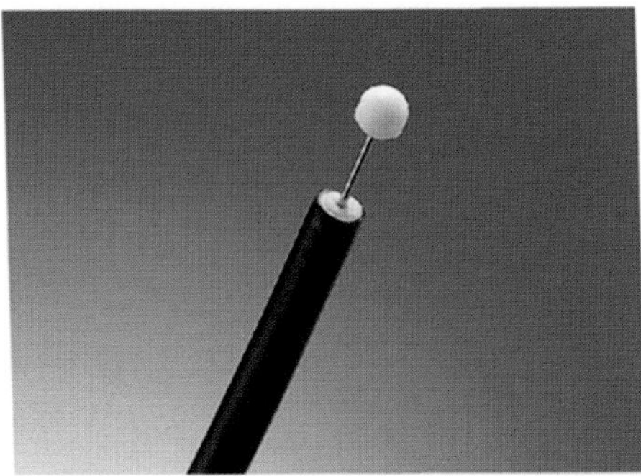

Fig. 1. Distal end of the IT knife

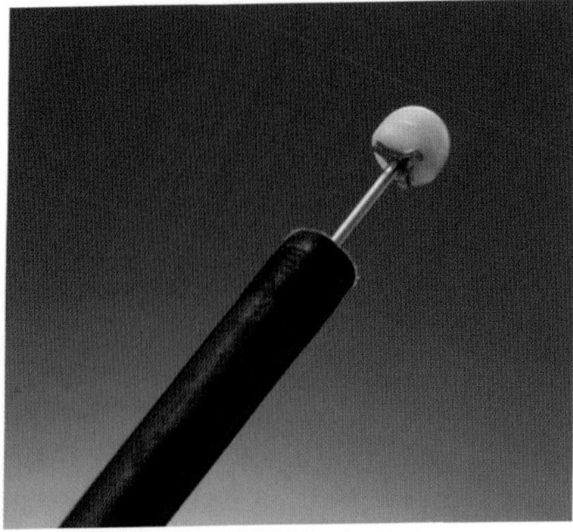

FIG. 2. Distal end of the IT knife 2

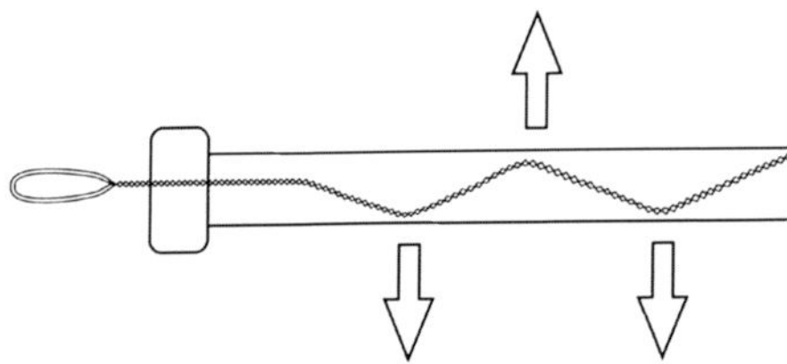

FIG. 3. Distal end of the flex knife

Flex Knife

A doctor's concept for the flex knife was a safe, smooth incision in all directions, dissection, and control of minor bleeding. By using a more flexible and thinner tube sheath and more flexible wire in the entire therapeutic device, the flexibility of the knife has been improved, and this has helped prevent a large stress concentration on the tissue to be dissected. This design has also facilitated an incision in the lateral direction, thus minimizing the damage to deep tissue. Furthermore, a new mechanism to adjust the extended length of the knife has improved its safety in incisions. When the knife is extended to its minimum length, it can be used as a hemostatic probe (Fig. 3).

A mechanism for adjusting the extended length of the knife has been realized by providing bending sections along the wire. Friction can be generated between the bending section and the inner wall of the sheath (see Fig. 1). The optimal friction has allowed adjustments to the length of the knife by the manipulation of the handle section without sacrificing the quality of the locking mechanism and the flexibility of the knife. The biggest problem in the design and mass production was how to achieve the optimal friction.

Hook Knife

A doctor's concept for the hook knife was the completion of the entire incision process using a high-frequency current, including marking and submucosal dissection, with the hook knife only.

To make this concept a reality, complete control of the hook was essential in order to achieve marking, as well as all incisions, including circumferential cutting and submucosal dissection, in all directions. Two control wires of different flexibility have been connected in as efficient a way as possible to transfer torque to the hook. This has helped to minimize a loss of torque in the bending section of the endoscope and provide a secure rotation of the hook. When the wire has been oriented in the desired direction and pushed out to its maximum length, the stopper of the control wire becomes engaged and locks in a hole within the sheath. This prevents undesired rotation of the hook during incision (Fig. 4).

The biggest problem we encountered was the selection of the two control wires and the position at which they are connected. In addition, high rotation ability cannot be obtained simply by providing the appropriate dimensions. Therefore, various innovative methods are used not only in the design, but also in the manufacture of the product.

Triangle Knife

The concept of a doctor for a triangle knife was ease of use and the completion of the entire incision process using high-frequency current, including marking and submucosal dissection, with the triangle knife only.

To realize this, we made the innovation of providing a conductive disk tip at the distal end of the cutting knife while lowering the electric current density. With this design, greater coagulation has been obtained while reducing the risk of perforation. For ease of use, we first made a disk-shaped and multiorientatable tip. However, this was not effective in catching tissue. We then adopted a triangular tip which was better able to catch tissue and had few orientational restrictions. The triangle tip has three peaks which are all effective at catching tissue, and a plate which is effective at coagu-

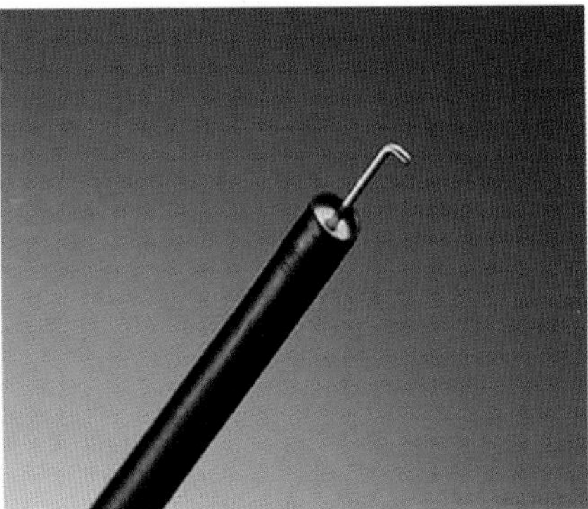

Fig. 4. Distal end of the hook knife

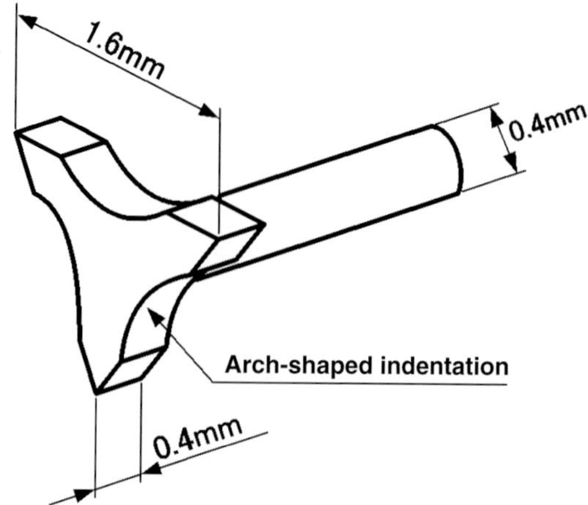

FIG. 5. Distal end of the triangle knife

lating tissue. What were also required were improved shapes for marking and a knife for precutting (Fig. 5).

The most difficult aspects were to combine the three peaks which could catch tissue easily and the plate for greater coagulation ability, and also to develop an optimal design for the marking and precutting knife. Other issues were how to establish a high-precision-process technology in mass production, how to obtain the shape of the disc as designed, and how to secure the adhesive quality and strength between the disc and the knife rod.

Hot Bite (Hemostatic) Forceps

The new Hot Bite forceps for ESD have been developed on the basis of a doctor's concept that the knife is the main player in the procedure, but that the Hot Bite is essential for performing it safely. The prolonged time of hemostasis should not be ignored because it can make up the longest portion of the entire procedure. When some inexperienced endoscopists perform ESD, they can spend the longest time in stopping bleeding. Therefore, the development of a Hot Bite which was reliable and easier to use was essential.

In order to realize this concept, it was necessary to develop the optimal design of the forceps cups in order to enable the endoscopist to confirm that the device is in contact with the target area of tissue, and to lift the tissue in order to minimize the thermal effect on a deeper area. We then needed to provide a corrugated surface on the outer edge of the cup to prevent slippage, and an indented surface in the center of the cups. The distal end of the forceps has been tapered so that it will not be lost in the endoscopic view. A new mechanism has been provided that allows each cup to regulate the opening width of the other cup when they both open to a preset width. This mechanism has given endoscopists a constant small opening width of the cup, resulting in an easer approach to target tissue and an easier location of the forceps.

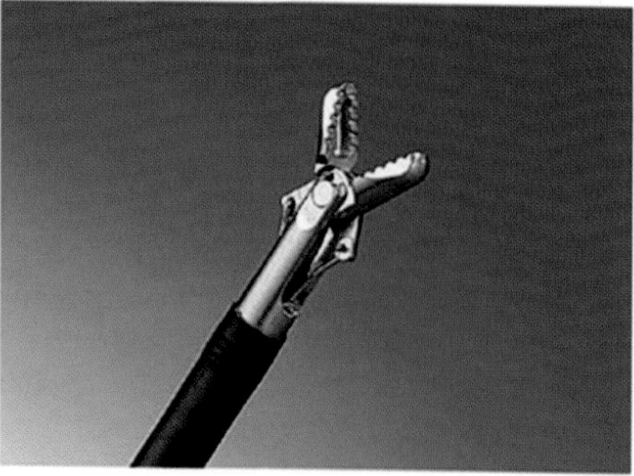

FIG. 6. Distal end of the Hot Bite forceps

In order to address the issue of the orientation of the forceps, it was necessary to control the orientation of both sides when they are positioned face to face. To improve the rotatability, we adopted a unique mechanism. A metal coil is connected to the forceps and the handle in the proximal section, but is not connected to the resin tube in the distal section. Any rotation given to the handle is not transferred to the tube, but only to the metal coil. This mechanism has made it possible for the metal tube only to rotate along with the distal forceps. This design has never been adopted in previous therapeutic devices (Fig. 6).

The most difficult problems faced in developing and manufacturing the forceps were how to establish a high-precision processing technology, and how to assemble the forceps because of their small size ($2 \times 1 \times 3.6$ mm) and the complex design with various functions at the distal end.

Future Prospects

Although ESD offers high-quality endoscopic treatment, it is still not easy to perform and requires endoscopists to acquire great skill in using the therapeutic devices. It is also a time-consuming procedure compared with other endoscopic procedures. These problems must be solved in order to advance the procedure still further. A key issue is how to offer better visibility of the target tissue. In surgical operations, right-handed surgeons use the left hand to improve visibility of the lesions. In the future, therapeutic devices for ESD must provide this traction ability in such a manner that the endoscope and the therapeutic devices can play the roles of both hands of the surgeon.

What is also important is the management of any perforation. There are two types of perforation: intraoperative perforation and postoperative perforation. The intraoperative perforation is most closely associated with mechanical applications of the therapeutic devices and the use of a high-frequency current. A postoperative perforation can be caused by damage to deeper tissue due to the thermal effects of a high-frequency current. In order to prevent these incidents, it is essential to develop a cutting device and injection solution that would minimize the risk of damage to tissue. Alternatively, it might be necessary to revise our way of thinking. A perforation is made for a purpose. This means that a new method or device could be developed which allows full-thickness resection. It may be necessary to study both how to minimize perforations and how to make a perforation.

Conclusion

Engineers do not have many chances of developing a new procedure that offers a highly effective medical advance. In the development of the ESD procedure, Olympus Medical Systems engineers have worked closely with doctors, and in particular with Dr. Hosokawa, in the development of the IT knife, with Dr. Yahagi for the flex knife, with Dr. Oyama for the hook knife, with Dr. Inoue for the triangle knife, and with Dr. Doi for the Hot Bite. It is quite an honor for Olympus Medical Systems to participate in these significant academic–industrial activities, and to disseminate the results from Japan to the rest of the world.

Small Intestine

Clinical Usefulness of Single-Balloon Enteroscopy for the Diagnosis and Treatment of Small-Intestinal Diseases

Kiyonori Kobayashi, Tomoe Katsumata, and Katsunori Saigenji

Summary. Double-balloon enteroscopy (DBE) requires a long preparation time, and scope insertion is often difficult because balloons have to be attached to both the endoscope and the overtube. We examined the clinical usefulness of a new model of single-balloon enteroscope (SBE). The study group comprised 40 patients who underwent enteroscopy with an SBE. The SBE does not require a balloon to be attached to the scope and has only a sliding tube. Therefore, examination preparations and scope insertion are easier than with DBE. Total enteroscopy was possible in 3 of 5 patients in whom the SBE was inserted deeply through both the mouth and the anus. There were no serious complications. In 10 of 16 patients who underwent enteroscopy for suspected small-intestinal bleeding, 6 had angiectasia and 4 had ulcers or erosions. In 5 patients, endoscopic hemostasis was performed successfully. In 7 of 8 patients in whom enteroscopy was performed for small-intestinal strictures, endoscopic diagnosis was possible. In 4 of 5 patients who underwent enteroscopy because protruding lesions were suspected on radiography, abnormal findings were observed. The SBE has many advantages, such as convenience and compatibility with conventional systems. An SBE is useful for the diagnosis and treatment of small-intestinal diseases.

Key words. Single-balloon enteroscopy, Small intestine, Diagnosis, Treatment, Narrow-band imaging

Introduction

Recently, the practical applications of capsule endoscopy (CE) and double-balloon enteroscopy (DBE) have led to remarkable advances in the endoscopic diagnosis of diseases of the small intestine [1–4]. In particular, DBE allows various types of endoscopic treatment, including the hemostasis of bleeding lesions and the balloon dilation of intestinal strictures. This procedure has therefore been widely used clinically for the diagnosis and treatment of diseases of the small intestine.

Department of Gastroenterology, Kitasato University East Hospital, 2-1-1 Asamizodai, Sagamihara, Kanagawa 228-8520, Japan

We had the opportunity to use a single-balloon enteroscope (SBE; SIF-Q260) developed by Olympus Medical Systems, Tokyo, Japan. This SBE is a new model endoscope with a balloon attached to the sliding tube only. In this study, we mainly examined the clinical usefulness of the SBE for the diagnosis and treatment of small-intestinal diseases.

Materials and Methods

Indications of Enteroscopy with an SBE

We performed enteroscopy with an SBE in 40 patients (27 men and 13 women), and the total number of sessions was 50. Their mean age was 61.3 ± 17.2 years, and 75% of the patients had systemic complications such as hypertension and chronic renal or liver disease. Frequent indications for enteroscopy with an SBE were to confirm suspected small-intestinal bleeding in 16 patients, to diagnose and treat small-intestinal strictures in 8 patients, and to confirm suspected small-intestinal protruding lesions in 5 patients. In all patients who underwent enteroscopy for suspected small-intestinal bleeding, upper gastrointestinal endoscopy and colonoscopy were performed before enteroscopy with an SBE to confirm the absence of bleeding lesions.

Characteristics of the SBE System

The SBE system consists of an enteroscope, a sliding tube, and a balloon controller. The effective length of the SBE is 2 m. The outer diameter is 9.2 mm. The instrument channel is 2.8 mm, which is similar to a conventional upper gastrointestinal endoscope, permitting the use of different types of devices, including various snares and forceps. The SBE system has a specialized sliding tube with a silicon rubber balloon attached to the tip. A radio-opaque chip is attached to the tip. The inner surface of the sliding tube is coated with a hydrophilic lubricant to facilitate sliding of the scope. The SBE system also has a balloon controller that can adjust the inflation and deflation of the balloon at the tip of the sliding tube.

The SBE provided high-quality "Q"-type endoscopic images. There is no magnifying function, but narrow-band imaging (NBI) can be performed. NBI permitted a clear evaluation of the vascular plexus of the small intestine (Fig. 1a,b). Close-up observation by NBI also permitted recognition of the villous architecture of the mucosal surface (Fig. 1c).

Enteroscopy with an SBE

Enteroscopy by the oral approach was performed after the patient had fasted overnight. Enteroscopy by the anal approach required bowel preparation, which is similar to that needed for colonoscopy. Before the procedure, the subjects received an intramuscular injection of scopolamine butylbromide (10 mg) to minimize peristalsis of the small intestine. For sedation, flunitrazepam or pethidine hydrochloride was administered intravenously. Propofol was given if needed, depending on the patients' level of consciousness. An SBE can be inserted through the mouth or anus. The route of insertion was determined on the basis of the findings of a radiographic examination of the small intestine performed before enteroscopy, or the color of bloody stools if

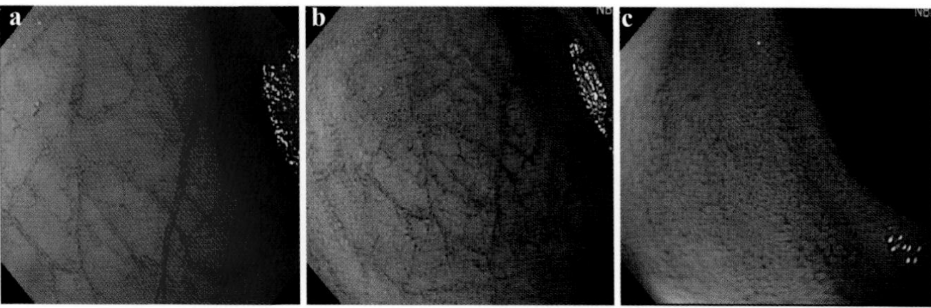

FIG. 1. Endoscopic findings obtained with a single-balloon enteroscope before and after narrow-band imaging (NBI). **a** Conventional endoscopic findings of the normal ileal mucosa were seen. **b** NBI permitted a clear evaluation of the vascular plexus of the small intestine. **c** Close-up observation by NBI also permitted recognition of the villous structure of the mucosal surface

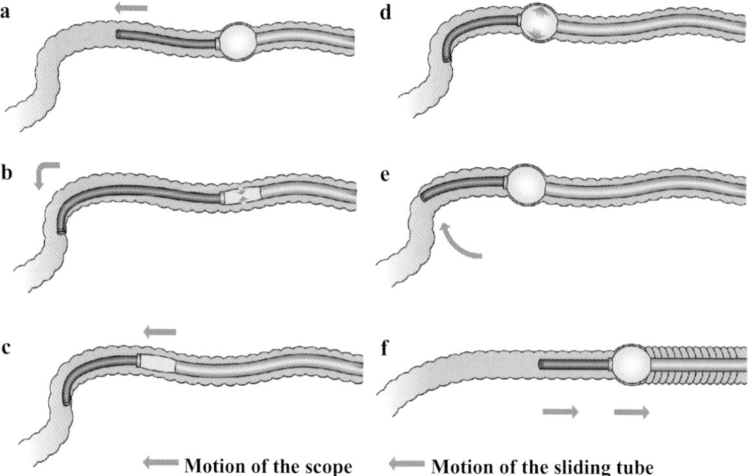

FIG. 2. Principles and methods of inserting the single-balloon enteroscope. **a** The scope was advanced as deeply as possible, while preventing intestinal distension by the balloon at the tip of the sliding tube around the scope. **b** When the scope could be advanced no further, the intestine was grasped with the angle of the scope tip, and the sliding tube balloon was deflated. **c,d** Next, the sliding-tube was advanced to near the scope tip, and then inflated again. **e,f** With the scope angle unlocked, the scope was pulled back along with the sliding tube, shortening the small intestine

small-intestinal bleeding was suspected but the lesion site was unclear. The SBE was inserted via the mouth for 22 sessions and via the anus for 28 sessions. The mean examination time in our hospital was 87.2 ± 34.3 min (range 18–186 min).

When the scope was inserted through the mouth, the patient was placed in the prone position. When the scope was inserted through the anus, the patient was first placed in the left lateral decubitus position and then in the ventral decubitus position. Before insertion of the SBE, the intestine was grasped with the balloon at the tip of the sliding tube around the scope. The scope was then advanced, while preventing intestinal distension (Fig. 2a). When the scope could be advanced no further, the intestine was grasped with the angle of the scope tip (Fig. 2b). Next, the sliding tube balloon was deflated, advanced to near the scope tip, and then inflated again (Fig. 2c,d). With the scope angle unlocked, the scope was pulled back along with the sliding tube, thus shortening the intestine (Fig. 2e,f). A similar procedure was then carried out to insert the SBE deeply into the small intestine. The positions of the scope and the loop formation were confirmed radiographically during insertion of the sliding tube and shortening of the intestine.

Results

Insertion Range and Safety of the SBE

For patients undergoing enteroscopy with an SBE, the scope was inserted deeply into the small intestine in 20 sessions. The routes of insertion were the mouth (8 sessions) and the anus (12 sessions). The insertion distance was difficult to measure accurately. In 17 sessions (85%), the scope was inserted at least 1.5 m into the small intestine, regardless of the insertion route. In 3 of the 5 patients in whom the SBE was inserted deeply through both the mouth and the anus, total enteroscopy was possible.

A few complications were associated with endoscopic examination with an SBE. Acute pancreatitis occurred in 2 patients, but responded to the intravenous administration of antibiotics and gabexate mesilate. The only complication associated with endoscopic treatment was bleeding after polypectomy in 1 patient. Endoscopic hemostasis by clipping was carried out immediately, resulting in complete hemostasis.

Diagnosis and Treatment of Small Intestinal Diseases by an SBE

Suspected Small-Intestinal Bleeding

Ten of the 16 patients who underwent enteroscopy for suspected small-intestinal bleeding had abnormal findings. These findings were angiectasia in 6 patients, ulcers or erosions in 4 patients, a bleeding polyp in 1 patient, and jejunal diverticula and a small submucosal tumor suspected to be a lipoma in 1 patient. In 3 of the 6 patients with angiectasia, the affected region was considered to be the bleeding source, and endoscopic hemostasis was carried out by clipping. In 1 of these patients, argon plasma coagulation was also performed. One patient who had an ileal ulcer with an exposed vessel underwent hemostatic treatment by argon plasma coagulation (Fig. 3). An ileal polyp with blood clots was removed by endoscopic polypectomy. There was no distinct rebleeding an average of 6 months after endoscopic treatment.

Small-Intestinal Strictures

In 7 of 8 patients in whom radiography revealed small-intestinal strictures, endoscopic observation of the strictures was possible. The underlying diseases of the strictures were Crohn's disease in 4 patients, ischemic enteritis in 2 patients, and adhesive strictures in 1 patient. The scope was difficult to insert in these strictures. However, the endoscopic findings and the histopathological findings of biopsy specimens allowed these diseases to be distinguished from malignant strictures. In 1

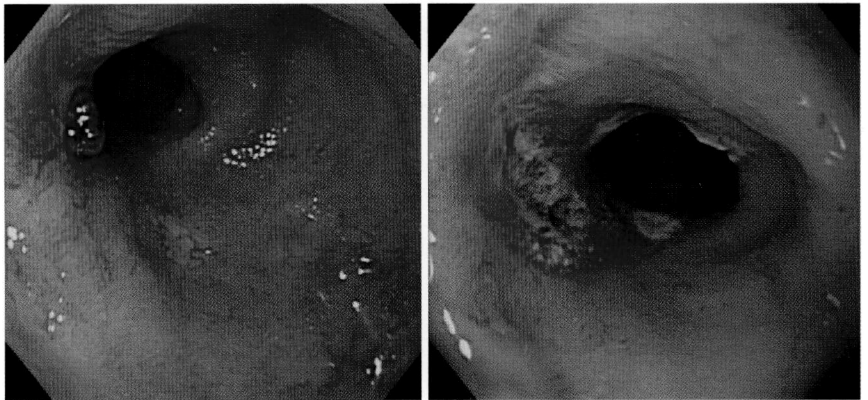

Fig. 3. A 77-year-old woman with NSAID ulcers. **a** Enteroscopic findings showed a small ulcer with an exposed vessel covered by clots in the middle part of the ileum. **b** Hemostatic treatment by argon plasma coagulation was performed for this lesion

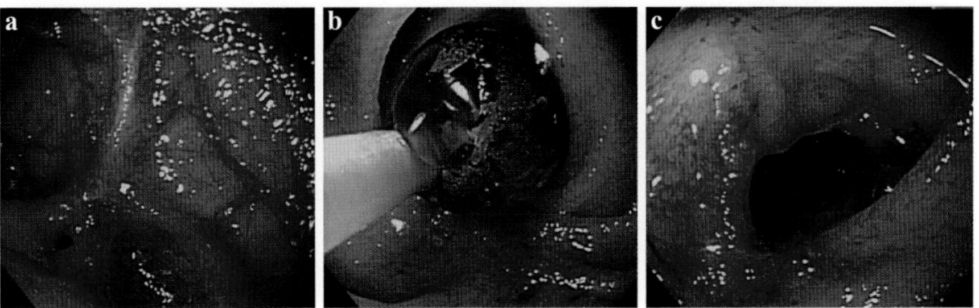

Fig. 4. A 33-year-old man with Crohn's disease. **a** Enteroscopic findings showed a severe stricture in the lower part of the ileum. **b** Endoscopic balloon dilation was performed 3 times for the stricture. **c** After endoscopic treatment, the enteroscope was able to pass though the stricture

patient who had an ileal stricture with Crohn's disease, endoscopic balloon dilation was performed, permitting passage of the scope (Fig. 4).

Suspected Small-Intestinal Protruding Lesions

Abnormal findings were confirmed in 4 of 5 patients who underwent enteroscopy with SBE because of suspected protruding lesions on a radiographic examination of the small intestine, a gastrointestinal stromal tumor in the jejunum, an advanced carcinoma in the jejunum, a carcinoid tumor in the ileum, and multiple jejunal polyps with Peutz–Jeghers syndrome. Multiple polyps were also removed by endoscopic polypectomy (Fig. 5).

Other Indications

In 1 patient in whom enteroscopy was performed because of multiple ulcers in the ileum, intestinal tuberculosis was suspected. The retrieval of a biliary stent that had

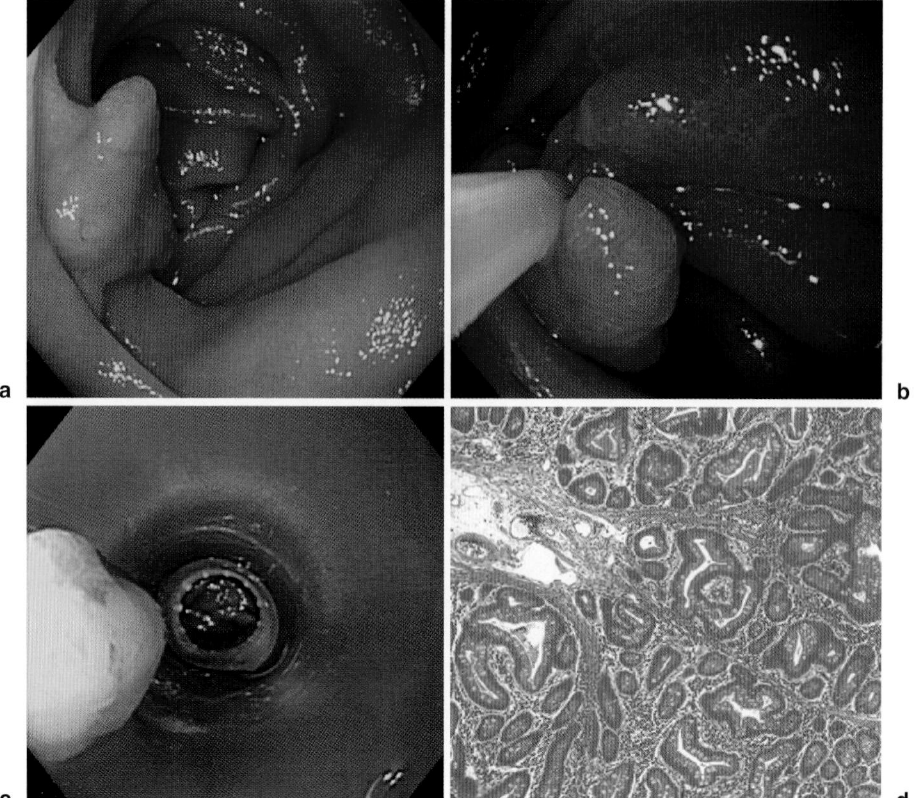

Fig. 5. A 29-year-old man with Peutz–Jeghers syndrome. **a** Enteroscopic findings showed a semipedunculated polyp in the middle part of the jejunum. **b** Three semipedunculated jejunal polyps were resected by endoscopic polypectomy. **c** For retrieval, the polyps were grasped with a tripod forceps inserted through the instrument channel of the endoscope. The enteroscope was then withdrawn, leaving the sliding tube in the small intestine. **d** Histopathological findings showed that all of the polyps were hamartomatous

been lodged in the jejunum, retrograde cholangiography after a Billroth II gastrectomy, and endoscopic lithotripsy of common bile-duct stones can be performed with an SBE. An SBE was also useful for a patient in whom a colonoscope was difficult to insert because of severe adhesion of the sigmoid colon caused by a total hysterectomy and radiotherapy. By straightening the sigmoid colon with the sliding tube, the SBE could be inserted. Total colonoscopy was thus successfully performed.

Discussion

Many studies in Japan and Western countries have reported that DBE is useful for the diagnosis and treatment of diseases of the small intestine [3–7]. With DBE, the intestine is grasped with a balloon attached to both the endoscope and the overtube, thereby preventing overextension of the intestine at the time of endoscope insertion and allowing the scope to be inserted deeply into the small intestine. The rates of successful enteroscopy of the entire small intestine differ depending on the center, and range from 8% to 86% [3,6–9]. The clinical use of DBE remains limited, but DBE is now acknowledged to be essential for enteroscopic diagnosis, along with CE. However, DBE has several limitations. Pre-examination preparations and the insertion procedure are somewhat troublesome because the balloon has to be attached to both the scope and the overtube. Efforts to solve such problems led to the development of the SBE, in which the balloon is attached to the sliding tube only. Therefore, pre-examination preparations, scope insertion, and cleaning and disinfection after examination are easier than with DBE. In addition, the endoscope can be removed and reinserted, leaving the sliding tube in the small intestine.

In our hospital, we used an SBE to perform enteroscopy in only 40 patients. There were no serious complications associated with these endoscopic examinations or endoscopic treatments. As for the performance of the SBE, visualization of the entire small intestine was possible in 3 of the 5 patients in whom the SBE was inserted deeply through both the mouth and the anus. This small number of patients is attributed to the fact that many patients had previously undergone radiography of the small intestine to evaluate small-intestinal lesions before enteroscopy. A larger series of patients should therefore be studied to assess the ease of inserting SBE into the small intestine.

Unlike a DBE, no balloon is attached to the tip of an SBE. Therefore, there is concern that the scope could be dislodged when the sliding-tube balloon is deflated and advanced to the scope tip. Dislodgment of the scope could usually be prevented by grasping the intestine with the angle of the endoscope. With DBE, the diameter of the balloon at the scope tip is smaller than that of the overtube. The overtube balloon is considered to play an important role in grasping the intestine when the intestine is shortened.

For the endoscopic diagnosis of small-intestinal diseases, enteroscopy with an SBE permitted the observation of vascular lesions such as angiectasia. In particular, radiography of the small intestine is often of limited value for the diagnosis of vascular diseases. Such diseases could be diagnosed only by enteroscopy. The SBE was useful for distinguishing intestinal lesions with strictures from neoplastic lesions. As for endoscopic treatment, the SBE allowed hemostasis by argon plasma coagulation or clipping, endoscopic balloon dilation, and endoscopic polypectomy to be performed safely. When small-intestinal polyps are endoscopically resected and retrieved, the removal of specimens via the overtube is not feasible with DBE because the balloon is attached to the scope tip. Therefore, multiple polyps are difficult to collect during examination. With the SBE, however, the scope can usually be inserted and removed, leaving the sliding tube in the small intestine. In our series, an SBE permitted the collection and histopathological examination of multiple polyps associated with Peutz–Jeghers syndrome.

Although our study group was small, enteroscopy with an SBE was found to be useful for the diagnosis and endoscopic treatment of small-intestinal diseases. The performance of the SBE should be compared with that of DBE to further define the advantages and limitations of these procedures. The safety of the SBE should also be further evaluated. Our results indicate that enteroscopy with an SBE is useful for both endoscopic diagnosis and various types of endoscopic treatment. We believe that clinically the SBE will be used more widely in the near future.

References

1. Costamagna G, Shah SK, Riccioni ME, et al. (2002) A prospective trial comparing small bowel radiographs and video capsule endoscopy for suspected small bowel disease. Gastroenterology 123:999–1005
2. Lewis BS, Swain P (2002) Capsule endoscopy in the evaluation of patients with suspected small intestinal bleeding: result of a pilot study. Gastrointest Endosc 56: 349–353
3. Yamamoto H, Kita H, Sunada K, et al. (2004) Clinical outcome of double-balloon endoscopy for the diagnosis and treatment of small-intestinal disease. Clin Gastroenterol Hepatol 2:1010–1016
4. May A, Nachbar L, Pohl J, et al. (2007) Endoscopic interventions in the small bowel using double-balloon enteroscopy: feasibility and limitations. Am J Gastroenterol 102:527–535
5. Manabe N, Tanaka S, Fukumoto A, et al. (2006) Double-balloon enteroscopy in patients with GI bleeding of obscure origin. Gastrointest Endosc 64:135–140
6. Heine GDN, Hadithi M, Groenen MJM, et al. (2006) Double-balloon enteroscopy: indications, diagnostic yield, and complications in a series of 275 patients with suspected small-bowel disease. Endoscopy 38:42–48
7. Di Caro S, May A, Heine DG, et al. (2005) The European experience with double-balloon enteroscopy: indications, methodology, safety, and clinical impact. Gastrointest Endosc 62:545–550
8. Akahoshi K, Kubokawa M, Matsumoto M, et al. (2006) Double-balloon endoscopy in the diagnosis and management of GI tract diseases: methodology, indications, safety, and clinical impact. World J Gastroenterol 12:7654–7659
9. Monkemuller K, Weigt J, Treiber G, et al. (2006) Diagnostic and therapeutic impact of double-balloon enteroscopy. Endoscopy 38:67–72

Cutting Edge Technology in Enteroscopy: Entero Pro, the Endo Capsule

HIDEO ITO[1] and RAIFU MATSUI[2]

Summary. A capsule endoscope had been desired for a long time. Olympus Medical Systems, Tokyo, Japan, launched a capsule endoscope in several countries in 2005. The image quality of the capsule endoscope, which contains CCD and LED, was designed to be identical to that of a conventional endoscope by using high-speed wireless transmission and advanced imaging processing technologies. Olympus Medical Systems is now planning to develop software which facilitates the diagnosis. In order to expand the application from the small intestine and improve the optics and the battery life, a self-propelling mechanism and a wireless therapeutic technology are being developed.

The other new technology is a single balloon enteroscope system. This allows a deeper intubation with conventional therapeutic ability. The system is composed of an endoscope, a disposable splinting tube, and a balloon control unit. The balloon is attached on the distal end of the tube, which is able to hold the small intestine by insufflation when shortening the intestine. The system has achieved great improvements in therapeutic enteroscopy.

The small intestine used to be called the "dark organ" because there was little chance of managing any diseases. Now Olympus Medical Systems has provided very efficient technologies in the enteroscopy field. The capsule endoscope can be used for a primary diagnosis, followed by the use of a single balloon enteroscope system as needed.

Key words. Enteroscopy, Capsule, Wireless, Single balloon enteroscope, Disposable tube

Introduction

The capsule endoscope had been conceived as the ultimate tool for endoscopic examination because of its painlessness and ease of use. However, there were many issues which had to be solved concerning the image sensor, battery, power consumption, and wireless technology during downsizing.

[1]Olympus Medical Systems Corp., Research and Development Division 1, Endoscope Department, 2951 Ishikawa-cho, Hachioji-shi, Tokyo 192-8507, Japan

[2]Olympus Medical Systems Corp., Research and Development Division 1, Future Endoscopic Department, Tokyo, Japan

Recent technological progress eventually led to its realization. The announcement of the world's first prototype, made by Given Imaging in Israel in 2000, inspired further technological progress. Olympus Medical Systems introduced the first capsule endoscope in Europe, Asia, and Oceania in October 2005, and launched it in North America upon FDA approval.

In Japan, an application to the Pharmaceutical Affairs Law has been submitted with the cooperation not only of EFJ affiliates, but also of carefully selected test laboratories. In October 2007, the approval is still pending.

Overview of the Capsule Endoscope

The capsule endoscope is a capsule-shaped camera that, after being swallowed like normal internal medicine, takes pictures of the inside of the body while passing through the intestinal tract. This procedure differs from conventional endoscopy. By simply swallowing the capsule endoscope, it moves through the intestinal tract by peristalsis, and allows gastrointestinal observations in a physiologically natural state. In particular, the small intestine can be observed with comparative ease.

As shown in Fig. 1, the system consists of a capsule endoscope for the small bowel (Figs. 2 and 3), a viewer (Fig. 4), a recorder unit and an antenna lead set (Fig. 5), and a workstation (Figs. 6 and 7). Because approval is still pending in Japan, the following explanations are focused on specifications for overseas countries.

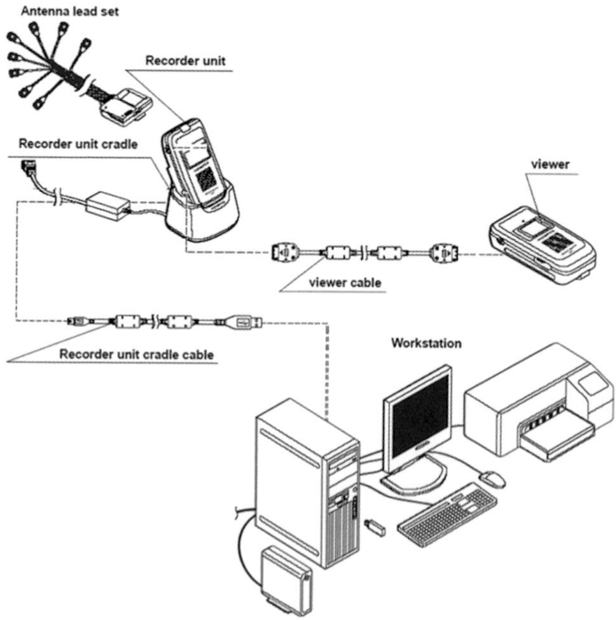

Fig. 1. Capsule endoscope system

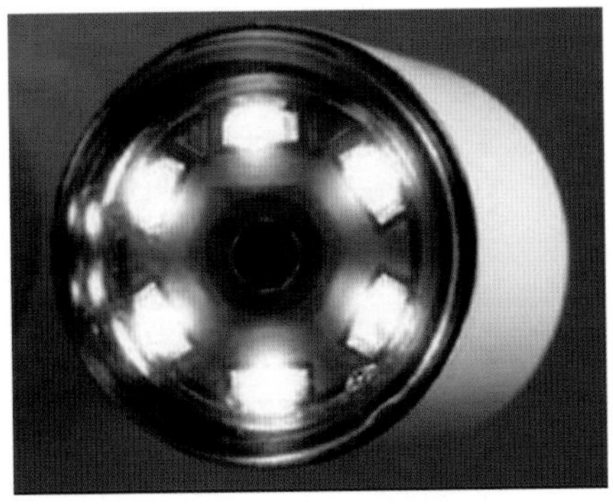

Fig. 2. Capsule endoscope for the small bowel

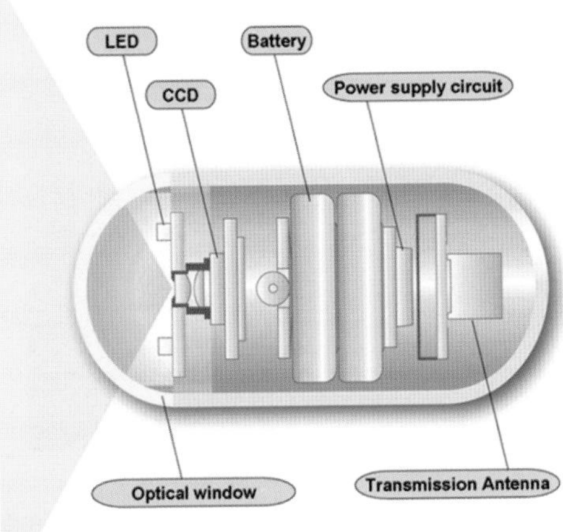

Fig. 3. Cross section of the capsule endoscope

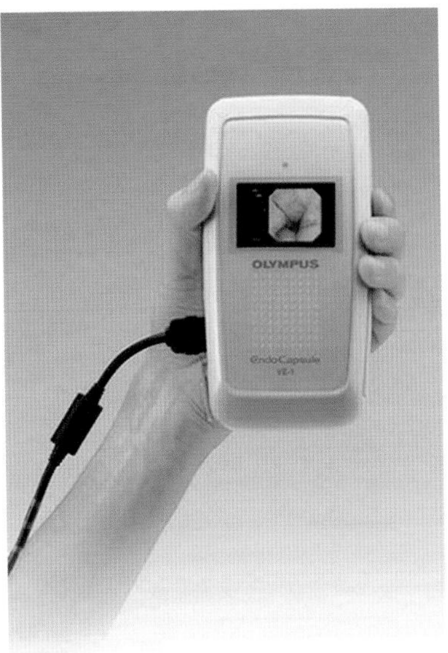

Fig. 4. Viewer

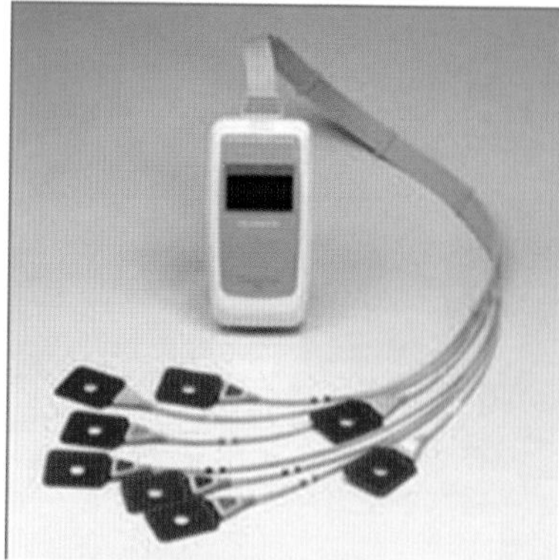

Fig. 5. Recorder unit and antenna lead set

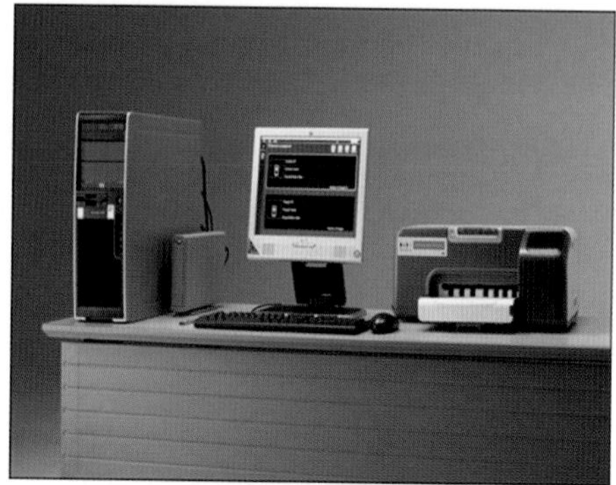

Fig. 6. Workstation

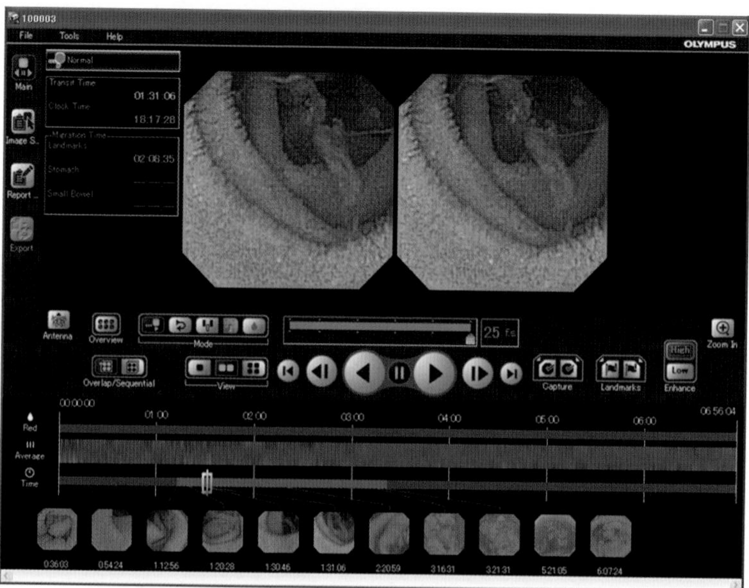

Fig. 7. Window as viewed on the monitor. Case provided by courtesy of Dr. J.F. Rey, Institut Arnault Tzanck

The camera is capsule-shaped, with an 11-mm outer diameter, and is 26-mm in length. It is made of biocompatible plastic and has a charge-coupled device (CCD) and six white light-emitting diodes (LEDs). Internally, it incorporates a wireless transmitter electrical circuit and small batteries to drive it.

The camera was successfully downsized by efficiently arraying the CCD, 6 LEDS, wireless transmitter, electrical circuits, and batteries in a small space. When connected to the receiver by a cable, the viewer displays the image that the recorder is receiving in real time. Images can be viewed before and/or during an examination as necessary.

The viewer is compact in size and fits snugly in the palm of the hand. The recorder runs on a detachable battery pack. When used in conjunction with a set of eight antenna leads, it picks up and records the image data from the capsule endoscope.

The workstation consists of purpose-specific software installed in a PC, a monitor, and a printer. Image data are transferred via a cradle, and are displayed continuously on the monitor at the preferred speed of the observers like a video. Images selected by the observer can be stored as thumbnails. Reports can be generated and printed out by the printer. Stored images can be exported into external storage devices or written onto DVD discs.

Features of the Capsule Endoscope

Improved Image Quality

The images look similar to ordinary endoscope images owing to the CCD, an appropriate optical system, and image processing. The system incorporates an automatic brightness control function using the technology developed with the video endoscope. The brightness of the image captured by a capsule endoscope is automatically detected and adjusted for the next frame if the previous one was excessively bright in order to prevent halation

Wireless Transmission of Image

The development of technologies for reliable transmission of images was made in conformity with broadcasting laws around the world. As a result, large volumes of data can be transmitted at high speed. In terms of information volume, the system is 10 times larger than the communication volume of one-segment broadcasting.

Future Development of the Capsule Endoscope

The capsule endoscope will probably evolve in the future in the following two ways.

1. Software improvements will make it much easier to read large volumes of image data.
2. System innovation.

These two directions are described in detail below.

Software Improvements

Currently, the capsule holds about 60 000 still images at each examination, and these all need to be diagnosed efficiently. Future software developments will target functional improvements to address this need. Currently, the supported functions include the detection of red colors and auto speed control that fast-forwards images of sluggish movement, and inversely slows images that contain movement.

We will be working on further developments targeting automatic diagnosis by expanding the support functions for diagnoses such as the detection of lesions.

System Innovation

The capsule endoscope was first developed for use in the small intestine, but will soon be developed for application to other organs. The optical system will be further improved to reduce oversights. The small battery will be improved and power consumption reduced to ensure a longer battery life. Then, although the current capsule endoscope moves passively through the intestinal tract by peristalsis, it is hoped that a self-propelled capsule endoscope that physicians can drive will be developed in the future.

Furthermore, by having this type of technology, i.e., movement control, at its core, in the future capsule endoscopes will be developed for administering medicines and performing treatments such as local injections.

Future developmental paths are outlined in Fig. 8. An Endo Capsule for use in the small intestine already exists under the name of the Entero Pro, and this is expected

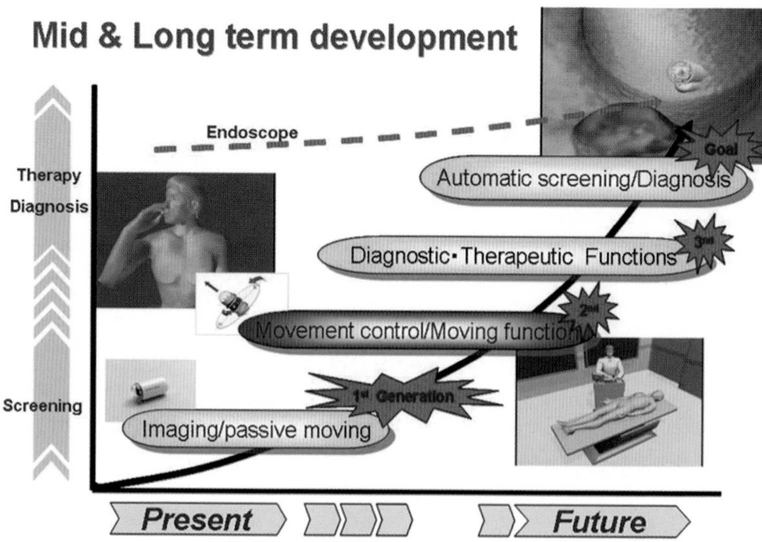

FIG. 8. Mid- and long-term development

to evolve alongside the endoscope. Future developments are expected to expand into various other fields by capitalizing on the convenience of using this device.

Single-Balloon Enteroscope System

Introduction

The development of enteroscopy started when the first fiberscopes were used. Pioneering doctors of that period invented unique approaches such as the Sonde-type scope and Ropeway-type scope [3,4], but deep intubation of the small intestine was still difficult. At that time, the small intestine was called the "dark organ" by endoscopists.

As a contribution to healthcare using enteroscopy, Olympus Medical Systems has successfully commercialized the single-balloon enteroscope system (Fig. 9), which allows deeper intubation. There follows a description of the single-balloon enteroscope system.

Components

The system consists of the endoscope, "SIF-Q260" (Fig. 10), a single use splinting tube, "ST-SB1" (Fig. 11), and a balloon control unit, "OBCU" (Fig. 12). The system is used with the Olympus Medical Systems' Evis system.

Endoscope: SIF-Q260

The SIF-Q260 (Olympus Medical Systems Corp.) has a high-quality CCD (Q-image) and a ϕ2.8 mm instrument channel. It provides high-quality images with various

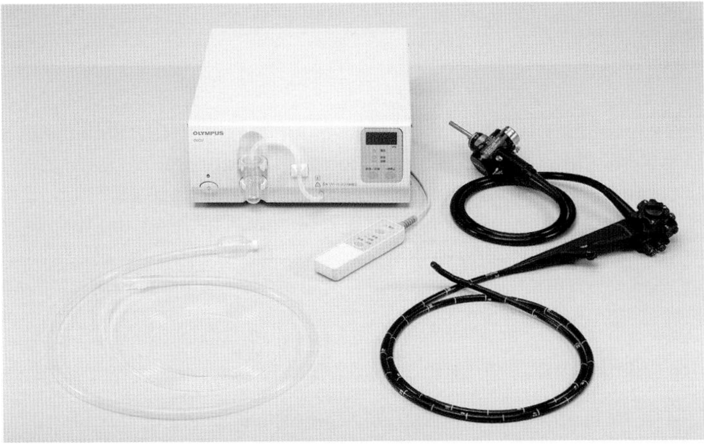

Fig. 9. Single-balloon enteroscope system

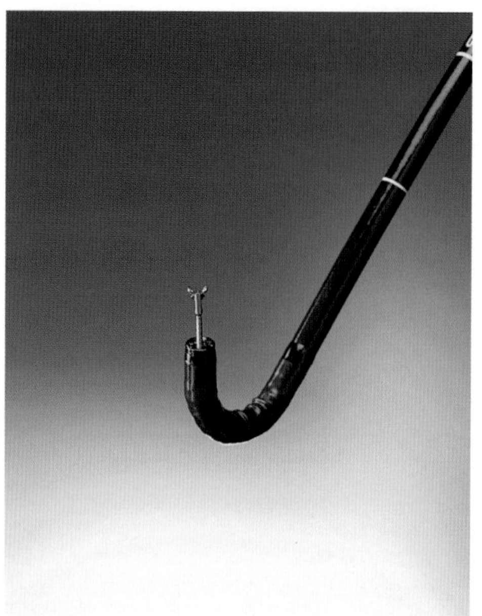

Fig. 10. Endoscope: SIF-Q260

Table 1. Specifications of SIF-Q260

Optics	Field of view	140°
	Depth of field	5~100 mm
Distal end outer diameter		9.2 mm
Insertion tube outer diameter		9.2 mm
Angulation range		U/D 180° R/L 160°
Insertion section working length		2,000 mm
Total length		2,345 mm
Instrument channel	Inner diameter	2.8 mm
	Minimum visible distance	3 mm
	Accessories enter	8 o'clock

therapeutic capabilities. In addition, narrow-band imaging (NBI) with the Evis Lucera spectrum system allows detailed observations of the mucosa.

The distal end and the insertion tube of the endoscope are ϕ9.2 mm in diameter. The working length of the insertion tube is 2000 mm. The insertion tube is very flexible in order to ensure ease of insertion. The basic structure of the SIF-Q260 is identical to that of a conventional endoscope, so that the cleaning, disinfection, and other handling operations are the same.

Single Use Spliting Tube: ST-SB1

The ST-SB1 is to facilitate the intubation. The tube is made of flexible silicone. The hydrophilic coating is applied inside the tube, and allows deep intubation even if there is a loop in intestine. The balloon which is attached to the distal end of the ST-SB1 is

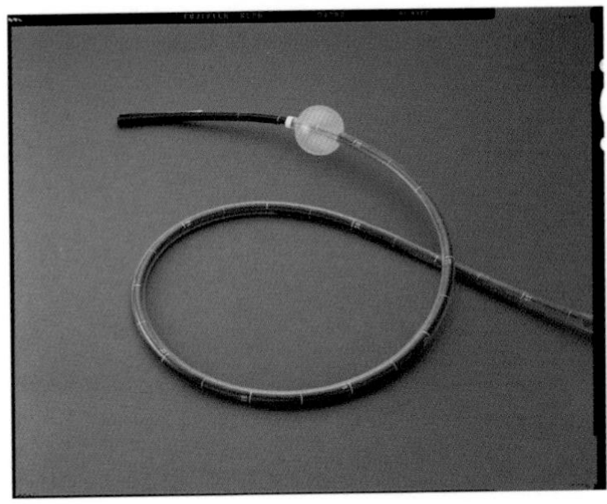

Fig. 11. Single use splinting tube: ST-SB1 (+SIF-Q260)

Table 2. Specifications of ST-SB1

Balloon	Outer diameter	40 mm
Insertion tube	Outer diameter	13.2 mm
	Inner diameter	11 mm
Working length		1,320 mm
Total length		1,400 mm
Material	Balloon	Silicone rubber
	Insertion tube	Silicone rubber

also made of silicone. It holds the small intestine safely when it is inflated. The tube is Latex-free because all materials, including the radio-opaque tip, are made of silicone.

Balloon Control Unit: OBCU

The purpose of the OBCU is to control the inflation and deflation of the balloon on the ST-SB1. When the balloon is inflated, the pressure is kept between 5.6 and 8.0 kPa by a sensor which monitors the pressure of the pump and the tubes. When the balloon is deflated, it is controlled at negative pressure. For additional safety, an alarm is set off if the pressure exceeds a certain level (8.2 kPa) during the procedure. Then the pressure is released in order to prevent it remaining high for a long time. The balloon can be operated either from a remote controller connected to the main unit, or from the buttons on the front panel of the main unit.

Features

Simple Setup

The setup is very easy. Connect one air tube between the OBCU and the ST-SB1. Then insert the SIF-Q260 into the ST-SB1 tube after water is fed inside of the tube. Deploy the disposable cover on the remote controller.

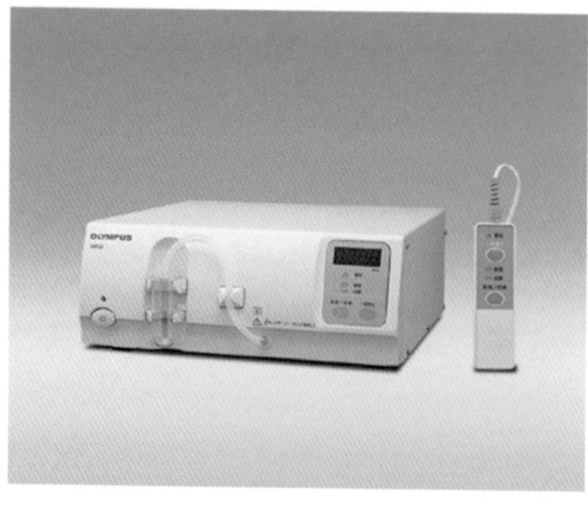

Fig. 12. Balloon control unit: OBCU

Table 3. Specifications of OBCU

Dimentions	370(W) × 139 (H) × 425 (D)
Weight	11 kg
Balloon control	Inflate, Deflate, Pause
Set pressure of Balloon	5.4 kPa $^{+2.6}_{-0}$ kPa
Pressure of opening air channel	8.2 kPa
Deflation pressure	–6.0 kPa $^{+0}_{-2.6}$ kPa

Deep Small-Intestinal Intubation

The simplicity of manipulation allows easy intubation from either the transoral or the transanal approach. The ST-SB1 easily holds the small intestine with the inflated balloon. The great slipperiness between the inside of the ST-SB1 and the SIF-Q260 facilitates good maneuverability through the complex loops in the stomach or colon.

After a Procedure

After a procedure has been completed, the ST-SB1, the air tube, and the remote controller cover are thrown away. The SIF-Q260 is reprocessed in the same way as a conventional endoscope. Because of the features described above, the single-balloon enteroscope system contributes to shortening the total procedure time.

Future Outlook

The commercialization of the single-balloon enteroscope system has resulted in the widespread use of deep intubation in the small intestine. More interest in enteroscopy is now expected. It would be possible to develop a better enteroscopy system with NBI observations, magnified observations, and other new observation technologies, or to combine these with endotherapy devices.

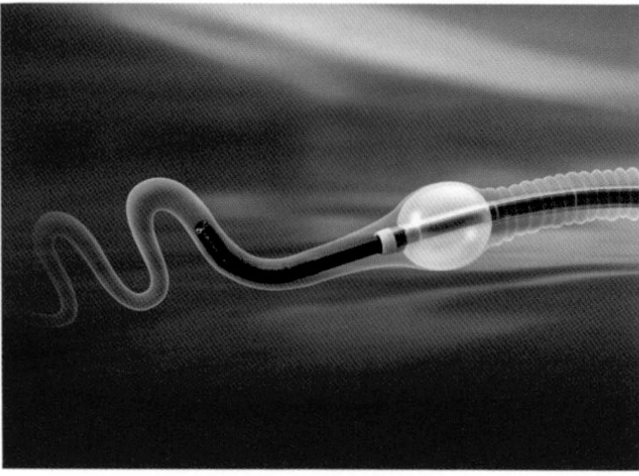

FIG. 13. SIF-Q260 + ST-SB1

However, nonfluoroscopic procedures, further improvements in the intubation, and a procedure which is less fatiguing for the patient are other important aspects that need to be addressed. There may be no end to the possible developments toward more safety, efficiency, and reliability in enteroscopy.

References

1. Hibi T, Ogata H, Otsuka K (2007) Capsule endoscopy atlas. p 2–8, Shindan to Chiryo sha Inc., Japan
2. Hibi T, Iwao T (2006) Endoscopic Diagnosis and Treatment of Large Intestinal Diseases. p 49–53, Shindan to Chiryo sha Inc., Japan
3. Hiratsuka H (1979) Present status and clinical application of small intestinal fiberscopy. J Nippon Med School 46:227–233, Medical Association of Nippon Medical School
4. Tada M, et al (1995) Up-to-date Enteroscopy for the Small Intestine. Stomach and Intestine (Tokyo) Vol.30 No.13:1647–1664

Future Perspectives of Small Bowel Capsule Endoscopy

James Daveson and Mark Appleyard

Summary. Since the advent of the first swallowable capsule designed to measure internal parameters from the small bowel 50 years ago, enormous advances in the ability to visualize the entire small bowel mucosa using a similar concept of a small swallowable capsule have been made. The incorporation of novel uses of light and other senses will lead to an expanded role for diagnostic capsules, as will the application of nanotechnologies to usher in new therapeutic indications for capsule endoscopy.

Key words. Capsule endoscopy, Small bowel, Optical biopsy, Biosensing, Nanosurgery

Introduction

2007 was the 50th anniversary of the development of a 2.8 cm by 0.9 cm capsule that was successfully swallowed and operated as it passed through the gastrointestinal tract. Using a sensing transducer and radio transmitter, it measured and relayed information, particularly concerning pressures generated from inside the small bowel [1]. In the year 2000, another capsule, 2.6 cm by 1.1 cm, was again swallowed, and using integrated circuit technology and advanced optical systems, it allowed wireless small bowel images to be relayed to an outside receiver [2]. In this new era inspired by the technology that is capsule endoscopy, new diagnostic and therapeutic visions will be realized.

Capsule endoscopy (CE) is now the diagnostic modality of choice for small bowel pathology. A number of clinical trials have demonstrated CE to be superior to other diagnostic modalities such as small bowel follow-through radiography, computerized tomographic enterography, magnetic resonance imaging (MRI) enteroclysis, and colonoscopy with ileoscopy in the diagnosis of small bowel disease. CE has demonstrated efficacy in a wide spectrum of disease, which includes obscure

Department of Gastroenterology, Royal Brisbane and Women's Hospital, Cnr Butterfield St and Bowen Bridge Rd, Herston, QLD, Australia 4029

gastrointestinal bleeding, nonstricturing Crohn's disease, small bowel tumors, and celiac disease [2].

Future potential advances in capsule endoscopy can be categorized under the broad headings of improved diagnostic capabilities and therapeutic applications. Advances in supportive technology such as improved software, wireless power, and capsule navigation systems will complement both these capabilities.

Diagnostic Capabilities

Diagnostic advancements will result from improvements in image quality as well as incorporating novel uses of light that will lead to improved screening and directed optical biopsies. Diagnostic capabilities are likely to be further expanded by combining light with tissue markers, whether they be injected or swallowed. Albeit currently less defined than light, other sensory markers such as temperature, noise, pressure, smell, and electrical impulses might add important information and lead to improved diagnoses and localization of small bowel pathology such as inflammation, ischemia, impaired motility, and possibly malignancy. The ability to biosense is likely to add to the capsule's diagnostic armamentarium.

Image Quality

Improvements in resolution will allow pathologies that are currently small and invisible to be seen. Current capsule imagers incorporate a field of view up to 150°, a depth of view of 1–30 mm, and 1:8 electronic magnification, allowing image detection to a minimum size of about 0.1 mm [2]. To obtain higher resolution, higher power consumption is required by the radiofrequency transmitter, and to date this has been a limiting factor. In the early 1990s these power concerns saw high-power consumption charge-coupled device (CCD) image sensors give way to complementary metal oxide semiconductor (CMOS) technology, thereby enabling sufficient battery life to support an 8-h capsule study.

Technological improvements in image quality continue to be pursued. In October 2005, the Endocapsule (Olympus Medical Systems, Tokyo, Japan) was launched, which saw a move back from CMOS technology to a CCD sensor camera [2]. However, both it and the CMOS technology, although able to transmit 2 images per second and delivering more 50,000 images to the sensor arrays, remain restricted to an 8- to 9-h battery life [2]. In 2007, the MiRO capsule was announced, which improves on the current magnification of 1.8 fold with digital zoom imaging allowing better mucosal resolution. It also incorporates a 150° field of view, 1.4–2.8 frames per second, and 9–11 h in battery time [3]. Recognizing power concerns, in 2006 a GICam pill was announced with a low power image compression processor [2] in an attempt to facilitate longer battery life.

Just as it will become possible to see more with improved resolution, larger areas could be visualized with the addition of multiple cameras within the one capsule. In 2004 Pill Cam ESO (Given Imaging, Yoqneam, Israel) was introduced with miniature cameras on both ends, capturing 14 images per second [2]. However, the sensitivity and specificity of small bowel imaging by CE is high, and although studies diagnosing additional lesions with repeat capsule studies exist, it remains unclear whether this translates to a need for multiple cameras with high frame rates per second within a single small bowel capsule. It may be more appropriate that additional cameras automatically activate when advanced software detects abnormalities.

Mesoscopic Imaging

The need for high-resolution optical technologies for imaging within the bowel is required for CE as it is for standard endoscopy. There is a need to be able to rapidly screen large segments of small bowel for areas of concern. Manipulated light, as seen with narrow-band imaging (NBI), is currently used to aid detection and diagnosis of dysplasia in the gastrointestinal (GI) tract, that is, to "red-flag" areas of concern [4]. Other red-flag technologies (RFT) include chromoendoscopy, biochromoendoscopy, and autoimmunofluorescence. An early forerunner of this type of technology is the "blue-light" technology introduced in the Rapid 5 software (Given Imaging) in 2007, which highlights areas of vascular anomalies. The two currently available capsule systems both have software that detects red colors which are most commonly associated with fresh blood.

However, light can also be manipulated [as in laser scanning confocal microscopy (LCM), optical coherence tomography (OCT), and ultrasound (USS)] to obtain true optical biopsies, thereby negating the need, expense, risk, and time required for traditional tissue biopsies. Although these new and exciting technologies have been used in other areas of medicine, conceivably it may be difficult to employ them successfully by CE. Their inherent limitations include (a) their difficulty in being contained within a single capsule, (b) their reliance on the need for stability and accurate placement along the bowel mucosa, with CE not yet mastering the ability to maneuver independently of peristalsis, and (c) the recent emergence of competing technologies such as balloon endoscopy that will be able to successfully incorporate these technologies.

Red-Flag Technologies

Chromoendoscopy

Chromoendoscopy (CME) is a technique in which stains are applied to the gastrointestinal mucosa to better characterize and highlight specific gastrointestinal findings. Studies have not been consistent in showing a benefit for chromoendoscopy for detecting adenomas [5]. The inability of a capsule to carry enough stain or to revisit the area of concern even with directed tissue staining currently limits its use in chromoendoscopy. Swallowed stains might be useful for aiding capsule detected mass lesions, but some stains can obscure vascular lesions, so it would be important to carefully select the patients for whom this technique is contemplated.

Biochromoendoscopy

Biochromoendoscopy (BCE) is a technique that combines the use of molecular imaging probes and CE to enhance the sensitivity and specificity in differentiating mucosal neoplasms. A near-infrared fluorescent probe injected intravenously and activated in vivo has been shown to be effective in mouse models in distinguishing adenomas from benign or inflammatory lesions in the intestines when using CE [6]. Again, the use of this technology as a rapid red-flag indicator in association with advanced automated detection software is conceivable.

Narrow-Band Imaging

Narrow-band imaging (NBI) allows the visualisation of defined mucosal surfaces and capillary vessels by adjusting the spectroscopic characteristics of the video-endoscopic system. Essentially the technology employs three optical filters for red-blue-green sequential illumination and narrows the bandwidth of the spectral transmittance. Some early data suggest that NBI might be useful for detecting dysplasia in the GI tract [4]. It is conceivable that NBI could be incorporated into a capsule endoscope and switched on to better characterize mass or vascular lesions.

Autoimmunofluorescence

In the technique of autoimmunofluorescence (AIF), low-power laser light is directed at a target tissue to induce endogenous tissue fluorescence without the use of photosensitizing agents. The induced autofluorescence has special characteristics that depend on the physicochemical composition of the tissue. It has been used by several groups to distinguish malignant or premalignant lesions from normal mucosa [7].

Optical Biopsy

Optical biopsy refers to the delineation of anatomical and/or pathological features without the conventional extraction of tissue. The development of this real-time interpretive technology is promising for CE as it does not require robotic equipment for capsule navigation and stability to coordinate directed tissue sampling, space for the storage and preparation of samples, or the retrieval of expelled capsules for tissue histology. Modalities for optical biopsy under development include reflectance LCM and OCT. Ultrasound (USS) is already being used to elucidate bowel pathologies.

Laser Scanning Confocal Microscopy

Laser scanning confocal microscopy (LCM) is a new noninvasive method of optical imaging designed to provide subsurface imaging. Focal laser illumination is combined with pinhole detection to geometrically reject out-of-focus light. A point is scanned in a raster pattern, and measurement of light returning to the detector from successive points is digitized so that an image of the scanned region can be constructed. Two LCM systems have been reported to examine GI lesions, reporting up to 97.4% sensitivity and 99.4% specificity in their ability to detect neoplastic change [8].

Optical Coherence Tomography

Optical coherence tomography (OCT) is a high-resolution, cross-sectional optical imaging technique that allows in situ imaging of tissue by measuring back-reflected light, and in real time provides a resolution approaching that for conventional histopathology. It is analogous to ultrasound although it uses light instead of acoustic waves. Ultrahigh-resolution OCT can visualize nuclei within single cells [7].

Ultrasound

A capsule could capture images by means of ultrasonic inspection. With less attenuation compared with images taken from outside the body, higher-resolution ultrasonic images could be obtained.

However, as stated, the translation of this technology into a capsule, given one does still need to be able to manipulate the capsule in the bowel, allowing it to be stabilized sufficiently for these images to be collected, will be challenging. Competing technologies such as balloon enteroscopy seem better placed to embrace it, particularly after diagnostic capsules containing red-flag technologies have identified a lesion.

Other Senses

Speculatively, the ability to derive information from other senses might allow the accurate diagnosis of small bowel pathologies at an early stage. In the 1950s, pressure and temperature could be sensed by a small capsule in the small bowel. Pressure was sensed by the motion of a diaphragm, which moved a piece of iron within the coil of a tuned circuit controlling the oscillator frequency. The transistor itself was quite sensitive to temperature, and as such was able to perform that function [1]. Promisingly, a wireless ingestible capsule endowed with three sensors for the monitoring of pH, temperature, and pressure was developed by the Smart Pill Corporation (Buffalo, NY, USA) and received FDA approval for sale and use in the United States in July 2006 [2]. The ability to record pressure will lead to a greater understanding of bowel motility and illnesses such as irritable bowel syndrome and will aid in manometric studies. Indirectly, wall compliance might be a marker for fibrosis or malignancy.

Increased temperature might foreseeably reflect inflammation and infection related to increased blood flow. Lack of an increase in temperature may provide clues toward small bowel ischemia. An acidic milieu may aid in the diagnosis of bacterial overgrowth, ischemia, or even certain tumors, while elasticity or its absence may give a clue to the neoplastic nature of underlying structures (an existing example is endoscopic ultrasound with pancreatic malignancies). Electrical impulses may, via CE, provide further insights into bowel motility in much the same way electrocardiography has provided insights into myocardial rhythm and ischemia. Furthermore, the ability to manipulate the electrical impulses of the bowel may also allow improved therapeutics in currently difficult-to-manage areas such as poor bowel motility. Noise, as a reflection of increased blood flow, in conjunction with increased temperature, may prove to reflect inflammation. Erythema and ulceration in the setting of reduced noise may indicate underlying ischemia with reduced electrical impulses.

Biosensing

Olympus Medical Systems, Tokyo, Japan, has developed a capsule with a negatively pressurized space controllable from outside the body for body fluid sampling [2].

Biosensing capsules might contain special sensors for oncological markers such as k-*ras* and be able to detect specific IgA antibodies in the bowel contents and to measure enzyme production from neuroendocrine tumors as well as luminal antigens.

Image Analysis and Software Development

Rapid 5 Software (Given Imaging) and Endo Capsule Software Light 2.0 (Olympus Medical Systems) already employ a tissue color bar that allows anatomical segmentation of the acquired images, permitting placement of the capsule position in the stomach, small bowel, or colon. Additional interpretive software should be able to complement this visual indicator to allow a global assessment of bowel preparation based on the clarity of the small bowel images.

The Olympus Medical Systems and Given software also employ viewing modes that reduce the number of images viewed, and hence improve reading times, by deleting images that are very similar. The sensitivity of this software analysis can be adjusted, and the optimal level of sensitivity that improves reading time, but does not miss significant findings, is currently unclear, although in these smart viewing modes one can follow the pace of the actual capsule through the small bowel. If the capsule marker moves quickly (in effect skipping multiple similar images of a study), then the implication is that the actual in vivo capsule is reasonably stagnant as it is seeing the same image over and over. Not withstanding the possibility of pathology causing mechanical holdup, this visual phenomenon should provide valuable insights into small bowel motility, possibly uncovering recurring patterns in illnesses such as irritable bowel syndrome. In addition, more accurate localization of the capsule should also be possible in the future. The current recorded small bowel transit time includes the stagnant periods when the in vivo capsule as just described is actually not moving much at all. Thus, the recorded period of movement of the capsule from the pylorus may be exaggerated. Software that can correctly delete stagnant phases and then recalculate the reduced time of actual movement through the small bowel will facilitate a more accurate localization of pathological abnormalities.

Other software developments might include some of the red-flag technologies already described that will allow rapid image scanning for areas of abnormality. Current software can identify images that contain certain reds, which can be associated with fresh blood. Other automatic computerized systems for the automatic detection of pathologies, such as that present in the ECG-Holter recording, are likely to be developed to overcome the drawback of time-consuming viewing [9].

Therapeutic Applications

Therapeutic applications will see advances in drug delivery and pathological localization. These developments will be supported by improved power supplies, capsule navigation systems, and nanotechnology that will allow therapeutic interventions at sites of abnormalities.

Drug Delivery

The ability to be able to direct the release of drugs such as chemotherapeutics, immunomodulators, or eventually antifibrotics into the bowel carries enormous potential. These drugs may be of use in nonoperative small bowel tumors or Crohn's disease. The NEMO project team, supported by Given Imaging, is studying biological markers including antibodies attached to nanocontainers to visualize gastrointestinal pathology. Olympus Medical Systems reports developing a capsule with a deflatable balloon that is controllable from outside the body to facilitate drug delivery. The Norika Project Team (RF SYSTEM Lab, Nagano, Japan) reports that they have developed a capsule with 40% of the capsule volume able to host reservoirs for drug delivery, sensors, or miniaturized knives and scissors for advanced diagnostic tasks [2].

Pathology Localization

A major problem in determining the site of pathology visualized by CE is its localization, given the length of the small bowel, lack of clear landmarks, and continuous free movement of the small bowel. Image analysis may aid in the localization of a capsule in relation to the distance through the small bowel, but localization within the abdomen is more challenging. Marking the small bowel at the site of pathology would be the most reliable method of localization within the abdomen. Improved capabilities of capsules may see them acquire the ability to offshoot biodegradable expanding bands from outside their body, enabling an accurate localization at subsequent laparotomy, or when followed by a therapeutic capsule. Equally, a small secondary capsule may be able to offshoot from the mother capsule and be externally controlled to attach onto the abnormal tissue or normal tissue close by, much the same way an endoclip can be attached to mucosa currently. The injection of a small amount of dye to tattoo the area may also be feasible.

Supportive Technology

Three current major limitations with CE include the following:

1. A restricted internal battery power supply.
2. The restrictions of movement only by peristalsis with consequent inability to halt the progression to examine areas of interest.
3. The current inability to use microelectromechanical systems to intervene therapeutically.

Addressing these issues are the concepts of wireless power, capsule navigation systems, and nanotechnology.

Wireless Power

The conventional wireless capsule uses a built-in battery for its power source, limiting it to only two frames/second for 8 h. In the 1950s, it was suggested a person could be placed within a coil, and then energy delivered to a secondary coil within the capsule [1]. Others have also suggested an external power source with coils outside the body being able to transmit energy to those coils inside the capsule by exploiting the principle of electromagnetic induction [2]. Biomedical devices to generate electricity from within the body are being devised, and it could be that current-generating bacteria could provide long-term power for capsules [2]. In a published experiment, the battery for power generation was derived from a gold and iron electrode, with the internal fluids of the subject acting as an electrode [1]. Improved power will assist with improved images and diagnostics as well as eventually providing the potential scope for unlimited power for maneuverability.

Capsule Navigation Systems

The Norika Project team reports developing a pill with an external controller, transmitter vest, and workstation. Three coils placed inside the capsule act as rotor coils, and three coils imbedded in a jacket act as stators. Rotator direction, which may enable enhanced image acquisition, is set by the direction of stator magnetic fields [2].

In a joint collaborative effort between Olympus Medical Systems and Arai & Nishigama Laboratory (Research Laboratory & Electrical Communication, Tohoku University), a capsule navigation system with an external magnetic field generator and permanent magnets built into the capsule is being developed. An external magnetic field generator using three pairs of opposing electromagnets creates a uniform magnetic field in any direction. By varying this magnetic field, the position, orientation, and posture of the pill can be controlled [2]. The NEMO project team is also looking at remotely controlling a capsule using magnetic fields.

Electrostimulation to move endoscopes in the small bowel have already been described. Ovoid devices with stainless steel electrodes mounted on the tapered sections with applied electrostimulation to one end have caused circular muscular contraction and propulsion of the device when tested in pigs and humans, with potential powering by a single button battery for more than 24 h [2].

Nanotechnology

The SSSA robotic capsule was developed by the research team of Scuola Superiore Sant' Anna (Pisa, Italy), which has developed a capsule with legs and a small balloon at its head (which can open the bowel, allowing the camera to focus on the largest area possible). When it comes to be tested in humans, the capsule body will be encased in a biocompatible and biodegradable layer to prevent accidental deployment in the mouth and esophagus. This layer will be dissolved by the gastric juices. Fine position control by varying the extension and orientation of the legs of the capsule will allow controlled passage over critical areas, as well as a reduced length of journey through the bowel [2]. It is likely that nanotechnology will progress to deliver the possibility of movable parts within a capsule.

Multiple Capsules

We suspect clinicians in the future will have multiple capsules at their disposal. They might be largely divided into diagnostic or therapeutic, possibly with reduced power and space being devoted to optics, instead allowing an increased capacity for therapeutic procedures and focused drug delivery. Our opinion is that diagnostic capsules will, for the immediate future, preside over therapeutic capsules in terms of clinical development and implementation. Although the development of additional power supplies and capsule navigation systems (both inherently important for therapeutic capsules) is ongoing, both remain firmly in the development phase. Moreover, balloon endoscopy is rapidly solidifying and broadening its role as the therapeutic extension of CE in the small bowel, and in the short term it would be difficult for a therapeutic capsule to compete with this technology.

Summary

Future indications for capsule endoscopy will be divided into diagnostic and therapeutic, and it may be that capsules also will develop along these two pathways. We believe the immediate focus will be on broadening the diagnostic capsule's armamentarium. Optical technologies, biosensing, and technologies extrapolating from a broad range of monitored senses incorporated into capsules are likely to be used to aid the diagnosis of early tumors, bowel ischemia, bacterial overgrowth, bowel inflammation, and enteric infections. Software development will also aid in the diagnosis and assessment of small bowel pathology and possibly altered bowel motility. Indeed, small bowel diseases currently not recognized might become so.

The therapeutic indications will be based on the development of remotely controlled capsules with more available power. Possibilities are not limited to photocoagulation for small bowel bleeding, but will possibly aid in definitive surgical interventions by tagging pathology. The ability to carry out therapy and deliver drugs will develop with advances in nanotechnology. Implantable or directed pulse generation in the bowel wall for altered motility may also become possible and useful.

The scope of capsule endoscopy will be limited only by the limitations of the clinicians' potential to recognize applications for it. Once a need of sufficient merit is recognized, the technology will follow at a rapid pace.

References

1. Mackay RS, Jacobson B (1957) Endoradiosonde. Nature (Lond) 4572:1239
2. Moglia A, Menciassi A, Schurr MO, et al (2007) Wireless capsule endoscopy: from diagnostic devices to multipurpose robotic systems. Biomed Microdevices 9:235–243
3. Kim TS, Song SY, Jung H, Kim J, Yoon ES (2007) Micro capsule endoscope for gastrointestinal tract. Engineering in Medicine and Biology Society. 29th Annual International Conference of the ICEE 22–26 Aug: 2823–2826
4. Hirata M, Tanaka S, Oka S, et al (2007) Magnifying endoscopy with narrow band imaging for diagnosis of colorectal tumors. Gatrointest Endosc 65:988–995
5. Hurlstone DP, Fujii T, Lobo AJ (2002) Early detection of colorectal cancer using high-magnification chromoscopic colonoscopy. Br J Surg 89:272–282
6. Alencar H, Funovics MA, Figueiredo J, Sawaya H, Weissleder R, Mahmood U (2007) Colonic adenocarcinomas: near-infrared microcatheter imaging of smart probes for early detection—study in mice. Radiology 244:232–238
7. Wang TD, Van Dam J (2004) Optical biopsy: a new frontier in endoscopic detection and diagnosis. Clin Gastroenterol Hepatol 2:744–753
8. Yoshida S, Tanaka S, Hirata M, et al (2007) Optical biopsy of GI lesions by reflectance-type laser-scanning confocal microscopy. Gastrointest Endosc 66:144–149
9. Fireman Z, Kopelman Y (2007) New frontiers in capsule endoscopy. J Gastroenterol Hepatol 22:1174–1177

Colon

Screening for Colorectal Cancer in the Asia-Pacific Region: Are We Ready Yet?

Jose D. Sollano, Jr.,[1] Ming-Shiang Wu,[2] and Joseph Sung[3]

Summary. The past two decades have witnessed a dramatic rise in colorectal cancer incidence and mortality in Asia. The Asia-Pacific Region represents a diversified population with disparities in disease prevalence, health belief attitudes, and health-care infrastructure. The public, in general, is poorly informed about the rising incidence of colorectal cancer and the benefits of screening tests. Financial constrains appear to be a major hurdle to implementing a screening program. Clinical studies showed that colonic neoplasms are predominantly found in the distal colon. However, 50% of patients with proximal colonic lesions have a normal distal colon. Large-scale studies from Asia using the fecal occult blood test have shown promising results. A risk stratification scoring system is in development to select high-risk subjects for screening colonoscopy. Asia needs to work together to stop the rising colorectal cancer mortality in this region.

Key words. Colorectal cancer, Screening, Colonoscopy, Asians, FOBT

Introduction

In 2005, the Asia-Pacific Working Group on Colorectal Cancer reported a dramatic increase in the incidence of colorectal carcinoma (CRC) in several countries in Asia [1]. Data from this region indicate that this incidence already approximates those reported from the West, especially among the more affluent populations. In men, the age-standardized rate for CRC is 49.3 in Japan, 44.4 in the United States, and 42.9 in western Europe [2]. In mainland China, along with lung and breast cancer, CRC is reported to be one of the three malignancies that has demonstrated a rapidly increasing incidence since 1991 [3]. In Singapore, it was the second most common cancer in both sexes at the turn of the century [4]. In the Philippines, colorectal cancer has

[1]University of Santo Tomas, Manila, Philippines
[2]National Taiwan University, Taipei, Taiwan
[3]Department of Medicine and Therapeutics, Prince of Wales Hospital, The Chinese University of Hong Kong, Hong Kong SAR

become the fourth most common cause of cancer mortality; it was sixth only 15 years ago [5].

There are a number of reasons attributable to these changes in epidemiology. Westernization in lifestyle, including dietary habits, has been implicated to increase the risks of CRC. The high consumption of meat and animal fat in Japan and preserved food in China is associated with the development of CRC. Interestingly, ethnicity and genetic factors appear to be a significant influence as well. In multiracial societies such as Singapore and Malaysia, a higher incidence of CRC is reported to be more common among the Chinese, compared to the Indians and Malays who are living in the same environment in those countries [6]. Two cross-sectional studies have been completed in Asia Pacific through a consortium in the Asia Pacific Working Group on Colorectal Cancer. From 10 Asian countries, a total of 7290 subjects had undergone colonoscopy in this study [7,8]. Among 5464 subjects with bowel symptoms referred for colonoscopy, advanced neoplasms (i.e., adenoma greater than 1 cm or with high-grade dysplasia or villous structure) was found in 512 (9.4%) subjects [7]. Factors associated with the presence of these lesions include male gender [relative risk (RR), 1.52], advanced age (RR, 1.05), and ethnicity. Japanese, Koreans, and Chinese are among the ethnic groups with the highest risk of developing advanced neoplasms. In this study, of 860 consecutive asymptomatic adults undergoing screening colonoscopy, 18.5% had colorectal neoplasms and 4.5% had advanced neoplasms [8]. When compared to the Chinese, Japanese and Koreans have an increased risk for CRC in Asia, at RR 2.65, 95% confidence interval (CI) 1.74–4.04 and RR 1.88, 95% CI 1.43–2.37, respectively.

Screening for Colorectal Cancer Leads to Decreasing Mortality in the West

Screening is a strategy that aims to ensure early diagnosis and prompt treatment of diseases to the ultimate advantage of the patients. According to the World Health Organization (WHO), screening is actively seeking to identify a disease or pre-disease condition in individuals who are presumed to be or consider themselves to be healthy [9]. According to the United Kingdom National Screening Committee (UK NSC), screening is the systematic application of a test or inquiry to identify individuals at sufficient risk of a specific disorder to warrant further investigation or direct preventive action among persons who have not sought medical attention on account of symptoms of that disorder [10]. The definition of screening has evolved since its first description by the U.S. Commission on Chronic Illness in 1958 to the latest UK NSC definition, which includes the risk-to-benefit concept of the many screening tools utilized in many diseases for which screening should be performed [11]. Screening for a certain condition is justified if the condition is an important health problem, its natural history is well understood, it has a recognizable latent, asymptomatic period, a suitable, safe, and acceptable screening test is available, an established treatment and its related facilities are widely available, and the cost of case-finding is affordable by the healthcare system of the given population. CRC is a disease that satisfies all these criteria. The recent report of decreased mortality related to CRC in the Unites States for the past 2 consecutive years represents a major triumph in this endeavor

[12,13]. Although several reasons have been proposed, the declining mortality has been largely attributed to the remarkable success of screening programs for colonic polyps and CRC in the United States. The legislative support to finance the CRC screening programs and the aggressive CRC information campaigns for the general population, with the help of prominent media personalities, had considerable impact on this effort.

Is Asia Ready for Colorectal Carcinoma Screening?

Asia, with its ethnical, geographic, and economic diversity, represents a very heterogeneous population. Is the Asia-Pacific region ready to implement a screening program for colorectal cancer? Can we repeat what was achieved with CRC in North America? According to a survey in Singapore that included 2000 randomly selected subjects, only 1.4%–2.7% of the interviewed subjects named colorectal cancer as a fatal disease, and less than 50% knew that the colon and rectum are part of the intestines [14]. Similarly, in a study that interviewed 1033 Hong Kong residents to determine their knowledge and attitude toward CRC screening, only 8.9% knew that CRC is a very common cause of death [15]. About half (49.7%) know that there is a screening venue nearby but only 29.5% are willing to join a free CRC screening program. Besides public awareness, financial consideration appears to be a major obstacle for a target population to access colorectal cancer screening tests [14]. It seems that even in a relatively affluent Asian population, cost is a major barrier to CRC screening. A positive family history and hence knowledge of CRC raise concern levels high enough to make respondents join even a paid screening program. A Singapore study also identified expense as a major reason for not submitting to a CRC screening in 56.6% of respondents. Among the Chinese in Singapore, knowledge about CRC is deficient; however, the influence of family and friends and prior experience with other screening programs will push them to submit to a CRC screening strategy [16]. There is a great need for an intensive campaign to raise the awareness of the Asian population regarding colorectal cancer. Information as to where to get the tests, clarifying issues of safety, ease, and diagnostic yield of current screening tests, impact of early detection and prompt treatment of precancerous polyps and/or early cancer, and strategies toward modifying culturally linked attitudes related to the screening tests need to be passed on to them. In addition, an overhaul of the healthcare funding allocation is necessary to make the tests affordable to the general population.

Who Should Be Screened for Colorectal Cancer?

The U.S. guidelines recommend that screening for CRC should be offered to all average-risk individuals above the age of 50 years [17,18]. The screening tests recommended for these individuals included fecal occult blood test (FOBT) annually, flexible sigmoidoscopy every 5 years, FOBT annually and flexible sigmoidoscopy every 5 years or colonoscopy every 10 years, or double-contrast barium enema every 5 years. None of these tests is recommended above the others as there is a lack of data in support of a particular choice. However, even in the United States it is well known that women have a lower risk of developing CRC and the incidence starts to climb at the age of 55 years instead of 50 [19]. On the other hand, African Americans have a higher risk of CRC than white Americans [20]. However, the guidelines have made no change regarding age and gender in the recommendations.

It has been pointed out earlier that several differences exist between the populations with CRC and its clinical presentation in Asia and the West. A study comparing an American cohort living in Florida versus a Chinese cohort in Guangzhou revealed that the mean age of diagnosis of CRC among the Chinese was significantly lower, that is, 48.3 years versus 69 years in the Americans. The distribution of colonic adenoma is also different comparing the East against the West. Lesions in the proximal colon were seen in 36.3% of Americans versus 26% in the Chinese. Distal CRC is significantly more common in the Chinese than in the Americans, 74% and 63.7%, respectively [21]. A Veterans Administration (VA) facility in New York City studied 2207 average-risk individuals above the age of 50 of varying ethnicity. Asians have a significantly higher prevalence of distal colonic neoplasia than other ethnic groups (24.7% in Asians, 12.6% in Caucasians, 11.2% in African Americans, and 15.9% in Hispanics). Proximal colonic lesions (found in follow-up colonoscopy when a distal lesion is noted on flexible sigmoidoscopy) as well as advanced neoplasms in the proximal colon were also lowest among Asians, 26.3% and 10.5%, respectively [22]. The predominant distal distribution of colonic neoplasms were also observed in 505 average-risk, asymptomatic individuals who were screened by colonoscopy in a community-based study in Hong Kong [23]. On the other hand, the distribution of advanced colonic neoplasms might be different in the younger cohorts. A recent study comparing younger subjects below the age of 40 years in Taiwan versus Americans revealed that there were more Taiwanese patients (52%) with proximal advanced lesions when a distal neoplasia was present than the Americans (30.8%) [24].

In the Asia Pacific Working Group on Colorectal Cancer studies, the distribution of advanced colonic neoplasms was analyzed [7,8]. In the symptomatic cohort, advanced proximal neoplasm was detected in 2.5%, but more than 60% of them had a normal distal colon [7]. Similarly, in the asymptomatic cohorts, 40% of patients with proximal neoplasms have a normal distal finding in colonoscopy [8]. Thus, using distal findings as a guide for referral to proximal lesions may not be appropriate. In view of the potential difference in risk factors associated with colorectal neoplasms in the East compared to the West, the Asia Pacific Working Group is working on a risk stratification scoring system to select the "higher-risk" individuals in the general population for (the) screening [25,26]. The risk stratification and prioritization of screening procedure is particularly important in areas with limited resources.

Which Test and Strategy Should Be Adopted in Asia?

With a wide range of screening tests available, the obvious question is which one is preferred. The fecal occult blood test (FOBT) has the lowest sensitivity and specificity but ironically is the only test that has been shown in a randomized study to reduce CRC incidence and mortality. On the other hand, colonoscopy is arguably the most accurate test, but there is no evidence to prove that it has reduced CRC incidence and mortality. Therefore, in all the available guidelines, none of these screening tests has been recommended over the others. Perhaps the best screening test for CRC is the one that could be offered by the healthcare system and be accepted by the population.

A population-based study in Beijing on 19 852 average-risk individuals older than 30 years of age showed that FOBT is quite an acceptable screening examination in China [27]; 74% of the target population complied to the test. Colonoscopy, performed for those who were tested positive for FOBT, revealed adenoma or colorectal malignancy in 55 of the 501 FOBT+ individuals. The strongest evidence of benefit of FOBT screening comes recently from Japan. A prospective study performed in 42,150 Japanese men and women aged 40–59 years showed that FOBT screening reduced the incidence of advanced CRC by 44% (OR, 95% CI –0.44, 0.28–0.69) and mortality from CRC by about one-third (OR, 95% CI –0.31, 0.14–0.69) [28]. These observations were noted in both men and women (advanced CRC, for males OR, 95% CI –0.32, 0.16–0.61, for females OR, 95% CI –0.62, 0.34–1.14; CRC deaths for males OR, 95% CI –0.30, 0.11–0.84, for females OR, 95% CI –0.24, 0.06–1.00). FOBT screening appears to be most advantageous for the Japanese population in the sixth decade of life.

A recent study performed among the ethnic Chinese in Hong Kong compared the accuracy and safety of FOBT, flexible sigmoidoscopy, and colonoscopy among individuals older than 50 years. FOBT was found to have a low sensitivity (14.3%) but a reasonable specificity (79.2%) of finding advanced colonic neoplasms [23]. However, the use of an immunochemical test has been shown to improve significantly the sensitivity and specificity of FOBT [29]; this is related to the fact that a dietary restriction is no longer required and compliance of this test may improve among Asian subjects.

Another interesting approach is to adopt an age-dependent two-step screening strategy for CRC. This approach was evaluated in a cohort of 2106 asymptomatic, average-risk Taiwanese 50 years or more of age who underwent colonoscopy as part of their regular health checks. Using a hypothetical mixed screening strategy, that is, performing colonoscopy for older individuals while performing sigmoidoscopy in younger individuals, the investigator suggested that a more cost-effective strategy can be implemented [30]. When a distal sentinel lesion was noted during sigmoidoscopy, a total colonoscopy followed. It is estimated that if colonoscopy is performed at 60 years, the detection rate for advanced proximal neoplasia is 80%–83% and that for advanced colonic neoplasia in the entire colon is 92%–93%. For every year over age 50, the risk for proximal advanced neoplasia increases by 7%. Distal adenoma (by histology) and distal polyps of 10 mm or larger are predictive of advanced proximal neoplasia. In average-risk Taiwanese, using a two-step screening strategy for CRC, that is, performing colonoscopy in individuals older than 60 years and in those with sentinel lesions detected after sigmoidoscopy, is an effective approach.

Quite clearly, screening strategies should be fitted to the demographic characteristics of the population, the incidence of colorectal cancer, and the available infrastructure and resources of the different countries in Asia. While many argue that colonoscopy should be the standard procedure for CRC screening, given the current disparity of incomes and diversity of healthcare systems in Asia, FOBT appears to be an attractive option for many countries who intends to start a screening program for CRC [31]. It is cheap, probably acceptable to almost all ethnic groups in the region, and has already shown its capability to decrease the incidence of advanced CRC, as well as reduce mortality. However, as the epidemiology of CRC in Asia unravels and becomes better understood, other strategies should be tested and validated so that a more cost-effective yet culturally acceptable screening algorithm can be offered to all Asian patients at risk for CRC.

Acknowledgment. This chapter is modified from the State-of-the-Art Lecture on "Colorectal Cancer Screening in Asia" from the Asia Pacific Digestive Week 2006, Cebu, Philippines.

References

1. Sung JJY, Lau JYW, Goh KL, et al (2005) Increasing incidence of colorectal cancer in Asia: implications for screening. Lancet Oncol 6:871–876
2. World Health Statistics Annual. Geneva, WHO Database. http://www-dep.iarc.fr/).
3. Lu JB, Sun XB, Dai DX, et al (2003) Epidemiology of gastroenterologic cancer in Henan province, China. World J Gastroenterol 9:2400–2403
4. Chia KS, Lee HP, Seow A, et al (1995) Trends in cancer incidence in Singapore 1968–1992. Singapore Cancer Registry report no. 4. Singapore Cancer Registry, Singapore
5. Philippine Cancer Society (2005) Philippine Cancer Facts and Estimates. Manila Cancer Registry, Rizal Cancer Registry and Department of Health—Philippine Cancer Control Program
6. Lim GCC, Lim TO, Yahaya H (eds) (2002) The first report of the National Cancer Registry: cancer incidence in Malaysia 2002. National Cancer Registry, Kuala Lumpur, Malaysia
7. Leung WK, Ho KY, Kim WH, et al (2006) Colorectal neoplasia in Asia: a multicenter colonoscopy survey in symptomatic patients. Gastrointest Endosc 64: 751–759
8. Byeon JS, Yang SK, Kim TI, et al (2007) Colorectal neoplasm in asymptomatic Asians: a prospective multinational multicenter colonoscopy survey. Gastrointest Endosc 65:1015–1022
9. Holland WW, Stewart S, Masseria C (2006) WHO policy brief: screening in Europe 2006. In behalf of the European Observatory on Health Systems and Policies. WHO, Geneva
10. Health Departments of the United Kingdom (2000) Second Report of the UK National Screening Committee
11. Commission on Chronic Illness (1957) Chronic illness in the United States. Commonwealth Fund, Harvard Medical Press, Cambridge
12. Washington Post Staff Writer (2007) Cancer deaths decline for second straight year: fewer smokers, more screening credited. Washington Post, Jan 18, A01
13. Grady D (2007) Second drop in cancer deaths could point to a trend, researchers say. New York Times, Jan 18
14. Wong NY, Nenny S, Seon-Cheon F (2002) Adults in a high-risk area are unaware of the importance of colorectal cancer: a telephone and mail survey. Dis Colon Rectum 45:946–950
15. Wong BCY, Chan AOO, Wong WM, et al (2006) Attitudes and knowledge of colorectal cancer and screening in Hong Kong: a population-based study. J Gastroenterol Hepatol 21:42–46
16. Ng EST, Tan CH, Teo DCL, et al (2007) The knowledge and perceptions regarding colorectal screening are unique in the Chinese: a community-based study in Singapore. Prev Med 45:332–335
17. Levin B, Bond J (1996) Colorectal cancer screening: recommendations of the US Preventive Service Task Force. Gastroenterology 111:1381–1384

18. Winawer S, Fletcher R, Rex D, et al (2003) Colorectal cancer screening and surveillance: clinical guidelines and rationale-update based on new evidence. Gastroenterology 124:544–560
19. Schoenfeld P, Cash B, Flood A, et al (2005) Colonoscopic screening of average-risk women for colorectal neoplasia. N Engl J Med 352:2061–2068
20. Agrawal S, Bhupinderjit A, Bhutani MS, et al (2005) Colorectal cancer in African Americans. Am J Gastroenterol 100:515–523
21. Qing SH, Rao KY, Jiang HU, et al (2003) Racial differences in the distribution of colorectal cancer: a study of differences between American and Chinese patients. World J Gastroenterol 9:721–725
22. Francois F, Park J, Bini EJ (2006) Colonic pathology detected after a positive screening flexible sigmoidoscopy: a prospective study of an ethnically diverse cohort. Am J Gastroenterol 101:823–830
23. Sung JJY, Chan FKL, Leung WK, et al (2003) Screening for colorectal cancer in Chinese: comparison of fecal occult blood test, flexible sigmoidoscopy, and colonoscopy. Gastroenterology 124:608–614
24. Soon MS, Kozarek RA, Ayub K, et al (2005) Screening colonoscopy in Chinese and Western patients: a comparative study. Am J Gastroenterol 100:2749–2755
25. Yeoh KG, Ho KY, Chiu HM, et al (2007) Development of a clinical risk score predictive of colorectal neoplasm. UEGW (United European Gastroenterology Week) 2007, Paris
26. Chiu HM, Lin JT, Wu MS, et al (2007) Prevalence and predictors of proximal advanced neoplasms in Asian subjects being screened for colorectal cancer. UEGW 2007, Paris
27. Li SR, Nie ZH, Li N, et al (2003) Colorectal cancer screening for the natural population of Beijing with sequential fecal occult blood test: a multicenter study Chin Med J 116:200–202
28. Lee, KJ, Manami I, Otani T, et al (2007) Colorectal cancer screening using fecal occult blood test and subsequent risk of colorectal cancer: a prospective cohort study in Japan. Cancer Detect Prevent 31:3–11
29. Wong BCY, Wong WM, Cheung KL, et al (2003) A sensitive guaiac fecal occult blood test is less useful than an immunochemical test for colorectal cancer screening in a Chinese population. Aliment Pharmacol Ther 18:94–106
30. Liou JM, Lin JT, Huang SP, et al (2007) Screening for colorectal cancer in average-risk Chinese population using a mixed strategy using sigmoidoscopy and colonoscopy. Dis Colon Rect 50:630–640
31. Sung JJY (2006) Does fecal occult blood test have a place for colorectal screening in China? Am J Gastroenterol 101:213–225

Establishment of a Standard Curriculum for Colonoscope Insertion Techniques

Masahiro Igarashi[1] and Sumio Tsuda[2]

Summary. This article introduces a standard training curriculum for beginners in colonoscopic examination. The purpose of this curriculum was the stable acquisition of techniques through short-term clinical experience, as compared with the learning curve for acquiring the techniques through conventional training methods. The curriculum was based on a three-step approach. Step 1 focuses on the acquisition of basic knowledge needed to perform colonoscopy. In step 2, basic techniques required for colonoscope insertion are acquired, using a colon model. Training with the use of a colon model has the most important role in this curriculum, which gives an overview of the technical skills required for colonoscope insertion and lists important points according to the segment of the colon. In step 3, the scope should pass through the sigmoid-desending junction (SDJ) within 15 min and reach the cecum within 20 min, with an insertion rate of 80%. The curriculum describes the details of training for beginners and provides specific goals. It also provides teaching doctors with guidelines for instruction and training. It is concluded that this curriculum should be useful for training of colonoscope insertion skills.

Key words. Colonoscopy, Training curriculum, Colon model, Colonoscope insertion skill, Manual compression

Introduction

There are two well-known basic techniques for colonoscope insertion: the two-man method developed by Tajima [1] and the one-man method developed by Shinya [2]. Recently, the one-man method has been used at most hospitals in Japan.

Education and training on techniques for colonoscope insertion are performed according to programs independently developed at individual hospitals. Teaching methods and curricula thus vary considerably. Only a small percentage of physicians who want to receive training in colonoscopy are actually trained at educational

[1]Department of Endoscopy, Cancer Institute, Ariake Hospital, 3-10-6 Ariake, Koto-Ku, Tokyo 135-8550, Japan
[2]Department of Gastroenterology, Chikushi Hospital, Fukuoka University, Fukuoka, Japan

institutions. At many hospitals, physicians independently acquire the necessary knowledge and skills by studying textbooks explaining insertion techniques, without receiving formal training in colonoscopy. Although about 40 years have passed since the advent of colonoscopy, standardized training curricula surprisingly have not been established. In 2004, a subcommittee for studying techniques for endoscope insertion was organized by the Coordinating Committee for the Promotion of Endoscopy. The purpose of the subcommittee was to develop a standard curriculum for education and training. About 3 years were required to establish such a curriculum. This chapter introduces the proposal.

Course of Preparation of the Curriculum

A study committee consisting of eight colonoscopists selected from different parts of Japan was organized in 2004. The goals of the education and training curriculum are shown in Fig. 1. The major objective was the stable acquirement of techniques through short-term clinical experience, as compared with the learning curve for the acquirement of techniques through conventional training methods. Basic knowledge and techniques required for the preparation of a curriculum on colonoscope insertion were extensively discussed. Basic knowledge and procedures required for colonoscopy were outlined in a stepwise approach. The need for the development of new educational materials (e.g., simulators and colon models) was proposed to facilitate training. Through trial and error, a new colon model (Colonoscope training model; KYOTOKAGAKU. Co. Ltd., Japan) was developed (Fig. 2).

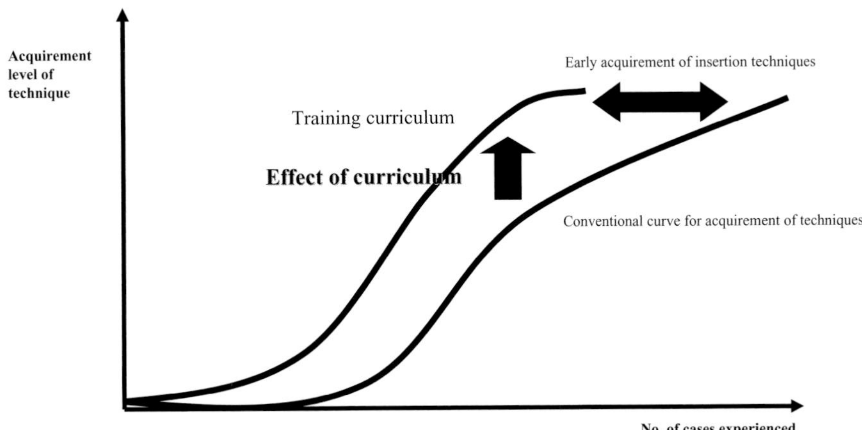

Aiming at stable acquirement of techniques through short-term clinical experience

Fig. 1. Schema of training curriculum

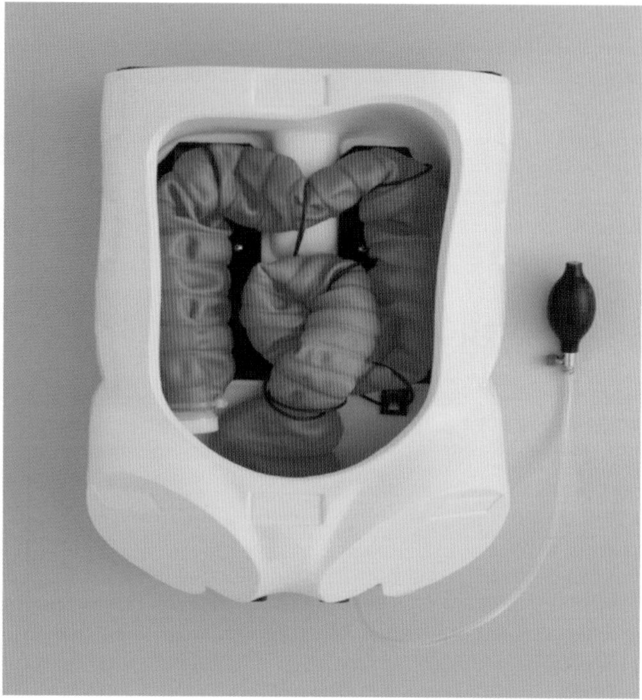

Fig. 2. New colon model

Contents of the Curriculum

The curriculum is targeted to physicians who want to acquire techniques for colonoscope insertion. The ultimate goal of the curriculum was to reach the cecum within about 20 min, with an insertion success rate of 80%. The curriculum was based on a three-step approach. A flowchart outlining the three steps is shown in Fig. 3. Step 1 focuses on the acquisition of basic knowledge needed to perform colonoscopy. In step 2, basic techniques required for colonoscope insertion are acquired, using a colon model. In step 3, techniques for insertion of a colonoscope in patients are acquired.

1. Step 1: Acquisition of basic knowledge (Table 1a)
   (1) Basic understanding of informed consent
   Understanding the need for informed consent and its significance.
   (2) Basic understanding of how to administer drugs related to examination
   Understanding the usage, side effects, and contraindications of drugs such as anticholinergic drugs, sedatives, analgesics, and antagonists.
   (3) Basic understanding of preparation
   Understanding the usage and contraindications of drugs used for preparation of colonoscopy and the treatment of complications.

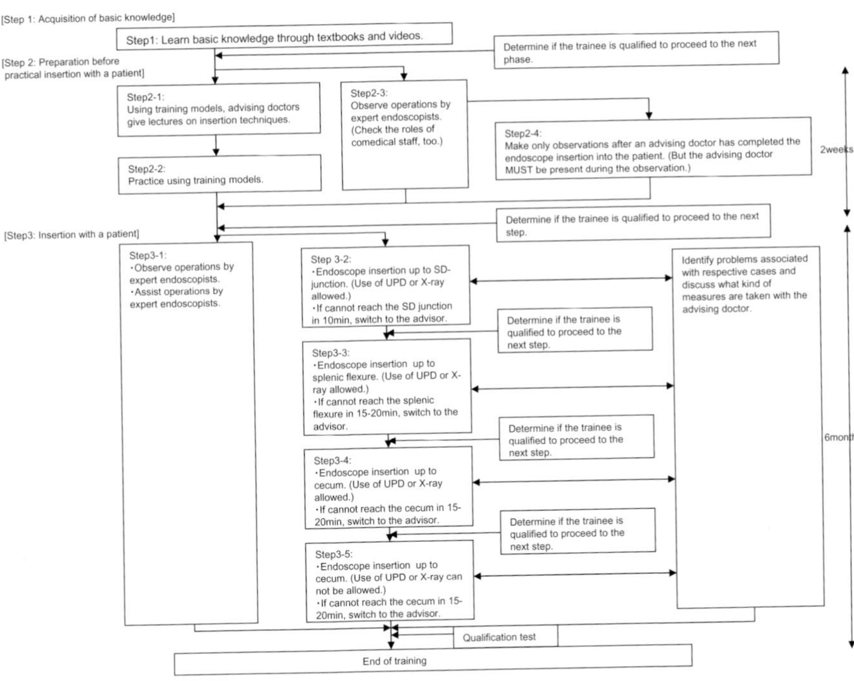

Fig. 3. Flowchart outlining the three steps. *UPD*, endoscope position detection unit; *SD junction*, junction of the sigmoid colon and the descending colon

(4) Basic understanding of disinfection and sterilization
Understanding methods used for disinfection and sterilization of endoscope and devices.

(5) Basic understanding of equipment and operation
Understanding the structures, types, handling, and operation of endoscopes, and what precautions are necessary. Understanding the usage and operation of various devices.

In addition to the foregoing points, acquisition of basic knowledge on scope insertion and diagnostics of lower gastrointestinal disease by means of textbook study. Such study must be done daily, parallel to training on colonoscope insertion.

2. Step 2: Acquisition of insertion techniques through use of a colon model
Step 2 encompasses the acquisition of two types of knowledge

One is visualization training in which trainees observe colonoscope insertion conducted by experts and thereby experience and understand the support work accompanying a colonoscopic examination (manually applied compression, supporting treatment devices, changes in patient position, preparation, pretreatment, observation of patients, etc.). Understanding the tasks of co-medical staff is also important. The other major subsection of step 2 is training on insertion using a colon model, including direct technical guidance by teaching doctors and

Table 1a. Details of step 1.

Step	Required knowledge	Details	Check
Step 1 Acquisition of basic knowledge through textbooks and videocassettes/DVDs	Basic understanding of informed consent	Understanding the need for informed consent and its significance	
	Basic understanding of how to administer drugs related to examination	Understanding the necessity, side effects, and contraindications of antispasmodic drugs and sedative drugs (calmatives, anodynes, and various antagonists)	
	Basic understanding of insertion	Understanding basic insertion techniques by studying insertion techniques in textbooks and by watching recordings of actual insertion techniques on videocassettes/DVDs	
	Basic understanding of diagnostics of the lower gastrointestinal tract	Acquiring knowledge about diagnostics of the lower gastrointestinal tract and recognizing the importance of diagnosis	
	Basic understanding of preparation	Acquiring knowledge about the items listed in the required knowledge column	
	Basic understanding of biopsy and treatment		
	Basic understanding of complications		
	Basic understanding of disinfection and sterilization		
	Basic understanding of equipment and operation	Learning the differences between the various types of scopes (narrow-diameter, standard-diameter, 2-channel, magnifying, Variable Stiffness, and UPD-compatible scopes), as well as how to use them and what precautions are necessary Gaining an overview of the internal structure of an endoscope Understanding the uses and operating methods of various devices (UPD, etc.) other than endoscopes	

TABLE 1b. Details of step 2.

Step	Required knowledge			Details	Check
Step 2-(1) Training using the colon model	Equipment layout			Understanding how equipment such as the monitor, examination table, endoscopy system, etc. is laid out and what is the purpose of each	
	Equipment setup			Knowing how to set up the equipment such as how to connect a scope with a processor/light source and how to start up the system	
	Standing position and posture			Learning the proper standing position and examination posture	
	Holding the insertion section			Knowing how to hold the insertion section at the proper distance from the anus and how much force to use	
	Holding the control section			Learning how to hold the control section so that angulation and operation of various buttons can be performed easily	
				Learning how to hold the control section so that a finger is not placed on the air button inadvertently (prevention of excessive air supply)	
	Acquisition of basic insertion patterns	General	No. 1	Operating the control section with the left hand and the insertion section with the right hand in a coordinated manner	
			No. 2	Ensuring a proper field of view by keeping the optimum distance from the colonic wall (to prevent so-called "red ball," which is a condition where the field of view is lost because the scope tip comes into contact with the colonic wall)	
			No. 3	Recognizing when the scope is warping	
			No. 4	Preventing the scope from warping by twisting the insertion section to the left and right, a maneuver referred to as "torque"	
			No. 5	Inserting the scope while visualizing the colon configuration	
			No. 6	Predicting the direction the scope will advance while recognizing various bends (R-S junction, S-D junction, splenic flexure, middle transverse colon, and hepatic flexure)	

TABLE 1b. *Continued.*

Step	Required knowledge		Details	Check
	Sigmoid colon	No. 7	Passing the S-D junction without making a loop at the sigmoid colon	
	↓	No. 8	Passing the S-D junction with push operation while making a loop at the sigmoid colon	
	Descending colon	No. 9	Straightening the insertion tube in accordance with the loop configuration and, after getting the feeling of freedom in maneuvering the insertion tube, confirming on the monitor that the insertion tube is straight	
	Transverse colon	No. 10	Shortening the transverse colon using the pull operation	
	Ascending colon	No. 11	Confirming the opening of the appendix and ileocecal valve	
	Ileum	No. 12	Advancing the scope to the ileum	
	Basics of observation during withdrawal		Recognizing the sites observed and performing observation during scope withdrawal while taking care at locations that are likely to be dead angles (e.g., behind folds and inner sides of bends)	
	Basic operation of the Variable Stiffness scope (applicable only to facilities that own one)		Using the Variable Stiffness function in accordance with the situation	
	Basic operation of the UPD (applicable only to facilities that own one)		Understanding how to operate the UPD	
			Learning how to confirm the loop configuration using the UPD and release the loop accordingly	
			Using images on the UPD monitor only when required such as releasing the loop (while maneuvering the scope primarily based on images on the endoscopic monitor and the feeling of the hand)	

Table 1c. Details of step 2 (*Continued*).

Step	Required knowledge	Details	Check
Step 2-(2) Attending clinical cases conducted by experts	Visualization training with clinical cases	Using visualization after watching teaching doctors demonstrate various techniques (points to watch: left-hand angulation operation, right-hand pushing and pulling of the insertion tube, left-right twisting operation or how to apply so-called "torque," coordinated movement of left and right hands, etc.)	
	Understanding the tasks of the staff	Understanding the tasks of co-medical staff by being present at clinical cases	
	Understanding the support work that accompanies an examination	Understanding the support work for biopsy	
		Learning what work is involved in supporting treatment (polypectomy, EMR, etc.) by attending clinical cases	
		Learning how to change patient positions	
		Learning how to administer drugs and what work is involved in supporting drug administration (such as monitoring)	
		Learning how to perform manual compression	
		Learning how to determine the condition of a patient and how to talk to the patient during the examination	
		Knowing how to disinfect and sterilize equipment (ideally, the trainee will be able to do this himself or herself)	
		Understanding other tasks related to endoscopy	

TABLE 1d. Details of step 3.

Step	Required knowledge			Details	Check
Step3-(1) Insertion of the scope into the deep parts of the patient's colon	Acquiring insertion techniques	General	No. 1	Comprehending the purpose of examination, surgical anamnesis, and past examination conditions (lesion location, treatment type, examination difficulty, etc.)	
			No. 2	Ensuring a proper field of view by keeping the optimum distance from the colonic wall (to prevent so-called "red ball," which is a condition where the field of view is lost because the scope tip comes into contact with the colonic wall)	
			No. 3	Inserting the scope while visualizing the colon configuration	
			No. 4	Adjusting the amount of air in the intestine appropriately while avoiding excessive insufflation	
			No. 5	Inserting the scope by utilizing the breathing of the patient as required	
			No. 6	Using manual compression at the trainee's own discretion (performing manual compression efficiently by taking advantage of the UPD marker when the UPD is used)	
			No. 7	Changing the patient position according to the situation	
		Before insertion	No. 8	Performing digital anal examination	
		Rectum	No. 9	Recognizing the regions of the rectum (upper rectum and lower rectum)	
			No. 10	After recognizing the R-S junction and predicting the direction of the sigmoid colon, advancing the scope to the sigmoid colon	
		Sigmoid colon	No. 11	Advancing the scope while avoiding excessive stretching and excessive looping	

		S-D junction ↓ Descending colon	No. 12	Recognizing the S-D junction and predicting the direction of the descending colon
			No. 13	Advancing the scope to the descending colon by maneuvering it according to the situation (twisting the insertion tube, sliding the scope tip, etc.)
			No. 14	Straightening the scope in accordance with the loop configuration, while using the right-turn shortening technique and confirming that the insertion tube has been straightened
		Splenic flexure	No. 15	After recognizing the splenic flexure and predicting the direction in which the transverse colon runs, advancing the scope to the transverse colon while keeping the warping of the insertion section to a minimum
		Transverse colon	No. 16	After recognizing the middle transverse colon and predicting the direction of the right transverse colon, advancing the scope to the right transverse colon
			No. 17	Shortening the transverse colon to reach the hepatic flexure
		Hepatic flexure	No. 18	After recognizing the hepatic flexure and predicting the direction of the ascending colon, advancing the scope to the ascending colon
		Ascending colon	No. 19	Confirming the opening of the appendix and ileocecal valve
		Ileum	No. 20	Advancing the scope to the ileum
		Target to be accomplished		20 minutes or less to reach the cecum on average 80% or higher insertion rate to reach the cecum on average
Step 3-(2) Observation during withdrawal	Capable of performing observation while withdrawing the scope from the patient in the presence of a teaching doctor	Performing observation while withdrawing the scope that has been inserted into the cecum by the teaching doctor to experience the feeling of freedom in maneuvering an insertion tube that is free from looping Recognizing the sites observed and performing observation during scope withdrawal while taking care at locations that are likely to be dead angles (e.g., behind folds and inner sides of bends) during observation		

self-study. Training with the use of a colon model has the most important role in this curriculum. Further details are described in Table 1b,c, which gives an overview of the technical skills required for colonoscope insertion and lists important points according to the segment of the colon.

Characteristics of the colon model

The colon model has three main characteristics. (1) The course of the intestine can be altered as needed into six patterns. Trainees can experience scope insertion for each of the patterns by altering the length, bends, and fixed sites of a tube simulating the intestine. The pattern can be easily changed by assembling the parts of the colon according to a schema outlined in the accompanying manual. (2) Air insufflation, water delivery, and aspiration can be performed. By applying pressure to the anal region, the intestine can be freely dilated and constricted by the insufflation and aspiration of air in the tube. (3) Trainees can experience inserting a scope with a model that closely simulates the clinical situation. The material is soft, and procedures such as hooking the fold [2] can be performed. Physicians can experience the sensation of inserting a scope into the intestine of patients.

Step 2-1. Layout and setup of equipment
Understanding how to lay out equipment such as the monitor, exami-nation table, and endoscopy system. Learning how to set up equipment, such as installation and connection of the scope, and how to start up the system.

Step 2-2. Basic techniques for colonoscope insertion
(1) Basic operation of a scope
Practice in operating the angle knob, air and water supply buttons, and the remote switch with the left hand. Practice in twisting the shaft of the scope and in push-and-pull operations with the right hand. Training in being able to smoothly perform right-hand and left-hand operations in a coordinated manner is extremely important.

(2) Basic operations at the time of insertion
The following basic precautions should be taken at the time of scope insertion: ① Air insufflation should be avoided. ② The tip of the scope should be advanced through the folds. ③ Excessive extension and bending of the intestine should be avoided. ④ The endoscope should be inserted slowly and carefully. ⑤ Push operations should not be performed when the colon is not visualized.

(3) Methods to facilitate insertion
Learning the following auxiliary procedures to facilitate insertion and the clinical significance of such techniques.

① Manual compression. The aim of manual compression is to provide a support point when the scope is pushed forward and thereby prevent the scope from warping [3]. The site of compression differs depending on the target region of the colon.

Lower abdomen: useful for preventing distension of the sigmoid colon and for procedures designed to shorten the sigmoid colon.

Right lower abdomen: useful when the scope is difficult to insert by push operation because of a large loop in the sigmoid colon and for the prevention of bends in the sigmoid colon.

Left lower abdomen: useful for reducing bends at the junction of the sigmoid colon and the descending colon (SDJ), facilitating scope insertion.

Left radial region: effective when the scope is difficult to insert from the splenic flexure to the transverse colon.

Right radial region: effective when the scope is difficult to insert from the transverse colon to the hepatic flexure.

② Changes in patient positions: inserting scopes with the patient in the left lateral position is basic position. We can change the position whenever useful position such as dorsal position, right lateral position, and prone position. Recognize the usefulness of each position.

③ Respiratory movement: deep breathing is often effective for inserting scopes from the hepatic flexure to the ascending colon.

④ Stiffness adjustable function: this function is useful for preventing scopes from warping.

⑤ Sliding tube: a sliding tube is useful when a loop formed in the sigmoid colon interferes with scope insertion.

⑥ Lubricants: lubricants are necessary for digital rectal examination and for inserting endoscopes into the anus. Unless lubricants are applied regularly, the scope is not smoothly inserted.

(4) Acquisition of basic insertion patterns

Inserting scopes into the rectum

While confirming the anal canal, the scope is advanced to the rectum. When the scope is pushed forward through the folds, a bend appears. This bend is the junction of the rectum and the sigmoid colon (RSJ). The scope should be slightly pushed to enter the sigmoid colon.

Inserting scopes from the sigmoid colon into the SDJ

Insertion of a scope from the sigmoid colon into the SDJ is most difficult. Physicians should use the colon model to master the following basic operations: (a) method for inserting the scope from the sigmoid colon while shortening the SDJ and (b) method for inserting the scope while creating a loop in the sigmoid colon.

(a) Method for inserting scopes from the sigmoid colon while shortening the SDJ
While confirming the lumen of the sigmoid colon, the scope is twisted to the right. Without exsufflation or extension of the lumen, the tip of the scope is pushed and pulled, facilitating passage through the SDJ (Fig. 4; N loop). This fundamental technique should be practiced repeatedly and is referred to as hooking the fold and right-turn shortening [2,4].

(b) Method for inserting the scope while creating a loop at the sigmoid colon. With the use of only the method described above, the scope cannot pass through the SDJ in some patients. When the scope cannot pass through the SDJ with the use of method (a), trainees learn how to create a loop (e.g., α-loop, N loop, and reverse α-loop) with

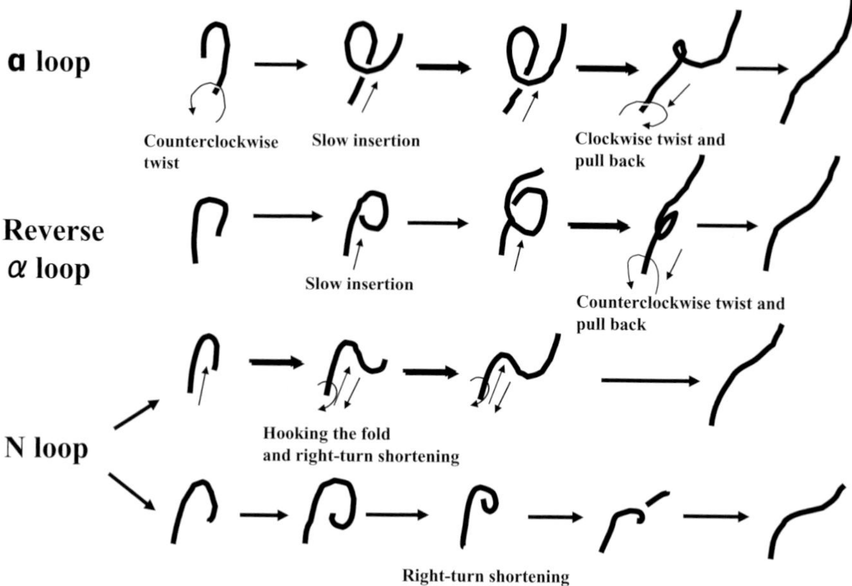

Fig. 4. Basic techniques for passing through the sigmoid colon

push operation and pass the scope through the SDJ [5]. When the scope passes through the sigmoid colon, the scope axis is twisted to the right and the scope is pushed forward, creating an α-loop and inserting the scope into the descending colon. When the scope is twisted from the top of the sigmoid colon to the right and is pushed forward, an N loop is formed and the scope is inserted into the descending colon. It is important to learn how to straighten the scope after forming a loop and inserting the scope into the descending colon. When the tip of the scope approaches regions without flexures, the scope is twisted to the right (in the case of an α-loop) and pulled out, straightening the scope. This technique should be acquired. In the case of a reverse α-loop, the scope is twisted to the left and pulled out. It is important for the right hand to sense straightening of the scope.

(5) Inserting the scope from the splenic flexure into the cecum

a. Passing through the splenic flexure

While confirming the lumen, the scope is advanced forward from the descending colon, facilitating passage through the splenic flexure. This procedure should be done when there are no bends or loops in the sigmoid colon (while straightening the scope).

b. Passing through the transverse colon

While confirming the lumen after passage through the splenic flexure, the scope is advanced forward, reaching the bends in the middle segment of the transverse colon. The scope is slightly pushed and angled to pass through the bends. When the lumen is seen, the scope is twisted to the left and pulled out. Exsufflation is effective at this time. While pulling out the scope, trainees should be able to sense when the tip of the scope approaches the hepatic flexure.

c. Passing through the hepatic flexure
While confirming the bend of the hepatic flexure, the tip of the scope is advanced toward the lumen side to enter the hepatic flexure. Passage is easy with the colon model, but may be difficult in humans. Trainees should learn that supporting measures such as changing the patient's position and the application of manual compression are useful at this time.

d. Insertion into the cecum
After passage through the hepatic flexure, the scope should be confirmed to be straight and then advanced further, reaching the cecum. In humans, the tip of the scope may sometimes not enter the cecum because of bends or adhesions of the transverse colon. Trainees should learn that deep breathing and changes in the patient's position are useful at this time.

These basic techniques for scope insertion should be repeatedly practiced with the colon model for at least 2 consecutive weeks. A teaching doctor should decide whether the trainee is qualified to start to insert the scope in humans. If permission is granted, the trainee advances to step 3. Even after entering step 3, the trainee should practice techniques for insertion with the colon model as needed.

Step 3-1. Scope insertion in humans
In principle, the scope should be inserted in humans under the guidance of a teaching doctor. Patients in whom the scope can be easily inserted (e.g., patients in whom experts judge that scope insertion is not difficult or those who have not undergone surgery) should be selected. If patients have severe pain and discomfort and the target time for scope insertion is exceeded, the teaching doctor should take over. The scope should pass through the SDJ within 15 min and reach the cecum within 20 min, with an insertion rate of 80%.

Step 3-2.
Parallel to point 1 (above), the trainee should practice observing the colon while withdrawing the scope in the presence of a teaching doctor.

After about 6 months of step 3, training is completed if the trainee has reached the goals of an insertion rate of 80% or higher within the target times (15 min or less to pass through the SDJ and 20 min or less to reach the cecum). Physicians who have successfully completed the program can work in clinical practice. If the target goals are reached in less than 6 months, the initial phase of training is completed.

Concluding Remarks

This chapter introduces a training curriculum for colonoscopic examination. Previously, a standard training curriculum for beginners was unavailable in Japan. With the present curriculum, trainees initially use a colon model to practice and acquire the basic techniques required for colonoscope insertion. After reaching a given level of proficiency, trainees are then allowed to perform colonoscopy in patients.

This progressive approach reduces the burden on patients and is close to ideal. The curriculum describes the details of training for beginners and proposes specific goals. It also provides teaching doctors with guidelines for instruction and training.

To facilitate self-study, explanations on techniques for colonoscopy are available on a DVD [6]. Such materials are expected to contribute substantially to improved education and training in colonoscopy.

Acknowledgments. We gratefully acknowledge the members of the subcommittee for the studying techniques for colonoscopy (Dr. Yusuke Saito, Asahikawa City Hospital; Dr. Hiro-o Yamano, Akita Red Cross Hospital; Dr. Eisai Chou, Ootsu City Hospital; Dr. Satoru Tamura, Kochi Medical University Hospital; Dr. Shinji Tanaka, Hiroshima University Hospital; and Dr. Osamu Tsuruta, Kurume University Hospital) and their participation in the establishment of this curriculum.

References

1. Tajima T (1987) Insertion method of colonoscopy. Gastroenterol Endosc 29:2950–2954
2. Shinya H (1982) Colonoscopy. Diagnosis and treatment of colonic disease. Igakushoin, Tokyo, pp 48–76
3. Williams CB (1990) Colonoscopy. In: Cotton PB, Williams CB (eds) Practical gastrointestinal endoscopy. Blackwell, London, pp 160–223
4. Kudo S (1993) How to insert the colonoscope into cecum. Igakushoin, Tokyo
5. Sakai Y (2000) Techniques in colonoscopy. In: Sivak M Jr (ed) Gastroenterological endoscopy. Saunders, Philadelphia, pp 1253–1280
6. Tsuda S (2007) Previous practice and object training: Igarashi M, Tsuda S (eds) Training of colonoscope insertion by DVD. Japan Medical Center, Tokyo, pp 104–142

Magnifying Endoscope Diagnosis and NBI Diagnosis in Colorectal Neoplasm

Hiroo Yamano, Kohei Kuroda, and Kenjiro Yoshikawa

Summary. Recently, endoscopic diagnosis has been developed with new endoscope techniques and equipment, and especially the magnifying function and the narrow-band imaging (NBI) system. The magnifying endoscope can observe the surface microstructure of colonic mucosa (pit pattern) after dye-spraying and enlarging 100 times or more. The pit pattern is divided into six categories, and we can distinguish between nonneoplasm/neoplasm, benign or malignant, and mucosal or invasive cancer. The newly available NBI system is based on the modification of spectral features with an optical color separation filter narrowing the bandwidth (415 nm and 540 nm) of spectral transmittance. The endoscopic image is reproduced in the processor with this information, and we can see the capillary network of superficial mucosa by using the magnifying endoscope. The capillary network patterns are divided into three categories, and correspond to pathological features. Many Japanese researchers are investigating capillary vessel patterns from various standpoints owing to the newly developed qualities of endoscopic diagnosis. In addition, NBI has enhanced the effectiveness of examinations to evaluate the mucous membrane, and helped the discovery of dysplasia and colitic cancer in inflammatory bowel disease. Both the magnifying endoscope and the NBI system are very important tools that have been researched and invented in Japan. These developments have greatly improved endoscopic diagnosis.

Key words. Endoscopic diagnosis, Magnifying endoscope, NBI (narrow-band image), Pit pattern, Capillary pattern

Introduction

Endoscopic diagnosis used to be based on the characteristics of a lesion, i.e., macroscopic shape, color, depression, and hardness. We then made a pathological diagnosis after examining a biopsy specimen taken from it. However, it is very

Department of Gastroenterology, Akita Red Cross Hospital, 222-1 Naeshirosawa-aza, Saruta, Kamikitade, Akita 011-1495, Japan

difficult to carry out endoscopic diagnosis until extensive experience has been acquired. Other problems are that there can be no common sense understanding about shape, color, hardness, etc., that the results of biopsies do not follow standard rules, and that pathologists have no agreed understanding about borderline lesions.

However, endoscope equipment has developed in recent years so that it is much easier to operate, has higher CCD, and the quality of the image and the data processing have considerably improved. In addition, in vivo observations of the surface of microstructures and the changes which take place in the blood vessels in the morbid state have become possible with the magnifying function and the narrow-band imaging (NBI) system. All these technologies were developed in Japan, and as a result endoscope diagnosis has greatly improved. In this chapter, we explain magnifying endoscopic diagnosis and NBI.

Magnifying Endoscope Diagnosis

From In Vitro to In Vivo

Magnified observation of colorectal neoplasia under a stereomicroscope was previously done with a fixed specimen which was excised during surgery. As a result, differences in the surface microstructure were discovered from changes in the morbid state in vitro [1,2].

Later, observations by a zoom-type magnifying endoscope (CF-200Z, Olympus Medical Systems, Tokyo, Japan, 1990) became possible, although attempts to observe the surface microstructure had to wait for advances in endoscope equipment which could be used in vivo. Kudo et al. [3,4] called the surface microstructure a "pit pattern," and they formulated a constant rule since the pit pattern has been found to correspond to the pathological features, and this has led to the establishment of magnifying endoscope diagnosis, i.e., the "pit pattern diagnosis."[5,6]

Magnifying Endoscope and Observations

The magnifying endoscope unit (Fig. 1) and the coloring agents (Fig. 2) are necessary to observe a pit pattern in vivo. We believe that our equipment gives the best results, although there are many other magnifying endoscopes now on the market. Electric magnification and the NBI system are installed to give high-pixel CCD, a Hi-vision signal, and a high level of image processing performance. We believe that this equipment gives the best observations and pictures of pit patterns. We use two types of coloring matter; one is a 0.2% indigo carmine solution as the contrast, and the other is a 0.04% crystal violet solution as the dye. We mix a small amount "Gascon (dimethylepolysiloxan)" in both solutions in order to prevent bubble generation when they are sprayed.

We now explain the observation procedure (Fig. 3). When a lesion is discovered, any dirt or mucus that adheres to it should first be removed with water. We then spray indigo carmine solution and observe the changes to a morbid state. It should be noted

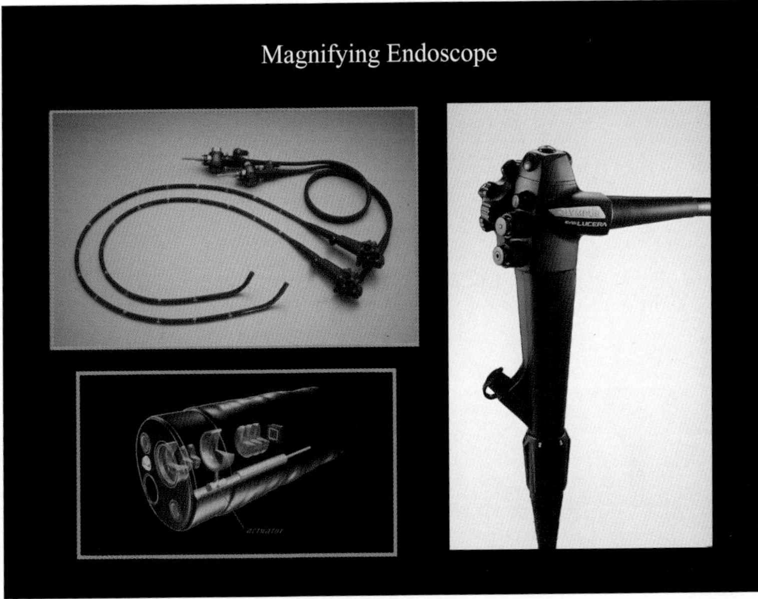

Fig. 1. Externals and internal structure of Magnifying Endoscope

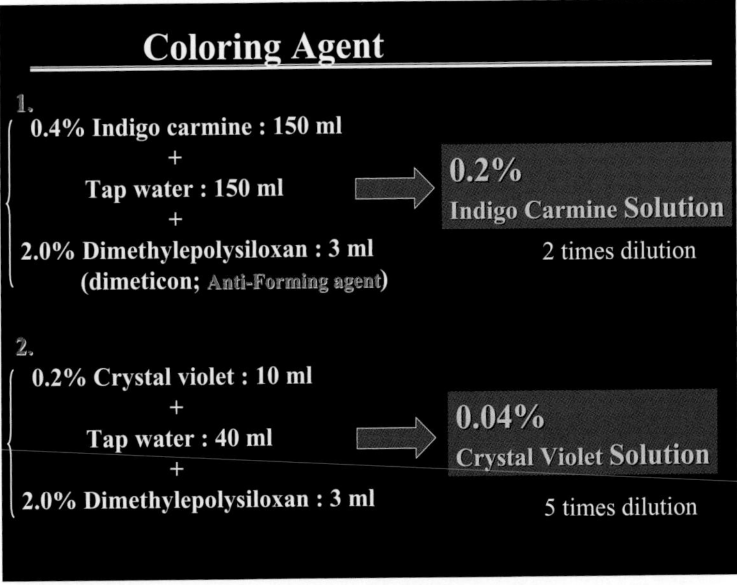

Fig. 2. The composition of Coloring Agents "Indigo Carmine" and "Crystal Violet"

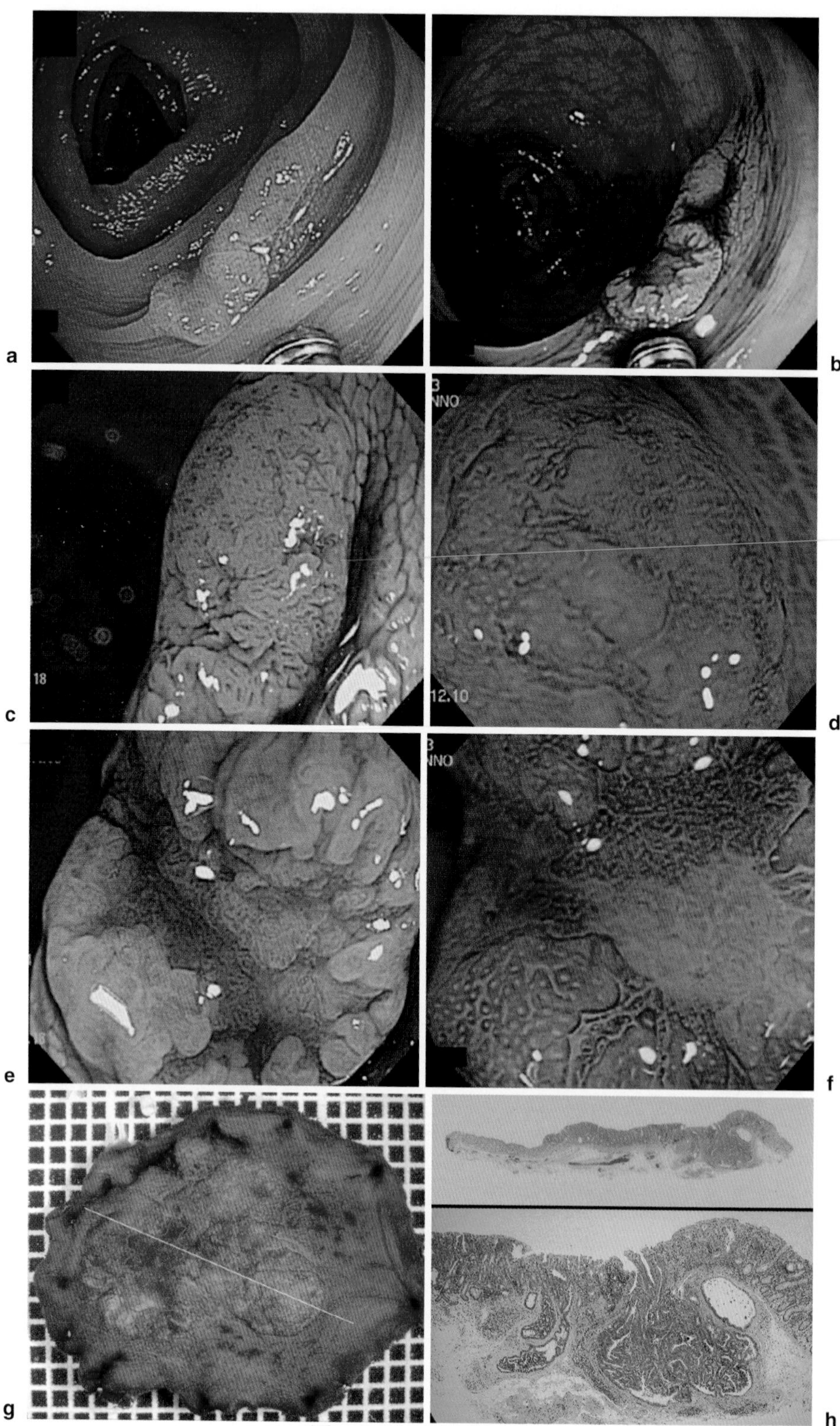

that it is better to make gradual observations and to take the first picture at a lower magnification after first noting its extent. If a more detailed examination is necessary, it should be dyed with a crystal violet solution.

Pit Pattern Classification (Fig. 4)

The pit patterns are divided into seven categories, from type I to type VN.

— Type I. This pattern consists of normal roundish pits, each 0.07 ± 0.02 mm in size. Pit shape and size vary slightly from site to site.
— Type II. This pattern consists of relatively large pits (0.09 ± 0.02 mm) with a star-like or onion-skin-like structure. This is the basic pit pattern of hyperplastic lesions.
— Type IIIs. This pattern consists of tubular or roundish pits which are smaller than normal ones (0.03 ± 0.01 mm). This is seen in depressed types of tumor.
— Type IIIL. This pattern consists of tubular pits which are larger than normal ones (0.22 ± 0.09 mm). This is the basic pit pattern of protruded-type adenoma.
— Type IV. This is a sulcus-, branch-, or gyrus-like pit pattern, although the gyrus-like pit pattern actually consists of an assembly of segmented grooves rather than pits. It is included in this category for convenience.
— Type VI. This pattern is similar to types IIIL, IIIs, and IV, but consists of a disordered array, a size disparity, and asymmetry, etc.
— Type VN. In this type the pattern disappears from the surface structure, and shows what is called "no structure." This can be seen in massive invading or advanced cancer-type tumors.

Histological Overview of Pit Pattern Analysis

We examined the accuracy of distinguishing a nonneoplasm from a neoplasm by using the pit-pattern diagnosis. It was assumed that types I and II pit patterns showed a nonneoplastic lesion in the magnifying endoscope, and the accuracy was 89.3%. It was then assumed that types IIIs, IIIL, IV, and V pit patterns showed a neoplastic lesion, and here the accuracy was 96.2% (Table 1).

We then examined the accuracy by assuming that types IIIs, IIIL, and IV showed adenoma, that type VI showed adenoma with severe atypia, mucosal cancer, and slightly invasive cancer (invading depth <1000 μm), and type VN showed invasive cancer, and especially a massively invasive one (invading depth >1000 μm). The results showed: type IIIs, 96.2% in 26 lesions; type IIIL, 96.0% in 2520 lesions; type IV, 88.9% in 686 lesions; type VI, 77.6% in 250 lesions; type VN, 93.0% in 43 lesions (Table 2).

It was unclear why type IV was less accurate. The first suggestion was that the assessment of type IV must be difficult, and the second was that pathologists

Fig. 3. The observation of Magnifying Endoscope and pathological feature

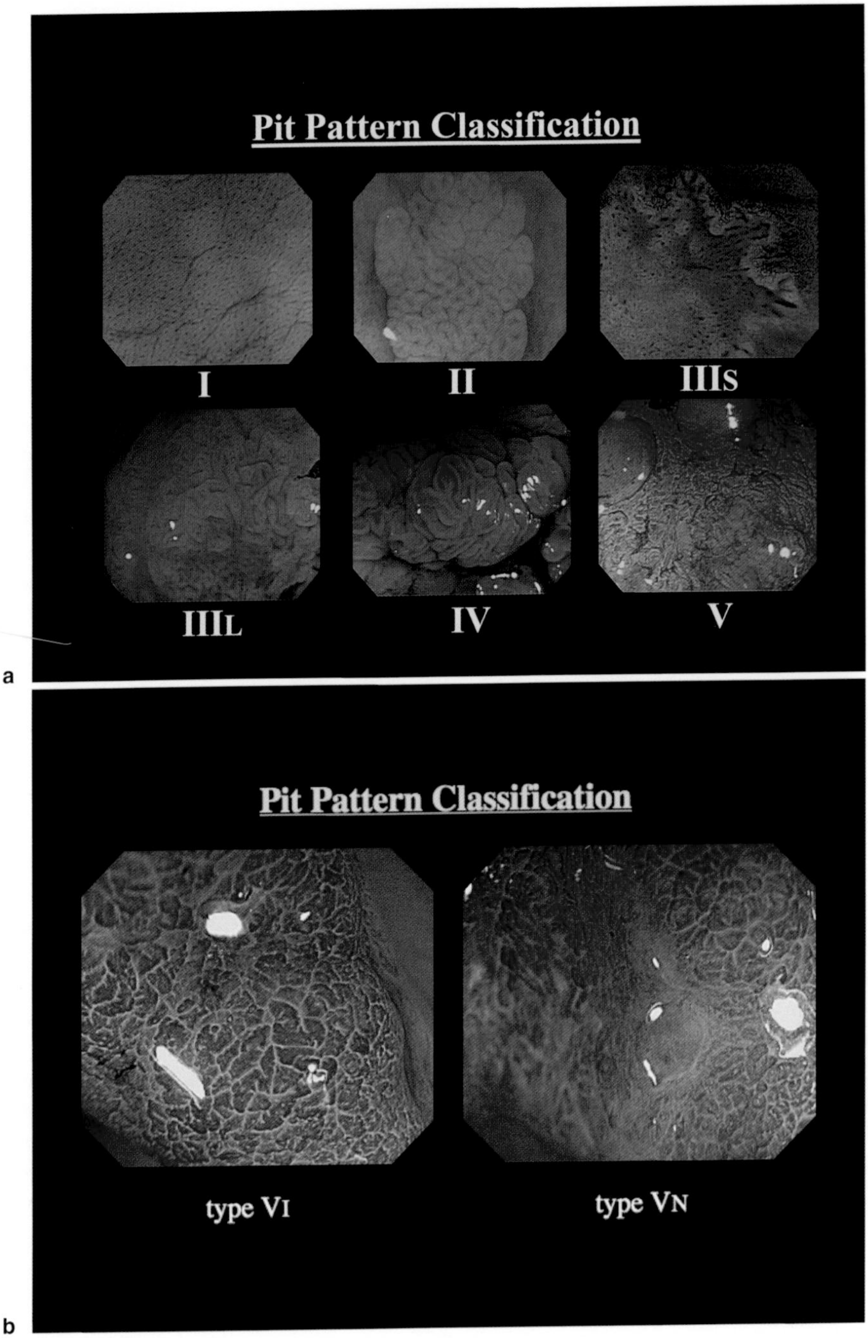

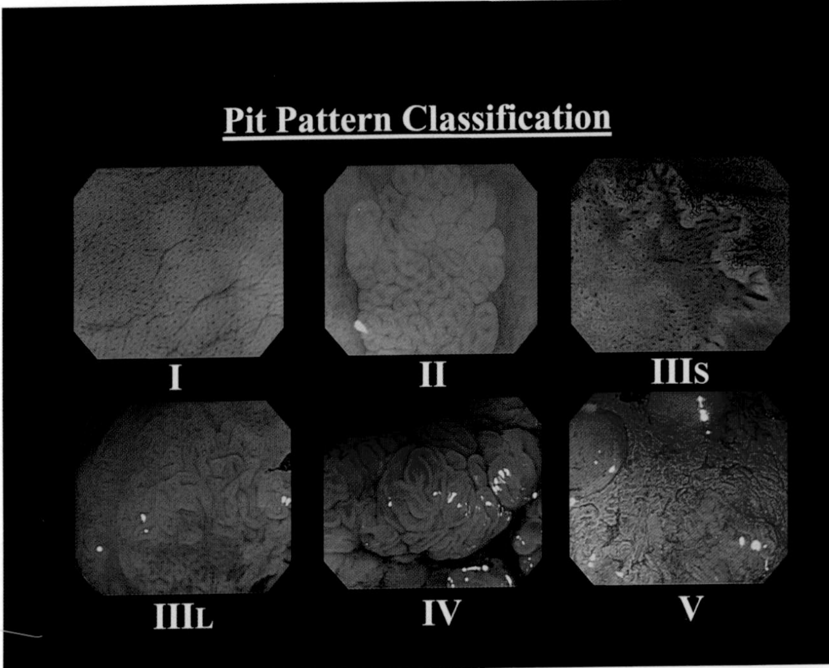

Fig. 4. Pit pattern classification

TABLE 1. Accuracy of neoplastic and non-neoplastic lesions.

	pit pattern		
	I, II	III-V	
non-neoplastic	117 (89.3)	46 →	normal 3 hyperplastic 9
neoplastic	14 ↓	1,151 (96.2)	inflamatory 31 juvenile 2 colitis 1
	adenoma mild	8	~5 mm:11
	mode.	4	
	focal sev	2 (LST)	

TABLE 2. Relationship Between Pit Pattern and Pathological Diagnosis.

	IIIs	IIIL	IV	VI	VN
Non-neoplasm	1	74	25		
adenoma					
mild-mode.	22	2162	488	45	
severe	3	256	122	58	
cancer in adenoma		27	45	97	
mucosal cancer			4	22	3
invasive cancer slight			1	17	3
massive		1	1	11	37
total	26	2520	686	250	43
Accuracy	96.2	96.0	88.9	77.6	93.0

do not have a common recognition of borderline lesions. However, based on these results, diagnosis using a magnifying endoscope is regarded as being very useful.

NBI Diagnosis

In general, we guide light onto the mucous membrane and observe it by reflection. An optical reflection is produced not only on the surface of the mucous membrane, but also at some depth. This light penetration differs depending on the wavelength of the light (Fig. 5). The newly available NBI system is based on the modification of spectral features, with an optical color separation filter narrowing the bandwidth of spectral transmittance. The NBI filter allows only two wavelengths to pass through, 415 nm and 540 nm (Fig. 6), and is placed inside the light source unit (Fig. 7). We can easily switch between a conventional and an NBI filter with a single button. The image is reproduced in the processor with information from both wavelengths, and we can see the capillary network of superficial mucosa by using a magnifying endoscope (Figs. 8 and 9).

Machida et al. reported that in distinguishing between nonneoplasms and neoplasms, the accuracy of a chromoendoscopic image and an NBI image in a magnifying

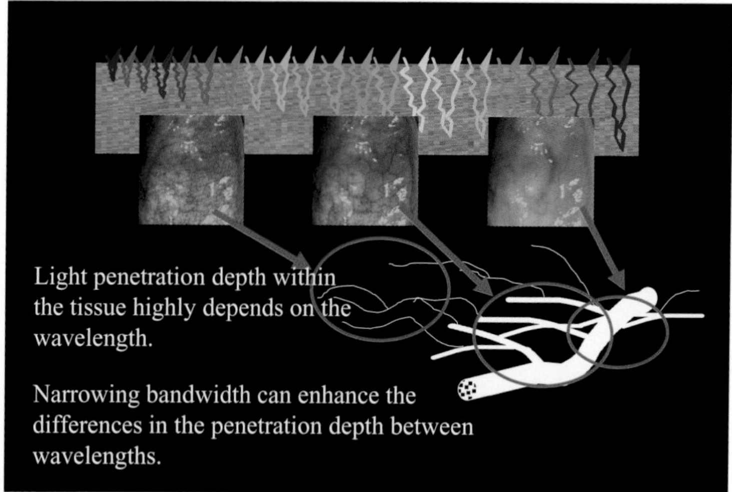

Fig. 5. Light penetration depth and wavelengths

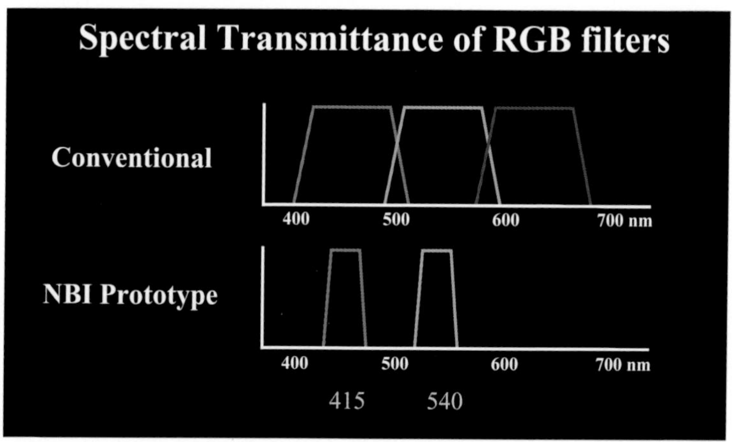

Fig. 6. Difference between conventional and NBI in RGB filters

endoscope was the same (Table 3) [5]. Sano et al. reported that capillary vessels were more than usually enhanced in colorectal neoplasm. He named the variations "capillary patterns" (CP), and divided them into major three classes. CP type I is an invisible or only faintly visible microvessel with the mucosal capillary network arranged in a honeycomb pattern around the normal or hyperplastic glands. CP type II is clearly visible, and has a loose density of slightly thicker capillaries. In this type, vascular casts showed that the microvasculature has a similar organization to that of the normal colon, but the capillaries are elongated and have larger diameters than normal ones. CP type III has clearly visible and uneven-sized thicker capillaries which are

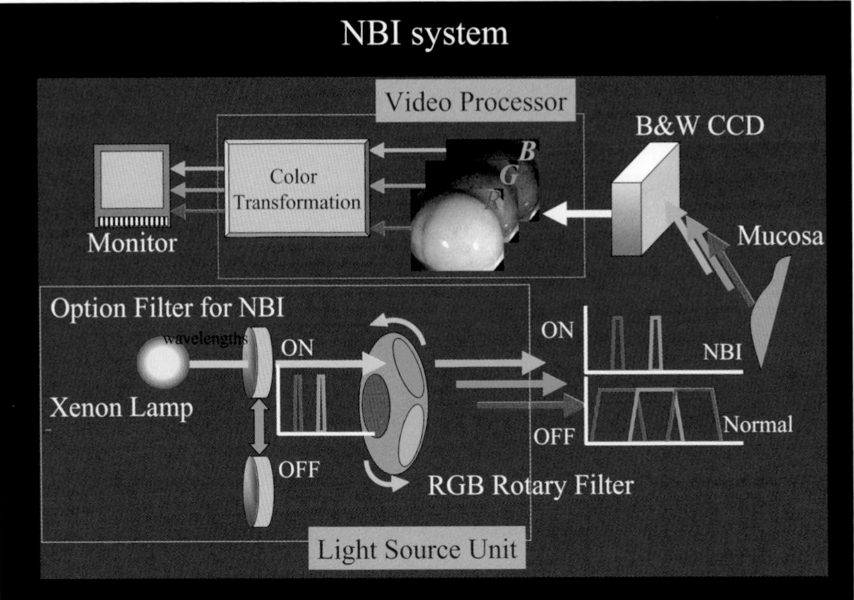

FIG. 7. Pattern diagrams of NBI system

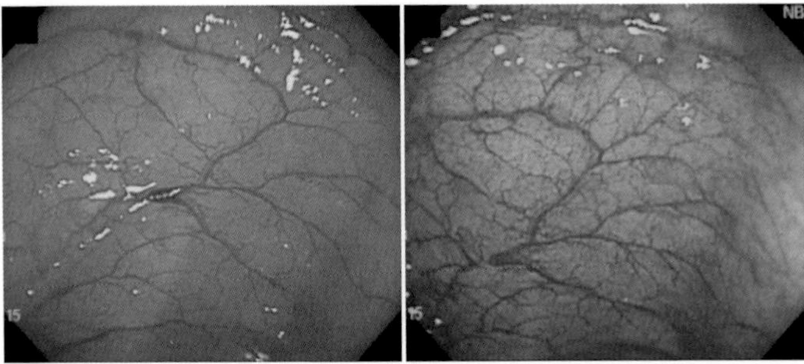

FIG. 8. Difference of vessels feature between conventional and NBI

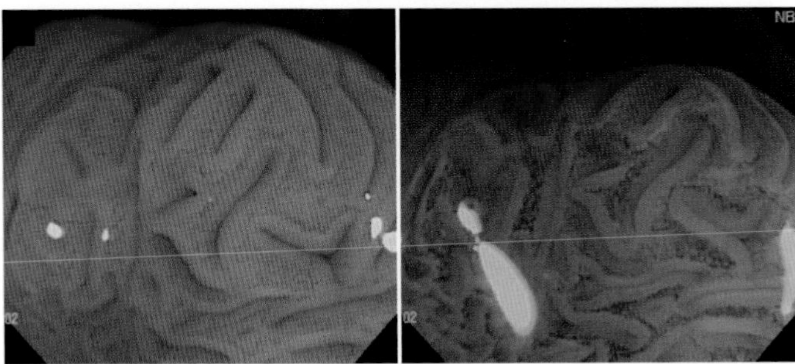

FIG. 9. Difference of surface view between conventional and NBI

TABLE 3. Discrimination of non-neoplasm/ neoplasm by MC vessel (NBI).

	Neoplastic	Non-Neoplastic
Meshed capillary positive	107	3
Meshed capillary negative	4	36
Sensitivity: 96.4%, Sepcificity: 92.3%		
Accuracy: 95.3%		
NPV (negative predict value): 90.0%		
PPV (positive predict value): 97.3%		

(Machida H, et al: Narrow-Band Imaging in the diagnosis of colorectal mucosal lesions: a pilot study. Endoscopy 36; 1094–1098, 2004)

branched, curtailed, irregular, and very dense. In this type, vascular casts of a colonic carcinoma are characterized by a disorganized structure and a density of microvessels. The increased number and density of microvessels results in the formation of nodular clusters of capillaries [6].

There has recently been an attempt to subclassify CP type III even further, and many Japanese workers are researching capillary vessel patterns from various standpoints using the latest developments in endoscopic diagnosis [7–9].)

In addition, NBI is being used very effectively in the examination and evaluation of the mucous membrane, and the discovery of dysplasia and colitic cancer in inflammatory bowel disease. NBI is an inspection method with great potential [10].

Conclusion

Both the magnifying endoscope and the NBI system have been researched and invented in Japan, and have greatly increased the scope of endoscope diagnosis.

References

1. Kosaka T (1975) Fundamental study on the diminutive polyps of the colon by mucosal stain and dissecting microscope. J Jpn Soc Coloproctol 28:218–228
2. Tada M, Kawai K, Akasaka Y, et al. (1978) Magnified observation of minute changes of polypoid lesions in the large intestine. Stomach Intestine 13:625–636
3. Kudo S, Kusaka N, Nakajima T, et al. (1992) Minute surface structure of depressed-type early colorectal cancer. Stomach Intestine 27:963–975
4. Kudo S, Hirota S, Nakajima T, et al. (1994) Colorectal tumors and pit pattern. J Clin Pathol 47:880–885
5. Machida H, Sano Y, Hamamoto Y, et al. (2004) Narrow-band imaging in the diagnosis of colorectal mucosal lesions: a pilot study. Endoscopy 36:1094–1098
6. Sano Y, Horimatsu T, Fu KI, et al. (2006) Magnifying observation of the microvascular architecture of colorectal lesions using the narrow-band imaging system. Dig Endosc 18:S44–S51
7. Kawano H, Tsuruta O, Toubaru T, et al. (2007) Diagnosis of colorectal lesions using the narrow-band imaging (NBI) system. Early Colorectal Cancer 11:119–124
8. Wada Y, Kashida H, Kudo S, et al. (2007) The surface microvasculature of colorectal lesions observed with the NBI zoom system; including comparison with pit pattern analysis. Early Colorectal Cancer 11:125–130

9. Tanaka S, Hirata M, Oka S, et al. (2007) Histological atypia/invasion depth diagnosis of colorectal tumors using narrow-band imaging (NBI) magnification. Early Colorectal Cancer 11:131–141
10. Matsumoto T, Kudo T, Iida M (2007) NBI colonoscopic findings concerning ulcerative colitis. Early Colorectal Cancer 11:143–148

Image Enhanced Endoscopy (IEE) Using NBI During Screening Colonoscopy: Usefulness and Application

Yasushi Sano

Summary. We review magnified observations of the microvascular architecture of colorectal lesions, and discuss the utility of detailed observations of this architecture for differential diagnosis during narrow-band imaging (NBI) colonoscopy. Angiogenesis is critical to the transition of premalignant lesions in a hyperproliferative state to the malignant phenotype. Therefore, diagnosis based on angiogenic or vascular morphological changes might be ideal for the early detection or diagnosis of neoplasms. In this review, we propose the term "meshed capillary" for nonneoplastic lesions in order to distinguish them from neoplastic lesions, and the capillary classification "capillary pattern" for the differential diagnosis of colorectal lesions. We believe that the combined use of NBI optical equipment-based image-enhanced endoscopy (IEE) and real chromoendoscopy decreases the time and cost of screening colonoscopy. To assess the feasibility and efficacy of using the NBI system, further studies are required for colorectal lesions and other lesions of the gastrointestinal tract.

Key words. Narrow-band imaging system, Colonoscopy, Microvascular architecture, Capillary pattern, Optical equipment-based image-enhanced endoscopy (IEE)

Introduction

The detection and subsequent removal of neoplastic colorectal lesions, including adenomatous polyps and early cancers, have been reported to reduce the incidence of colorectal cancers, based on the concept of the adenoma–carcinoma sequence [1]. Therefore, the roles of screening colonoscopy and polypectomy are becoming more important because colorectal cancer is the third most common cause of cancer mortality, and the incidence of colorectal cancer in Japan is increasing [2]. Although efficacious colonoscopy is recommended, it has been reported that 10% to 30% of resected polyps are nonneoplastic lesions that did not need to be removed [3]. Therefore, distinguishing between nonneoplastic lesions and neoplastic lesions

Sano Hospital, Department of Gastrointestinal Center, Kobe, Japan

can increase the efficiency of treatment by eliminating the time and cost of unnecessary polypectomy [4,5]. The narrow-band imaging (NBI) system is based on modifying spectral features by narrowing the bandwidth of spectral transmittance with optical filters. Since 1999, we have been developing our own NBI system with support from a Grant for Scientific Research Expenses for Health and Welfare Programs, Japan. NBI modification provides a unique image emphasizing the capillary pattern and the surface structure [6–8]. In our pilot study, the NBI system was sufficient to distinguish between nonneoplastic lesions and neoplastic lesions, and had a special feature allowing otherwise invisible endoscopic findings to be visualized without a dye solution. [8–11].

In this chapter, we describe the usefulness of NBI in screening colonoscopy and target optical IEE, and discuss the utility of detailed observations of the microvascular architecture for differential diagnosis during colonoscopy.

Improvement of Visibility

Our pilot study found that, compared with normal observations, clearer observation of the capillary vessels in the network on the surface layer of the mucosa is possible using the NBI system. [9] Therefore, recognizing the lesion becomes easier, since the permeable image of the vessels is interrupted. On normal mucosa, a regular hexagonal or honeycomb-like pattern is found around the crypt of the gland. On the other hand, in a neoplastic lesion these vessels become thicker, and disruption of the vessels, differences in the diameters of the vessels, and a rise in vessel density can be found when the abnormality gets worse. Since the filter of NBI is adjusted to Hb absorption characteristics, a brownish area can be found if the observation area contains a large number of capillary vessels (Fig. 1). Contrast enhancement of the lesion makes the disruption of the normal vessel network in colonic lesions obvious, and improves the visualization [11,22].

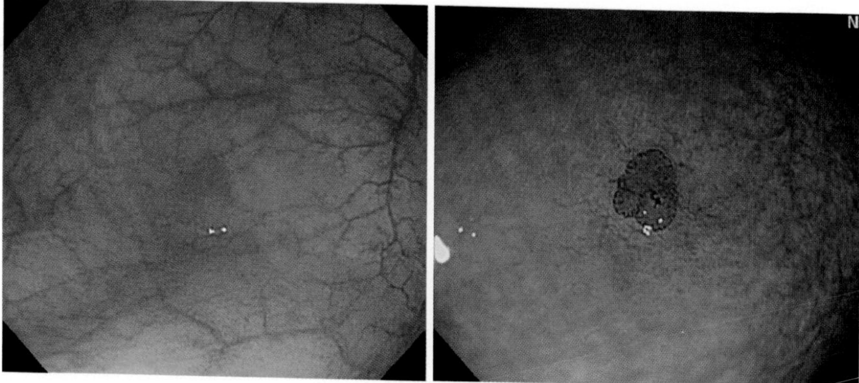

Fig. 1. Brownish area and typical endoscopic features of a flat adenomatous polyp on narrow-band imaging (NBI). **a** Standard colonoscopy. A 0–IIa type lesion, 4 mm in size, can be seen in the rectum. **b** NBI without any dye spraying. The lesion can be seen as a dark brown lesion (*brownish area*)

Improvement in the Observation of the Surface Structure (Pit Pattern) and the Microcapillaries (Capillary Pattern [CP])

Several studies have reported that observations using chromoendoscopy, as well as chromoendoscopy with a magnifying function, is helpful for differentiating neoplasia from nonneoplasia. In our pilot study [9], the accuracy of endoscopic diagnosis was 79.1% with conventional colonoscopy and 93.4% with NBI colonoscopy. This was similar to that with chromoscopy. Therefore, by combining the NBI system with the magnifying function, it is expected that it will be possible to infer the pit pattern on the surface layer of the mucosa without any staining, and obtain as accurate a diagnosis as that obtained with optical chromoendoscopy.

The NBI modification provides a unique image which emphasizes the capillary pattern as well as the surface structure. Angiogenesis is critical to the transition of premalignant lesions in a hyperproliferative state to the malignant phenotype [12–14]. Therefore, a diagnosis based on the angiogenic or vascular morphological changes might be ideal for the early detection or diagnosis of neoplasms. We have described the utility of detailed observations of microvascular architecture for differential diagnosis during NBI colonoscopy [10,15]. We named the mucosal capillary meshwork which is arranged in a honeycomb pattern around the mucosal glands "meshed capillary" (MC), and using NBI colonoscopy with magnification we classified the microvascular architecture into 3 types, i.e., capillary pattern (CP) types I, II, and III [15,20,21,22]. These capillary vessels, which can be observed clearly by NBI, are thought to be similar to observations of capillary vessels of around 300 μm, according to the Monte Carlo simulation that we conducted [16]. The definition of each CP is summarized in Fig. 2 and described in detail below.

Normal Colonic Mucosa (CP: Type I)

Using NBI colonoscopy without magnification, not only thick veins and capillaries but also fine capillaries can be seen as a brown color. The vessel network of the mucosa is well visualized in much finer detail on NBI colonoscopy than on standard colonoscopy. However, the mucosal capillary meshwork (MC) arranged in a honeycomb pattern around the mucosal glands is invisible, or only faintly visible, under magnifying observations using NBI colonoscopy (Fig. 3a), because the endoscopic resolution is not sufficient to visualize the network. The diameter of the vessels was reported to be from 8.6 ± 1.8 μm to 12.4 ± 1.9 μm (range 6.4–20.9 μm) [13,14].

Hyperplastic Polyp (CP: Type I)

Most hyperplastic polyps can be seen as light brown lesions without neovascularization on NBI colonoscopy. A Kudo's type II pit pattern can be seen by magnifying observations using NBI without any dye solution [17]. In many cases the mucosal capillary meshwork is invisible, or only faintly visible, under magnifying observations using NBI colonoscopy because the endoscopic resolution is not sufficient to visualize

	Schematic micro-vessel architecture	Capillary characteristics	Vessel diameter (μm) (minimum – maximum)	Visibility using NBI (Capillary pattern classification)
Normal mucosa	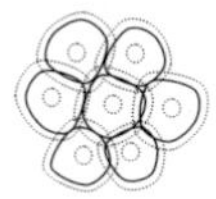	Mucosal capillary network (meshwork) arranged in a honeycomb pattern around the mucosal glands.	8.6±1.8 to 12.4±1.9 (6.4 - 20.9)	MC vessel: Invisible ~ faintly visible (Capillary pattern type I)
Hyperplastic	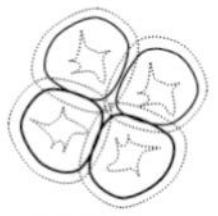	Mucosal capillary network (meshwork) arranged in a honeycomb pattern around the mucosal glands.	< 10	MC vessel: Invisible ~ faintly visible (Capillary pattern type I)
Adenoma	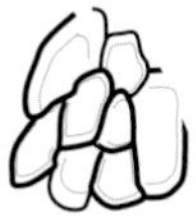	Vascular casts showed that the microvasculature have a similar organization to the normal colon. However, capillaries are elongated and have increased diameters compared to normal.	13.1+3.3	MC vessel: Clearly visible Slightly thicker capillary Capillary density: loose (Capillary pattern type II)
Carcinoma	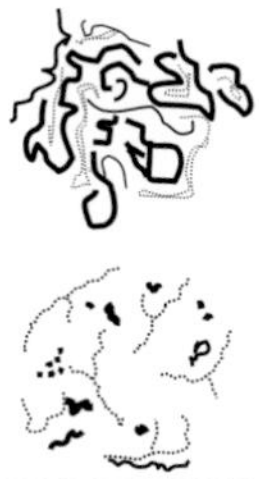	Vascular casts of colonic carcinoma is characterized by a disorganized structure and increased density of microvessels. The increased number and density of microvessels results in formation of nodular clusters of capillaries.	18.3±0.1 to 19.8±7.6 (2.2 – 84.5)	MC vessel: Clearly visible thicker capillaries, unevenly sized with branching and curtailed irregularity. (Capillary pattern type IIIA) MC vessel: Presence of a nearly avascular or loose microvascular area due to histological desmoplastic changes in the stromal tissue (Capillary pattern type IIIB)

FIG. 2. Sano's endoscopic microvascular classification of colorectal lesions using NBI (Sano's classification of capillary patterns)

the network (Fig. 3b). We have previously reported that intratumor microvessel density in a small hyperplastic polyp was significantly higher than that in normal mucosa, but that the vessel diameter was not significantly larger than in normal mucosa [18]. However, MC vessels are sometimes recognized in parts of hyperplastic polyps such as large hyperplastic polyps [5,15] or hyperplastic polyps with serrated adenomatous changes [5,15].

Adenomatous Lesion (CP: Type II)

Adenomatous lesions, including the flat and depressed types, can be seen as dark brown neovascular lesions (a brownish area) on NBI colonoscopy without magnification, and are easily detected while withdrawing from NBI colonoscopy. A Kudo's type III or IV pit pattern, demarcated by the appearance of MC vessels, can be seen by magnifying observations using NBI without the application of any dye solution [8,15]. MC vessels are clearly visible because the capillaries are elongated and have increased diameters compared with normal capillaries (Fig. 3c). The vessel diameter has been reported to be 13.1 ± 3.3 μm [13,14].

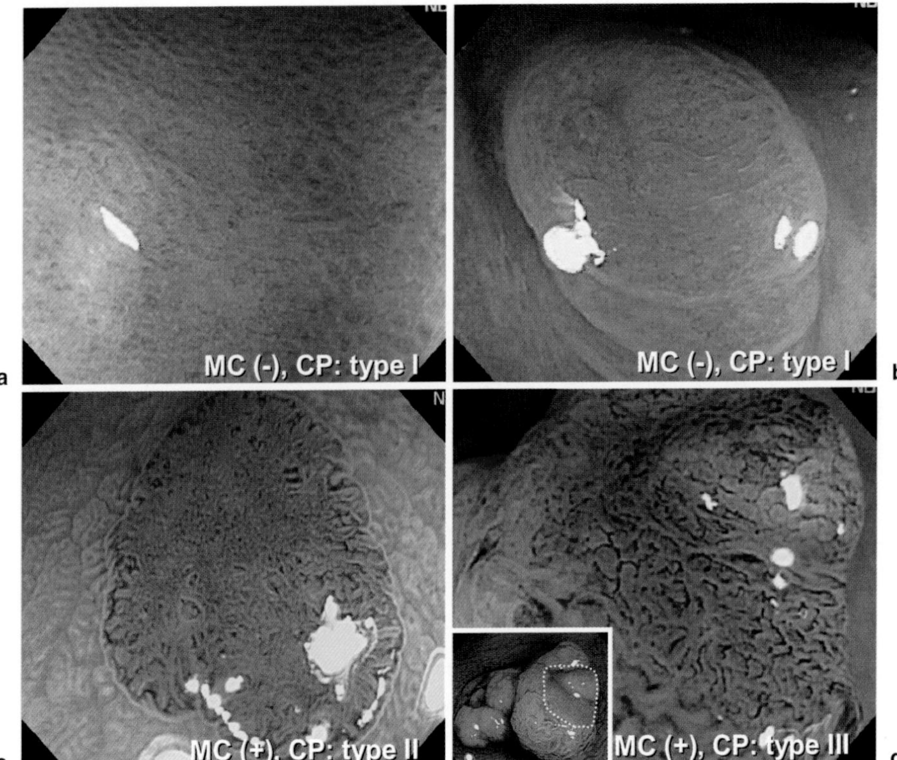

Fig. 3. Magnifying endoscopic findings of macrocapillary vessels using NBI in normal colonic mucosa, hyperplastic polyps, adenomas, and carcinomas. **a** Normal colonic mucosa. In many cases the mucosal capillary meshwork arranged in a honeycomb pattern around the mucosal glands is invisible, or only faintly visible, with magnifying observation using NBI colonoscopy, because the endoscopic resolution is not high enough to visualize the network (MC (−), CP: type I). **b** Hyperplastic polyps. In many cases the mucosal capillary meshwork is invisible, or only faintly visible, with magnifying observation using NBI colonoscopy, because the endoscopic resolution is not high enough to visualize the network (MC (−), CP: type I). **c** Adenomatous polyps. MC vessels are clearly visible, because these capillaries are elongated and have larger diameters than normal capillaries. The honeycomb-like pattern of capillaries on the surface of the tumor is retained (MC (+), CP: type II). **d** Carcinoma in adenomas (magnified view of the demarcated area *lower left*, chromoendoscopic view). The microvascular architecture of colonic carcinoma is characterized by a disorganized structure and an increased density of microvessels. MC vessels are clearly visible and show unevenly sized, thicker capillaries which are branching, curtailed, and irregular (MC (+), CP: type IIIA)

Intramucosal and Superficial Submucosal Cancer (CP type IIIA)

The MC vessels are clearly visible and show unevenly sized thicker capillaries (diameter: >18 μm) with branching and curtailed irregularity when compared to adenomatous polyps. MC vessels of intramucosal and superficial submucosal cancer (Sm1) are characterized by a lack of uniformity (blind ending, branching) and an increased density of microvessels. Therapeutically, lesions diagnosed as CP type IIIA should be resected by snare polypectomy, EMR or ESD (Fig. 3d).

Deep Submucosal Invasive Cancer (CP type IIIB)

Microvascular observation of colorectal cancer lesions under magnifying NBI has demonstrated that, in addition to the characteristics shown by CP type III lesions, a lesion showing a clear distinction between normal/cancerous mucosa on the surface and, presence of a nearly avascular or loose microvascular area due to histological desmoplastic changes in the stromal tissue, are highly associated to deep submucosal invasion or beyond [23,24]. Therapeutically, lesions diagnosed as CP type IIIB should be removed surgically.

Recently, Katagiri et al. reported that capillary patterns observed by NBI with magnification provided high accuracy for distinction between low grade dysplasia (CP-II) and high grade dysplasia/invasive cancer (CP-III). Sensitivity and specificity were 90.3% and 97.1% respectively. The overall accuracy was 95.5% [20].

Histological Findings of Microvascular Proliferation

We evaluated microvascular proliferation with CD-31 immunohistochemical staining in normal colonic mucosa, hyperplastic polyps, adenomas, and carcinomas (Fig. 4). Many microcapillary vessels measuring less than 10 μm could be seen in the stroma at the surface of normal colonic mucosa and hyperplastic polyps. However, adenomatous and cancerous lesions with thicker capillary vessels (20–30 μm) could be seen surrounding glands just under the basal membrane at the surface. These findings suggest that MC vessels were histologically confirmed to be dilated, with increased microvasculature and vessel diameters in the superficial portion of adenomatous and cancerous lesions, by immunohistochemical staining with antihuman monoclonal CD-31 antibody [19].

A Bench Study: Comparison Between Endoscopic Resolution and MC Vessels

MC vessels in normal colonic mucosa and hyperplastic polyps are invisible, or only faintly visible, under magnifying observation using NBI colonoscopy. To evaluate the correlation between endoscopic resolution and the visibility of MC vessels, a square plate (TOPPAN-TEST-CHART-NO1) was used in this bench study. As previously reported, the diameter of MC vessels ranges from 8 to 12 μm in normal colonic

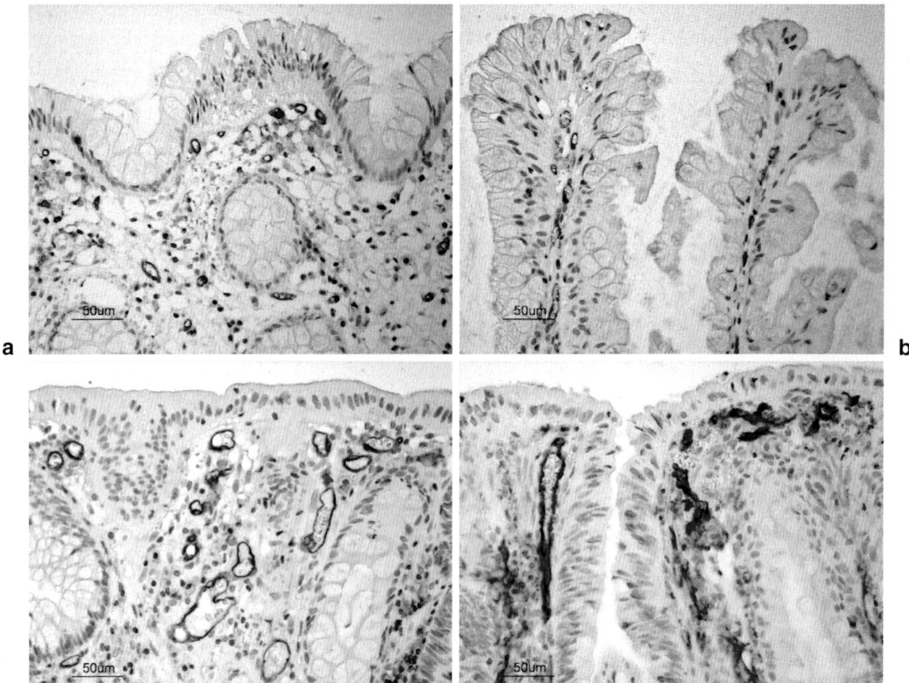

Fig. 4. Histological findings of macrocapillary vessels in normal colonic mucosa, hyperplastic polyp, adenoma, and carcinoma. All specimens are stained for endothelial cells with an anti-CD31 antibody (clone JC/70A, DAKO, dilution 1:20). Original magnification ×100. **a** The superficial portion of normal colonic mucosa. Many microcapillary vessels, measuring approximately 10 μm, can be seen in the stromal tissue. **b** The superficial portion of a hyperplastic polyp. Many microcapillary vessels, measuring approximately 10 μm, can be seen in the stromal tissue as in normal mucosa. **c** The superficial portion of an adenomatous polyp. Thicker capillary vessels can be seen surrounding the adenomatous glands. **d** The superficial portion of a well-differentiated adenocarcinoma. Thicker capillary vessels can be seen surrounding the cancerous glands

mucosa and hyperplastic polyps [12–14]. As shown in Fig. 5a, the bars on the square plate, which are approximately 8–12 μm when adjusted to the same scale as the polyp, are not clearly visible or distinguishable owing to the endoscopic resolution. On the other hand, MC vessels in adenomatous or cancerous lesions are in the range 13–20 μm [12–14]. These vessels are clearly visible on NBI colonoscopy with magnification (Fig. 5c). In this bench study, the bars on the square plate, which are approximately 14–20 μm when adjusted to the same scale as the polyp, are clearly visible. Therefore, the presence of MC vessels on magnifying endoscopy using NBI is a useful indicator for distinguishing between hyperplastic polyps and adenomatous polyps.

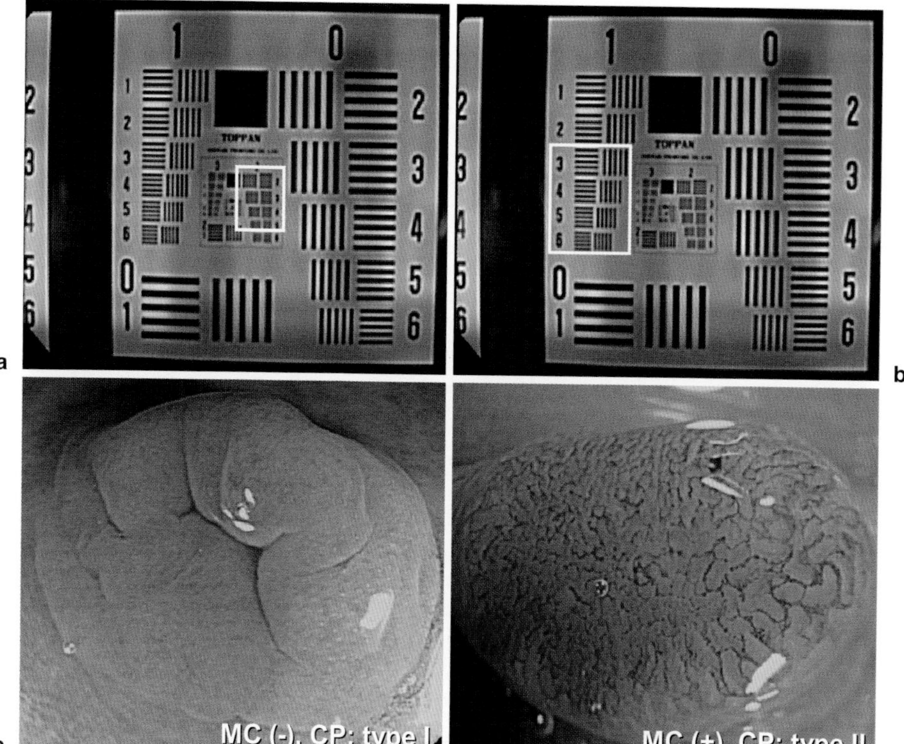

FIG. 5. Comparison between endoscopic resolution and meshed capillary vessels. **a** Magnified observation of a square plate (TOPPAN-TEST-CHART-NO1), 3 mm in size. The area highlighted relates to the bars, which are approximately 8–12 µm, which are not clearly visible or distinguishable due to the endoscopic resolution. **b** Magnified observation of a hyperplastic polyp, also 3 mm in size, MC (–), CP: type I. At this magnification, it is not possible to identify the MC vessels which are only 8–12 µm in diameter, as shown in FIG. 6a. **c** Magnified observation of a square plate (TOPPAN-TEST-CHART-NO1), 3 mm in size. The area highlighted relates to the bars, which are approximately 14–20 µm, which are clearly visible at this magnification. **d** Magnified observation of an adenomatous polyp, also 3 mm in size, MC (+), CP: type II. It is possible to identify the MC vessels which are 14–20 µm, as shown in FIG. 5c

Future Prospects

Diagnoses on the basis of mucosal patterns have been reported to be correlated with histological diagnoses. Chromoendoscopy is often used, as it is a contrast staining method using a biocompatible dye agent such as indigo carmine. In mucosa with glands, the dye agents accumulate within crypt orifices. Although chromoendoscopy is effective in many applications, it is still only an optional diagnostic method because of the time needed, the additional cost, and the necessity of complete mucus removal. In this review, we have described the utility of detailed observations of the microvas-

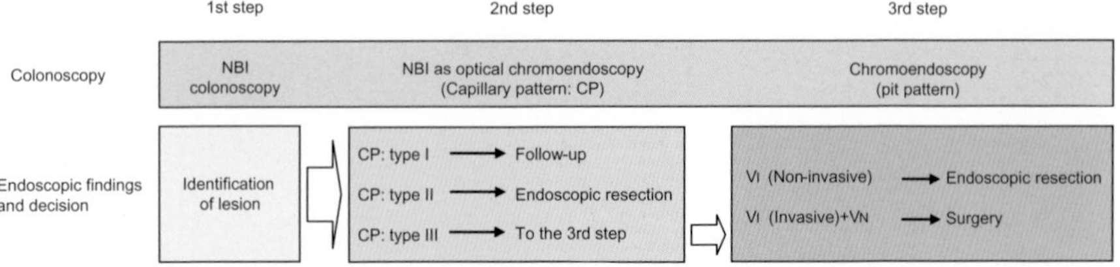

FIG. 6. Three-step strategy for the management of colorectal lesions using conventional colonoscopy, NBI colonoscopy, and chromoendoscopy. When you find a lesion in a normal observation, observe it with NBI mode. If the result is CP: Type I, follow-up is recommended, if it is CP: Type II, resection is recommended, and if it is CP: Type III, conduct chromoendoscopy and observe the pit pattern (VI or VN) carefully before deciding on the treatment policy

cular architecture for differential diagnosis during NBI colonoscopy. An NBI modification provides a unique image that emphasizes the capillary pattern and the surface structure. Our initial data indicate that NBI may be as effective, or more effective, than chromoscopy without the same problems [9].

Angiogenesis is critical to the transition of premalignant lesions in a hyperproliferative state to a malignant phenotype. Therefore, a diagnosis based on the angiogenic or vascular morphological changes might be ideal for the early detection or diagnosis of neoplasms. In this review, we have proposed the term "meshed capillary" (MC) to distinguish between nonneoplastic and neoplastic lesions, and the capillary classification "capillary pattern" (CP) for the differential diagnosis of colorectal lesions. On the basis of previous investigations, the surface microvascular architecture in colorectal lesions can be divided into three patterns: (1) honeycomb-like capillaries in the normal mucosa and hyperplastic polyps (8–12 μm); (2) elongated meshwork capillaries with a greater diameter in adenomatous lesions (approximately 13 μm); (3) disorganized meshwork capillaries with an increased density of microvessels in cancerous lesions (18–19 μm) [12–14]. These capillary patterns can easily be recognized using NBI colonoscopy, and we believe that the combined use of NBI and real chromoendoscopy decreases the time and cost of screening colonoscopy. The three-step strategy for the management of colorectal lesions using these procedures is shown in Fig. 6. However, at the present time, NBI colonoscopy may not be superior to chromoendoscopy for distinguishing between endoscopically treatable early invasive cancers and untreatable cancers. We should use the three different procedures without getting them confused.

In the near future, we hope that NBI procedures will become standard for screening and surveillance colonoscopy. To assess the feasibility and efficacy of using the NBI system, further studies are required for colorectal lesions and other lesions of the gastrointestinal tract.

References

1. Winawer SJ, Zauber AG, Ho MN, et al. (1993) Prevention of colorectal cancer by colonoscopic polypectomy. National Polyp Study Workgroup. N Engl J Med 329: 1977–1981

2. Saito H (2000) Screening for colorectal cancer: current status in Japan. Dis Colon Rectum 43:S78–84
3. Vatan MH, Stalsbert H (1982) The prevalence of polyps of the large intestine in Oslo: an autopsy study. Cancer 40:819–825
4. Fu KI, Sano Y, Kato S, et al. (2004) Chromoendoscopy using indigo carmine dye spraying with magnifying observation is the most reliable method for differential diagnosis between non-neoplastic and neoplastic colorectal lesions: a prospective study. Endoscopy 36:1089–1093
5. Sano Y, Saito Y, Fu KI, et al. (2005) Efficacy of magnifying chromoendoscopy for the differential diagnosis of colorectal lesions. Dig Endosc 17:105–116
6. Sano Y, Kobayashi M, Hamamoto Y, et al. (2001) New diagnostic method based on color imaging using a narrow-band imaging (NBI) system for the gastrointestinal tract. Gastrointest Endosc 53:AB125
7. Gono K, Obi T, Yamaguchi M, et al. (2004) Appearance of enhanced tissue features in narrow-band endoscopic imaging. J Biomed Opt 9:568–577
8. Sano Y, Muto M, Tajiri H, et al. (2005) Optical/digital chromoendoscopy during colonoscopy using a narrow-band imaging system. Dig Endosc 17:S60–S65
9. Machida H, Sano Y, Hamamoto Y, et al. (2004) Narrow-band imaging for differential diagnosis of colorectal mucosal lesions: a pilot study. Endoscopy 36: 1094–1098
10. Sano Y, Horimatsu T, Fu KI, et al. (2006) Magnified observation of microvascular architecture using narrow-band imaging (NBI) for differential diagnosis between non-neoplastic and neoplastic colorectal lesion: a prospective study. Gastrointest Endosc 63:AB102
11. Tanaka S, Kaltenbach T, Chayama K, et al. (2006) High-magnification colonoscopy (with videos). Gastrointest Endosc 64:604–613
12. Konerding MA, Fait E, Gaumann A, et al. (2001) 3D microvascular architecture of pre-cancerous lesions and invasive carcinomas of the colon. Br J Cancer 84: 1354–1362
13. Fait E, Malkusch W, Gnoth SH, et al. (1998) Microvascular patterns of the human large intestine: morphometric studies of vascular parameters in corrosion casts. Scanning Microsc 12:641–651
14. Skinner SA, Frydman GM, O'Brien PE (1995) Microvascular structure of benign and malignant tumors of the colon in humans. Dig Dis Sci 40:373–384
15. Sano Y, Horimatsu T, Kuang I Fu, et al. (2006) Magnified observation of microvascular architecture of colorectal lesions using a narrow-band imaging system. Dig Endosc 18:S44–S51
16. Gono K, Yamazaki K, Doguchi N, et al. (2003) Endoscopic observation of tissue by narrow-band illumination. Opt Rev 10:1–5
17. Kudo S, Hirota S, Nakajima T, et al. (1994) Colorectal tumours and pit pattern. J Clin Pathol 47:880–885
18. Sano Y, Maeda N, Kanzaki A, et al. (2005) Angiogenesis in colon hyperplastic polyp. Cancer Lett 218:223–228
19. Muto M, Nakane M, Katada C, et al. (2004) Squamous cell carcinoma in situ at oropharyngeal and hypopharyngeal mucosal sites. Cancer 101:1375–1381
20. Katagiri A, Fu KI, Sano Y, Ikematsu H, Horimatsu T, Kaneko K, Muto M, Yoshida S. Narrow band imaging with magnifying colonoscopy as a diagnostic tool for predicting the histology of early colorectal neoplasia. Aliment Pharmacol Ther. 2008 Feb 14 [Epub ahead of print]
21. Yasushi Sano, Hiroaki Ikematsu, Kuang I Fu , Fabian Emura, Atsushi Katagiri, Takahiro Horimatsu, Kazuhiro Kaneko, Roy Soetikno, Shigeaki Yoshida. Meshed capillary vessels using narrow band imaging for differential diagnosis of small colorectal polyps. Gastrointes Endosc (in press)

22. Toshio Uraoka, Yasushi Sano, Yutaka Saito, Hiroshi Saito, Takahisa Matsuda, and Kazuhide Yamamoto Narrow-band imaging for improving colorectal adenoma detection: Appropriate system function settings are required. GUT (in press)
23. Fukuzawa M, Saito Y, Matsuda T, Uraoka T, Horimatsu T, Ikematsu H et al. The Efficiency of Narrow Band Imaging with Magnification for the Estimation of Invasion Depth Diagnosis in Early Colorectal Cancer. -A Prospective Study [Abstract]. Gastrointest Endosc 2007;65:342
24. Horimatsu T, Ikematsu H, Sano Y, Katagiri A, Fu KI, Ohtsu A. A Micro-Vascular Architecture with NBI Colonoscopy Is Useful to Predict Invasiveness and Allow Patients to Select for Endoscopic Resection Or Surgical Resection [Abstract]. Gastrointes Endosc 2007;65:270

The Efficacy of Narrow-Band Imaging (NBI) and Autofluorescence Imaging (AFI) Colonoscopy for Patients with Ulcerative Colitis

Kenji Watanabe, Nobuhide Oshitani, and Tetsuo Arakawa

Summary. We investigated the efficacy of surveillance colonoscopy using narrow-band imaging as a handy method of optical pancolonic chromoendoscopy, and the potential of autofluorescence imaging colonoscopy for patients with ulcerative colitis.

Key words. Autofluorescence imaging (AFI), Narrow-band imaging (NBI), Ulcerative colitis

Introduction

The main purposes of colonoscopic examinations for patients with ulcerative colitis (UC) are an observation of activity and the detection of complications, including surveillance colonoscopy (SC) for colitis-associated cancer or dysplasia (CC/D). Usually, conventional colonoscopy using white light (WL) observation is used to observe the mucosal activity of UC and perform SC. In addition, magnifying chromoendoscopy is useful to detect the mucosal healing of UC in detail [1,2]. On the other hand, CC/D is important because it is one lethal complication of UC. Several important articles about surveillance colonoscopy have been published in the last few years [3–5]. These articles proved the efficacy of magnifying chromoendoscopy and targeted biopsy to detect CC/D in surveillance colonoscopy.

Recently, image-enhancing technology, narrow-band imaging (NBI), and autofluorescence imaging (AFI) has been used for gastrointestinal endoscopy. Most of the articles about colonoscopy using NBI and AFI were describing the detection of neoplasms [6,7]. Rutter et al. [4] reported the efficacy of magnifying colonoscopy, pancolonic chromoendoscopy, and targeted biopsy for CC/D, but in practice it is difficult to perform pancolonic chromoendoscopy for all patients diagnosed with UC.

In a prospective study, we aimed to investigate the efficacy of NBI for SC (NBI–SC) to detect CC/D as a handy optical method of pancolonic chromoendoscopy [8]. We also aimed to reveal the efficacy and potential of AFI colonoscopy for patients with ulcerative colitis, and we therefore performed preliminary studies [9].

Department of Gastroenterology, Osaka City University Graduate School of Medicine, 1-4-3 Asahi-machi, Abeno-ku, Osaka 545-8585, Japan

Materials and Methods

Study Design and Patient Population

All patients in our hospital were recruited for these studies. UC was diagnosed based on clinical history, and endoscopic and histological findings. Patients were prepared by giving them 2 l electrolyte lavage solution orally.

Each patient gave informed consent in accordance with the Helsinki Declaration before the study began.

SC Using NBI

We performed a prospective study of NBI–SC on about 80 patients from April 2005 to March 2006. All patients were in the clinical remission stage, or with pancolitis type or left-sided colitis type UC, and their disease duration was more than 7 years. We observed the whole colon using NBI after insertion into the cecum with a magnifying colonoscope (CF-Q240ZI, CF-H260AZI; Olympus Medical Systems, Tokyo, Japan). NBI could provide a pit-pattern diagnosis for CC/D indirectly (Fig. 1). If we found a suspicious lesion for CC/D, we magnified the lesion and made a decision whether or not to perform a target biopsy. We compared the results of NBI–SC and surveillance colonoscopy by using conventional magnifying chromoendoscopy (CHR–SC) carried out for about 60 patients as a prospective study.

A pathological diagnosis of CC/D was performed by two independent pathologists using hematoxylin–eosin staining and additional p53 or Ki-67 immunohistochemical staining.

Colonoscopy Using AFI

During the 8-month period between July 2006 and November 2006, 18 UC patients underwent colonoscopy with AFI (CF-FH260AZI; Olympus Medical Systems). The UC activity of all patients was in clinical remission. After insertion into the cecum and with white-light observation, AFI was used to observe abnormal lesions and remission mucosa as necessary. The AFI was carried out in such a way as to observe the target as perpendicularly as possible. If the target was a magenta color, we decided that the target was positive for AFI. If a biopsy was taken, a pathological diagnosis was determined by using hematoxylin–eosin staining. Histological UC activity was graded at three levels, severe, moderate, or mild, depending on the extent of infiltration of inflammatory cells (Fig. 2).

Results

The Efficacy of NBI–SC as Handy Optical Pancolonic Chromoendoscopy

The accuracy of the detection of neoplastic lesions and CC/D was equivalent for NBI–SC and CHR–SC (neoplastic lesions, NBI–SC 14%, CHR–SC 13%; dysplastic lesions, NBI–SC 7%, CHR–SC 5%). Both methods reduced the number of biopsies

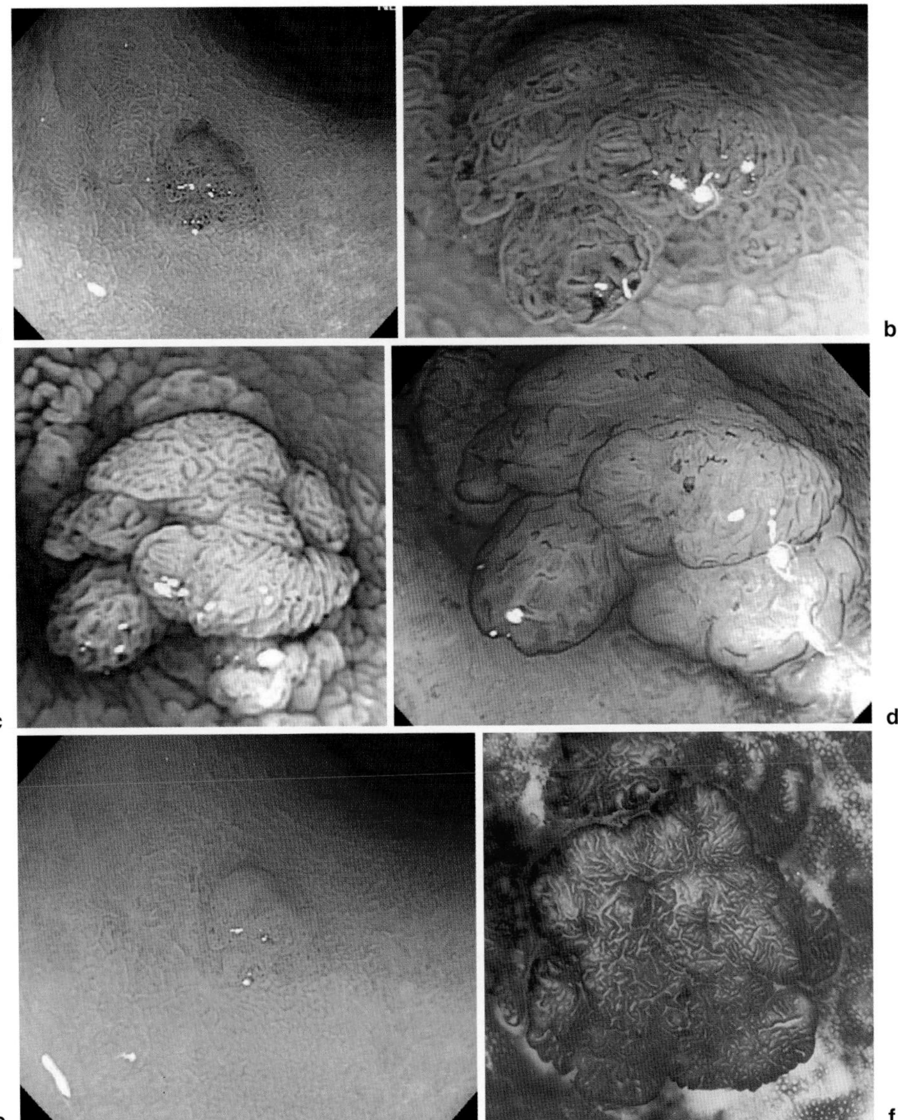

Fig. 1. Male patient, 61 years old, with pancolitis-type ulcerative colitis (UC) of 21 years duration. We performed optical pancolonic chromoendoscopy using narrow-band imaging surveillance colonoscopy (NBI–SC), and detected a small slightly elevated lesion in the sigmoid colon (**a**). NBI observation was easy compared with white light (WL) for this lesion (**e**). We also carried out magnifying observations and immediately found an indirect diagnostic pit pattern in the structural architecture of the surface of this lesion (**b**). If we need more information for colitis-associated cancer or dysplasia (CC/D), we can also perform chromoendoscopy using an indigo carmine dye solution (**c**) or a crystal violet dye solution (**d**) after NBI observations. We performed a total colectomy on this patient because we had detected multiple dysplasias in the colon. The stereoscopic miscroscopic findings for this dysplasia were shown to be type III- or type IV-like pits (**f**)

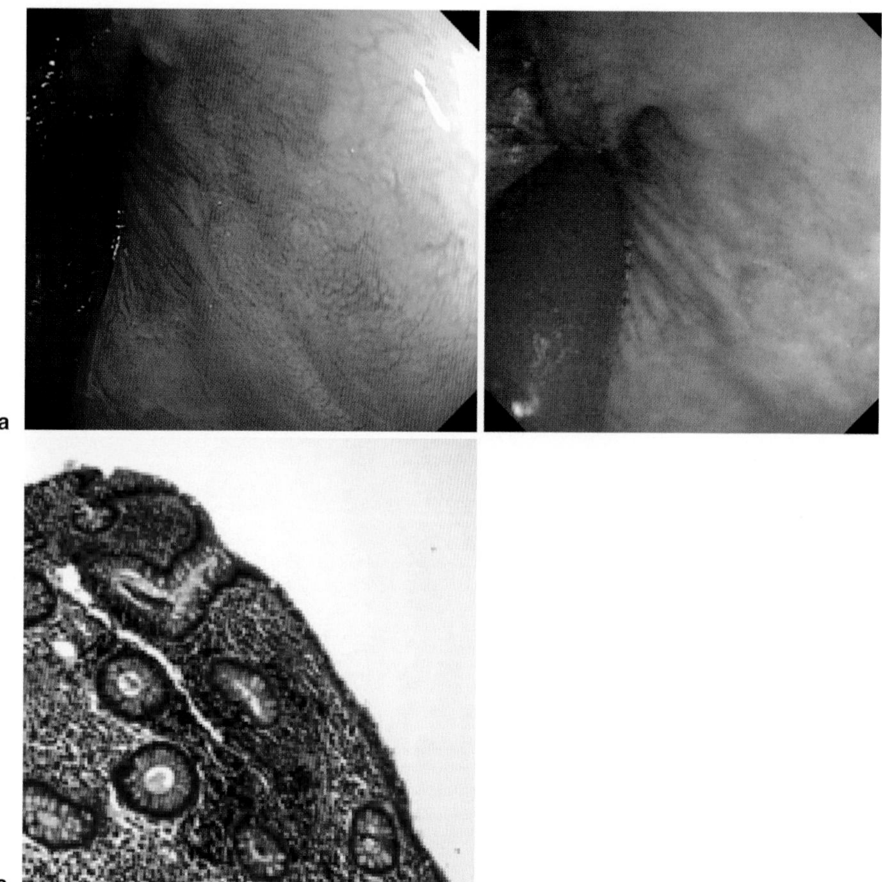

Fig. 2. Female patient, 46 years old, with pancolitis-type UC. We observed endoscopic remission with WL (**a**), but the AFI finding was positive (magenta) (**b**). This AFI diagnosis depended on histological UC activity in a biopsy specimen (**c**)

needed to compare the methods of surveillance colonoscopy by using random biopsies (NBI–SC 2.1 pieces/patient; CHR-SC 1.8 pieces/patient). The largest difference was in the total time taken for surveillance colonoscopy (NBI–SC 11 min 38 s; CHR–SC 16 min 48 s; Student's *t*-test $P < 0.05$). NBI–SC could change an NBI observation and a conventional observation easily and immediately, so that it was possible to carry out an indirect pit-pattern diagnosis rapidly.

The Relation of AFI Observations and Histological Activities of UC

Twenty-one biopsies specimens were taken from endoscopic remission colonic mucosa that was diagnosed using white-light observations. Twelve specimens were

AFI-positive (not strongly positive) and 9 specimens were negative. While most histological activity findings for AFI-positive samples showed moderate activity (10/12, 83.8%), most findings for AFI-negative samples showed mild activity (7/9, 77.8%) (Fig. 2).

Discussion

Endoscopy using image-enhancing technology is now carried out by NBI and AFI. An NBI or AFI videoscope is very easy to use for standard clinical colonoscopy. Both examinations are very suitable for gastrointestinal neoplastic lesions. In particular, Kara et al. [10] have reported the efficacy of three-color observations (white light, AFI, and NBI) for detecting early neoplasia in Barrett's esophagus. In contrast, the efficacy of NBI and AFI for patients with UC has still not been confirmed. The colonic mucosa of patients with UC can present several different appearances.

NBI can visualize the microvascular architecture of neoplasms by magnifying observations. Recently, the efficacy of these findings for esophageal and pharyngeal cancer has been confirmed in Japan. However, these findings are not helpful for patients with UC because remission mucosa in UC usually shows severe dilatation of the vessels. On the other hand, NBI can detect the structural architecture of the surface of neoplasms. These findings are provided indirectly by surface microvessels between crypts. It is easy to perform of optical chromoendoscopy to detect CC/D with recently developed high-resolution colonoscopy, especially by using magnifying colonoscopy.

Rutter et al. [4] reported the efficacy of magnifying colonoscopy, pancolonic chromoendoscopy, and target biopsy for CC/D, but in practice it is difficult to perform pancolonic chromoendoscopy for all UC patients. NBI gives us a convenient way to perform optical pancolonic chromoendoscopy easily. The accuracy of NBI–SC is similar to that of CHR–SC. Recent studies of SC have revealed the efficacy of magnifying chromoendoscopy for CC/D [3–5], but in this study we have shown that NBI–SC has a similar efficacy to CHR–SC. Dekker et al. [7] also reported similar results recently. We could reduce the number of biopsies taken by targeted biopsies during the NBI–SC procedure. Most importantly, the efficacy of NBI–SC was found to shorten the total time needed for surveillance colonoscopy compared with CHR–SC. The shorter times needed for NBI–SC will encourage the use of surveillance colonoscopy and increase the number of such studies in regular clinical work.

Residual stools are shown in a red color in NBI observations, which makes it easier to confirm the presence of such stools. Washing residual stools out of the colon is important in order to perform high-quality SC.

Our preliminary study has revealed the relation of AFI observations and the histological activities of UC. The mechanism for increasing the autofluorescence intensity is not yet established, but we have proved the relation between AFI findings (magenta) and inflammation of the mucosa with UC.

Recently, the clinical endpoints of the treatment of patients with UC have been changed in order to achieve endoscopic remission, but even though patients achieve endoscopic remission, recurrences still sometimes occur. An AFI-negative finding means more complete histological remission. We need further prospective studies to investigate the relation between autofluorescence findings and recurrence rate. Even though colonoscopic findings have achieved endoscopic remission by using WL observations, in an AFI-positive case, the patient might have to continue the same remission maintenance therapy. However, in an AFI-negative case, the patient might be able to decrease the dosage of drugs for remission maintenance therapy.

We also need further examinations of the efficacy of surveillance colonoscopy by using AFI although, as we revealed, colonic remission mucosa of patients with UC can be seen as AFI-positive. If CC/D can be seen as AFI-positive, it results in a problem of detecting magenta-colored lesions in the magenta-colored background of colonic mucosa in cases of surveillance colonoscopy. This means that AFI may have limitations for surveillance colonoscopy, as the resolution of an AFI scope is relatively blurred. We hope to develop a higher-resolution AFI scope in the next generation.

Conclusion

NBI-SC will be of practical use in surveillance colonoscopy as a handy optical pancolonic chromoendoscope. UC is very varied in its clinical course and in the part of the colon which is affected. We expect to provide efficient diagnosis to patients with UC by the use of three-color colonoscopy (WL, NBI, and AFI).

References

1. Matsumoto T, Kuroki F, Mizuno M, et al. (1997) Application of magnifying chromoscopy for the assessment of severity in patients with mild to moderate ulcerative colitis. Gastrointest Endosc 46:400–405
2. Fujiya M, Saitoh Y, Nomura M, et al. (2002) Minute findings by magnifying colonoscopy are useful for the evaluation of ulcerative colitis. Gastrointest Endosc 56: 535–542
3. Keisslich R, Fritsch J, Holymann M, et al. (2003) Methylene blue-aided chromoendoscopy for the detection of intraepithelial neoplasia and colon cancer in ulcerative colitis. Gastroenterology 124:880–888
4. Rutter MD, Sounders BP, Schofield G, et al. (2004) Pancolonic indigo carmine dye spraying for the detection of dysplasia in ulcerative colitis. Gut 53:256–260
5. Matsumoto T, Nakamura S, Jo Y, et al. (2003) Chromoscopy might improve diagnostic accuracy in cancer surveillance for ulcerative colitis. Am J Gastroenterol 98:1827–1833
6. Uedo N, Iishi H, Tatsuta M, et al. (2005) A novel videoendoscopy system by using autofluorescence and reflectance imaging for diagnosis of esophagogastric cancers. Gastrointest Endosc 62:521–528
7. Dekker E, van den Broek FJ, Reitsma JB, et al. (2007) Narrow-band imaging compared with conventional colonoscopy for the detection of dysplasia in patients with long-standing ulcerative colitis. Endoscopy 39:216–221
8. Watanabe K, Machida H, Oshitani N, et al. (2006) The efficacy of surveillance colonoscopy for ulcerative colitis-associated cancer or dysplasia by using NBI (narrow-band imaging). Gut 55:A231
9. Watanabe K, Yamagami H, Oshitani N, et al. (2007) Potential of autofluorescence colonoscopy for patients with ulcerative colitis. Dig Endosc 19:s150–s152
10. Kara MA, Peters FP, Fockens P, et al. (2006) Endoscopic video-autofluorescence imaging followed by narrow-band imaging for detecting early neoplasia in Barrett's esophagus. Gastrointest Endosc 64:176–185

The Value of Narrow-Band Imaging Colonoscopy and Autofluorescence Imaging Colonoscopy for Ulcerative Colitis

Takayuki Matsumoto, Tetsuji Kudo, and Mitsuo Iida

Summary. Narrow-band imaging (NBI) and autofluorescence imaging (AFI) colonoscopy are procedures which show gastrointestinal neoplasia and inflammation as colored areas distinctive from the surrounding normal tissue. By means of NBI colonoscopy, colorectal mucosa of ulcerative colitis (UC), especially in apparently inactive disease, is classified into two types according to the mucosal vascular pattern. In contrast, AFI colonoscopy can divide active mucosa under conventional colonoscopy into high-AF and low-AF patterns. When compared with histology, the vascular pattern under NBI colonoscopy is representative of epithelial damage, and the AF pattern is representative of inflammatory infiltrates. It is, therefore, suggested that the severity of UC can be classified by NBI and AFI colonoscopy. The procedures also seem to be applicable to cancer surveillance for UC, because the tortuous pattern determined by magnifying NBI colonoscopy and the sharply demarcated dark purple areas shown under AFI colonoscopy are suggestive of dysplastic lesions. Based on these findings, it is suggested that NBI and AFI colonoscopy are promising procedures for the diagnosis and management of UC.

Key words. Ulcerative colitis, Colonoscopy, Narrow-band imaging, Autofluorescence imaging, Dysplasia

Introduction

Narrow-band imaging (NBI) endoscopy is a technology which enhances specific depth and color tone. By means of NBI with a filter that has the absorption property of hemoglobin, the vascular architecture and the surface structure outlined by vessels in the gastrointestinal mucosa are enhanced [1].

When tissues are exposed to light of short wavelengths, some endogenous biological substances emit fluorescent light with a longer wavelength, i.e., autofluorescence (AF). Nonneoplastic and neoplastic tissues have different AF characteristics [2,3].

Department of Medicine and Clinical Science, and Department of Anatomic Pathology, Graduate School of Medical Sciences, Kyushu University, 3-1-1 Maidashi, Higashi-ku, Fukuoka 812-8582, Japan

This has led to the development of light-induced fluorescence endoscopy, a technique in which the mucosa is excited with blue light and real-time AF endoscopic images (AFI) are produced.

Although the roles of NBI and AFI colonoscopy have mainly been considered with regards to their accuracy for the diagnosis of colorectal cancer, our recent analyses have revealed that these procedures may be diagnostic of disease activity and neoplastic lesions in patients with ulcerative colitis (UC) [4–7]. In this chapter, the details of our experience of these procedures in patients with UC are presented.

Assessment of Disease Activity

NBI Colonoscopy

In the active phase of UC, the mucosa observed under conventional colonoscopy shows a lack of the mucosal vascular pattern (MVP), fine granulations, and spontaneous bleeding (Fig. 1A,B), while in NBI observations it is depicted as a brownish color (Figs. 1B and 2B). Vessels in the deep layer, which are observed as linear, green structures, are obscure in active UC. In contrast, NBI occasionally depicts vessels in the deep layer which cannot be discerned by conventional colonoscopy. NBI can detect the patchy and skipped involvement that is found in approximately 30% of patients with active UC. By means of magnifying NBI observation, circular pits of crypt openings and mucosal surface patterns, which have a coral-reef-like or villous appearance, can easily be observed in active UC. While conventional colonoscopy is superior to NBI for the determination of small yellowish spots, crypt openings are emphasized by NBI.

In the inactive phase of UC, NBI is useful for the assessment of the MVP. The MVP under NBI shows two distinctive patterns, one being a deep vasculature which is shown as green in color, and the other superficial vasculature which is brown in color. When UC has completely healed, conventional colonoscopy depicts an MVP as seen in normal subjects. In this situation, both green vessels in the deep layer and brownish vessels in the superficial layer are observed clearly by NBI. The MVP is divided into two types. In one type the superficial brown vessels are enhanced (Fig. 3A,B), and in the other the brownish vessels become obscure with obvious crypt openings (Fig. 3C,D). When the histological findings were investigated and compared, there were trends toward more severe inflammatory infiltrates, and more frequent goblet cell depletion and basal plasmacytosis in the latter pattern than in the former [4].

AFI Colonoscopy

Under AFI colonoscopy, the mucosa of UC is generally classified into three types of colored area: green, white, and purple. When the green and white colors are regarded as high AF and the purple color as low AF, segments with mucosa of normal appearance and those with inactive UC are regarded as high AF. In contrast, segments with active UC are divided into two patterns under AFI; approximately half of those show high AF (Fig. 1C) while the remaining segments show low AF (Fig. 2C).

In our retrospective analysis, the incidence of low AF was significantly higher in active mucosa than in normal or quiescent mucosa. When the AFI findings were

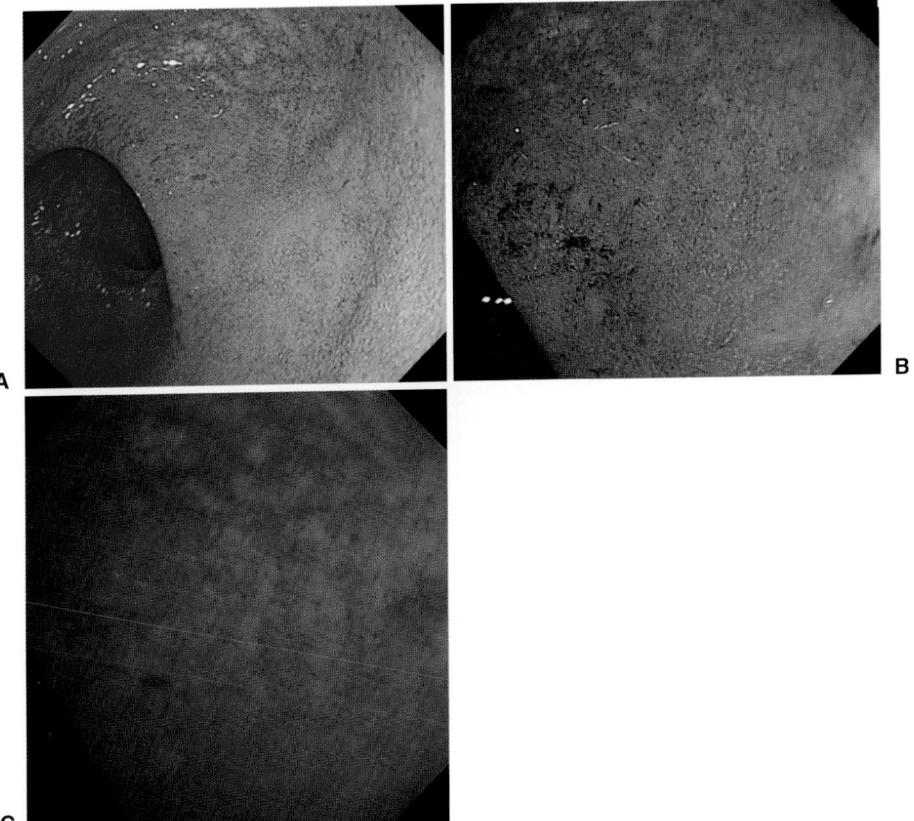

Fig. 1. Conventional, NBI, and AFI colonoscopic findings in active ulcerative colitis. **A** Conventional colonoscopy shows fine granular mucosa with friability and white spots. **B** NBI colonoscopy shows brownish mucosa with obvious spots, which are white in color. **C** AFI colonoscopy depicts the mucosa as a green-colored area

compared with the histological findings, the inflammatory infiltrates were more severe and crypt distortion was more frequent in the latter than in the former segments [5]. Furthermore, when active segments under conventional colonoscopy were assessed, there was a trend toward a higher grade of inflammatory cell infiltrates in segments with low AF than in those with high AF [5]. It therefore seems likely that the mucosal thickness, determined by the degree of inflammatory infiltrates, is the major factor which determines AF status in active UC. It seems likely that high AF in active UC may be a consequence of resolving processes even in the active disease. From this perspective, AFI colonoscopy may contribute to the identification of mucosal healing in patients with UC.

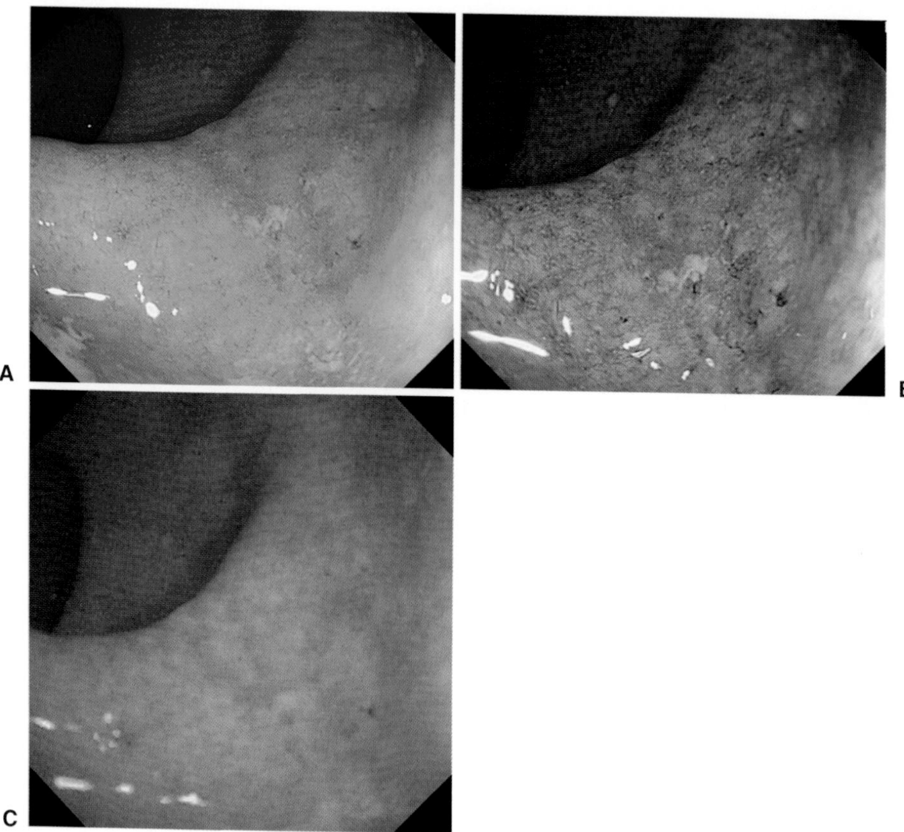

FIG. 2. Conventional, NBI, and AFI colonoscopic findings in active ulcerative colitis. **A** Conventional colonoscopy shows active mucosa with mucous exudates. **B** NBI colonoscopy shows the villous structure clearly. **C** Under AFI colonoscopy, the mucosa is shown to be purple in color

Diagnosis of Dysplasia

NBI Colonoscopy

It has been confirmed in various clinical trials that chromoscopy with target biopsy can be recommended as a strategy for cancer surveillance in UC. In a prospective trial from The Netherlands, however, NBI colonoscopy did not increase the sensitivity in the detection of dysplastic lesions in patients with longstanding UC [8].

In our pilot study with magnifying NBI colonoscopy, we used a gross configuration of the target area, either protruding or flat, and magnifying NBI findings, either honeycomb-like, villous, or tortuous, for the hallmark in the diagnosis of dysplastic lesions in UC. As a result, the relative frequency of occurrence of dysplasia was significantly higher in protruding lesions (10%) than in flat mucosa (1.1%). Furthermore, the relative frequency of occurrence of dysplasia was significantly higher in

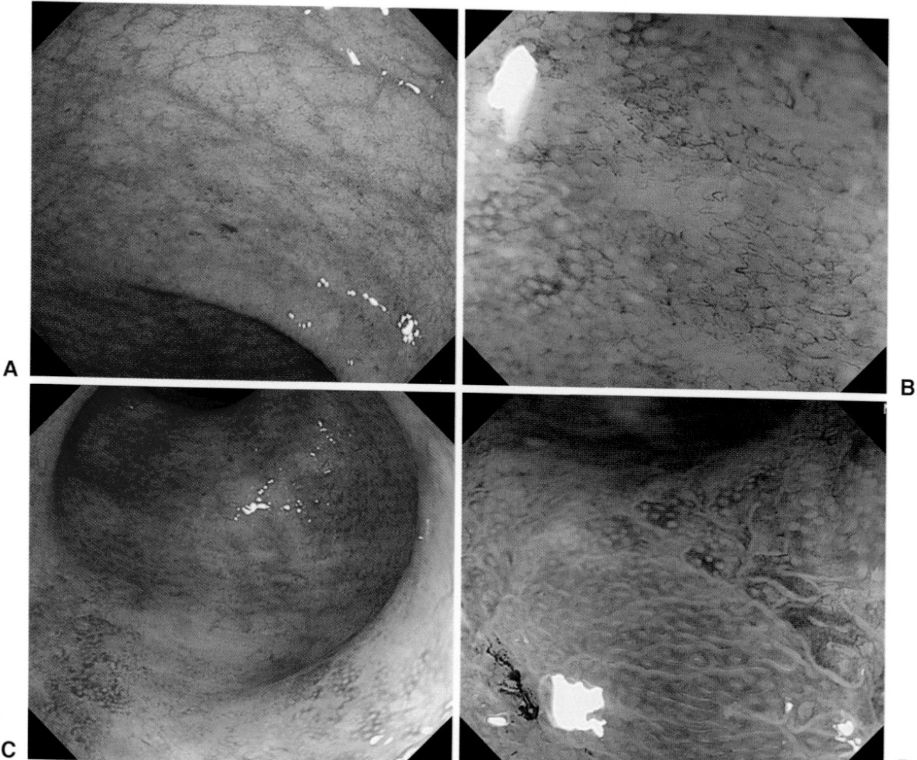

Fig. 3. Conventional and NBI colonoscopic findings in inactive ulcerative colitis. **A** Conventional colonoscopy shows mucosa with a slightly distorted vascular pattern. **B** NBI colonoscopy shows a regular, honeycomb-like vascular structure in the mucosa indicated in Fig. 3A. **C** Conventional colonoscopy shows a mucosa with a distorted vascular pattern. **D** Under NBI observation, the mucosa indicated in Fig. 3C is composed of obvious cryptal openings

areas of tortuous pattern (8%) (Fig. 4) than in those of honeycomb-like or villous patterns. The sensitivity and specificity of protruding lesions under conventional colonoscopy for the diagnosis of dysplasia were 40.0% and 93.8%, respectively, and those of tortuous pattern under NBI colonoscopy were 80% and 84.2%, respectively [6]. Based on these observations, magnifying NBI colonoscopy seems to be an easily applicable procedure for the identification of target areas for cancer surveillance in UC. The diagnostic yield of NBI colonoscopy in our study seemed to be increased by the application of the magnifying facility.

AFI Colonoscopy

Fluorescence endoscopy with 5-aminolaevulinic acid (5-ALA) sensitization has been shown to be a promising procedure for the detection of dysplasia in patients with UC [9]. By means of this procedure, dysplastic lesions can be detected as reddish areas

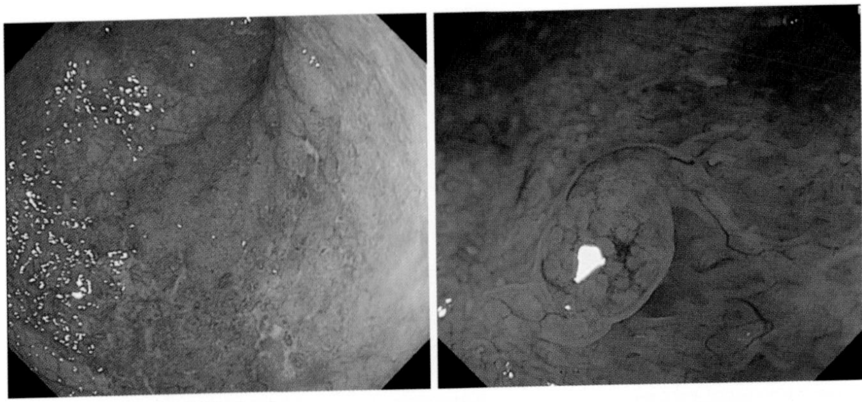

Fig. 4. NBI colonoscopic findings in a case of high-grade dysplasia. **A** Conventional colonoscopy reveals a slightly elevated mucosa. **B** Under magnifying NBI colonoscopy, the surface of the lesion is characterized by tortuous structures. The lesion was diagnosed as high-grade dysplasia

under blue light. However, the diagnostic value of the procedure has been questioned by another group of investigators from Germany, where dysplasia was not detected in areas positive for 5-ALA fluorescence [10].

We applied AFI colonoscopy to patients with UC in whom dysplasia was histologically verified. We regarded sharply demarcated areas of dark purple color to be AFI-positive lesions, and obscure areas of green or light purple to be AFI-negative areas. In one patient, there were distinctive flat areas which were dark purple in color. A total of 10 biopsy specimens, 7 from AFI-positive areas and 3 from AFI-negative areas, were obtained during the surveillance. As a result, 3 of 7 AFI-positive lesions (43%) and none of 3 AFI-negative lesions (0%) were diagnosed as dysplasia. In another patient, there were four AFI-positive areas in the distal colon and the rectum. Fourteen specimens were obtained, 4 from the AFI-positive areas and 10 from AFI-negative areas. In this case, 3 of 4 areas positive for AFI (75%) and 3 of 10 AFI-negative areas (30%) were diagnosed as either dysplasia or adenoma. One of the three AFI-positive dysplastic lesions was high-grade dysplasia. Although a prospective study with a large number of subjects with UC is warranted, our experience suggests that AFI colonoscopy may be a procedure which is applicable to cancer surveillance in patients with UC.

References

1. Gono K, Obi T, Yamaguchi M, et al. (2004) Appearance of enhanced tissue features in narrow-band endoscopic imaging. J Biomed Opt 9:568–577
2. Haringsma J, Tytgat GN (1999) Fluorescence and autofluorescence. Baillieres Best Pract Res Clin Gastroenterol 13:1–10
3. Vo DT, Panjehpour M, Overholt BF, et al. 1995) In vivo cancer diagnosis of the esophagus using differential normalized fluorescence (DNF) indices. Lasers Surg Med 16:41–47

4. Matsumoto T, Kudo T, Iida M, et al. (2005) Findings obtained by narrow-band imaging colonoscopy in patients with ulcerative colitis (in Japanese with English abstract). Stomach Intestine 40:1425–1428
5. Matsumoto T, Kudo T, Esaki M, et al. (2007) Auto-fluorescence imaging colonoscopy in ulcerative colitis: comparison with conventional and narrow-band imaging colonoscopy. Digest Endosc 19:S139–144
6. Matsumoto T, Kudo T, Jo Y, et al. (2007) Magnifying colonoscopy with narrow-band system for the diagnosis of dysplasia in ulcerative colitis. A pilot study. Gastrointest Endosc 66:957–965
7. Matsumoto T, Moriyama T, Jo Y, et al. (2007) Autofluorescence colonoscopy for the diagnosis of dysplasia in ulcerative colitis. Inflamm Bowel Dis 13:640–641
8. Dekker E, van den Broek FJC, Reitsma JB, et al. (2007) Narrow-band imaging compared with conventional colonoscopy for the detection of dysplasia in patients with longstanding ulcerative colitis. Endoscopy 39:216–221
9. Messmann H, Endlicher E, Freunek G, et al. (2003) Fluorescence endoscopy for the detection of low- and high-grade dysplasia in ulcerative colitis using systemic or local 5-aminolaevulinic acid sensitization. Gut 52:1003–100
10. Ochsenkühn T, Tillack C, Stepp H, et al. (2006) Low frequency of colorectal dysplasia in patients with long-standing inflammatory bowel disease colitis. Detection by fluorescence endoscopy. Endoscopy 38:477–482

Autofluorescence Imaging Makes It Easy to Differentiate Neoplastic Lesions from Nonneoplastic Lesions in the Colon

Shoichi Saito[1], Hiroyuki Aihara, Hisao Tajiri[1,2], and Masahiro Ikegami[3]

Summary. The autofluorescence imaging (AFI) system is a newly developed videoscope system which is incorporated with another charge coupled device (CCD) for white light (WL) mode. The purpose of this study was to differentiate neoplastic from nonneoplastic lesions by using the AFI system. This prospective study covered 190 lesions which had been examined by WL and AFI before endoscopic or surgical resection was performed. In the AFI observations, the intensity of the change to a magenta color was classified into levels 0–3. Level 0 means no change, and the color remains the same dark green as the surrounding mucosa. Level 1 is a weak color change toward magenta in the tumor area. In contrast, level 3 is a strong color change in the area of the tumor. Level 0 was found in 25 cases. In the 190 cases which were in levels 1–3, there were 27 hyperplastic polyps (HP), 12 serrated adenomas (SA), 46 tubular adenomas (TA), 61 intramucosal cancers (M-Ca), and 44 submucosal invasive cancers (SM-Ca). Under the diagnostic criteria that neoplastic lesions were at grade 1 or above, the sensitivity, specificity, and accuracy were 97.6%, 92.0%, and 98.8%, respectively. These results suggested that AFI might be easily be used to distinguish neoplastic from nonneoplastic lesions in the colon.

Key words. Autofluorescence imaging, AFI, Conventional white light endoscopy, Submucosal invasive cancer, Image-enhanced endoscopy

Introduction

It has been found that autofluorescence imaging (AFI) is produced by short-wavelength light exposed to intestinal mucosa [1]. This short-wavelength light is known as excitation light, and changes to a different color when exposed to neoplastic or nonneoplastic tissue. Lam et al. [2] reported that the autofluorescence intensity has

[1]Department of Endoscopy, Jikei University School of Medicine, Minato-ku, Tokyo 105-8461, Japan

[2]Division of Gastroenterology and Hepatology, Department of Internal Medicine, Jikei University School of Medicine, Tokyo, Japan

[3]Department of Pathology, Jikei University School of Medicine, Tokyo, Japan

been shown to decrease markedly on tumor tissue under bronchoscopic examination using a helium–cadmium laser light source (442 nm wavelength). Since then, Xillix Technology Co. (Vancouver, Canada) and Olympus Medical Systems, Tokyo, Japan, have developed a new autofluorescence endoscopic imaging system. This system facilitates the detection of tiny lesions by endoscopic examination, and has also been used with considerable success in the diagnostic assessment of lesions in the gastrointestinal tract [1,3].

The new AFI system which we used for this research came onto the market in 2006, and was produced in Japan by Olympus Medical Systems. This system is composed of a light-source system (CLV-260SL), a processor (CV-260SL), a liquid-crystal video monitor, and a dedicated videoendoscope (CF-FH260AZI). This fiberscope consists of two different charge-coupled devices (CCD), one for conventional WL mode and the other for AFI mode. In autofluorescence mode, excitation light (395–475 nm) to induce autofluorescence, and green light (550 nm) and red light (610 nm) for taking reflective images, are provided by a light source equipped with a 300-W xenon arc lamp through a rotation filter. An excitation light filter is incorporated with the CCD for the AF mode to permit only 490–625-nm light to act on the CCD. The image processor artificially colors the AFI to green, the green reflectance image to red, and the red reflectance image to blue, and then composite images are displayed on the screen. Therefore, with AFI, gastrointestinal mucosa is depicted as green or white, and that with attenuated AFI is depicted as magenta [4].

The first report about this AFI system was in the detection and diagnosis of early superficial esophageal cancers and gastric cancers [4]. In this report, it was concluded that AFI was not as sensitive as chromoendoscopy, but that it did have advantages over standard conventional WL imaging.

However, the usefulness of AFI for colon disease is still unknown because few reports have been published. The aim of this study was to evaluate the usefulness of the AFI system for the diagnosis of colon tumors.

Patients and Methods

Patients

We investigated 155 patients with 190 lesions who had undergone endoscopic or surgical resections after WL mode and AFI observations at our department during the period from September 2005 to September 2007. The AFI images of these 190 lesions were diagnosed by two endoscopists with more than 10 years' experience before being included in this prospective study. The study protocol was approved by the institution's ethics committee, and all the patients provided written informed consent.

Grades for the Fluorescence Intensity of Colon Tissue

The intensity of the change of the lesion to a magenta color when observed with the AFI system was classified into 4 levels from grade 0 to grade 3 (Figs. 1 and 2). Grade 0 is dark green, which is similar to that of the mucosa surrounding the tumor and means that there is no change in the colon next to the tumor lesion. Grade 1 is a

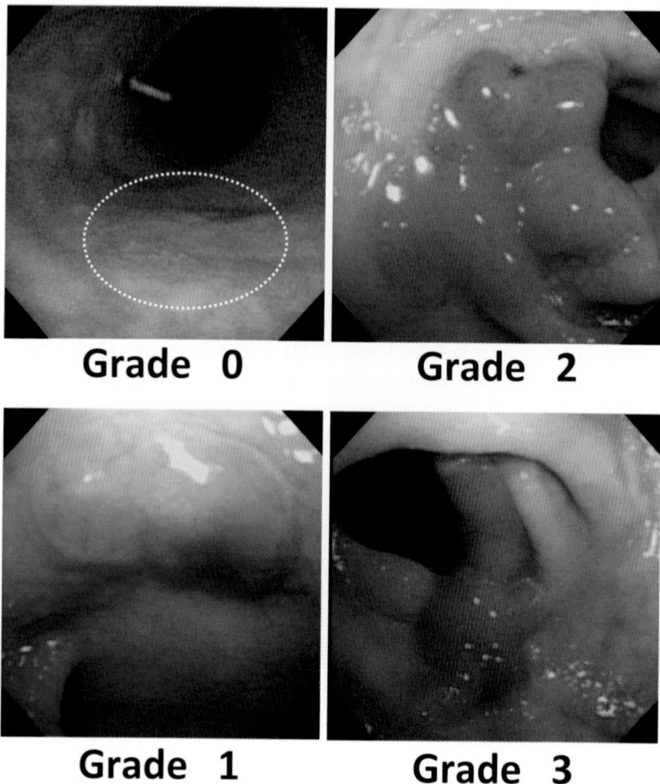

Fig. 1. Classification of the intensity of the color change using autofluorescence imaging (AFI) of the superficial type for a colon tumor. Grade 0, there is no difference in color between a neoplastic lesion and the surrounding mucosa. The *circle* shows the existence of a tumor. Grade 1, a slight change in the magenta color at the tumor lesion. Grade 2, an intermediate change in the magenta color at the tumor lesion. Grade 3, a strong change in the magenta color at the tumor lesion

change into the weakest magenta color at the tumor lesion. In contrast, grade 3 is a strong change at the tumor lesion, and grade 2 is an intermediate color change between grades 1 and 3 at the tumor lesion.

Histological Assessment

All the resected specimens were immersed in 10% buffered formalin for 24 hour and then embedded in paraffin. Sections cut from the paraffin blocks were stained with hematoxylin and eosin, and immunohistochemical staining for desmin. The histological findings were evaluated by two pathologists who were expert in digestive disease and who were unaware of the endoscopic findings. Tumor lesions diagnosed as low-grade dysplasia of category 3 according to the revised Vienna classification were classified as adenoma, and lesions of category 4 were defined as carcinoma. The

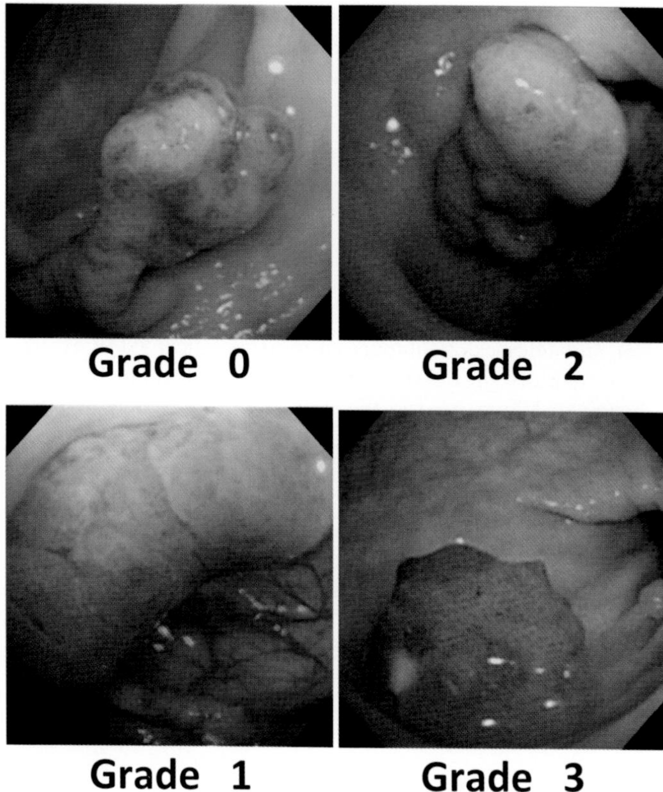

Fig. 2. Classification of the intensity of the change in color using AFI of the protruded type for a colon tumor. Grade 0, there is no difference in color between a neoplastic lesion and the surrounding mucosa. Grade 1, a slight change in the magenta color at the tumor lesion. Grade 2, an intermediate change in the magenta color at the tumor lesion. Grade 3, a strong change in the magenta color at the tumor lesion

method for measuring SM-Ca depth was in accordance with that described previously in a Japanese article [5].

Results and Discussion

Recently, the clinical performance and value of AFI observations for the diagnosis of colonic neoplasia have been reported in relation to studies of colon tumors. Using surgical specimens from the colon, Izushi et al. [6] reported that the reason for decreased fluorescence in neoplastic lesions was the decrease in collagen fluorescence. Nakaniwa et al. [7] reported that their findings using the AFI system were superior to those from observations of autofluorescence using a fiberscope because it was possible to highlight small lesions without dye-spraying or magnification. However, the benefits of AFI observations, and in particular those relating to the differentiated findings from neoplastic and nonneoplastic lesions, remain largely unknown [8]. We have shown the benefits of AFI observations in a prospective double-blind study where AFI observations were compared with WL observations in the detection of early gastric cancer [9]. Here, we have investigated and shown the benefits of using AFI observations in cases of colon tumor.

The Change to a Magenta Color is Different in Histological Findings

We observed 190 colon tumors (27 cases of hyperplastic polyp [HP], 12 cases of serrated adenoma [SA], 46 cases of tubular adenoma [TA], 61 cases of intramucosal cancer [M-Ca], and 44 cases of submucosal invasive cancer [SM-Ca]) using the AFI system. We first examined the differences in the results of AFI images compared with those from histology. Figure 3 shows the intensity of the change to a magenta color for various histological types. For HPs, 85% showed a dark green color which was similar to that of the surrounding mucosal area, and just four HPs (14.8%) showed a mild to moderate (grade 1 to 2) magenta color. In contrast, the results of the color changes in TAs, M-Cas, and SM-Cas were in almost the same ratio. In particular, more than 90% of cases of M-Cas and SM-Cas showed a strong change to the magenta color (grade 2 to 3). However, in SAs, more than 90% of lesions showed a magenta color which was not a strong change (grade 1 to 2). These results suggest that only neoplastic lesions can be detected with confidence. This also applies to SAs, which are intermediate in position between HPs and TAs using the AFI system.

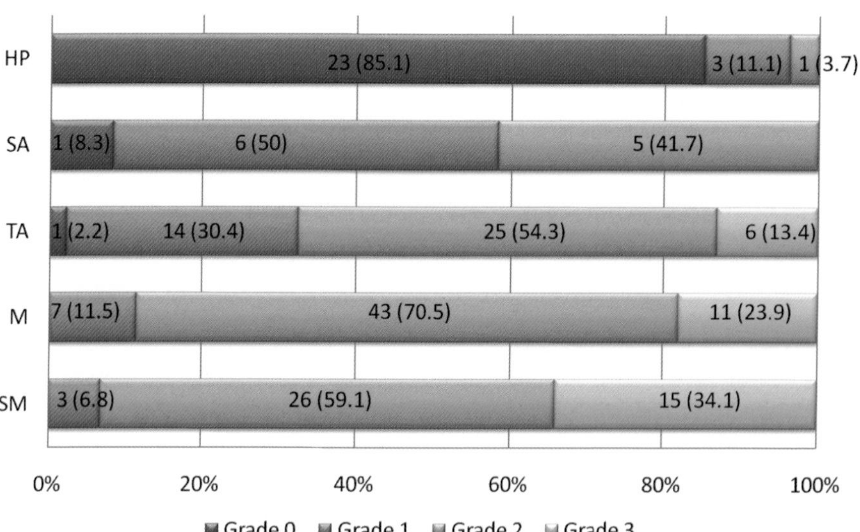

Fig. 3. Comparison of various histological types and AFI findings for a colon tumor. *HP*, hyperplastic polyp; *SA*, serrated adenoma; *TA*, tubular adenoma; *M*, intramucosal cancer; *SM*, submucosal invasive cancer. Case number (%)

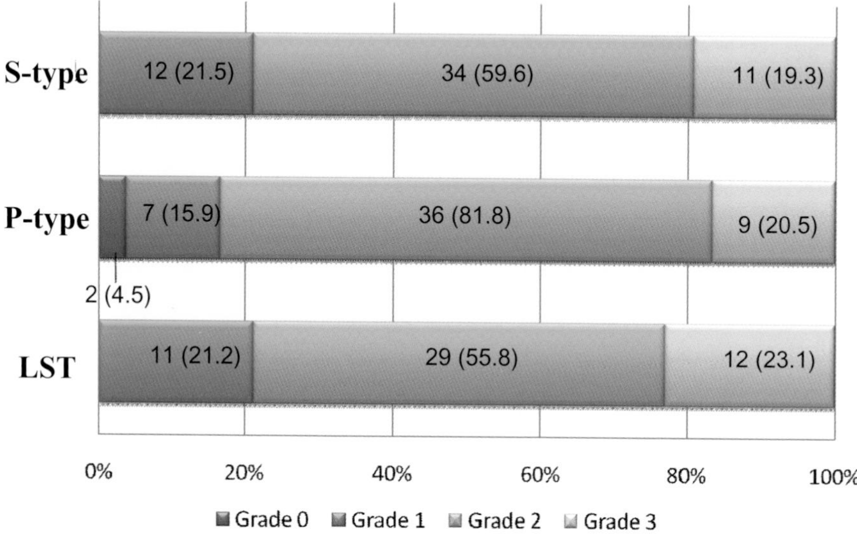

FIG. 4. Comparison of macroscopic figures and AFI findings for a neoplastic tumor. *S-type*, superficial type; *P-type*, protruded type; *LST*, lateral spreading tumor. Case number (%)

Macroscopic Figures Do Not Influence the Change to a Magenta Color

We studied macroscopic figures of endoscopic images and classified them into three types. Pedunculated and semipedunculated polyps were defined as the protruded type (P-type), and sessile polyps were also defined as the P-type. Lesions which were less than 20 mm in size and either the flat elevated type or the depressed type were defined as the superficial type (S-type). Only tumors more than 20 mm in size were defined as lateral spreading tumors (LST) [10]. Not including HP cases, 163 lesions were examined. As shown in Fig. 4, no marked differences were found on macroscopic figures. This result indicates that the intensity of the color change is not affected by the tumor figures. However, in our experience, flat lesions such as LST have tended to show a strong change into the magenta color. Therefore, it is necessary to establish the original substances which did change color, except for the collagen in the physical structures of the tissue.

Tumor Size Does Not Influence Changes into a Magenta Color

It was also necessary to investigate whether tumor size is connected to the intensity of the color change. Not including HP cases, 163 lesions were examined. We show that the intensity of the color change was similar at any tumor size (Fig. 5). This result indicates that the magenta color is not affected by tumor size. Moreover, it is suggested that because small-sized depressed-type tumors with a neoplastic character tended to show the magenta color, this would be expected to make it easy to detect even a small lesion by using the AFI system.

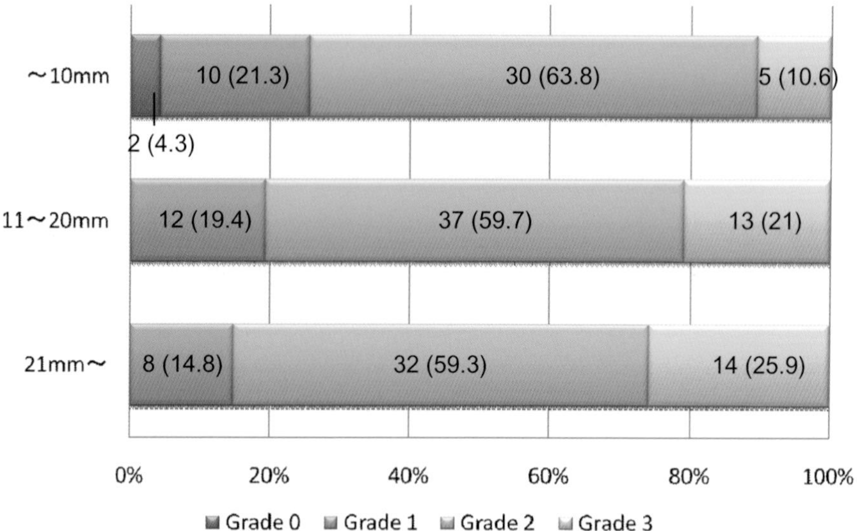

Fig. 5. Comparison of tumor size and AFI findings for a neoplastic tumor. Case number (%)

Table 1. Diagnostic accuracy in colon tumor

	Sensitivity	Specificity	Accuracy
Neoplastic Lesion ↕ Non-neoplastic Lesion	97.6%	92.0%	98.8%

AFI System Might Be Able to Distinguish Neoplastic from Nonneoplastic Lesions

Nakaniwa et al. [7] reported that adenoma and hyperplasia could be distinguished from each other by using the AFI system. To identify colon tumors, especially flat lesions such as LST, it is necessary to differentiate an adenoma, including an M-Ca, from a large-sized hyperplastic polyp. As shown Table 1, if the findings observed at level 1 or above were assumed to be from a neoplastic lesion, the sensitivity, specificity, and accuracy for a differentiated diagnosis of a neoplastic lesion (SA, TA, M-Ca, and SM-Ca) from a nonneoplastic lesion (HP) were 97.6%, 92.0%, and 98.8%, respectively. These data are slightly better than those of a previous report [7] in which 168 colon polyps were studied, and the sensitivity and specificity were 89% and 81%, respectively. It is supposed that it was the pathological criteria used by pathologists [11,12] which made the difference between HP and SA. However, even if HP was over-diagnosed as a neoplastic tumor because the sensitivity was superior to the specificity in our data, it could still be concluded that the AFI system might be a useful method because of the possibility of differentiating neoplastic from nonneoplastic lesions immediately. In particular, in order to diagnose a colon tumor, such a large-sized flat hyperplastic polyp in which the neoplastic character may or may not be clear, the AFI system will be particularly helpful as the modality to use with confidence to select either endoscopic or surgical resection according to the change to the magenta color.

References

1. Haringgsma J, Tygat GNJ (1999) Fluorescence and autofluorescence. Baillieres Best Pract Res Clin Gastroenterol 13:1–10
2. Lam S, MacAulay C, Hung J (1991) Mechanism of detection of early lung cancer by ratio fluometry. Lasers Life Sci 4:67–73
3. Du Vall A, Kost J, Scheider D, et al. (1996) Laser-induced fluorescence (LIF) endoscopy (E): a pilot study of a real-time (RT) auto-fluorescence imaging system for early detection of dysplasia and carcinoma in the gastrointestinal (GI) tract. Endoscopy 28:S45
4. Uedo N, Iishi H, Tatsuta M, et al. (2005) A novel videoendoscopy system by using autofluorescence and reflectance imaging for diagnosis of esophagogastric cancers. Gastrointest Endosc 62:521–528
5. Kitajima K, Fujimori T, Fujii T, et al. (2004) Correlations between lymph node metastasis and depth of submucosal invasion in submucosal invasive colorectal carcinoma. J Gastroenterol 39:534–543
6. Izushi K, Tajiri H, Fujii T, et al. (1999) The histological basis of detection of adenoma and cancer in the colon by autofluorescence endoscopic imaging. Endoscopy 31:511–516
7. Nakaniwa N, Namihisa A, Ogihara T, et al. (2005) Newly developed autofluorescence imaging videoscope system for the detection of colonic neoplasms. Dig Endosc 17:235–240
8. Mashiko T, Imazu H, Saito S (2007) Novel autofluorescence imaging system is useful for detection of colorectal neoplastic lesions (in Japanese). Tokyo Jikeikai Med J 122:143–153
9. Kato M, Kaise M, Yonezawa J (2007) Autofluorescence endoscopy versus conventional white light endoscopy for the detection of superficial gastric neoplasia: a prospective comparative study. Endoscopy 39:937–941
10. Kudo S (1993) Endoscopic mucosal resection of flat and depressed types of early colorectal cancer. Endoscopy 25:455–461
11. Longacre TA, Fenoglio-Preiser CA (1990) Mixed hyperplastic adenomatous polyps/serrated adenoma: a distinct form of colorectal neoplasia. Am J Surg Pathol 14: 524–537
12. Snover DC, Jass JR, Fenoglio-Preiser CA, et al. (2005) Serrated polyps of the large intestine: a morphological and molecular review of an evolving concept. Am J Clin Pathol 124:380–391

Endoscopic Ultrasonography Diagnosis for Colorectal Diseases

Eisai Cho[1], Masatoshi Miyata[1], and Masatsugu Nakajima[2]

Summary. We have used endoscopic ultrasonography (EUS) for all the colorectal diseases. For cancer, we determined the treatment method by evaluating the depth of cancer invasion. Moreover, we have applied EUS for submucosal cancer to decide whether the depth of submucosal invasion was superficial and thus to estimate the indication of endoscopic resection. Lymph node metastasis has been examined for staging in cases with invasive cancer. We have performed EUS for active ulcerative colitis in observing the depth of inflammation and determined treatment strategy by diagnosing clinical severity. Submucosal tumorous lesions and extramural lesions have been examined to clarify the site and inner condition. EUS is an essential method that leads to accurate diagnosis of any colorectal disease by delineating pathological conditions precisely. With improvement of the instrumentation, EUS can be used as a routine diagnostic tool as is colonoscopy.

Key words. Endoscopic ultrasonography (EUS), Cancer, Submucosal cancer, Ulcerative colitis, Submucosal tumor

Introduction

We have attempted performing endoscopic ultrasonography (EUS) in all sites in the colon and rectum for more than 2000 patients beginning in 1984. EUS can make the target lesion apparent in the vertical direction of the wall. The colorectal diseases to which we have applied EUS include cancer, submucosal tumor, and inflammatory bowel disease. In this chapter, we describe the usefulness of EUS for colorectal diseases.

[1]Department of Gastroenterology, Otsu Municipal Hospital, 2-9-9 Motomiya, Otsu, Shiga 520-0804, Japan
[2]Department of Gastroenterology, Kyoto Second Red Cross Hospital, Kyoto, Japan

Instruments and Techniques

The instruments of EUS used for colorectal lesions are echo-colonoscopes and ultrasonic probes. The most improved dedicated forward-viewing echo-colonoscope (XCF-UMPQ230; Olympus Medical Systems) provides a 360° circular image at 20 or 7.5 MHz [1,2]. This scope could be handled from the anus to the terminal ileum. The ultrasonic probe is a through-the-scope catheter with 20 MHz. The anorectal ultrasonic probe is used only for the anorectal region because it has no endoscopic function.

Patients undergoing EUS of the colon are prepared with oral lavage solution. Before the examination, antispasmodic agents are used intravenously or intramuscularly. EUS is performed by the deaerated water filling method after a lesion is observed endoscopically.

EUS Images of the Normal Colon and Rectum

The normal colorectal wall is constantly visualized by EUS as a five-layered structure (Fig. 1). From the colonic lumen inward, the first, third, and fifth layers are hyperechoic and the second and fourth layers are hypoechoic. Comparing with the appearance of the histological layers, it was confirmed that the first hyperechoic and second hypoechoic layers corresponded to the mucosa, the third hyperechoic layer to the submucosa (SM), the fourth hypoechoic layer to the muscularis propria

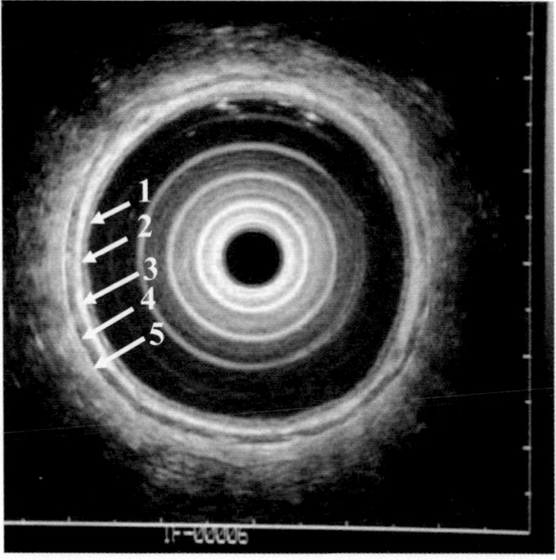

Fig. 1. Endoscopic ultrasonography (EUS) image of the normal colon with a five-layered structure

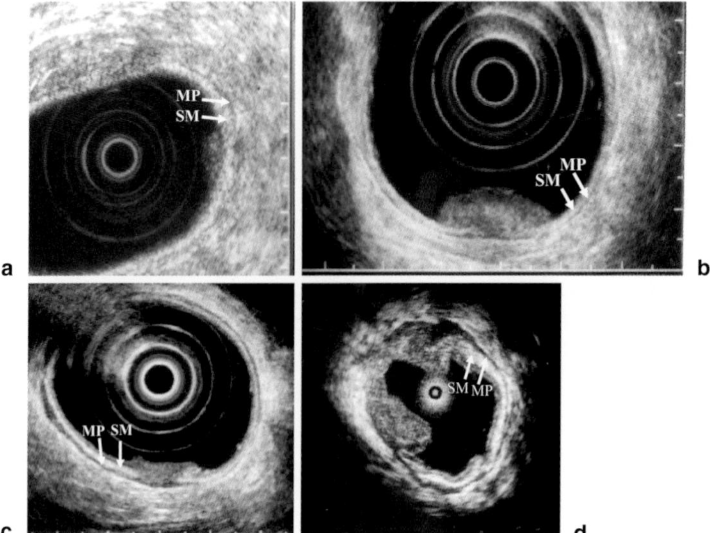

Fig. 2. **a** EUS image of mucosal cancer demonstrated as a hypoechoic mass within the first and second layer. **b** EUS of submucosal cancer shown as a hypoechoic mass destroying first and second layers. **c** EUS of cancer extending into the muscularis propria delineated as a hypoechoic mass interrupting first, second, and third layers. **d** EUS of cancer with penetration into the subserosa described as a hypoechoic mass penetrating through first, second, third, and fourth layers. *SM*, submucosa; *MP*, muscularis propria

(MP), and the fifth hyperechoic layer to the subserosa and serosa (or adventitia) [3]. The target lesions are evaluated by comparison with the five-layered wall structure.

EUS Diagnosis of Cancer Invasion

By EUS, cancer of the colon is demonstrated as a hypoechoic mass whose echo level is intermediate between the hyperechoic level of the third layer and the hypoechoic level of the fourth layer. Mucosal cancer is visualized as a hypoechoic mass that is localized within the first and second layers (Fig. 2a). Submucosal cancer is shown as a hypoechoic mass that destroys the first and second layers and extends into the third layer (Fig. 2b). Cancer extending into the muscularis propria is shown as a hypoechoic mass that interrupts the wall structure of the first three layers and spreads into the fourth layer (Fig. 2c). Cancer with penetration into the subserosa is visualized as a hypoechoic mass that interrupts the first four layers (Fig. 2d) [2,3]. Based on these criteria, we can diagnose cancer invasion preoperatively.

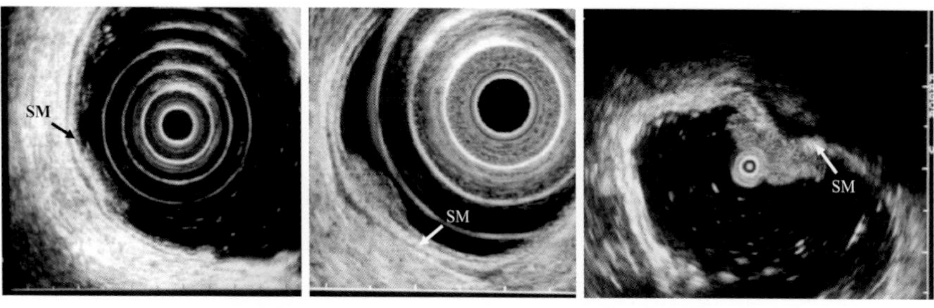

Fig. 3. **a** EUS image of SM1 shown as a hypoechoic mass limited within superficial layer of the third layer. **b** EUS image of SM2 described as a hypoechoic mass located at the middle portion of the third layer. **c** EUS image of SM3 delineated as a hypoechoic mass located near the fourth layer. *SM*, submucosa

EUS Diagnosis of Submucosal Cancer Invasion

It has been confirmed that cancers localized within the mucosa or the submucosa less than 1000 μm in depth have no risk of spread to lymph nodes. There is a greater risk of spread to the lymph nodes when the tumor deeply invades the submucosa. Histologically, the depth of submucosal tumor invasion is regulated by the submucosa (sm), equally divided into three levels in the vertical direction. Tumors of sm1 are defined as those remaining within the superficial one-third of the submucosal layer, sm2 those extending to the middle one-third of the submucosal layer, and sm3 as those reaching the deeper one-third of the submucosal layer near the muscularis propria. Endoscopic treatment can be curative for sm1 because the probability of lymph node metastasis is almost nil. Surgical resection with lymphadenectomy should be considered for sm2 and sm3. Therefore, preoperative differential diagnosis as to whether the depth of tumor invasion of submucosal cancer is within sm1 or beyond sm2 is vital for selection of the treatment method. EUS diagnosis of submucosal cancer invasion is classified as SM1, SM2, and SM3 corresponding to the histological classification. An EUS image of SM1 is defined such that the deepest portion of a hypoechoic mass is localized within the superficial one-third of the third layer (Fig. 3a). An EUS image of SM2 is defined such that the deepest portion of the hypoechoic mass is located between one-third and two-thirds of the third layer (Fig. 3b). An EUS image of SM3 is defined such that the deepest portion of the hypoechoic mass extends between two-thirds of the third layer and the fourth layer (Fig. 3c) [2]. The EUS classification can help us select the treatment method for submucosal cancer.

EUS Diagnosis of Lymph Nodes Metastasis

Normal lymph nodes cannot be detected by EUS. EUS images of enlarged lymph nodes appear as discrete round or oval hypoechoic masses that are not contiguous to blood vessels (Fig. 4) [2]. It is difficult to differentiate malignant lymph nodes from

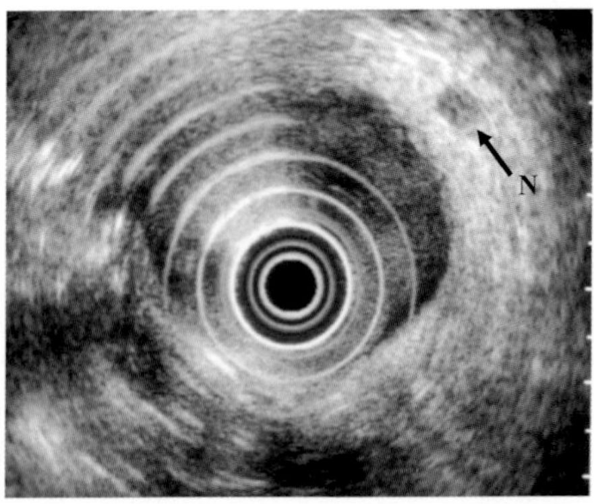

Fig. 4. EUS image of metastatic lymph node (*N*) shown as a round mass that is not contiguous to a blood vessel

lymphadenitis by size, shape, echo level, or border appearance. It is, therefore, considered that any of these hypoechoic masses detected by EUS might be malignant lymph nodes in cases of invasive colorectal cancer [3].

EUS Diagnosis of Ulcerative Colitis

Diagnosing the activity of ulcerative colitis (UC) is crucial for therapeutic strategy. We have used the criteria of clinical severity and endoscopic grades in evaluating the severity of inflammation. Especially, endoscopic observation is indispensable in assessing the extent of the disease and mucosal changes. The severity of inflammation has a close relationship to the depth of inflammation. However, there are some difficulties in colonoscopy in estimating the depth of inflammation because endoscopic observation is restricted to the internal surface of the colorectal wall. The ultrasonograms of UC in the active stage show hypoechoic changes in the colorectal wall [4]. These EUS changes of the wall that are recognized in the active stage disappear or normalize in the stage of remission. When the stage of UC is exacerbated, the hypoechoic changes of the wall extend from the mucosal layer to the deeper layers with thickening of the whole wall.

These EUS images of active UC are classified into the following types. In UC-M, the wall becomes thickened with its structure preserved (Fig. 5a); in UC-SM, hypoechoic changes reach the superficial portion of the third layer with thickening of the whole wall (Fig. 5b); in UC-SM deep, hypoechoic changes reach the deeper portion of the third layer with thickening of the whole wall (Fig. 5c); in UC-MP, hypoechoic changes extend into the fourth layer with thickening of the whole wall (Fig. 5d); and in UC-SS/SE, hypoechoic changes penetrate through the fourth layer with thickening of the whole wall (Fig. 5e). By using

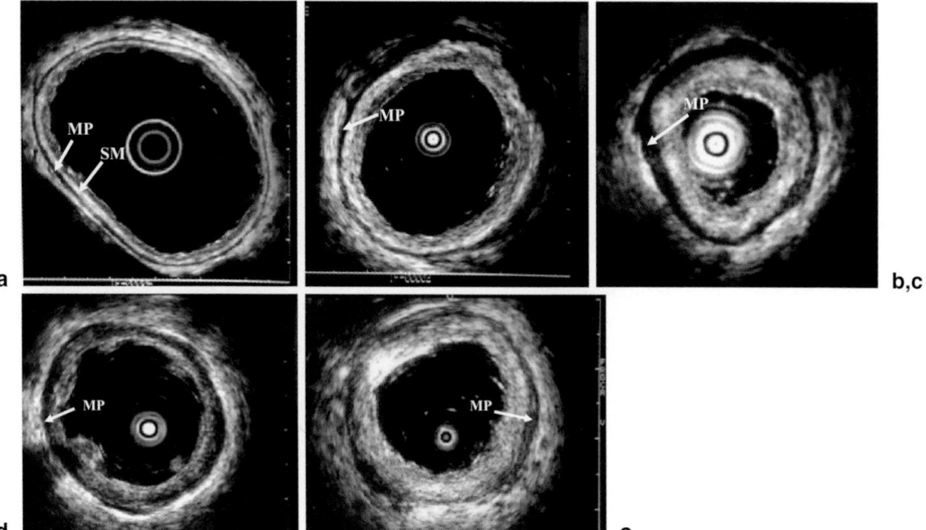

Fig. 5. EUS images of cases of ulcerative colitis (UC). **a** EUS of UC-M showing the wall thickened with its structure preserved. **b** EUS of UC-SM indicating hypoechoic changes reach the superficial portion of the third layer with thickening of the whole wall. **c** EUS of UC-SM deep demonstrating hypoechoic changes reach the deeper portion of the third layer with thickening of the whole wall. **d** EUS of UC-MP presenting hypoechoic changes reach the fourth layer with thickening of the whole wall. **e** EUS of UC-SS/SE revealing hypoechoic changes penetrate the fourth layer with thickening of the whole wall. *SM*, submucosa; *MP*, muscularis propria

EUS for active cases with UC, we can evaluate the severity by grading the depth of inflammation [5].

EUS Diagnosis of Submucosal Tumorous Lesions

Submucosal tumorous lesions of the colon and rectum are often difficult to diagnose by conventional endoscopic observation. EUS can differentiate submucosal tumors from extramural lesions by identifying the wall and adjacent organs. Submucosal tumors can be assessed by observing the location and inner condition. The location of submucosal tumors can be demonstrated comparing the wall structure. The echo level is expressed by comparing echo free, hyperechoic fourth layer, and hyperechoic third layer. The internal echo sometimes becomes heterogeneous when the size of the tumor increases. EUS images of various submucosal tumors are shown in Fig. 6. The echo levels of submucosal tumors are described in Table 1.

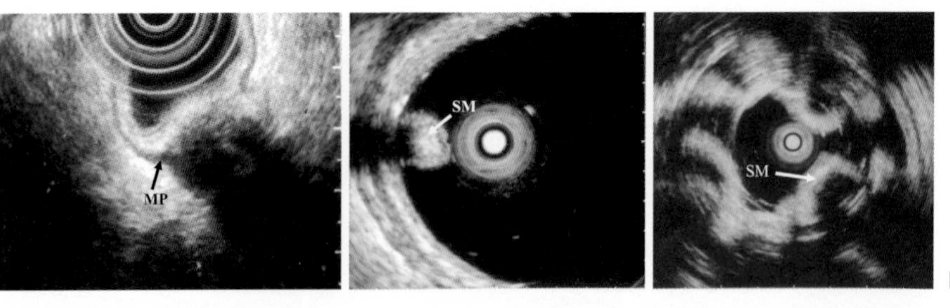

Fig. 6. EUS images of submucosal tumorous lesions. **a** EUS of a case of endometriosis shown as a hypoechoic mass mainly extending outside from muscularis propria (*MP*). **b** EUS of a case of lipoma shown as a hyperechoic mass in the third layer. *SM*, submucosa. **c** EUS of a case of pneumatosis cystoides intestinalis visualized as masses in the third layer with acoustic shadows. *SM*, submucosa

Table 1. Echo level of Submucosal tumors.

	Echo level				
Histology	echo free	—	hypoechoic	—	hyperechoic
Lymphangioma	●				
Hemangioma	●				
Malignant lymphoma		●			
Carcinoid tumor			●		
Endometriosis			●		
Myogenic tumor			●		
Lipoma					●
PCI					★

PCI, pneumatosis cystoides intestinalis
★: acoustic shadow

EUS Diagnosis of Carcinoid Tumor

Carcinoid tumors tend to infiltrate from the deeper portion of the mucosa to the submucosa. EUS reveals carcinoid tumor as a hypoechoic mass in the submucosa at an early stage (Fig. 7). Carcinoid tumors should be treated because of their malignant potential. When the tumor reaches the muscularis propria, it should be removed surgically. EUS can determine the treatment method by diagnosing whether the tumor is located within the submucosa or has invaded the muscularis propria.

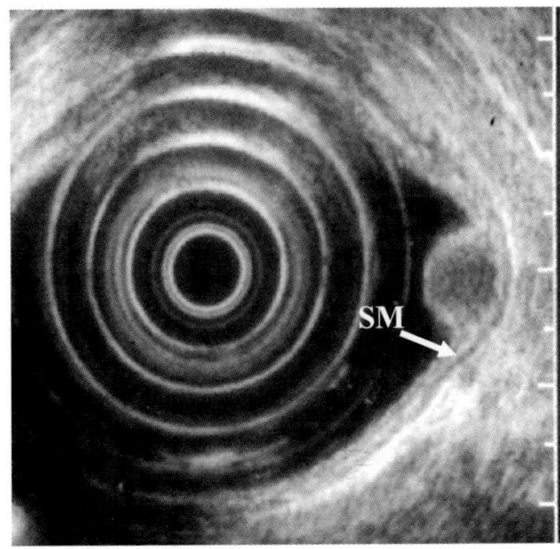

Fig. 7. EUS image of a case of carcinoid tumor shown as a hypoechoic mass within the third layer. *SM*, submucosa

Conclusion

EUS is a useful and reliable method for staging of cancer and in determining the indication of endoscopic resection for submucosal cancer. EUS allows us to evaluate the severity of patients with ulcerative colitis and to clarify the location and inner condition of submucosal tumors. With advances and improvement of the instruments, EUS can be an essential method for diagnosing colorectal diseases more accurately. We can understand the pathological conditions of any colorectal disease by observing the mucosal surface with colonoscopy and changes in the wall with EUS.

References

1. Cho E, Kawabata H, Kohri Y, et al (2003) Newly developed echo-colonoscope for colorectal diseases. Dig Endosc 14:S91–S92
2. Cho E, Hasegawa K, Okabe Y, et al (2001) Endoscopic ultrasonography for colorectal cancer. Dig Endosc 13:S19–S21
3. Cho E, Nakajima M, Yasuda K, et al (1993) Endoscopic ultrasonography in the diagnosis of colorectal cancer invasion. Gastrointest Endosc 39:521–527
4. Cho E, Mochizuki N, Ashihara T, et al (1998) Endoscopic ultrasonography in the evaluation of inflammatory bowel disease. Endoscopy 30:A94–A96
5. Cho E, Yasuda K, Nakajima M (2004) EUS in the diagnosis of ulcerative colitis. Dig Endosc 16:S182–S184

Endoscopic Mucosal Resection and Endoscopic Piecemeal Mucosal Resection for Colorectal Neoplasia

Yusuke Saitoh[1], Mikihiro Fujiya[1], and Jiro Watari[2]

Summary. Endoscopic mucosal resection (EMR), including endoscopic piecemeal mucosal resection (EPMR), allows a less invasive treatment option, especially for flat and depressed type (F&D type) colorectal neoplasia, and can provide specimens for histopathological analysis. EMR should be applied for colorectal adenomas, carcinoma in situ, and focally extended submucosal cancers (equivalent to submucosal cancers with less than 1000 μm invasion distance) without lymph node metastasis. To determine the indication of EMR, invasion depth diagnosis is important, with the use of the indigo carmine dye spray method and also high-frequency ultrasound probes (HFUP) or magnifying colonoscopy with the narrow-band imaging system (NBI). If the lesion requires piecemeal resection, especially for larger lesions 21 mm or more in size, intentional EPMR is recommended. Larger-sized high nodules, or a region with the histological estimation of high malignant potential by magnifying colonoscopy, should be resected en bloc, followed by other resection procedures for residual lesion. EMR including EPMR provide a 95% or more success rate and fewer complications for the treatment of F&D type early colorectal neoplasia. As the detection of F&D type tumors increases, EMR and EPMR will become a more essential treatment for colorectal neoplasia, including early carcinomas.

Key words. Endoscopic mucosal resection, Endoscopic piecemeal mucosal resection, Flat and depressed type colorectal neoplasia, Granular type laterally spreading tumors

Introduction

The endoscopic mucosal resection (EMR) technique was initially developed and conducted for curative endoscopic treatment of the flat or depressed type early gastric adenomas and intramucosal carcinomas [1]. In the 1990s, it was also conducted for

[1]Digestive Disease Center, Asahikawa City Hospital, Kinsei 1-1-65, Asahikawa, 070-8610, Japan

[2]Third Department of Internal Medicine, Asahikawa Medical College, Asahikawa, Japan

the colorectal lesions [2] with increasing detection of the flat and depressed lesions (F&D lesions) in Japan, which are difficult to resect by conventional polypectomy [3]. EMR allowed a less-invasive treatment option for the patients and good quality of life compared to surgical resection and has now become a popular method for all superficial lesions of the gastrointestinal (GI) tract. There is an advantage when using EMR compared with other therapeutic modalities, such as an argon-plasma coagulator (APC), laser ablation, heater probe, and irradiation, because resected specimens and histological diagnosis with lateral and vertical margins can be obtained, and vessel permeation can also be determined. Definitive therapeutic strategy can be determined based on histological diagnosis obtained by EMR. In the past several years, the endoscopic submucosal dissection (ESD) technique, which was widely used for gastric lesions, has been used for colorectal lesions as well. A large en bloc specimen can be obtained using ESD, and a precise histological diagnosis can be made with a very low incidence of positive lateral margin by marginal mucosal cut. However, the ESD technique is difficult in the colorectum because of twisting and the haustra folds of the colon, and it carries a high risk of perforation of the colonic wall, which has a relatively thinner muscle layer compared with the stomach; also, a longer procedure time, sometimes more than 3 h, is required. Moreover, strict indicative colonic lesions for ESD are relatively rare. In this chapter, the usefulness of conventional EMR, including the endoscopic piecemeal mucosal resection (EPMR) technique and results, is described.

Indication of EMR

Basically, EMR should be applied for superficial lesions of the GI tract as curative endoscopic resection. There are two essential factors for curative EMR. The first factor is that the lesion should be removed completely, which implies that the lesion is disease free not only in the lateral margin but also in the vertical margin. The second factor is the more important issue: that EMR must be indicated for lesions without lymph node metastasis, which are usually intramucosal lesions (adenomas and carcinoma in situ) in the GI tract. Differing from the indication for gastric and esophageal lesions, not only intramucosal lesions but some submucosal cancers are amenable to EMR in the colorectum. Submucosal cancers have been divided into three subtypes according to the degree of cancer extent into the submucosa: sm1 is focally extended submucosal cancers, that is, cancer limited within the upper third of the submucosa; sm2 is moderately extended submucosal cancers, cancer limited to the middle third of the submucosa; and sm3 is massively extended submucosal cancers, cancer that has invaded into the lower third of the submucosa. Subsequent studies have shown that lymph node metastasis was frequent in moderately and massively extended submucosal cancers (sm2-3 cancers), whereas it was rare in intramucosal and focally extended submucosal cancers (m-sm1 cancers). Recent pathological study has revealed that sm1 cancer is equivalent to lesions of submucosal invasion distance of less than 1000 μm and sm2–3 cancer corresponds to the lesions of submucosal invasion distance of 1000 μm or more. Current indications for EMR are flat and depressed (F&D) type adenomas, intramucosal carcinoma, and submucosal cancers satisfying all four of these following factors:

(1) negative submucosal vertical margin; (2) histological type is well or moderately differentiated adenocarcinoma; (3) submucosal invasion distance is less than 1000 μm; and (4) negative vessel permeation, ly0 and v0. Submucosal cancers that do not satisfy all four of these factors should be considered for treatment by surgical resection [4].

Invasion Depth Diagnosis for the Determination of EMR

To determine a precise therapeutic strategy, as to whether EMR or a surgical operation should be chosen, it is essential to differentiate intramucosal lesions and submucosal cancers with less than 1000 μm invasion distance from invasive (submucosal cancers with 1000 μm or more invasion distance) carcinomas. However, preoperative diagnosis of invasion depth is sometimes difficult by routine examinations such as barium enema [5], colonoscopy, and conventional endoscopic ultrasonography (EUS). To enhance the details of the lesions, chromoendoscopy using 0.08% to 0.1% indigo carmine solution in addition to conventional video-colonoscopy is recommended. By using chromoendoscopy, we and other authors have described various colonoscopic findings useful for invasion depth diagnosis [3,6]. HFUP and magnifying colonoscopy if also available for the precise invasion depth diagnosis, and is also useful for the discrimination of m and sm carcinomas with less than 1000 μm submucosal invasion distance and invasive sm carcinomas of 1000 μm or more submucosal invasion distance [7]. Recently, the narrow-band imaging (NBI) system has been available as digital chromoendoscopy, and its usefulness for invasion depth diagnosis using the surface microvascular pattern of the lesions has been reported. However, studies using NBI are still pending. In the meantime, NBI will be a promising diagnostic modality for precise invasion depth diagnosis [8].

EMR and EPMR Techniques

EMR technique is known as the strip biopsy technique; it lifts the lesion by submucosal saline (glycerol, hyaluronic acid, etc.) injection, followed by snare resection. For larger lesions, lifting with a grasping forceps allows for a wider resection (lift and cut technique) using a dual-channel colonoscope.

To obtain a precise pathological diagnosis, it is important to resect the lesion en bloc. However, en bloc resection becomes difficult according to the size of the lesions. Figure 1 shows the en bloc resection rate in each size of the flat elevated and granular type of laterally spreading tumor (LST-G). The en bloc resection rate obtained was a high value of 92.9% for lesions less than 10 mm in size, and 86.0% for lesions of 11–15 mm. In contrast, the en bloc resection rate becomes a lower value, 77.4%, for lesions of 15–20 mm and 40.0% for 21 mm or more. En bloc resection is difficult especially for lesions of 21 mm or more. For larger LST-G lesions for which en bloc resection seems to be difficult, intentional EPMR is recommended. There are two subtype of LST-G, homogeneous type and nodular mixed type. The homogeneous type is composed of uniformly gathered nodules, and the nodular mixed type has larger-sized high nodules in the lesion. A higher incidence of concomitant

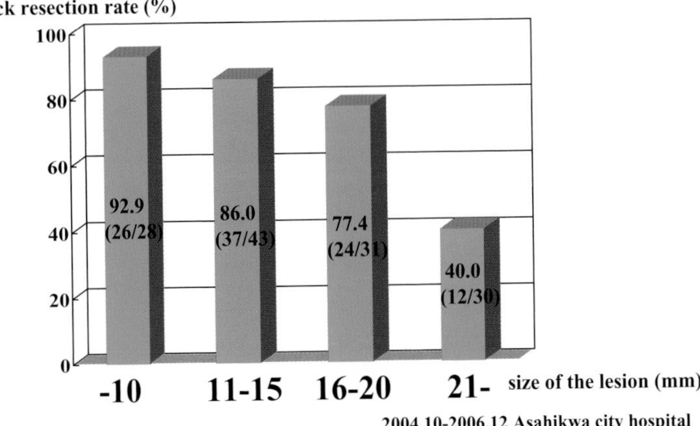

FIG. 1. En bloc resection rate for each tumor size [flat, elevated, and granular type of laterally spreading tumor (LST-G), 132 lesions]

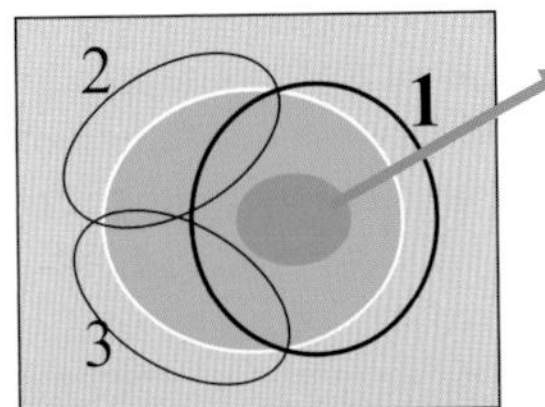

Estimated malignant region

Estimated malignant region should be resected enblockly first: 1, followed by the resection of residual lesion. 2, 3

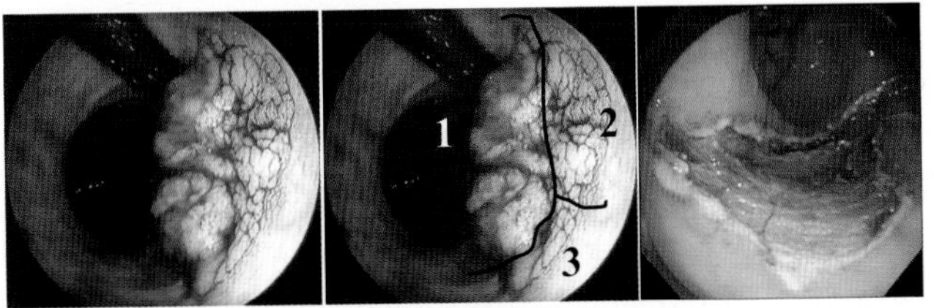

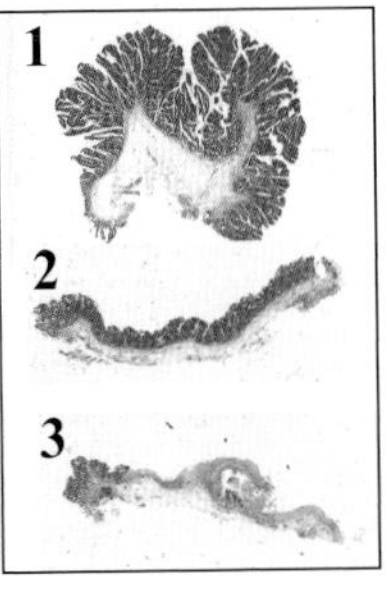

Rectal lesion with 30mm in size. The lesion had to do piecemeal resection. Intentional EPMR was proceeded. Large nodule was firstly resected enblockly followed by other 2 resection for residual flat lesion. Histologic diagnosis was intramucosal tubular adenocarcinoma with adenoma.

FIG. 2. Intentional endoscopic piecemeal mucosal resection (EPMR)

intramucosal and submucosal carcinomas has been reported in nodular mixed type than in homogeneous type, and carcinoma is usually included in larger-sized high nodules. So, if the lesion requires piecemeal resection, larger-sized high nodules, or a region with an estimation of histological high malignant potential by magnifying colonoscopy, should be resected en bloc followed by other resection procedures for any residual lesion. A case of EPMR is described in Fig. 2.

EMR and EPMR Techniques

Confirmation of the Margin of the Lesion

The margin of the lesion should be carefully confirmed using indigo carmine and marked with the cautery tip about 1 mm from the margin. For larger F&D lesions 21 mm or more in size, which it is obligatory to resect in piecemeal fashion, intentional EPMR should be performed, as already mentioned.

Submucosal Saline Injection

After confirmation of the margin of the lesion, physiological saline was injected into the submucosal layer beneath the lesion. Submucosal injection is most important, and the success of EMR depends on this procedure. A submucosal injection site is recommended at the oral border of the lesion to obtain an adequate position of the lesion for EMR. The lesion will protrude toward the colonoscope and will easily be snared by this technique. Another important technique is that the saline should be injected into the shallow portion of the submucosal layer to make a good bulge easy to be strangulated by the snare. If a good bulge cannot be obtained at the beginning of injection, the injection needle should be gradually pulled back with some lifting up of the scope to inject the saline into the shallow portion of the submucosa and to obtain a good bulge for EMR. The total volume of injected saline is dependent on the lesion size, but enough saline, usually more than 10 ml, is required to lift up the whole lesion.

Snaring and Cutting

After a good bulge is made by submucosal injection, the lesion should be resected with some surrounding normal mucosa. After getting a good bulge, a prompt procedure should take place to avoid flattening of the bulge, which makes it difficult to snare the lesion because of slipping of the snare. Collapse of the colonic lumen with suction will be useful during strangulation with the snare, and a stiffer snare is better for snaring and strangulation to avoid slipping. It is important to confirm before cutting that the proper muscle is not being squeezed by jiggling the snare. If the snare and strangulated lesion move well, the proper muscle layer is not strangulated with it. For cutting, we use about a 40 W cutting current; we do not use blended current, to avoid insufficient histological evaluation of the lateral margin of the resected specimen as a result of burning.

Confirmation After Resection

Confirmation should be recommended, especially in the post-EMR ulcer margin, by using dye spray or magnifying colonoscopy, to prevent any residual lesion. It is reported that residual lesions after incomplete EMR may have a higher growth potential than the tumors before resection [9]. Pre-EMR marking is important to avoid incomplete resection. If residual lesion is suspected, another EMR procedure including the submucosal injection should be done.

Retrieval

For small lesions resected by conventional polypectomy, retrieval with suction and suction trap will be enough. However, in the case of retrieval of EMR specimens, the use of retrieval devices such as basket forceps (five pad), retrieval forceps, or retrieval net is recommended to prevent destruction of the resected specimens in the suction channel.

Success Rate and the Incidence of Relapse in EMR and EPMR

During the past 10 years, 945 F&D type of colorectal neoplasia (adenomas and early cancers) were treated by EMR and EPMR in our department. Figure 3 shows the results of EMR. Of a total of 945 lesions, 915 lesions (96.6%) could be cured with only EMR, 13 lesions (1.4%) required surgery followed by EMR because of a positive cut end or vessel permeations, and 19 lesions (2.0%) relapsed after the initial EMR procedures. Of the 19 lesions that relapsed after EMR, the macroscopic type were all LST-G, and 5 lesions were pathological cut end unclear or positive by piecemeal resection. For the relapsed lesions, only 2 lesions were sent to surgery and another 17 lesions were endoscopically treated (re-EMR for 11 lesions, APC for 6 lesions). The other reported success rates in Japan are about 90% with minimal complications [10]. EMR and intentional EPMR obtain a high success rate of complete resection for

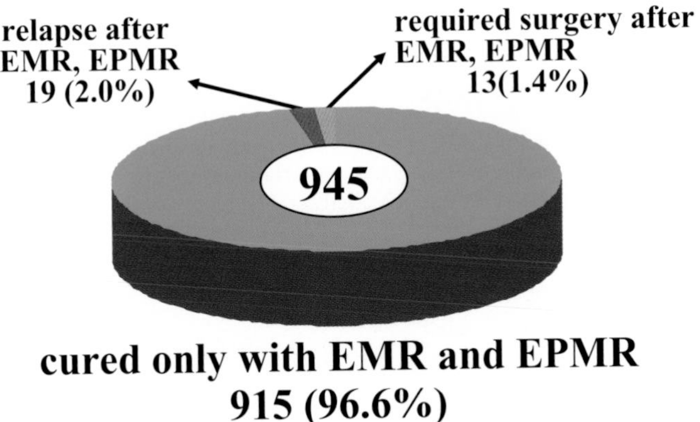

Fig. 3. Results of endoscopic mucosal resection (EMR) and EPMR for flat and depressed (F&D) type colorectal lesions

colorectal larger lesions with minimal complications and procedure time compared with the ESD technique.

Conclusion

EMR, including EPMR, is a suitable, less-invasive treatment, especially for F&D type early colorectal cancers including larger LST-G. Invasion depth diagnosis using dye spray, HFUP, or magnifying colonoscopy with NBI is the most important for the determination of EMR and scheduled EPMR.

References

1. Takemoto T, Tada M, Yanai H, et al (1989) Significance of strip biopsy with particular references to endoscopic "mucosectomy." Digest Endosc 1:4–9
2. Kudo S (1993) Endoscopic mucosal resection of flat and depressed types of early colorectal cancer. Endoscopy 25:455–461
3. Saitoh Y, Waxman I, West AB, et al (2001) Prevalence and distinctive biological features of flat colorectal adenomas in a North American population. Gastroenterology 120:1657–1665
4. Japanese Research Society for Cancer of the Colon and Rectum (2006) General rules for clinical and pathological studies on cancer of the colon, rectum and anus: histopathological classification, 7th edn. Kanehara Syuppan, Tokyo
5. Watari J, Saitoh Y, Obara T, et al (1997) Early nonpolypoid colorectal cancer: radiographic diagnosis of depth of invasion. Radiology 205:67–74
6. Saitoh Y, Obara T, Watari J, et al (1998) Invasion depth diagnosis of depressed type early colorectal cancers by combined use of videoendoscopy and chromoendoscopy. Gastrointest Endosc 48:362–370
7. Saitoh Y, Obara T, Einami K, et al (1996) Efficacy of high-frequency ultrasound probes for the preoperative staging of invasion depth in flat and depressed colorectal tumors. Gastrointest Endosc 44:34–39
8. Hirata M, Tanaka S, Oka S, et al (2007) Evaluation of microvessels in colorectal tumors by narrow band imaging magnification. Gastointest Endosc 66:945–952
9. Tanaka S, Haruma K, Tanimoto T, et al (1996) Ki-67 and transforming growth factor alpha (TGF-α) expression in colorectal recurrent tumors after endoscopic resection. In: Recent advances in gastroenterological carcinogenesis, vol I. Monduzzi Editore, Bologna, pp 1079–1083
10. Igarashi M, Yokoyama K, Takahashi H, et al (1998) A study on the indication for and limitations of EMR for the problems associated with remnant lesions. Early Colorectal Cancer 2:639–645 (in Japanese with English abstract)

Strategy of Endoscopic Treatment for Colorectal Tumor: Recent Progress and Perspective

Shinji Tanaka, Shiro Oka, and Kazuaki Chayama

Summary. In the *Colorectal Cancer Treatment Guidelines*, the 2005 edition published by the Japanese Society for Cancer of the Colon and Rectum, curative conditions of radical cure based on endoscopically resected specimens of tumors and the selection of treatment methods for colorectal adenoma and early carcinoma were explained in detail. Mucosal lesions can be cured by complete endoscopic resection. On the other hand, submucosal carcinoma showing a positive submucosal (SM) stump, SM invasion for a distance of more than 1000 μm, positive vessel involvement, or poorly differentiated adenocarcinoma/undifferentiated carcinoma should undergo additional surgical resection. In relation to these, we assessed the present situation and perspective of endoscopic submucosal dissection (ESD). The indications for colorectal ESD are as follows. (1) Large size, in which en bloc resection using snare endoscopic mucosal resection is difficult, although it is indicative for endoscopic treatment [laterally spreading tumor of the nongranular type, particularly those of the pseudo-depressed type, lesions with VI type pit pattern, carcinoma with submucosal infiltration, and large lesion with elevated type suspected to be cancer]; (2) mucosal lesions with fibrosis caused by biopsy, peristalsis of the lesions, or chronic inflammation; and (3) local residual early cancer after endoscopic resection.

Key words. Endoscopic mucosal resection (EMR), Endoscopic submucosal dissection (ESD), Colorectal tumor, Submucosal carcinoma, Lymph node metastasis

Introduction

Factors that are important and should be considered while selecting endoscopic treatment for colorectal tumor are tumor size, histological type, and invasion depth. In recent times, the technology applied for endoscopic resection has advanced, and the range of the afflicted area that can be resected endoscopically has extended considerably. Metastasis of intramucosal (M) carcinoma of the colorectum has not been

Department of Endoscopy and Gastroenterology, Hiroshima University Hospital, 1-2-3 Kasumi, Minami-ku, Hiroshima 734-8551, Japan

reported to date [1]. Therefore, a patient who has undergone complete endoscopic resection of intramucosal colorectal carcinoma can be evaluated as completely cured. On the other hand, 10%–20% of submucosal (SM) carcinomas are reported to metastasize to the lymph node [1,2]. Therefore, even after complete endoscopic resection of SM carcinoma, an additional surgery is required in some cases. Under these circumstances, evaluation of radical cure based on the resection of the tumor becomes extremely important. In the summer of 2005, the *Colorectal Cancer Treatment Guidelines*, the 2005 edition was published by the Japanese Society for Cancer of the Colon and Rectum [1]. In this section, based on the contents of this guideline, we have outlined the treatment guidelines for early colorectal carcinoma and the criteria for radical cure evaluation after endoscopic treatment. We have also described the present situation and the future prospects of colorectal endoscopic submucosal dissection (ESD), as these have progressed in recent years.

Endoscopic Treatment for Early Colon Carcinoma

In principle, endoscopic treatment should be applied only to a tumor with almost no risk of metastasis to the lymph node, and the size and location of the tumor should be suitable for en bloc resection. To perform endoscopic treatment, information regarding the size, predicted invasion depth, and the histological type of the tumor is essential [3,4]. Because there are many adenomatous lesions in the colon and rectum, preoperative discrimination among adenoma, adenocarcinoma in adenoma, and cancer without adenomatous components is very important for selecting an appropriate therapy. In addition, magnifying colonoscopic examination and optical-digital method such as narrow-band imaging (NBI) are useful for the aforementioned preoperative discrimination [5]. Various modalities such as barium enema, conventional endoscopic examination, magnifying colonoscopic examination, optical-digital method including NBI, and endoscopic ultrasound (EUS) are available for determining the invasion depth of early colorectal carcinoma [5]. The invasion depth should be accurately determined preoperatively by selecting an appropriate modality.

Based on the guideline [1], the lesions with following conditions can be treated endoscopically (Fig. 1): (1) adenoma, mucosal (M) carcinoma, or SM carcinoma without massive invasion; (2) tumors of maximum diameter less than 2 cm; and (3) any macroscopic types. The average diameter of lesions that can be treated with en bloc snare endoscopic mucosal resection (EMR) is approximately 2 cm; hence, for the tumor to be treated endoscopically, its maximum diameter should be less than 2 cm. Because the aim is to perform en bloc resection, detailed histological analysis is essential for appropriate endoscopic resection while considering the limit of diagnostic accuracy before treatment.

However, many adenomatous lesions exist in the colorectum, and carcinoma can be discriminated from adenoma by magnifying colonoscopic examination or pit pattern diagnosis using NBI, as already mentioned (Fig. 2). A majority of large tumors with diameters exceeding 2 cm are classified as laterally spreading tumors (LSTs) (Fig. 3), and most granular-type LSTs (LST-G) are adenomatous lesions [3,4]. In the granular-homogeneous type LSTs, carcinoma and SM invasion are infrequent. In granular-nodular mixed type LSTs, SM invasion may exist in a greater nodule. As

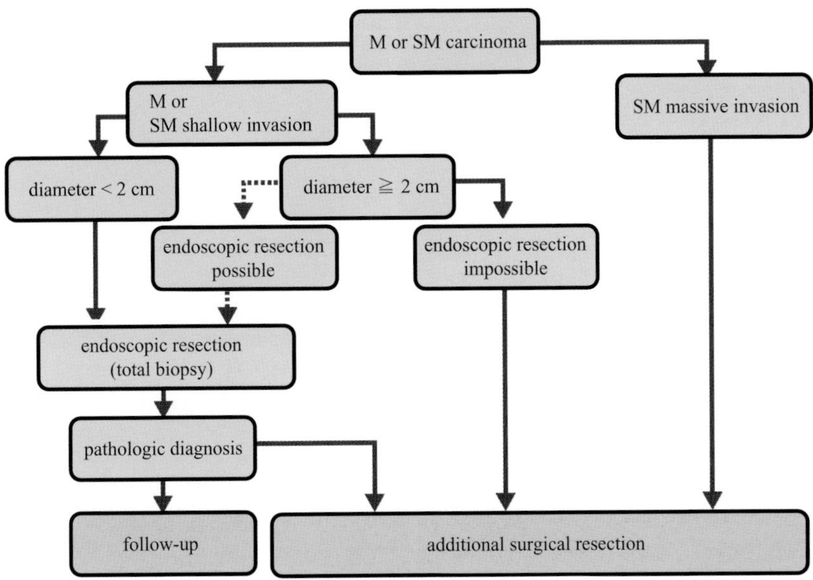

Fig. 1. Treatment strategy for lesions diagnosed as mucosal (M) or submucosal (SM) carcinoma

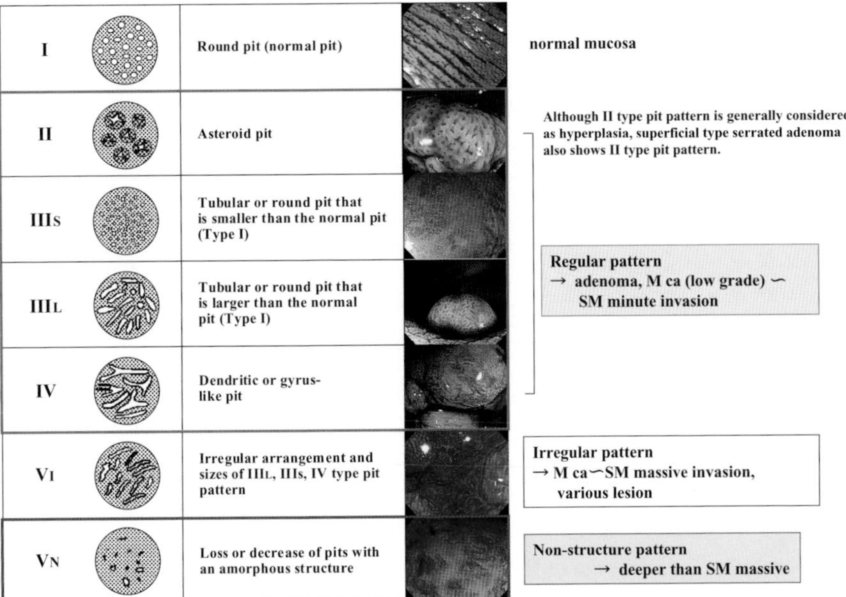

Fig. 2. Pit pattern classification for colorectal tumor (Kudo and Tsurura, 2001)

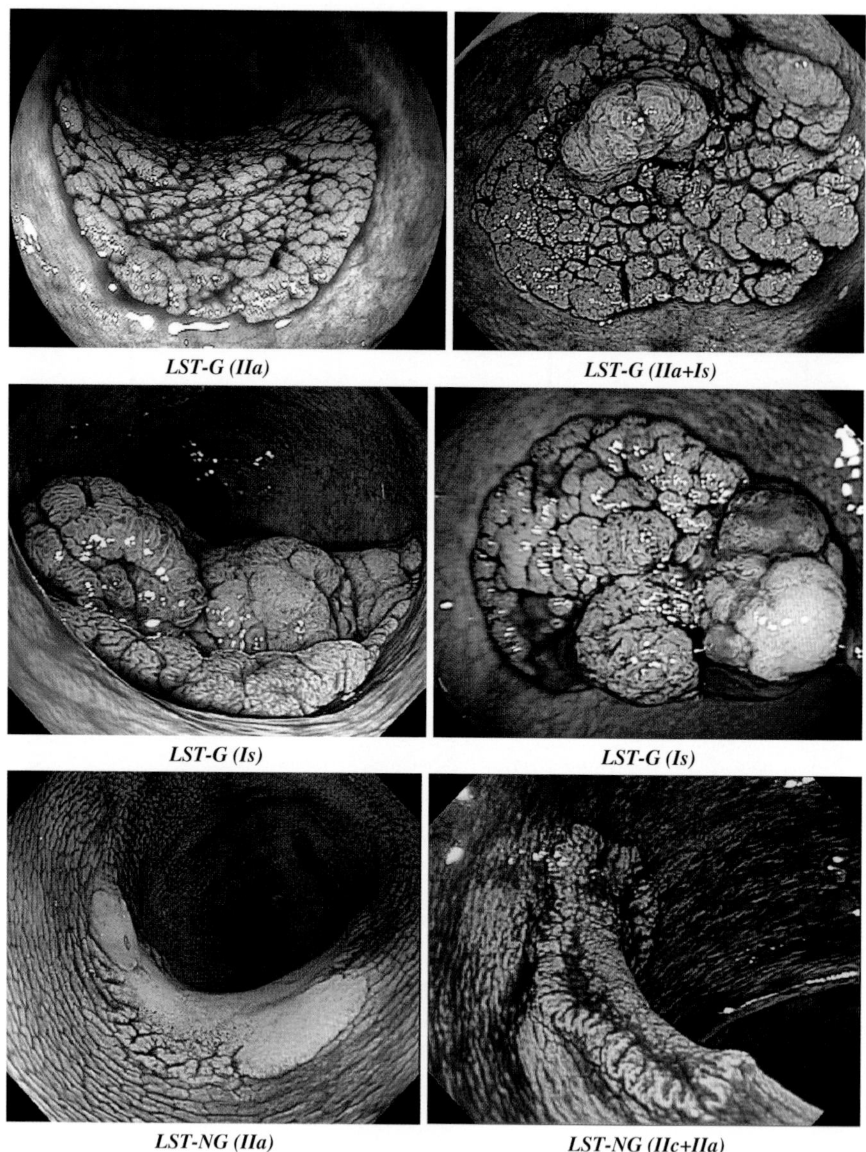

Fig. 3. Various types of laterally spreading tumor (LST). *LST-G*, granular type of spreading tumor; *LST-NG*, nongranular type of spreading tumor

LST-G is either an adenoma or focal adenocarcinoma in an adenoma, the carcinomatous portion may form a greater nodule, and the pit pattern diagnosis can be reached. In addition, prearranged piecemeal resection without excising the carcinomatous portion in pieces can also be applied. On the other hand, because nongranular-type LST (LST-NG) has higher rates of carcinoma occurrence and invasion than LST-G, LST-NG should be treated carefully. In particular, pseudo-depressed type LST-NG will be the first step toward the standardization of colorectal ESD, and it may gradually become popular [8]. Sufficient training and experience for this method are obviously indispensable.

The colon and rectum is a long hollow viscous organ. With the exception of the rectum, which lies below the peritoneal reflection, dysfunction induced by local resection of a part of the colon is not grave, in contrast to resection in the esophagus or the stomach. Moreover, the rectal region can be surgically resected through the anus. Regarding a large benign lesion, when ESD is presumed to require more time than laparoscopic resection, the applicability of ESD should be questioned. Moreover, even if the lesion can be treated by ESD, there are high chances of requiring additional surgical resection after postoperative pathological diagnosis. In actual clinical settings, to avoid any medical accidents that may impede the progress of ESD, treatments such as EMR (including piecemeal resection), ESD, and laparoscopic surgery should be appropriately selected depending on the characteristics of the lesion, skill of the colonoscopist, size of the lesion, expected time required for ESD, and the hospital facilities. Regarding colorectal ESD, efficient use of the colonoscope is more important than the size of the lesion and the macroscopic type of the tumor. If the colonoscope cannot be controlled, unreasonable ESD should not be attempted. Moreover, it is essential to select the best medical treatment for a patient after considering the skills of the endoscopist or a laparoscopist.

The peculiarities of the colorectum and a colorectal tumor should be adequately understood to avoid performing unnecessary ESD for reasons of incorrect diagnosis [8]. The application of endoscopic treatment should be based on a well-balanced consideration of the outcome of radical cure evaluation, safety, convenience, and economical efficiency. At present, the application of colorectal ESD has not yet been based on a well-balanced consideration. As progress in equipment and technology is ongoing, difficult tasks are rendered easy and impossible tasks are made possible. However, such progress in older techniques or in development of new techniques and equipment is a systematic and gradual process. Colorectal ESD can be considered to have reached the midway point in this process. In contrast to early gastric carcinoma, ESD for early colorectal carcinoma has not been standardized. In the colon and rectum, a majority of small lesions can be radically cured using snare EMR. Therefore, snare EMR will be used even in the future. Parallel to the standardization of ESD, standardization and improvement of snare EMR, which is the basic technique for colonoscopic treatment, is imperative. Presently, to avoid any complication and medical accidents that may result in social criticism of ESD, treatments such as EMR (including piecemeal resection), ESD, transanal endoscopic surgery, laparoscopic surgery, and open surgery should be appropriately selected depending on the skill of the colonoscopist and surgeon [8].

Colorectal ESD is used only in a limited number of facilities, and with regard to technical progress, it is currently at the clinical study stage [8,9]. Even in pioneer facilities, assistant colonoscopists cannot perform colorectal ESD as the standard method. For prospective standardization, the establishment of safety and handiness of ESD is essential, and this will occur only gradually. Colorectal ESD should not be performed for inappropriate cases by colonoscopists with insufficient experience and knowledge only satisfy their personal ambition of performing a colorectal ESD or doing something exciting. Such an action may be registered as a criminal case.

Conclusion

In this chapter, the application of colonoscopic treatment to colorectal tumor, radical cure evaluation after treatment, EMR, piecemeal EMR, the current situation and complications of ESD, and future perspectives have been explained. The use of colonoscopic treatment is continuously increasing. Further, the extension of the indication of colonoscopic treatment and the development of new technologies for treatment, such as ESD, are expected in the near future.

References

1. Japanese Society for Cancer of the Colon and Rectum (2005) Colorectal cancer treatment guidelines: the 2005 edition, 1st edt. Kanahara-Shuppan, Tokyo
2. Tanaka S, Oka S, Tamura T, et al (2006) Molecular pathologic application as a predictor of lymph node metastasis in submucosal colorectal carcinoma: Implication of immunohistochemical alteration as the deepest invasive margin. In: Muto T, Mochizuki H, Masaki T (eds) Tumor budding in colorectal cancer: recent progress in colorectal cancer research. NOVA, Hauppauge, NY, pp 171–180
3. Tanaka S, Haruma K, Oka S, et al (2001) Clinicopathologic features and endoscopic treatment of superficially spreading colorectal neoplasms larger than 20 mm. Gastrointest Endosc 54:62–66
4. Uraoka T, Saito Y, Matsuda T, et al (2006) Endoscopic indications for endoscopic mucosal resection of laterally spreading tumours in the colorectum. Gut 55:1592–1597
5. Tanaka S, Kaltenbach T, Chayama K, et al (2006) High-magnification colonoscopy. Gastrointest Endosc 64:604–613
6. Tanaka S, Igarashi M, Kobayashi K, et al (2007) Surveillance of cases with submucosal colorectal carcinoma resected endoscopically without additional surgery. In: Sugihara K, Tada M, Fujimori T, Igarashi M (eds) Colorectal disease (in Japanese). Nippon Medical Center, Tokyo, pp 112–120
7. Tanaka S, Oka S, Hirata M, et al (2007) Curative conditions of endoscopic resection for colorectal tumor: recent progress, problems and perspective (in Japanese with English abstract). Stomach Intest 42:1443–1451
8. Tanaka S, Oka S, Kaneko I, et al (2007) Endoscopic submucosal dissection for colorectal neoplasia: possibility of standardization. Gastrointest Endosc 66:100–107
9. Saito Y, Uraoka T, Matsuda T, et al (2007) Endoscopic treatment of large superficial colorectal tumors: a case series of 200 endoscopic submucosal dissections (with video). Gastrointest Endosc 66:966–973
10. Tsuda S (2006) Complications and related to endoscopic submucosal dissection (ESD) of colon and rectum and risk management procedures (in Japanese with English abstract). Early Colorectal Cancer 10:539–550

Pancreatobiliary Diseases

EST vs EPBD

Endoscopic Sphincterotomy and Endoscopic Papillary Balloon Dilatation for Bile Duct Stones

Naotaka Fujita, Yutaka Noda, and Kei Ito

Summary. Since its development in the early 1970s, endoscopic sphincterotomy (EST) has been playing a pivotal role in the treatment of bile duct stones. With various advances in technology, nearly 100% of patients with bile duct stones can be successfully treated by EST. Its major drawback is that hemorrhage, perforation, or pancreatitis can develop, and minimizing procedure-related complications is of great concern for biliary endoscopists. Endoscopic papillary balloon dilatation (EPBD) was developed 10 years after EST as a possible solution to these issues. Although the success rate of duct clearance with EPBD is comparable to that of EST, postprocedure pancreatitis is more frequent than in EST, as has been shown by several randomized controlled trials. Whether or not EPBD lowers the risk of recurrent stones in the long term by avoiding disruption of the sphincter of Oddi is the crucial point for this procedure to be widely accepted. Recently, the combined use of EST with large balloon dilation has been receiving attention. The benefit of this combination should be clarified by randomized controlled trials with appropriate patient selection. In addition, an increasing number of alternatives to EST and EPBD have been reported in recent years, and these will expand the role of endoscopists in the management of bile duct stones.

Key words. Endoscopic sphincterotomy (EST), Endoscopic papillary balloon dilatation (EPBD), Bile duct stones, Endoscopic retrograde cholangiopancreatography (ERCP), Endoscopic biliary drainage

Transpapillary Approach to Bile Duct Stones

Since its development by Kawai et al. [1] in 1973 and by Classen and Demling [2] in 1974, endoscopic sphincterotomy (EST) has been playing a pivotal role in the treatment of bile duct stones. EST creates a sufficient outlet for bile duct stones following selective cannulation of the bile duct by extending the orifice of the papilla of Vater. With various advances in technology, nearly 100% of patients with bile duct stones can be successfully treated by EST. EST has been evolving in terms of increased safety

---

Department of Gastroenterology, Sendai City Medical Center, 5-22-1 Tsurugaya, Miyagino-ku, Sendai, Miyagi 983-0824, Japan

and improved success rate with the development of accessories such as wire-guided sphincterotomes [3], auto-regulator-assisted electrosurgical units [4], needle knife sphincterotomy in combination with pancreatic stenting, and so forth. However, EST requires the use of electrocautery, and drawbacks such as hemorrhage, perforation, or pancreatitis can develop [5,6]. Minimizing procedure-related complications is of great concern for biliary endoscopists.

Although the short-term outcomes are satisfactory, another concern with EST is a substantial incidence of recurrence, the prevalence of recurrent bile duct stones following EST being reportedly 10% to 15% [7–10]. Risk factors for recurrent bile duct stones after EST have been analyzed [8,9,11], including a dilated bile duct, pigment stones, the gallbladder status, peripapillary diverticula, the application of lithotripsy, and the development of pneumobilia.

As a possible solution to these issues, endoscopic papillary balloon dilatation (EPBD) was developed. Staritz et al. [12] first reported the use of EPBD as a treatment for bile duct stones, but it was not widely employed because of a high incidence of postprocedural acute pancreatitis. After the report by MacMathuna et al. [13] in 1995, the use of EPBD revived. In 1998, Komatsu et al. [14] reported that in 226 cases which underwent EPBD, complete duct clearance was achieved in 95% and the incidence of complications was only 8.0%. Several studies, mainly from Asian countries, have also reported excellent duct clearance with acceptable complication rates. Tsujino et al. [15] recently reported on the immediate and long-term outcomes of EPBD in 1000 patients with bile duct stones. In their article, they reported the rate of complete duct clearance as being 96% in 1.5 sessions, and that of short-term complications to be 4.8%, including one case of a severe form of acute pancreatitis. As for long-term complications, stone recurrence was observed in 8% of the patients during a follow-up period of 5 years. Postprocedure pancreatitis is a great concern with EPBD, and a nondilated bile duct, a history of post-ERCP pancreatitis [16], contrast medium injection into the pancreatic duct [17], edema of the papilla, and microstone fragments [18] are all considered to be possible risk factors.

The expected clinical impact of EPBD on the treatment of bile duct stones is a minimization of the recurrence of stones in the long term by preserving the sphincter of Oddi function, since this acts as a valve to prevent regurgitation of the duodenal contents. Therefore, some researchers expect that the preservation of the sphincter of Oddi may contribute to a reduction in the recurrence of bile duct stones. However, it has been shown by Yasuda et al. [19] that EPBD causes a certain degree of damage to the sphincter of Oddi. Further long-term follow-up data over 10 years are awaited to allow a comparison with EST data.

Randomized Controlled Trials of EST vs EPBD

There have been several randomized controlled trials (RCTs) [20–28] in which the results of EST and EPBD as treatments for bile duct stones were compared (Table 1). All studies except one showed equivalent results for successful duct clearance between EST and EPBD. On the other hand, postprocedure pancreatitis was more frequent with EPBD than with EST, while bleeding was encountered more often following EST. Although they are reported in an RCT style, the power of some studies is insufficient

TABLE 1. Early complications of endoscopic sphincterotomy (EST) and endoscopic papillary balloon dilatation (EPBD) reported in randomized controlled trials.

	EST		EPBD		
Ref.	*N*	Compl. (%)	*N*	Compl. (%)	Pancreatitis
20	20	10	20	10	ns
21	101	24	101	17	ns
22	55	5.6	55	2	ns
23	30	16.4	30	30	ns
24	70	11.4	70	10	ns
25	144	11.9	138	13.4	$P = 0.0132$
27	114	4.4	118	14	$P < 0.01$
26	99	3.0	103	6.8	ns
28	90	3.3	90	14.4	$P < 0.05$

TABLE 2. EPBD vs EST in bile duct stones: duct clearance.

Ref.	*N*	Initial success	Total success
29	EPBD 552	70 } $P = 0.01$	94
	EST 554	80	96
30	EPBD 878	73.5 } #1	90.1 } #2
	EST 890	80.9	95.3

	RR	95% CI
#1	0.90	0.84, 0.97
#2	0.96	0.93, 0.98

for a conclusion to be drawn since the method of determining the sample size was not adequately described. Some researchers find the effectiveness of the two methods to be identical, while others conclude that EST is superior to EPBD from the viewpoint of complications. These differences may be due to the degree of experience in the two procedures of each endoscopist before participation in a study, the regimen of EPBD (pressure, balloon size, duration of dilation, number of dilation), and so on. Amazingly, in the study by DiSario et al. [27], there were two deaths due to severe post-ERCP pancreatitis among 118 patients in the EPBD group. Such events are extraordinary even in clinical practice. There is a possibility that the endoscopists involved in the study were unfamiliar with this technique, even though they were experts in EST. Whether this result is truly attributable to the EPBD procedure itself or not, the cause should be carefully analyzed in order to avoid recurrence of such an outcome.

Two articles on a meta-analysis of the results of a comparison of EST and EPBD in the treatment of bile duct stones have been published (Tables 2 and 3). An article by Baron and Harewood in 2004 [29] reported a statistically significant difference between the two methods with respect to the initial success rate of duct clearance and the incidence of bleeding. According to an article by Weinberg in 2006 [30], as well as the initial success rate and the total success rate of complete duct clearance, the incidences of pancreatitis, bleeding, and biliary infection are also significantly different. However, even meta-analysis cannot clarify all the features of the procedures, as the conditions of the studies included are not always identical.

TABLE 3. EPBD vs EST in bile duct stones: complications.

Ref.	*N*	Pancreatitis	Bleeding	Perforation	Infection	Mortality
29	BD 552					
	ST 554	7.4	0 } $P = 0.01$	0.4	2.7	0.18
		4.3 }	2.0 }	0.4	3.6 }	0.18
		#1			#3	
30	BD 878	8.6 }	0.1 } #2	0.3	2.5 }	0.7
	ST 890	4.3	4.8 }	0.5	5.0	0.3

	RR	95% CI
#1	1.98	1.34, 2.90
#2	0.15	0.06, 0.39
#3	0.55	0.31, 0.96

These two meta-analyses did not refer to the long-term outcome of the procedures. The efficacy of EPBD in terms of its preservation of the sphincter of Oddi function (to some degree), and in the prevention of the recurrence of stones or biliary infections, as suggested by Tanaka et al. [31], should be carefully evaluated and clarified to justify the application of this technique.

The indications for EPBD in cases of bile duct stones have not been fully established. As shown in the literature, it is possible to remove bile duct stones in most cases by this technique. However, the high incidence of an immediate complication of acute pancreatitis makes endoscopists hesitate to consider EPBD as the first choice of treatment. At present, cases with a history of Billroth II reconstruction [32] and those with hemorrhagic diathesis such as liver cirrhosis [33,34] are considered to be good candidates for EPBD. Cases with a small number of small stones can be treated by EPBD as safely and successfully as with EST.

Combined Use of EST and EPBD

Recently, some articles have been published [35–38] on the combined use of EST and EPBD with a large dilator balloon, and this technique is now drawing attention. The basic idea of the combined use of EST and large balloon dilation is to avoid or lessen the risk of bleeding and perforation in full-length EST and the prevalence of postprocedure pancreatitis in EPBD by establishing a large opening of the papilla of Vater, which renders the application of mechanical lithotripsy unnecessary without consideration of the preservation of the sphincter of Oddi function. In 2003, Ersoz et al. [35] reported their results on the performance of EST plus dilation with a large balloon for difficult bile duct stones in 58 patients. They used a balloon of 10–20 mm diameter to extend the orifice of the papilla of Vater following EST. Complete duct clearance was achieved in one session, two sessions, or with the combined use of a mechanical lithotriptor in 85%, 93%, and 100% of patients, respectively. Complications such as cholangitis, pancreatitis, and bleeding were encountered in 15.5% of cases. In their article, Lee et al. [36] also reported excellent results in 55 cases of bile duct stones treated by this method with an acceptable complication rate. The complete disappearance of the notch on the balloon located at the level of the papilla of Vater was observed in 69.1% of cases. In spite of the high prevalence of large stones (mean 20.8 ± 5.6 mm), mechanical lithotripsy was required in only 3 cases (5.5%). One case developed a recurrence of stones in 6 months during a follow-up period of 6–12 months. As contraindications, they listed those patients with a common bile duct <10 mm or with stricture at the distal common bile duct due to repeated cholangitis. Heo et al. [38] conducted a randomized controlled trial of a comparison of EST plus large balloon dilation with EST alone involving 200 consecutive patients, and concluded that EST plus large balloon dilation is an effective alternative to EST alone based on similar rates of successful stone removal and complications.

Endoscopic Drainage of the Bile Duct in Acute Cholangitis with Bile Duct Stones

Another way to manage bile duct stones endoscopically is endoscopic biliary drainage. Complete duct clearance is ideal in cases with bile duct stones. However, some clinical factors, including the patients' general condition and tolerance, can prohibit completion of the treatment. In such cases, endoscopic biliary drainage (EBD) is a substitute. EBD is also recommended in cases with incomplete duct clearance. There are two types of EBD, endoscopic nasobiliary drainage (ENBD) and endoscopic biliary stenting (EBS). ENBD is performed for the purpose of temporary drainage. It allows an evaluation of the volume, color, and turbidity of the drained bile, lavage of the bile duct, the administration of antibiotics directly into the bile duct, and repeat cholangiography. Patient discomfort is a major problem with ENBD, especially in elderly patients, and sometimes leads to self-removal of the drainage tube. EBS also allows the temporary drainage of infected bile. In contrast to ENBD, EBS maintains the physiological flow and circulation of bile, and there is no patient discomfort immediately after the procedure. There have been two studies [39,40] comparing ENBD and EBS for bile duct stones with severe acute cholangitis in an RCT manner. According to the results of these studies, the efficacy of biliary drainage is the same in the two procedures. In clinical practice, the evacuation of thick pus is sometimes encountered following endoscopic biliary drainage in acute cholangitis. On such occasions, the risk of stent occlusion by dense infected bile is more likely to occur in EBS.

Recently, consensus guidelines for the management of acute cholangitis have been published. In these guidelines, the significance of endoscopic procedures is emphasized [41], and these procedures discussed in the present article are considered to be the mainstay of treatment.

Alternatives to EST and EPBD

There have been many nontranspapillary procedures to manage bile duct stones. As a counterpart of EPBD, dilatation of the orifice of the papilla of Vater has also been performed via the transhepatic route [42]. Even EST is feasible via the transhepatic route using a cholangioscope akin to conventional EST [43]. Artifon et al. [44] developed a puncture needle for suprapapillary puncture of the bile duct and reported the results of a pilot study. Although the feasibility of gaining access to the bile duct was well proven, improvements in the procedure are necessary to lessen the incidence of complications.

In cases with cholecystocholedocholithiasis, the simultaneous treatment of both stones at the time of laparoscopic surgery has been reported [45–47]. Completing all treatment in the same session sounds ideal, but at present the need for relevant expertise is an obstacle to the widespread use of this treatment.

Current advances in interventional endoscopic ultrasound (EUS) have allowed the removal of bile duct stones via an artificial fistula in the duodenum created under EUS guidance. Puspok et al. [48] carried out stone extraction from the common bile duct in two cases via a fistula created by the placement of three 10-Fr stents and two 7-Fr stents, respectively, following puncture under endosonographic guidance. Although further study is needed, this technique may expand the role of endoscopists in the management of bile duct stones.

References

1. Kawai K, Akasaka Y, Hashimoto Y, et al. (1973) Preliminary report on endoscopic papillotomy. J Kyoto Pref Univ Med 82:353–355
2. Classen M, Demling L (1974) Endoscopische Sphincterotomine der Papilla Vateri und Stein-extraction aus Ductus Choledocus. MedWschr 99:496–497
3. Fujita N, Lee S, Kobayashi G, et al. (1989) A newly developed papillotomy knife with a channel for guidewire (in Japanese with English abstract). Gastroenterol Endosc 31:417–421
4. Perini RF, Sadurski R, Cotton PB, et al. (2005) Post-sphincterotomy bleeding after the introduction of microprocessor-controlled electrosurgery: does the new technology make the difference? Gastrointest Endosc 61:53–57
5. Freeman ML, Nelson DB, Sherman S, et al. (1996) Complications of endoscopic biliary sphincterotomy. NEJM 336:909–918
6. Ito K, Fujita N, Noda Y, et al. (2007) Risk management of endoscopic sphincterotomy for choledocholithiasis. Dig Endosc 19: S44–S48
7. Tanaka M, Takahata S, Konomi H, et al. (1998) Long-term consequence of endoscopic sphincterotomy for bile duct stones. Gastrointest Endosc 48:465–469
8. Pereira-Lima JC, Jakobs R, Winter UH, et al. (1998) Long-term results (7 to 10 years) of endoscopic papillotomy for choledocholithiasis. Multivariate analysis of prognostic factors for the recurrence of biliary symptoms. Gastrointest Endosc 48:457–464
9. Sugiyama M, Atomi Y (2002) Risk factors predictive of late complications after endoscopic sphincterotomy for bile duct stones: long-term (more than 10 years) follow-up study. Am J Gastroenterol 97:2763–2767
10. Costamagna G, Tringali A, Shah SK, et al. (2002) Long-term follow-up of patients after endoscopic sphincterotomy for choledocholithiasis, and risk factors for recurrence. Endoscopy 34:273–279
11. Ando T, Tsuyuguchi T, Okugawa T, et al. (2003) Risk factors for recurrent bile duct stones after endoscopic papillotomy. Gut 52:116–121
12. Staritz M, Ewe K, Meyer zum Bruschenfelde KH (1983) Endoscopic papillary balloon dilatation (EPD) for treatment of common bile duct stones and papillary stenosis. Endoscopy 15:197–198
13. MacMathuna P, White P, Clarke E, et al. (1995) Endoscopic balloon sphincteroplasty (papillary dilatation) for bile duct stones: efficacy, safety and follow-up in 100 patients. Gastrointest Endosc 42:468–474

14. KomatsuY, Kawabe T, Toda N, et al. (1998) Endoscopic papillary dilation for the management of common bile duct stones: experience of 226 cases. Endoscopy 30:12–17
15. Tsujino T, Kawabe T, Komatsu Y, et al. (2007) Endoscopic papillary balloon dilation for bile duct stone: immediate and long-term outcomes in 1000 patients. Clin Gastroenterol Hepatol 5:130–137
16. Sugiyama M, Abe N, Izumisato Y, et al. (2003) Risk factors for acute pancreatitis after endoscopic papillary balloon dilation. Hepatogastroenterology 50:1796–1798
17. Tsujino T, Isayama H, Komatsu Y, et al. (2005) Risk factors for pancreatitis in patients with common bile duct stones managed by endoscopic papillary balloon dilation. Am J Gastroenterol 100:38–42
18. Sato D, Shibahara T, Miyazaki K, et al. (2005) Efficacy of endoscopic nasobiliary drainage for the prevention of pancreatitis after papillary balloon dilatation: a pilot study. Pancreas 31:93–97
19. Yasuda I, Tomita E, Enya M, et al. (2001) Can endoscopic papillary balloon dilation really preserve sphincter of Oddi function? Gut 49:608–609
20. Minami A, Nakatsu T, Uchida N, et al. (1995) Papillary dilation vs papillotomy for bile duct stones. A randomized trial with manometric function. Diag Dis Sci 40: 2550–2554
21. Bergman JJ, Rauws EAJ, Fockens P, et al. (1997) Randomized trial of endoscopic balloon dilatation versus endoscopic sphincterotomy for removal of bile duct stones. Lancet 349:1124–1129
22. Ochi Y, Mukawa K, Kiyosawa K, et al. (1999) Comparing the treatment outcomes of endoscopic papillary dilation and endoscopic sphincterotomy for removal of bile duct stones. J Gastroenterol Hepatol 14:90–96
23. Arnold JC, Benz C, Martin WR, et al. (2001) Endoscopic papillary balloon dilation vs. sphincterotomy for removal of common bile duct stones: a prospective randomized pilot study. Endoscopy 33:563–567
24. Natsui M, Narisawa R, Motoyama H, et al. (2002) What is an appropriate indication for endoscopic papillary balloon dilation? Eur J Gastroenterol Hepatol 14:635–640
25. Fujita N, Maguchi H, Komatsu Y, et al. (2003) Endoscopic sphincterotomy and endoscopic papillary balloon dilatation for bile duct stones: a prospective randomized controlled multicenter trial. Gastrointest Endosc 57:151–155
26. Vlavianos P, Chopra K, Mandalia S, et al. (2003) Endoscopic balloon dilatation versus endoscopic sphincterotomy for the removal of bile duct stones: a prospective randomised trial. Gut 52:1165–1169
27. DiSario JA, Freeman ML, Bjorkman DJ, et al. (2004) Endoscopic balloon dilation compared with sphincterotomy for extraction of bile duct stones. Gastroenterology 127:1291–1299
28. Watanabe H, Yoneda M, Tominaga K, et al. (2007) Comparison between endoscopic papillary balloon dilatation and endoscopic sphincterotomy for the treatment of common bile duct stones. J Gastroenterol 42: 56–62
29. Baron TH, Harewood GC (2004) Endoscopic balloon dilation of the biliary sphincter compared to endoscopic biliary sphincterotomy for removal of common bile duct stones during ERCP: a metaanalysis of randomized, controlled trials. Am J Gastroenterol 99:1455–1460
30. Weinberg BM, Shindy W, Lo S (2006) Endoscopic balloon sphincter dilation (sphincteroplasty) versus sphincterotomy for common bile duct stones. Cochrane Database Syst Rev 18:CD004890
31. Tanaka S, Sawayama T, Yoshioka T (2004) Endoscopic papillary balloon dilation and endoscopic sphincterotomy for bile duct stones: long-term outcomes in a prospective randomized controlled trial. Gastrointest Endosc 59:614–618

32. Bergman JJ, van Berkel AM, Bruno MJ, et al. (2001) A randomized trial of endoscopic balloon dilation and endoscopic sphincterotomy for removal of bile duct stones in patients with a prior Billroth II gastrectomy. Gastrointest Endosc 53:19–26
33. Kawabe T, Komatsu Y, Tada M, et al. (1996) Endoscopic papillary balloon dilatation in cirrhotic patients: removal of common bile duct stones without sphincterotomy. Endoscopy 28:694–698
34. Park DH, Kim MH, Lee SK, et al. (2004) Endoscopic sphincterotomy vs endoscopic papillary balloon dilation for choledocholithiasis in patients with liver cirrhosis and coagulopathy. Gastrointest Endosc 60:180–185
35. Ersoz G, Tekesm O, Ozutemiz AO, et al. (2003) Biliary sphincterotomy plus dilation with a large balloon for bile duct stones that are difficult to extract. Gastrointest Endosc 57:156–159
36. Lee DK, Lee BJ, Hwhang SJ, et al. (2007) Endoscopic papillary large balloon dilation after endoscopic sphincterotomy for treatment of large common bile duct stone. Digestive Endosc 19:S52–S56
37. Minami A, Hirose S, Nomoto T, et al. (2007) Small sphincterotomy combined with papillary dilation with large balloon permits retrieval of large stones without mechanical lithotripsy. World J Gastroenterol 13:2179–2182
38. Heo JH, Kang DH, Jung HJ, et al. (2007) Endoscopic sphincterotomy plus large-balloon dilation versus endoscopic sphincterotomy for removal of bile-duct stones. Gastrointest Endosc 66:720–726
39. Lee DW, Chan AC, Lam YH, et al. (2002) Biliary decompression by nasobiliary catheter or biliary stent in acute suppurative cholangitis: a prospective randomized trial. Gastrointest Endosc 56:361–365
40. Sharma BC, Kumar R, Agarwal N, et al. (2005) Endoscopic biliary drainage by nasobiliary drain or by stent placement in patients with acute cholangitis. Endoscopy 37:439–443
41. Nagino M, Takada T, Kawarada Y, et al. (2007) Methods and timing of biliary drainage for acute cholangitis: Tokyo Guidelines. J Hepatobiliary Pancreat Surg 14:68–77
42. Berkman WA, Bishop AF, Palagallo GL, et al. (1988) Transhepatic balloon dilation of the distal common bile duct and ampulla of Vater for removal of calculi. Radiology 167:453–455
43. Itoi T, Shinohara Y, Takeda K, et al. (2004) A novel technique for endoscopic sphincterotomy when using a percutaneous transhepatic cholangioscope in patients with an endoscopically inaccessible papilla. Gastrointest Endosc 59:708–711
44. Artifon EL, Sakai P, Ishioka S, et al. (2007) Suprapapillary puncture of the common bile duct for selective biliary access: a novel technique. Gastrointest Endosc 65:124–131
45. Jacobs M, Verdeja JC, Goldstein HS (1991) Laparoscopic choledocholithotomy. J Laparoendosc Surg 1:79–82
46. Sackier JM, Berci G, Paz-Partlow M (1991) Laparoscopic transcystic choledocholithotomy as an adjunct to laparoscopic cholecystectomy. Am Surg 57:323–326
47. Nathanson LK, O'Rourke NA, Martin IJ, et al. (2005) Postoperative ERCP versus laparoscopic choledochotomy for clearance of selected bile duct calculi: a randomized trial. Ann Surg 242:188–192
48. Puspok A, Lomoschitz F, Dejaco C, et al. (2005) Endoscopic ultrasound guided therapy of benign and malignant biliary obstruction: a case series. Am J Gastroenterol 100:1743–1747

Strategy for the Endoscopic Treatment of Common Bile Duct Stones: Should We Cut or Dilate the Papilla?

Ichiro Yasuda, Takuji Iwashita, and Hisataka Moriwaki

Summary. Endoscopic sphincterotomy (EST) is a well-established standard technique for treating common bile duct stones. However, endoscopic papillary balloon dilation (EPBD) has recently been introduced as an alternative to avoid bleeding and perforation. In addition, this procedure can also help preserve the papillary function. However, the occurrence of postprocedure pancreatitis remains an important problem with EPBD. Indeed, EPBD has been abandoned in the United States owing to concerns about the increased risk of pancreatitis. On the other hand, it is still widely performed in Japan, and various measures have been taken to prevent the occurrence of postprocedure pancreatitis. In patients for whom EST is unsuitable, such as those with coagulopathy and those with a prior Billroth II gastrectomy, EPBD is considered to be indicated. Patients with a single stone or only a few small stones may also be considered for this procedure, because neither mechanical lithotripsy nor repeated cannulations will be necessary. Using a relatively small balloon and inflation with a low pressure for short durations is currently the most popular treatment strategy for EPBD in Japan. Nevertheless, in order to expand the number of patients considered for this treatment modality, special medication and treatment, such as an intravenous drip infusion of isosorbide dinitrate and stent placement in the pancreatic duct, are considered to be necessary.

Key words. Bile duct stone, Endoscopic sphincterotomy, Endoscopic papillary balloon dilation, Endoscopic treatment

Introduction

Endoscopic sphincterotomy (EST) is a well-established standard treatment for common bile duct stones, but it has potential risks, such as bleeding and perforation, and it can also result in injury to the function of the sphincter of Oddi. Recently, endoscopic papillary balloon dilation (EPBD) has been introduced as an alternative

First Department of Internal Medicine, Gifu University Hospital, 1-1 Yanagido, Gifu 501-1194, Japan

Table 1. Comparisons of the success rate and early complications in EST and EPBD.

	Ref. 1		Ref. 2		Ref. 3		Ref. 4		Ref. 5		Ref. 6	
	EST	EPBD	EST	EPBD	EST	EPBD	EST	EPBD	EST	EPBD	EST	EPBD
No. of patients	20	20	101	101	55	55	35	35	30	30	70	70
Indications	None		None		<15 mm, No. <10		None		<20 mm, No. <5		None	
Successful clearance rate (%)	100	100	91	89	92.7	98.1	100	100	100	77*	98.6	92.9
Early complications (%)	10	10	24	17	5.6	2.0	8.6	5.7	16.7	30.0	11.4	10.0
Pancreatitis (%)	10	10	6.9	6.9	3.7	0	5.7	5.7	10.0	20.0	4.3	5.7
Mild (%)					0	0	5.7	5.7	10.0	13.3	4.3	5.7
Moderate (%)					3.7	0	0	0	0	0		
Severe (%)					0	0	0	0	0	6.7		
Cholecystitis (%)												
Cholangitis (%)									0	10.0	4.3	2.9
Aggravation of jaundice (%)			1.0	2.0	0	2.0						
Fever (%)			5.0	4.0								
Abdominal pain (%)			4.0	0								
Bleeding (%)			4.0	0			2.9	0	6.7	0	2.9	0
Perforation (%)			1.0	2.0	1.9	0						
Basket impaction (%)											0	1.4
Bile leakage (%)			1.0	1.0								
Cardiopulmonary (%)			1.0	1.0								

No, number of stones; $^{*}P < 0.05$

to EST in order to avoid such undesirable effects while also preserving the papillary function. However, EPBD has currently been abandoned in the United States, and it is performed on only a small number of carefully selected patients in Europe owing to concerns related to an increased risk of pancreatitis. On the other hand, it is still widely performed in Japan, where various measures have been taken to prevent the occurrence of postprocedure pancreatitis. We describe the current indications and appropriate techniques for performing EPBD.

Comparisons of the Early Outcomes Between EST and EPBD

Comparisons of the success rates for bile duct clearance and for the occurrence of early complications between EST and EPBD are shown in Table 1 [1–14]. The data include 14 previously published findings, including 13 randomized controlled trials (RCT) [1–8,10–14] and one meta-analysis [9] of 8 RCTs [1–8]. From these data, the success rates for bile duct clearance were found to be similar for the two procedures, except for the findings in one RCT [5]. However, mechanical lithotripsy was required more frequently in EPBD than in EST [2,4,9,14]. No statistically significant difference was observed in the total number of complications between EST and EPBD. However, EPBD carried a higher risk of pancreatitis in 3 RCTs [8,10,14] and in one meta-analysis [9], while EST carried a higher risk of bleeding in 2 RCTs [10,11] and in one meta-analysis [9].

Ref. 7		Ref. 8		Ref. 9		Ref. 10		Ref. 11		Ref. 12		Ref. 13		Ref. 14	
EST	EPBD	EST	EPBD	EST	EPBD	EST	EPBD	EST	EPBD	EST	EPBD	EST	EPBD	EST	EPBD
99	103	144	138	554	552	120	117	53	51	45	46	16	16	90	90
None		<14 mm		Meta-analysis		<10 mm, No. <4		<20 mm		None		None		None	
86.9	87.4%	100	99.3	96	94	92.5	97.4	100	94.1	100	100	100	100	95.6	86.6
3.0	6.8	11.8	14.5	10.3	10.4	3.3	17.9*			0	0	25.0	18.8	3.3	14.4*
1.0	4.9	2.8	10.9*	4.3	7.4*	0.8	10.3*	0	0			18.8	18.8	2.2	10.0*
0	1.9	2.1	8.7											0	8.9
1.0	1.9	0.7	2.2											2.1	1.1
0	1.0	0	9			0	5.1								
		4.2	2.2			0.8	0								
1.0	1.9	4.2	1.4	3.6	2.7	0.8	0.9					12.5	0	0	3.3
		1.4	0	2.0*	0	27.0*	10.5	26.4*	2.0					1.1	0
				0.4	0.4	0.8	0	0.8	0						
		0.7	0.7											0	1.1
								0	1.7						

Post-EPBD Pancreatitis

Postprocedure pancreatitis is the most serious problem associated with EPBD. A multicenter RCT from the United States reported a higher incidence of pancreatitis and two subsequent deaths in the EPBD group [10]. Because the results of this report were so impressive, EPBD is no longer performed in the United States. On the other hand, most of the RCTs from Japan have demonstrated similar rates of pancreatitis between EST and EPBD [1,3,4,6], and therefore many Japanese endoscopists remain skeptical regarding the increased risk of pancreatitis associated with EPBD. However, a multicenter RCT in Japan showed the incidence of postprocedure pancreatitis to be significantly higher in the EPBD group than in the EST group [8], and a higher incidence of pancreatitis in EPBD is now also widely recognized in Japan. Several Japanese endoscopists have tried to identify the causes of this phenomenon in order to take measures to prevent it.

How to Prevent Post-EPBD Pancreatitis

As shown in Table 2, a previous history of pancreatitis and a nondilated bile duct have been reported to be risk factors for post-EPBD pancreatitis [15,16]. Therefore, special attention should be paid to such high-risk patients, or they should be excluded from consideration for EPBD. The use of a mechanical lithotriptor, prolonged procedures, and the injection of contrast medium into the pancreatic duct are also risk factors for post-EPBD pancreatitis [17–19]. As a result, the injection of contrast

TABLE 2. Risk factor for post-EPBD pancreatitis.

Prior history of acute pancreatitis [15,16]
Nondilated bile duct (≤9 mm) [16]
Use of a mechanical lithotriptor [17,18]
Prolonged procedure (≥30 min) [17]
Contrast medium injection into the pancreatic duct [19]

medium into the pancreatic duct should be avoided whenever possible. Patients with large stones, and cases in which stone extraction tends to be difficult, such as cases with multiple stones, should also be treated with extreme care. Mechanical lithotripsy and/or the repeated insertion of either a basket or a balloon catheter are required in such cases, and such treatment can cause papillary edema. The misinsertion of the catheter into the pancreatic duct can also easily occur under such conditions, thus possibly causing pancreatitis. If the procedure time becomes extended and papillary edema occurs, then the procedure should either be discontinued after the placement of a biliary drain or be converted to EST.

Regarding the appropriate balloon diameter for the EPBD, an 8-mm balloon is generally used in Japan, but a 6-mm balloon is sometimes useful, especially in cases with a nondilated bile duct. It is important to choose an appropriate balloon size, and the diameter of the balloon should never be larger than that of the bile duct. Currently, the balloon is inflated at a relatively low pressure, and it is deflated again after a short time of full expansion. To be specific, the balloon is gradually inflated until the disappearance of the balloon waist, and then it is immediately deflated after reaching its full expansion. The maximum pressure during the balloon inflation is usually below 4 atm. This is because a gradual inflation at a low pressure is considered to prevent papillary edema. Using a relatively small balloon (either 8 mm or 6 mm in diameter) and inflation with a low pressure for short durations is now the standard technique for performing EPBD in Japan.

Several kinds of medication and additional procedures have also been tried to prevent complications. The intravenous drip infusion of isosorbide dinitrate relaxes the sphincter of Oddi, and it is considered to reduce the occurrence of papillary edema after EPBD [20,21]. Epinephrine spray on the papilla after EPBD has also been tried in an attempt to prevent papillary edema [22], and the efficacy of stent placement in the pancreatic duct has also been reported [23]. The application of endoscopic nasobiliary drainage after EPBD may reduce the incidence of pancreatitis by preventing pancreatic duct obstruction due to either residual stones or papillary edema. However, to date these measures have only been attempted at a few institutions, and there is insufficient evidence to demonstrate the efficacy of such preventive procedures.

Sphincter of Oddi Function After EST and EPBD

One of the supposed advantages of EPBD rather than EST is the better preservation of papillary function after the treatment. Histopathological findings after EPBD have demonstrated the architectural preservation of the sphincter of Oddi in animal models, and also in clinical samples of patients with a prior history of EPBD, based on the findings of both surgical operations and autopsies. Several manometric studies have demonstrated the better preservation of papillary function after EPBD [1,3,4], and quantitative cholescintigraphy has also further confirmed this finding. Therefore, EPBD is considered to preserve the papillary function successfully. In contrast, EST results in a permanent loss of the sphincter function, while also causing chronic duodenobiliary reflux with bacterial colonization and inflammation of the biliary system, thereby leading to a recurrence of bile duct stones, cholangitis, and cholocystitis [4], and also possibly increasing the potential risk of a malignant degeneration of the epithelium in the biliary system. However, to date no severe late complications have been revealed in long-term follow-up studies.

Proposed Indications for EPBD

EPBD is considered to be a good alternative for patients for whom EST is not indicated, such as patients with liver cirrhosis or other coagulopathies. EST is also not indicated for patients with a prior Billroth II gastrectomy since the procedure is more difficult, thereby increasing the risk of complications in such patients. However, the routine use of EPBD still remains controversial. Patients with either a single stone or a few smaller stones, normally less than 10 mm in diameter, can generally be treated easily and safely because neither mechanical lithotripsy nor repeated cannulations are necessary. However, careful consideration is called for before recommending any further expansion of the indications for this procedure.

Conclusions

Owing to the fact that post-EPBD pancreatitis remains a problem and the clinical benefits of EPBD based on long-term follow-up studies have yet to be demonstrated, EST still continues to be the standard treatment for bile duct stones. EPBD should be attempted based on the appropriate indications, and the procedure must be performed in an appropriate manner. In addition, the use of several kinds of special medication and treatment before and/or after the procedure may also be necessary to prevent the occurrence of complications.

References

1. Minami A, Nakatsu T, Uchida N, et al. (1995) Papillary dilation vs sphincterotomy in endoscopic removal of bile duct stones. A randomized trial with manometric function. Dig Dis Sci 40:2550–2554
2. Bergman JJGH, Rauws EAJ, Fockens P, et al. (1997) Randomised trial of endoscopic balloon dilation versus endoscopic sphincterotomy for removal of bile duct stones. Lancet 349:1124–1129
3. Ochi Y, Mukawa K, Kiyosawa K, et al. (1999) Comparing the treatment outcomes of endoscopic papillary dilation and endoscopic sphincterotomy for removal of bile duct stones. J Gastroenterol Hepatol 14:90–96
4. Yasuda I, Tomita E, Enya M, et al. (2001) Can endoscopic papillary balloon dilation really preserve sphincter of Oddi function? Gut 49:686–691

5. Arnold JC, Benz C, Martin WR, et al. (2001) Endoscopic papillary balloon dilation vs. sphincterotomy for removal of common bile duct stones: a prospective randomized pilot study. Endoscopy 33:563–567
6. Natsui M, Narisawa R, Motoyama H, et al. (2002) What is an appropriate indication for endoscopic papillary balloon dilation? Eur J Gastroenterol Hepatol 14:635–640
7. Vlavianos P, Chopra K, Mandalia S, et al. (2003) Endoscopic papillary balloon dilatation versus endoscopic sphincterotomy for the removal of bile duct stones: a prospective randomised trial. Gut 52:1165–1169
8. Fujita N, Maguchi H, Komatsu Y, et al. (2003) Endoscopic sphincterotomy and endoscopic papillary balloon dilation for bile duct stones: a prospective randomized controlled multicenter trial. Gastrointest Endosc 57:151–155
9. Baron TH, Harewood GC (2004) Endoscopic balloon dilation of the biliary sphincter compared to endoscopic biliary sphincterotomy for removal of common bile duct stones during ERCP: a metaanalysis of randomized, controlled trials. Am J Gastroenterol 99:1455–1460
10. DiSario JA, Freeman ML, Bjorkman DJ, et al. (2004) Endoscopic balloon dilation compared with sphincterotomy for extraction of bile duct stones. Gastroenterology 127:1291–1299
11. Lin CK, Lai KH, Chan HH, et al. (2004) Endoscopic balloon dilatation is a safe method in the management of common bile duct stones. Dig Liver Dis 36:68–72
12. Takezawa M, Kida Y, Kida M, et al. (2004) Influence of endoscopic papillary balloon dilation and endoscopic sphincterotomy on sphincter of Oddi function: a randomized controlled trial. Endoscopy 36:631–637
13. Tanaka S, Sawayama T, Yoshioka T (2004) Endoscopic papillary balloon dilation and endoscopic sphincterotomy for bile duct stones: long-term outcomes in a prospective randomized controlled trial. Gastrointest Endosc 59:614–618
14. Watanabe H, Yoneda M, Tominaga K, et al. (2007) Comparison between endoscopic papillary balloon dilatation and endoscopic sphincterotomy for the treatment of common bile duct stones. J Gastroenterol 42:56–62
15. Sugiyama M, Izumisato Y, Abe N, et al. (2003) Predictive factors for acute pancreatitis and hyperamylasemia after endoscopic papillary balloon dilation. Gastrointest Endosc 57:531–535
16. Sugiyama M, Abe N, Izumisato Y, et al. (2003) Risk factors for acute pancreatitis after endoscopic papillary balloon dilation. Hepato-Gastroenterology 50:1796–1798
17. Yasuda I, Enya M, Tomita E, et al. (2003) Indications for endoscopic papillary balloon dilation for common bile duct stones for the prevention of pancreatitis and the preservation of papillary function after the procedure. Pancreas 27:93–94
18. Shim CS (2003) Endoscopic papillary balloon dilation for removal of common bile duct stones. Dig Endosc 15:1–6
19. Tsujino T, Isayama H, Komatsu Y, et al. (2005) Risk factors for pancreatitis in patients with common bile duct stones managed by endoscopic papillary balloon dilation. Am J Gastroenterol 100:38–42
20. Minami A, Maeta T, Kohi F, et al. (1998) Endoscopic papillary dilation by balloon and isosorbide dinitrate drip infusion for removing bile stone. Scand J Gastroenterol 33:765–768
21. Nakagawa H (2004) Comparing balloon diameter on performing endoscopic papillary balloon dilatation with isosorbide dinitrate drip infusion for removal of bile duct stones. Dig Endosc 16:289–294
22. Ohashi A, Tamada K, Tomiyama T, et al. (2001) Epinephrine irrigation for the prevention of pancreatic damage after endoscopic balloon sphincteroplasty. J Gastroenterol Hepatol 16:568–571
23. Aizawa T, Ueno N (2001) Stent placement in the pancreatic duct prevents pancreatitis after endoscopic sphincter dilation for removal of bile duct stones. Gastrointest Endosc 54:209–213

TABLE 2. Procedure-related complications of EPBD and EST from Prospective Randomized Trials.

	Bergman [3]	Ochi [4]	Arnold [4]	Yasuda [4]	Natsui [4]	Fujita [4]	Viavianos [4]	Tanaka [5]	Disario [6]	Watanabe [7]	Total
Pancreatitis (EPBD)	7/101 (7%) (2 severe)	0/55 (0.0%)	6/30 (20%) (2 severe)	—	4/70 (5.7%)	15/138 (10%)	5/103 (4%) (1 severe)	3/16 (18%)	18/117 (15%) (8 severe)	15/90 (16%)	73/720 (10%)
Pancreatitis (EST)	7/101 (7%) (1 severe)	2/55 (3%)	3/30 (10%)	—	3/70 (4.3%)	4/144 (2%)	1/99 (1%)	3/16 (18%)	1/120 (0.8%)	6/90 (6%)	30/725 (4%)
Bleeding (EPBD)	0/101 (0.0%)	0/55 (0.0%)	0/30 (0.0%)	—	0/70 (0.0%)	0/138 (0.0%)	—	0/16 (0.0%)	—	0/90 (0.0%)	0/500 (0%)
Bleeding (EST)	4/101 (4%)	0/55 (0.0%)	2/30 (6%)	—	2/70 (2.9%)	2/144 (1%)	—	0/16 (0.0%)	—	1/90 (1%)	11/506 (2%)
Cholangitis (EPBD)	—	2/55 (3%)	3/30 (10%)	0/35 (0.0%)	2/70 (2.9%)	2/138 (1%)	2/103 (2%)	0/16 (0.0%)	1/117 (0.8%)	3/90 (3%)	15/654 (2%)
Cholangitis (EST)	—	2/55 (3%)	0/30 (0.0%)	0/35 (0.0%)	3/70 (4.3%)	6/144 (4%)	1/99 (1%)	2/16 (12.5%)	1/120 (0.8%)	0/90 (0.0%)	15/659 (2%)
Perforation (EPBD)	2/101 (2%)	0/55 (0.0%)	0/30 (0.0%)	—	0/70 (0.0%)	0/138 (0.0%)	—	0/16 (0.0%)	0/117 (0.0%)	0/90 (0.0%)	2/617 (0.3%)
Perforation (EST)	1/101 (1%)	1/55 (2%)	0/30 (0.0%)	—	0/170 (0.0%)	0/144 (0.0%)	—	0/16 (0.0%)	1/120 (0.8%)	0/90 (0.0%)	2/626 (0.3%)
Death (EPBD)	—	—	—	—	—	0/138 (0.0%)	0/103 (0.0%)	—	2/117 (1.7%)	—	2/358 (0.5%)
Death (EST)	—	—	—	—	—	0/144 (0.0%)	1/99 (1%)	—	0/120 (0.0%)	—	1/363 (0.3%)

which a severe morbidity of 7% (including two deaths following EPBD) was reported, also remain unanswered by this meta-analysis. The mean age of all the patients across the eight prospective randomized studies of EPBD and EST was 65.6 years. Younger patients appear to have a higher risk of post-ERCP pancreatitis. In contrast to the younger age group, older patients with atrophied pancreas parenchyme have a lower chance of pancreatitis after ERCP. Thus, this meta-analysis does not address the risk of EPBD and pancreatitis in patients less than 50 years of age, i.e., the group for which there is the most concern about the long-term complications of EST.

The causes of pancreatitis after EPBD are variable. Compression of the pancreatic duct and orifice due to biliary ballooning is suspected to be the most influential cause other than ballooning itself, but the process of selective cannulation, the to-and-fro passage of the basket catheter into the bile duct to remove the stone, and edema or tissue spasm that is developed by irritation of the pancreas orifice could also be to blame. It is presumed that the size of the balloon and the duration of ballooning does not greatly affect the incidence of pancreatitis. In a study of endoscopic papillary large balloon dilatation (EPLBD) that will be described later, the incidence of pancreatitis was negligible even though the size of the EPLBD balloon was much larger than that of the EPBD balloon. If pancreatitis occurs after EPBD because of compression of the pancreatic duct and orifice due to biliary ballooning, it can be asserted that the risk of pancreatitis is higher in difficult cases of selective cannulation or bile duct stone removal.

Preservation of the SOD following EPBD may prevent the long-term consequences of the permanent loss of the biliary sphincter that may follow EST. Both manometric and histopathological studies in animals and humans suggest that sphincter function and architecture are maintained after EPBD. Biliary sphincter function was lost in almost all patients in the EST group, but it was variably maintained in the EPBD group. In one study, basal biliary SOD pressure was significantly higher 1 year after EPBD, although it was still significantly lower than pre-EPBD sphincter pressure. Although the preservation of biliary sphincter function is much more likely following EPBD, this may not apply to all patients. In addition, the failure of selective bile duct cannulation, a failure to remove stones using EPBD and the resultant "rescue" sphincterotomy, or EST for the treatment of recurrent common bile duct (CBD) stones after EPBD could all be reasons for the failure of sphincter preservation in one-third of patients who undergo EPBD.

Does the preservation of biliary sphincter integrity and function justify the risk? Maintaining a barrier between the duodenal contents and the biliary tree is an important goal. There are data to suggest that after EPBD, the sphincter regains at least partial function. Loss of sphincter competence results in bacterial colonization of the biliary tree, which is considered to be a risk factor for the formation of primary bile duct stones, making new stone formation in the bile duct less common after EPBD than after EST. However, the results of short-term follow-up studies do not show that bile duct stone formation is reduced after EPBD. It is unclear whether the reported stone recurrence represents true de nove bile duct stone formation or the persistence of retained stone fragments. The stone recurrence rate after EST is higher in patients with gallbladder preservation than in cholecystectomy patients. This means that many patients have recurrent stones due to secondary migrated choledocholithiasis rather than de nove stone formation in the CBD. In contrast to EPBD, EST creates a wide and persistent opening through which small stones can pass spontaneously.

This might be an advantage that outweighs the disadvantages of bacterial colonization. Long-term follow-up data regarding stone recurrence after EPBD are not available. When mechanical lithotripsy is used, tiny crushed, fragmented stones can the reason for recurrent stones after EPBD. The all-important question "Is chronic exposure of the biliary epithelium to duodenal contents a cancer risk?" remains unanswered. To date, there have been no reports that EST increases the risk for biliary tract cancer.

Bleeding significantly decreased after EPBD compared with EST. Clinically significant post-EST bleeding is relatively rare (less than 2%) in patients with coagulopathy, but patients requiring anticoagulation therapy within 3 days of the procedure are at increased risk of bleeding, including delayed bleeding. In these patients, EPBD is a useful alternative to EST. Another group for whom EPBD may be an attractive option are patients who refuse blood transfusions because of religious beliefs.

Another exclusion criterion in five of the eight studies was the presence of acute cholangitis or acute cholecystitis. Although this should not prevent the successful clearance of bile duct stones using EPBD, there are insufficient data in published randomized trials to draw conclusions about the suitability of EPBD for patients with cholangitis or cholecystitis. In patients with cholangitis, EST is better than EPBD as a one-step treatment. Biliary drainage may be necessary before EPBD in order to prevent a worsening of the cholangitis.

EPBD has technical advantages over EST because the enlargement of the biliary orifice by EPBD is easy and simple. EPBD can be performed safely even on patients with an unsuitable anatomy for EST, such as a Billroth II gastrectomy. As mentioned above, EST and EPBD both have their strong and weak points, and it is important to choose the procedure that is most beneficial for both the patient and the surgeon.

EPLBD After EST for Treatment of Large Common Bile Duct Stones

Endoscopic mechanical lithotripsy (EML) is used when stone removal is not possible by EST owing to the large size of a bile duct stone. It has been reported that the success rate of removing bile duct stones using EML ranges from 80% to 98% (see Table 1). The disadvantages of EML are its lengthy procedure time, possible injury of the EST site or bile duct as a result of using accessories, and impaction of the stone-capturing basket. Full incision of the sphincter causes many complications, such as bleeding, perforation, and pancreatitis, in 5%–10% of cases (see Table 2).

The earlier EPBD method did not include EST in order to preserve SOD function. However, EPLBD requires a midincision EST (m-EST) rather than a full incision. After m-EST, large balloon dilation (diameter 15–20 mm) is performed and the removal of the bile duct stone is completed (Table 3). EPLBD is believed to have a lower risk of bleeding and perforation than full EST, as well as a lower risk of serious pancreatitis than EPBD (Table 4). One possible reason why pancreatitis does not often occur is that the preceding m-EST may shift the expansive force more toward the CBD rather than the pancreas orifice. Ersoz et al. [8] first introduced this method in 2003, but it did not attract attention at that time. It seemed that surgeons were worried about serious complications such as severe pancreatitis and bile duct perforation caused after large balloon inflation. However, recent data from various institutes in

TABLE 3. Outcome of EST plus EPLBD and EST from Pospective Random Trial.

	Heo 2007 [9]	Minami 2007 [10]	Lee 2007 [11]
EST + EPLBD (n)	100	88	55
EST (n)	100		
Sex (M/F) (EST + EPLBD)	48/52	47/41	21/34
Sex (M/F) (EST)	50/50		
Mean age (EST + EPLBD)	64.4 ± 12.8	74 ± 17	70.8 ± 11.8
Mean age (EST)	62.8 ± 15.7		
Stone number (EST + EPLBD)	2.7 ± 2.7	2.5 ± 3.5	2.4 ± 0.4
Stone number (EST)	2.2 ± 1.9		
Stone D. (mm) (EST + EPLBD)	16 ± 0.7	14 ± 3.4	20.8 ± 5.6
Stone D. (mm) (EST)	15 ± 0.7		
Success on 1st sess (EST + EPLBD)	83/100 (83%)	87/88 (99%)	—
Success on 1st sess (EST)	87/100 (87%)	—	—
Overall success (EST + EPLBD)	97/100 (97%)	87/88 (99%)	55/55 (100%)
Overall success (EST)	98/100 (98%)		
Mech lithotripsy (EST + EPLBD)	8/100 (8%)	0/88 (0%)	3/55 (5%)
Mech lithotripsy (EST)	9/100 (9%)		

TABLE 4. Procedure-related Complications EST plus EPLBD and EST from Prospective Randomized Trial.

	Heo 2007 [9]	Minami 2007 [10]	Lee 2007 [11]
Pancreatitis (EST + EPLBD)	4/100	1/88	0/55
Pancreatitis (EST)	4/100		
Bleeding (EST + EPLBD)	0/100	1/88	2/55
Bleeding (EST)	2/100		
Cholecystitis (EST + EPLBD)	1/100	1/88	—
Cholecystitis (EST)	1/100		

Korea [9,11] suggest that it is an effective procedure that does not cause complications if performed under strictly established guidelines.

The main purpose of this procedure is to avoid or lessen the use of EML for removing a large common bile duct stone. The additional aims of this method are to reduce the complication rate by avoiding full-incision EST, shorten the time required for the procedure, and minimize the complications associated with EML.

The patients targeted for this method are those who already have a dilated CBD due to a large CBD stone. Patients with a CBD diameter of less than 10 mm because of a small stone would not be suitable candidates for the procedure. For the same reason, patients with stricture at the distal CBD due to repeated cholangitis would be excluded because of the possibility of perforation because of the large balloon dilation required.

The m-EST is performed up to the transverse fold of the papilla using a pull-type sphincterotome. Using the guidewire, the large balloon dilator (controlled radial expansion dilatation (CRE) balloon, Boston Scientific Microvasive, Cork, Ireland) is inserted into the bile duct. This balloon was originally used as an esophageal and pyloric dilator. We used 15–18-mm balloons, and their diameter was adjusted by the amount of pressure applied. A 15-mm balloon was expanded to the maximal diameter of from 15 mm (45 Psi) to 18 mm (150 Psi), and an 18-mm balloon from 18 mm (45 Psi) to 20 mm (90 Psi). The ability to alter the balloon pressure helps to adjust the balloon size according to the size of the stone and the bile duct. After the midportion of the balloon is positioned in the papilla orifice, balloon expansion is started gradually, and contrast media diluted with saline is used to slowly fill the balloon while monitoring the inflation process via fluoroscopy. To complete balloon dilation, only a small amount of pressure should be applied relative to the balloon's maximum pressure. A large balloon dilator is capable of the three distinct diameters listed on the package and hub labels. Inflation of the balloon to the pressure corresponding to the smallest balloon diameter is performed, and this should be maintained until the desired dilation is achieved. To achieve a larger balloon diameter, the pressure should be increased as indicated. If the balloon notch cannot be resolved with a pressure that is 80% of the maximum inflation pressure listed on the catheter hub, there is no need to increase the balloon pressure further to avoid perforation. The balloon notch readily disappears in the process of inflation of the CBD diameter as for the large balloon diameter. When the notch disappears, the inflation reached should be maintained for 30–60 s.

After inflation is complete, the papilla orifice will have been shaped into a large round hole. In many cases, the hole becomes large enough to observe the mucosa of the distal CBD, but if this is the case it indicates that the distal CBD and papillary orifice are dilated as much as the CBD. Ultimately, the bile duct gains a uniform cylindrical shape from the upper part of the bile duct to the papillary orifice, and when it is in this state a bile duct stone can easily be removed by balloon or basket (Fig. 1). If the size of the stone is small, it can easily be removed using endoscopic suction after the deflation of the balloon. After performing EST, the shape of the papillary orifice will be triangular and the distal CBD will be narrow. After inflating the balloon, however, the papillary orifice will take the shape of a large round hole and gain a cylindrical configuration without a narrowing of the distal CBD (Fig. 2).

The safety of this procedure is very great in patients with dilated bile ducts due to the prolonged existence of a stone because the distal bile duct, including papilla, has already been enlarged.

During the initial trials of this procedure, the occurrence of pancreatitis was of much concern because such a large balloon was used, but in practice not a single case of pancreatitis was observed. One possible reason why pancreatitis did not occur is that the preceding m-EST procedure may shift the expansive force more toward the CBD rather than the pancreas orifice. The inflation time was set at about 30–70 s, but within this time, pancreatitis was not induced. However, once the notch of the balloon disappears, there is no need to maintain inflation.

The most serious complication in EPLBD is perforation, and to prevent this, patients receiving the procedure must be very carefully screened. For patients undergoing EPLBD, their CBD must be dilated sufficiently by the stone, and the CBD should have no tight and/or long stricture. During the procedure, if the balloon notch does not easily widen because of considerable stricture of the bile duct, additional pressure should not be applied to the balloon. In such a case, it would be wise to use EML (Fig. 3). Furthermore, in some patients, the stone cannot be removed even with a fully

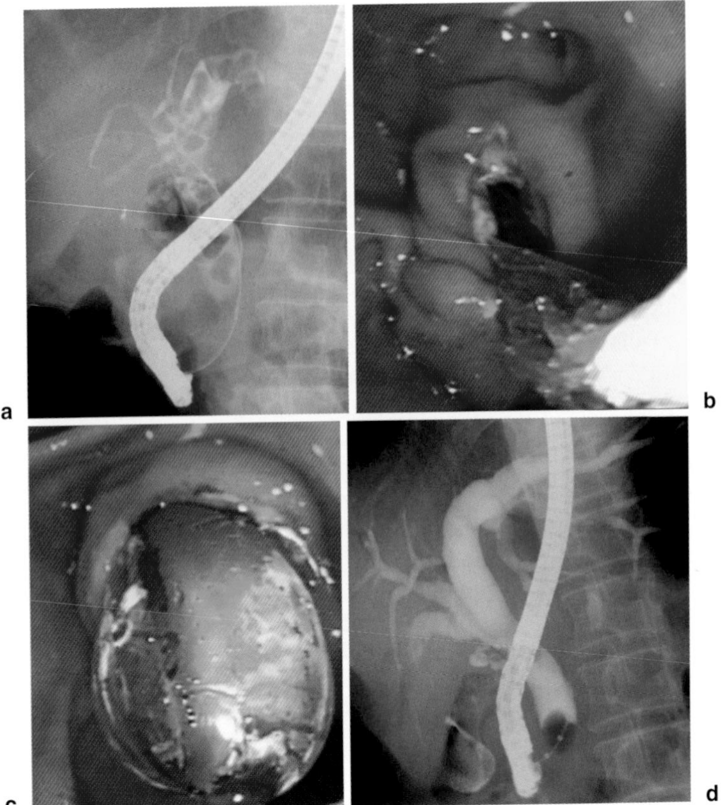

Fig. 1. **a** Multiple large stones in the common bile duct (CBD) and left intrahepatic duct. **b,c** Dilation of ampulla by an 18-mm balloon after mid-endoscopic sphincterotomy (mid-EST). **d** Multiple stones can easily be removed by balloon and basket in a short time without using endoscopic mechanical lithotripsy (EML)

dilated balloon owing to the excessive size of the stone. Again, for the safety of the patient, stone fragmentation should be used in such a case to break up the stones prior to removal. Because the balloon is used after m-EST, and with continuous observation of the intact unincised papillary tissue throughout the procedure, there is minimal risk of retroperitoneal perforation if the application of high balloon pressure can be avoided. If retroperitoneal perforation occurs after the procedure, an immediate operation is required in most cases owing to major complications.

There is no need to worry about bleeding during an m-EST. Even if a small amount of bleeding does occur, the subsequent balloon inflation will easily control it. The m-EST ballooning itself cannot fully remove the risk of bleeding, but compared with a full EST, it is assumed that an accident such as cutting a major vessel of the papilla roof would be very rare. In our experience, there was no major bleeding while EPLBD took place. However, after the use of m-EST and EPLBD, there is a possibility of delayed bleeding. Delayed bleeding may occur if the procedure is terminated without

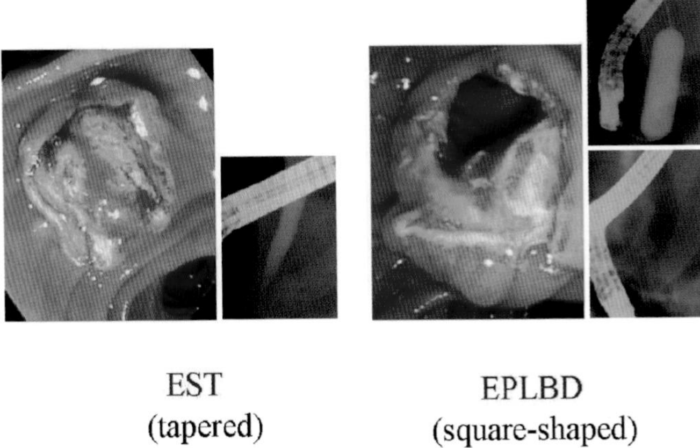

Fig. 2. *Left* Ampulla and distal CBD. The distal CBD is still in a tapered shape after an ampulla incision. *Right* Ampulla and distal CBD after mid-EST and 18-mm balloon dilation. The ampulla is wide open and the distal CBD is in a tubular shape. The endoscopic retrograde cholangiopancreatography (ERCP) picture shows an air biliarygram after endoscopic papillary large balloon dilatation (EPLBD)

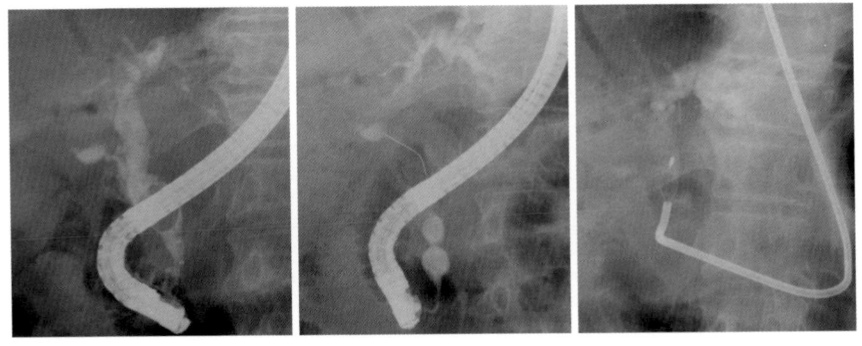

Fig. 3. **a** A large stone in the CBD. **b** Full inflation of the balloon was not possible owing to the stricture of the distal CBD. **c** The stone was removed by MLT, since EPLBD was not an appropriate way to remove the stone in this case

confirming complete hemostasis when there is bleeding during ERCP, or if the injured vessel is compressed for a certain period of time with a ballooning effect. In order to avoid delayed bleeding, careful observation of the source of the delayed bleeding around the dilated papillary orifice should be carried out after the procedure.

It has not yet been determined whether EPLBD can be used safely on patients with a bleeding tendency or liver cirrhosis. Compared with EST, EPLBD with a small balloon was found to be safe on patients with a bleeding tendency, but there is no guarantee that EPLBD will always be safe for patients with an increased bleeding risk. One report, by Ki et al. [12], showed that a large CBD stone could be removed by

EPLBD alone without m-EST. Complete stone clearance was possible in 28 patients without EST. These important data demonstrate that the application of a large balloon is possible without EST. Therefore this method would be feasible for patients with large bile duct stones who are at risk of bleeding.

SOD function is not preserved after ELPBD, and results in an even worse condition than after EST. The pressure gradient between the CBD and the duodenum is believed to be eliminated after EPLBD, as it is after surgical sphincteroplasty. However, it seems that ascending cholangitis induced by the reflux of the duodenal contents into the bile duct is not likely to occur after the procedure. Bile flow and the minimal pressure gradient between the CBD and the duodenum appear to recover some time after the procedure.

In our experience, EPLBD can be safely carried out on patients with anatomic alterations, such as periampullary diverticulum, and on patients who have had Billroth II operations. An additional incision in the remaining papillary roof is required to remove the stone when there is a recurrence of large stones in patients with a history of EST. In many cases it is hard to decide on the upper margin of this incision, but even in this type of situation EPLBD can be applied. There is a possibility in every case that complete resolution of the balloon notch cannot be achieved in the course of ballooning because of a scarring change of the incised orifice. Forceful contrast media injection is not recommended in this situation.

This procedure is performed to treat benign disease. Although it is effective, it is important to ensure that there are no procedure-related complications, especially any that could be lethal. Strict candidate screening, the avoidance of forced procedures, and immediate conversion to an alternative procedure, such as EML, should be undertaken if any difficulty is encountered during surgery.

References

1. Staritz M, Ewe K, Myer zum Buschenfelde KH (1982) Endoscopic papillary dilatation: a possible alternative to endoscopic papillotomy. Lancet 1:1306–1307
2. May GR, Cotton PB, Edmunds SE, et al. (1993) Removal of stones from the bile duct in ERCP without sphincterotomy. Gastrointest Endosc 39:749–754
3. Bergman JJGHM, Rauws EAJ, Fockens P, et al. (1997) Randomized trial of endoscopic balloon dilation versus endoscopic sphincterotomy for removal of bileduct stones. Lancet 349:1124–1129
4. Baron TH, Harewood GC (2004) Endoscopic balloon dilation of the biliary sphincter compared to endoscopic biliary sphincterotomy for removal of common bile duct stones during ERCP: a metaanalysis of randomized, controlled trials. Am J Gastroenterol 99:1455–1460
5. Tanaka S, Sawayama T, Yoshioka T (2004) Endoscopic papillary balloon dilation and endoscopic sphincterotomy for bile duct stones: long-term outcomes in a prospective randomized controlled trial. Gastrointest Endosc 59:614–618
6. Disario JA, Freeman ML, Bjorkman DJ, et al. (2004) Endoscopic balloon dilation compared with sphincterotomy for extraction of bile duct stones. Gastroenterology 127:1291–1299
7. Watanabe H, Yoneda M, Tominaga K, et al. (2007) Comparison between endoscopic papillary balloon dilation and endoscopic sphincterotomy for the treatment of common bile duct stones. J Gastroenterol 42:56–62

8. Ersoz G, Tekesin O, Ozutemiz AO, et al. (2003) Biliary sphincterotomy plus dilation with a large balloon for bile duct stones that are difficult to extract. Gastrointest Endosc 57:156–159
9. Heo JH, Kang DH, Jung HJ, et al. (2007) Endoscopic sphincterotomy plus large-balloon dilation versus endoscopic sphincterotomy for removal of bile-duct stones. Gastrointest Endosc 66:720–726
10. Minami A, Hirose S, Nomoto T, et al. (2007) Small sphincterotomy combined with papillary dilation with large balloon permits retrieval of large stones without mechanical lithotripsy. World J Gastroenterol 13:2179–2182
11. Lee DK, Lee BJ, Hwang SJ, et al. (2007) Endoscopic papillary large balloon dilation after endoscopic sphincterotomy for treatment of large common bile duct stone. Dig Endosc 19:S52–S56
12. Ki SH, Jeong SJ, Lee DH, et al. (2006) Large balloon sphincteroplasty without preceding endoscopic sphincteroplasty for the treatment of large bile duct stone. Gastroenterology 63:AB290 (Abstract W1407)

Future Prospects of ERCP from the Product Development Standpoint

Yasuo Miyano

Introduction

Endoscopic retrograde cholangiopancreatography (ERCP) is primarily aimed at the management of biliary stones and the treatment of jaundice, and is a procedure performed using endoscopic therapeutic devices with varied technical features and functions because they need to overcome clinical and anatomical variations. Therefore, it is necessary for physicians and nurses to acquire great skill and knowledge about how to use these various devices.

Concept and Design of Typical Therapeutic Devices

The V-system is a complete ERCP system that integrates the endoscope and various therapeutic devices. The concepts of the V-system are to "simplify catheter exchange," "realize complete control by the endoscopist," and "improve efficiency."

As a means to put these concepts into practice, we have adopted mechanisms of "fixation of the guidewire to the scope," "fixation of the catheter to the scope," and "improvements in the basic performance of individual therapeutic devices."

The mechanism of locking the guidewire has helped to minimize the need for the physician and assistant to work in close collaboration no matter what kind of catheter is used. The mechanism of locking the catheter has enabled the endoscopist to control the guidewire or sphinctectome completely, and adjust the balloon size even in difficult cases where fine manipulations of the guidewire are required.

Future Prospects

In ERCP, many challenges remain to be overcome in order to make progress in the development of the endoscope and related therapeutic devices. This requires enhanced efficiency and solving difficult problems. It is because of the functional limitations of the therapeutic devices that so many kinds of devices exist. When new devices that offer more reliable procedures can be developed, both the procedures and the devices can be standardized. For example, a tube stent and a metal stent exist for the treatment of jaundice. The tube stent is easy to exchange but has short-term patency. On the other hand, the metal stent has long patency but is

Therapeutic Products Development Department, Olympus Medical Systems Corp., 2951 Ishikawa-cho, Hachioji, Tokyo 192-8507, Japan difficult to exchange. To improve the quality of life (QOL) of patients still further, a new stent must be developed that facilitates device exchange and offers long-term patency. Such a stent will be developed in the near future, whether on a tube, metal, or other basis. It is also known that research will move forward to develop more curative treatments of cancers using advanced drug eluting techniques.

In the mean time, ERCP is a procedure which is difficult to perform and takes time and effort on the part of physicians and assistants to acquire the necessary skills and techniques. The development of a simulation device would help them to do so.

Papillectomy

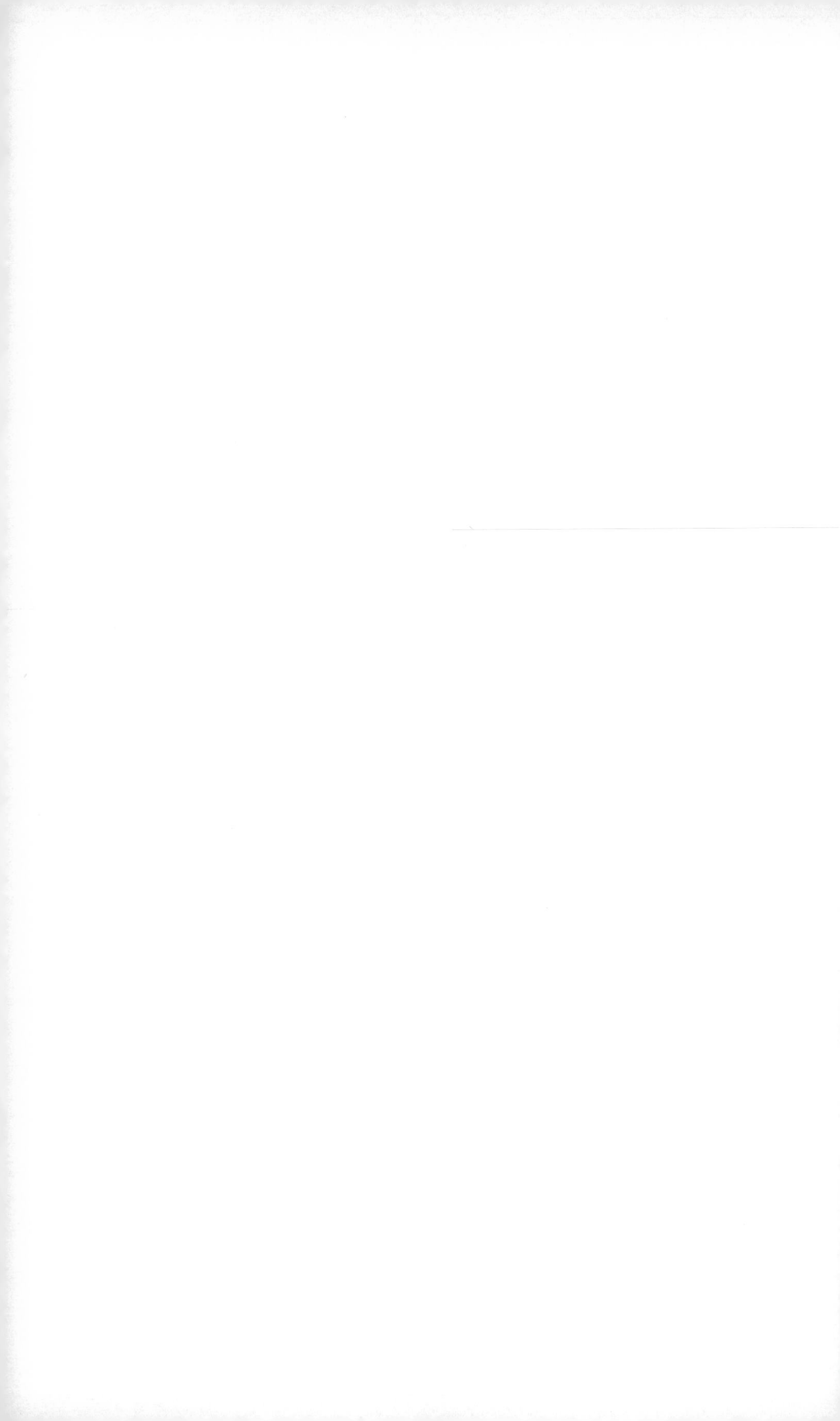

Endoscopic Diagnosis and Resection Therapy of the Tumor of the Major Duodenal Papilla

Akihiro Itoh[1], Yoshiki Hirooka[2], and Hidemi Goto[1]

Summary. Endoscopic ultrasonography and intraductal ultrasonography (IDUS) are useful for diagnosing tumor extension of the major duodenal papilla. Especially, IDUS makes it possible to diagnose early cancer that has never been correctly diagnosed by other modalities. On the other hand, we think that endoscopic resection therapy of the tumor that is benign adenoma or early cancer may be initially selected as a curative treatment similar to endoscopic mucosal resection for early gastric or colonic cancer. Between 1993 and 2007, 91 patients with tumor of the duodenal major papilla underwent endoscopic resection therapy at our institute. The indication for this therapy was defined as a case with adenoma or early cancer without infiltration into the bile and pancreatic ducts. The tumors were resected in a radical fashion using pure cutting current. Temporary endoscopic pancreatic duct stenting could prevent acute pancreatitis, which is important as an early complication. We have a few cases with late complications, but they were improved conservatively in all cases. We think that endoscopic resection therapy can be assessed as a safe and curative treatment of adenoma of the major duodenal papilla. In addition, it is occasionally estimated as a curative therapy for early cancer.

Key words. Duodenal papilla, Diagnosis, Endoscopic resection, IDUS, EUS

Introduction

The tumor of the major duodenal papilla is not a tumor that we meet clinically with high frequency. However, we often find patients with early cancer or adenoma of the major papilla, because the number of people having medical checkups and of endoscopists with awareness of such tumors are presently increasing. In addition, endoscopic resection therapy for these conditions is receiving much attention.

As diagnostic methods for the tumor of the papilla, we have endoscopy (duodenoscopy), roentgenography (duodenography), extracorporeal ultrasonography (US),

[1]Department of Gastroenterology, Nagoya University Graduate School of Medicine, 65 Tsuruma-cho, Showa, Nagoya 466-8550, Japan

[2]Department of Endoscopy, Nagoya University Hospital, Nagoya, Japan

computed tomography (CT), endoscopic ultrasonography (EUS), endoscopic retrograde cholangiopancreatography (ERCP), intraductal ultrasonography (IDUS), and so on. The development of these modalities improves the precision of diagnosing the tumor. Especially, IDUS is the only modality that makes it possible to diagnose early cancer of the papilla, and it is very useful for determining the indication of endoscopic resection therapy.

Endoscopic resection therapy of the tumor was reported as palliative therapy for advanced cancer cases long ago, and some reports of this as curative therapy for adenoma have appeared recently. This therapy has not become widespread yet because the prevalence of disease at the duodenal major papilla is relatively low. Therefore, sufficient evidence has not yet been obtained about the indications or safety of this procedure.

In addition, the reason why this procedure is not estimated as equal in position to endoscopic mucosal resection therapy in other gastrointestinal tract locations has resulted from the lack of establishment of safety and of diagnostic strategy.

We have tackled diagnosing tumors of the papilla more precisely by using IDUS and performing endoscopic resection of the tumor since 1993 [1,2]. We show how to diagnose the tumor of the papilla in the first half of this chapter and how to resect the tumor in the latter half.

Diagnosis

Endoscopy

Adenoma and cancer account for the majority of tumors of the major duodenal papilla. Cancer of the papilla is classified into four types (mass-forming type, ulceration type, mixed type, and others) according to the endoscopic findings in the Japanese rules [3]. There are two subtypes (tumor-exposed type, nonexposed type) in tumors of the mass-forming type. The mixed type indicates a mass-forming tumor with ulceration.

Tumors of the papilla are often detected in cases without jaundice as well as cases with obstructive jaundice. We see these tumors when we perform endoscopy or upper gastrointestinalgraphy as a medical checkup or screening, or with ERCP for other purposes. Most such asymptomatic cases are adenoma or early cancer, which we can resect endoscopically. Close observation with the endoscope is important to detect those tumors.

We have to distinguish a tumor from a nontumor lesion endoscopically, because it is not always easy to diagnose lesions of the duodenal papillary region accurately using biopsy specimens. Furthermore, we also need to distinguish adenoma from cancer. The tumor surface of adenoma shows discoloration or a reddish color, and a typical adenoma shows discoloration (Fig. 1). On the other hand, that of cancer shows a reddish color in almost all cases, so we can recognize that the discolored tumor indicates adenoma. The case with adenoma, whose surface shows reddish, is not always distinguished easily from cancer. We can sometimes find a small reddish part or a small erosion in the discolored tumor. It is a point to notice because there is a strong probability that those findings show the existence of cancer in the lesions. In addition, it is important information when we obtain the biopsy specimens.

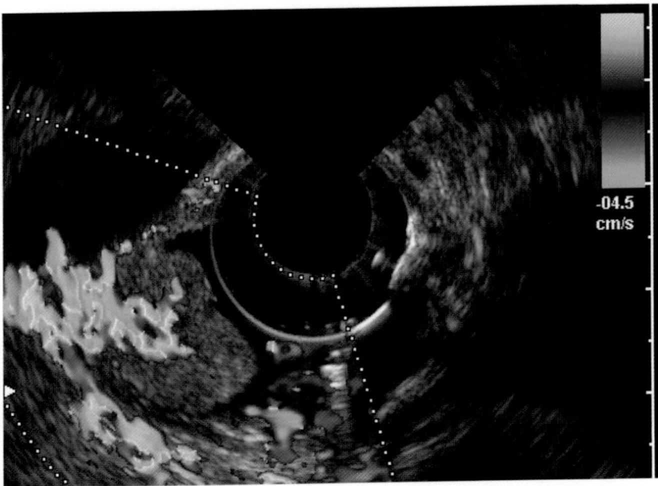

Fig. 6. Contrast-enhanced endoscopic ultrasonography (CE-EUS) image of the adenoma case clearly shows the vessels flowing into the tumor

oral side of the tumor in most cases. It is important to observe the outflow of the bile and pancreatic juice carefully around this areas before first touching with the catheter. Generally, a filling defect or irregularity and stenosis of the papillary bile or pancreatic duct on the ERCP image show tumor ductal infiltration and invasion to the bile duct or pancreatic parenchyma, respectively.

We usually perform ERCP followed by IDUS. We previously reported the clinical usefulness of the IDUS system, which was developed to visualize arterial structures, in diagnosing tumors of the major duodenal papilla [1,2]. IDUS images of the major papillary region can be obtained by inserting the IDUS probe into the bile or pancreatic duct via the major papilla. Because IDUS has a higher frequency than EUS, Oddi's muscle layer is demonstrated as a hypoechoic layer around the bile duct and the pancreatic duct. The tumor depth of invasion is diagnosed according to the spatial relationship between the tumor echo and the basic structures, which include Oddi's muscle layer and the duodenal muscularis propria layer visualized as hypoechoic layers. Eighty-five cancer patients who received IDUS performed preoperatively underwent surgical resection in our institute. Diagnosing accuracy in evaluating tumor extension was 82.5% (66/85). IDUS is the only modality that can demonstrate Oddi's muscle layer as one layer. Therefore, IDUS made it possible to diagnose early cancer of the major duodenal papilla. It is clear that IDUS has an advantage on this point compared with EUS. Furthermore, tumor infiltration into the bile or pancreatic duct is clearly demonstrated as an echogenic papillary tumor in the duct (Figs. 7, 8). IDUS also has a higher accuracy rate than EUS in diagnosing tumor infiltration beyond the common duct. We think that IDUS is a most reliable modality in diagnosing tumor extension, and it is a indispensable modality in determining the indication of endoscopic resection therapy for a tumor of the major duodenal papilla.

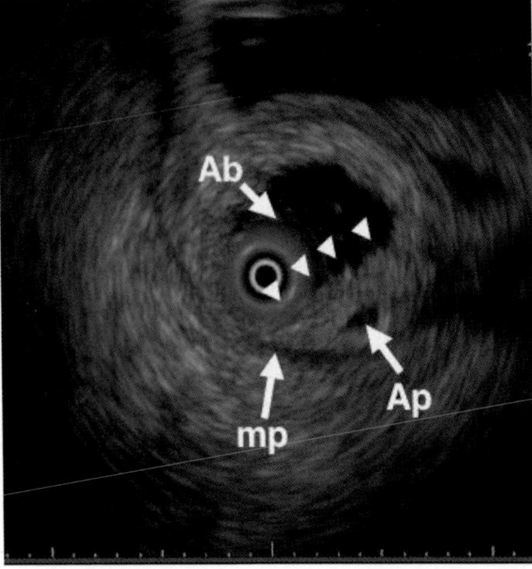

Fig. 7. Intraductal ultrasonography (IDUS) image of the same case as in Fig. 2 shows the minute papillary projections (*arrowheads*) in the ampullary bile duct (*Ab*). *Ap*, ampullary pancreatic duct; *mp*, muscularis propria

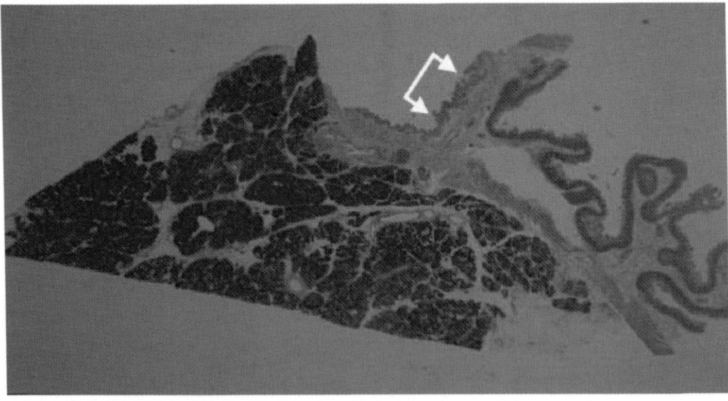

Fig. 8. Histopathological findings of the same case as Fig. 7 show that a small papillary cancer is spreading along the ampullary bile duct (*arrows*)

Endoscopic Resection Therapy

Indication

Tumor ductal infiltration into the bile duct or the pancreatic duct limited to the site where the ducts penetrate the muscularis propria layer is a necessary condition, because endoscopic resection is limited to this level in theory. The idea that the indication of endoscopic resection therapy for the tumor of the major duodenal papilla is limited to adenoma without tumor infiltration into the bile or pancreatic duct is generally accepted at present. However, the indication is set for adenoma or early cancer without ductal infiltration in our institute. We think that the case with adenoma or cancer in adenoma derived from the ampullary duodenum is a good indication.

Standard Procedure

The standard procedure of endoscopic resection therapy in our institute is shown below. We usually carry out the therapy in the roentgen room under the same premedication as ERCP. Normal duodenoscopes are usually used for this procedure. We use the normal snare with hooks or the special-order hard snare made of monofilament for excision. In late years we have mainly used the latter, with which we can obtain a larger and thicker resected specimen. First, we look up at the tumor and hang the snare into the anal side from the oral side on the occasion of excision (Fig. 9). Next, we usually try to resect the tumor en bloc with cutting current during cauterization (Fig. 10). One of the reasons we use a cutting current is that long-time exposure to electricity can cause acute pancreatitis.

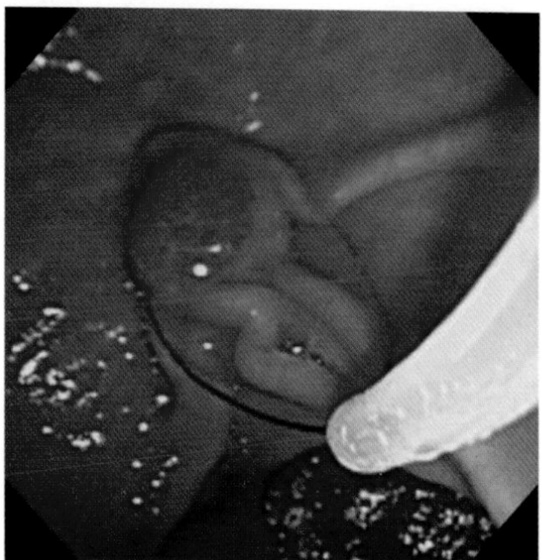

Fig. 9. Endoscopic finding on the occasion of an excision shows that the snare, made of monofilament, is hung into the anal side from the oral side

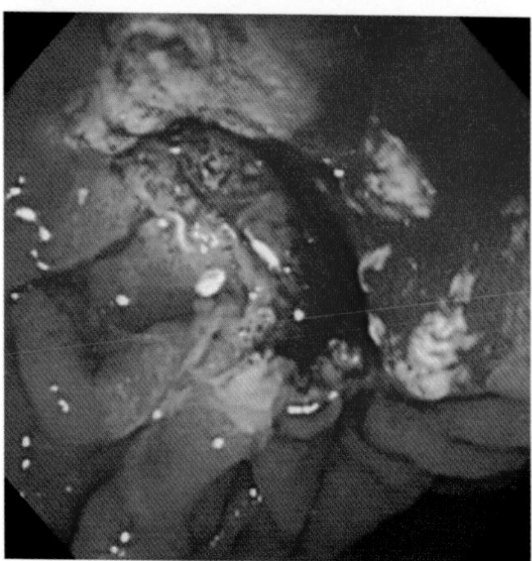

Fig. 10. Endoscopic finding just after the excision shows hemorrhage from the anal side of the excision plane

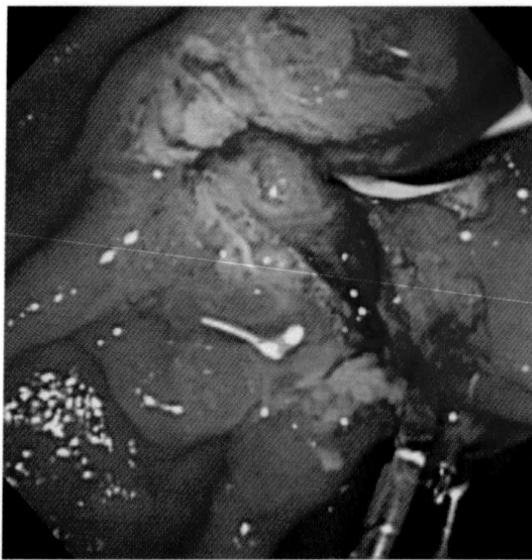

Fig. 11. Endoscopic finding shows that hemostasis is performed with clipping, and the guidewire is inserted into the pancreatic duct. The orifice of the bile duct is also seen on the posterior side close to the orifice of the pancreatic duct

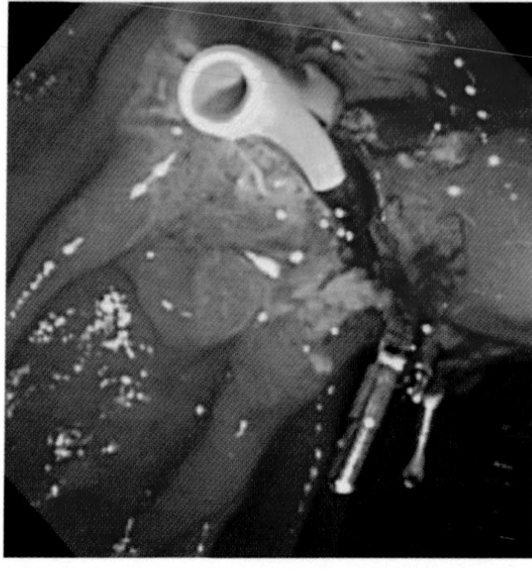

Fig. 12. Endoscopic finding showing the pancreatic tube stent placed sequentially

Local injection of materials such as physiological saline into the submucosa is not recommended, because only the surrounding mucosa, but not the lesion, is lifted and the procedure becomes rather difficult at the duodenal papillary region. We can usually see the orifices of the bile and the pancreatic ducts separately at the oral side of the section and perform pancreatic stent placement sequentially. Unless the stent is placed into the pancreatic duct, acute pancreatitis occurs at a high rate in cases with poor function of the minor papilla in our experience. Hemostasis is followed by stent placement if the bleeding is observed. Injection therapy of hypertonic saline with epinephrine is effective for slight bleeding. Clipping is more effective for spurting hemorrhage (Figs. 11, 12).

Outcome

Between September 1993 and September 2007, we performed endoscopic resection therapy for 91 patients with tumor of the major duodenal papilla. Among 91 excision cases, the results of 86 cases, except for 5 that were not tumorous lesions as final diagnosis, are shown below.

The complete resection rate was 69.8% when we defined the case with no tumor tissue at both the horizontal and vertical edge as complete excision on the resected specimen. Sixteen of the patients were not indicated as cases that had bile duct or pancreatic duct infiltration or advanced cancer. The true complete resection rate, excluding these, was evaluated as 85.7%. Finally, the tumor-free rate was 96.6% of all patients with neoplasms.

Three cases of serial observations demonstrated local recurrences in 6 months, 5 years 5 months, and 5 years 7 months after endoscopic resection, surgical resection, or endoscopic therapy was performed, respectively. We think that it may be controversial to regard our indication criteria as optimal from these results.

Safety

Early Complication

Perforation, bleeding, pancreatitis, and cholangitis are early complications. The results in our institute were 0%, 27.5%, 6.6%, and 3.3%, respectively. Endoscopic hemostases were successful, and blood transfusion was not required in any bleeding cases. The occurrence rate of acute pancreatitis has been decreasing since we tried pancreatic duct stenting in 1997.

Late Complication

As late complications, we had cholangitis (4.4%), bile duct stones (2.2%), acute cholecystitis (1.1%), bile duct obstruction (1/1%), and pancreatic duct stricture (1/1%). These cases were improved conservatively or endoscopically in all cases.

From the analysis of both early and late complications, endoscopic resection therapy may be evaluated as being a safe procedure.

Conclusion

The major duodenal papilla is a part of the intestine and the pancreatobiliary tract. Therefore, endoscopic and ultrasonographic approaches similar to those for intestinal lesions and pancreatobiliary lesions are required for diagnosing tumor of the papilla precisely. Especially, endoscopic findings and IDUS accurate diagnosis of the tumor extent are very important for determination of endoscopic resection therapy.

Our procedure of endoscopic resection therapy can be assessed as a safe and curative treatment of tumor of the major duodenal papilla.

References

1. Itoh A, Tsukamoto Y, Naitoh Y, et al (1994) Intraductal ultrasonography for the examination of duodenal papillary region. J Ultrasound Med 13:679–684
2. Itoh A, Goto H, Naitoh Y, et al (1997) Intraductal ultrasonography in diagnosing tumor extension of cancer of the papilla of Vater. Gastrointest Endosc 45:251–260

3. Japanese Society of Biliary Surgery (2003) General rules for surgical and pathological studies on cancer of the biliary tract (in Japanese). Kanehara Shuppan, Tokyo
4. Gono K, Yamazaki K, Doguchi N, et al (2003) Endoscopic observation of tissue by narrow band illumination. Opt Rev 10:1–5
5. Itoh A, Hirooka Y, Goto H, et al (2007) Endoscopic approach to the pancreatobiliary tract using narrow band imaging. Dig Endosc 19:S115–S120
6. Yasuda K, Mukai H, Cho E, et al (1988) The use of endoscopic ultrasonography in the diagnosis and staging of carcinoma of the papilla of Vater. Endoscopy 20:218–222
7. Mitake M, Nakazawa S, Tsukamoto Y, et al (1990) Endoscopic ultrasonography in the diagnosis of depth invasion and lymph node metastasis of carcinoma of the papilla of Vater. J Ultrasound Med 9:645–650
8. Niwa K, Hirooka Y, Itoh A, et al (2003) Preclinical study of endoscopic ultrasonography with electronic radial scanning echoendoscope. J Gastroenterol Hepatol 18:825–835
9. Kanamori A, Hirooka Y, Itoh A, et al (2006) Usefulness of contrast-enhanced endoscopic ultrasonography in the differentiation between malignant and benign lympadenopathy. Am J Gastroenterol 101:45–51

have four distal and proximal flaps to prevent the stent from migration. Reportedly, conventional stents can become occluded in the side hole of the PS or in the flap hole [3], but the DLS does not have a side hole, even in the flap portion. In addition, because there is no difference in the duration of stent patency between the 10 Fr. gauge and the 12 Fr. gauge [4], we used DLS with a bore diameter of 10 Fr. JF-260V, TJF-240, and TJF-260V (Olympus Medical Systems) scopes are used for placing the duodenal bend type.

Indications for EBS

In cases of malignant biliary stricture, various types of diagnostic imaging such as computed tomography (CT) and ultrasonography (US) are performed before endoscopic retrograde cholangiopancreatography (ERCP). In cases indicated for surgery (Table 1), ENBD or PS capable for extubation is placed for a short period before the surgery. An MS or PS is inserted when surgery is difficult or impossible for reasons such as aging or patient refusal. In cases of benign biliary stricture (including postoperative biliary damage), a PS capable of extubation is placed. Although a method of placing a MS has been reported, uncovered MS cannot be removed. Thus, the lumen in an uncovered MS stent becomes occluded by mucosal proliferation caused by hyperplasia [5], making an uncovered MS placement contraindicated in principle. A covered MS, which can be removed, is sometimes placed, but long-term placement produces a high frequency of proliferation caused by hyperplasia in the MS or complications such as cholecystitis or dislocation or migration of the MS [6]. Expansion using a large-caliber stent or placing multiple PS may be safer [7]. Thereby, a DLS, because of its shape, may be indicated for malignant or benign middle and distal common bile duct strictures.

TABLE 1. The indications of EBS.

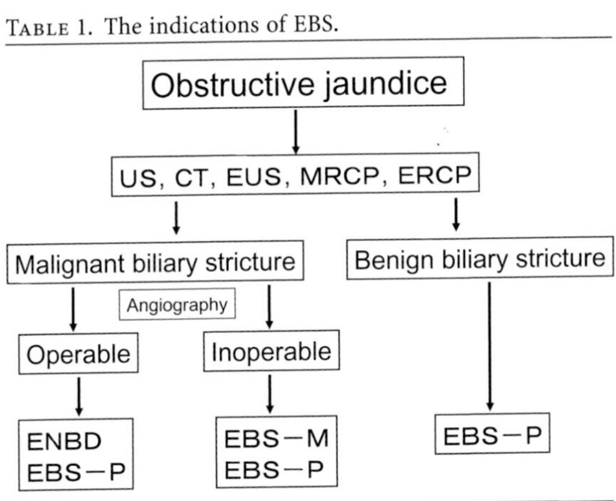

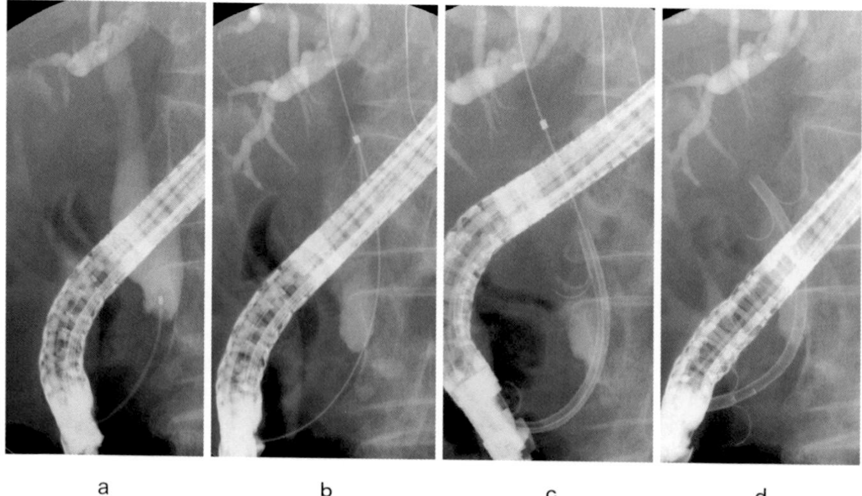

Fig. 2. Insertion methods of the Doublelayer stent (DLS). **a** The stricture in the lower common bile duct (CBD) caused by pancreatic head cancer. **b** The guiding tube inserted into CBD. **c** The DLS inserted into the CBD through guidetube. **d** The insertion of DLS was succeeded

How to Insert a DLS

Before an ERCP, abdominal CT, magnetic resonance cholangiopancreatography (MRCP), and so on are performed to determine the patient's status. Pharyngeal anesthesia and sedation are given in the same manner as for ERCP. Scopes such as the TJF-240 or TJF-260V are used. A cannula that can accept a 0.035-inch guidewire is selected. First, ERC is performed to determine the condition of the stricture (Fig. 2a). The guidewire and papillotome are then inserted together, and endoscopic sphincterotomy is performed in the major papilla.

In cases of severe stricture in the common bile duct, the biliary duct is first dilated using a biliary dilation catheter with a diameter of 5 to 10 Fr. The length of the stricture is measured, and a DLS that is slightly longer than the stricture's length is selected. As an example, for a stricture with a length of 45 mm, select a 50-mm DLS.

First, the DLS is loaded into the stent insertion device. The guidewire and guiding tube are then inserted (Fig. 2b). The DLS is then inserted, forwarding the pushing tube, fixing the guiding tube (Fig. 2c). During insertion of the DLS, a separate scope should be used for observing the duodenum so that the duodenal scope can follow (not apart from) the major papilla. When the DLS leaves the scope, the elevator of the duodenal scope is lowered and the DLS is pushed forward. Then, the DLS is inserted using the scope's up-angulation mechanism. When it is fluoroscopically confirmed that the tip of the DLS has passed over the edge of the stricture on the hepatic side, the guidewire and guiding tube are removed while keeping the pushing tube forward. This step completes DLS placement (Fig. 2d).

Table 1. Patient characteristics.

	CMS	UMS	
Cases	237	100	ns
Sex (M/F)	137/100	51/49	ns
Mean age	70.2	71.1	ns
Causative disease			ns
Pancreas ca.	161	59	
Bile duct ca.	35	18	
Metastatic nodes	24	11	
Gallbladder ca.	7	8	
Papillary ca.	9	4	

CMS, covered metallic stent; UMS, uncovered metallic stent; ca, cancer

Table 2. Results of covered metallic stent according to cancer type.

	Panc	BDC	MN	GBC	Papillary
Cases	161	35	24	7	9
Mean stent patency	160	168	207	200	271
Complications	71 (44%)	15 (43%)	3 (13%)	0 (0%)	3 (33%)
Stent obstruction	40 (25%)	11 (31%)	2 (8%)	0 (0%)	3 (33%)
Mean patency	139	216	147	—	175
Cause					
Tumor ingrowth	0	0	0	0	0
Tumor overgrowth	11 (7)	7 (20)	0	0	0
Sludge	14 (9)	2 (6)	2 (8)	0	1 (11)
Food scraps	11 (7)	2 (6)	0	0	2 (22)
Kink	4 (3)	0	0	0	0
Unknown	0	0	0	0	0
Other complications	31 (19%)	4 (11%)	1 (4%)	0 (0%)	0 (0%)
Cholecystitis	7 (4)	1 (3)	0	0	0
Pancreatitis	8 (5)	2 (6)	1 (4)	0	0
Migration	15 (9)	1 (3)	0	0	0

Panc, pancreas cancer; BDC, bile duct cancer; LNM, lymph node metastasis; GBC, gallbladder cancer; papillary; papillary cancer

occlusion by tumor overgrowth in bile duct cancer (20%) was higher than those of other types of cancer ($P = 0.02321$, pancreas cancer; $P = 0.0345$, metastatic nodes) (Table 2). We thought that pancreas cancer and metastatic nodes had a tendency to progress expansively, but that bile duct cancers progress longitudinally. Therefore, pancreas cancer and metastatic nodes were good indications for CMS. However, for bile duct cancer cases, we should treat with antitumor therapy, such as radiation or chemotherapy.

Resectable cases and benign stricture cases are considered to be a contraindication because of UMS embedded into bile duct wall and tumor tissues; the UMS cannot be removed. However, CMS could be removed as previously reported [7,8]. Then, indications were changed to include resectable and benign stricture cases using CMS.

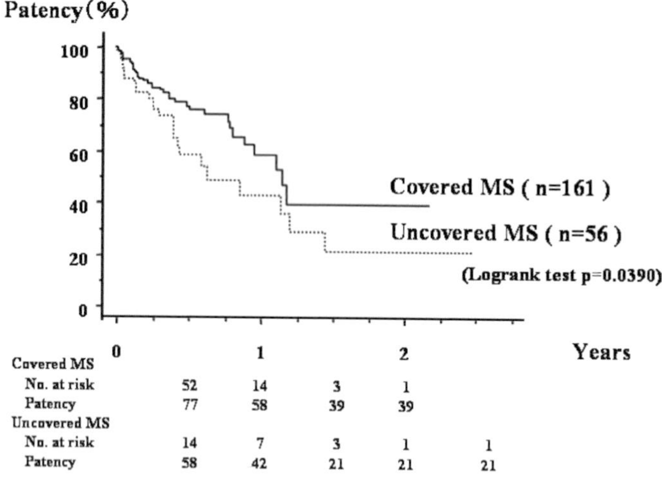

FIG. 2. Cumulative stent patency of pancreas cancer cases. *MS*, metallic stent

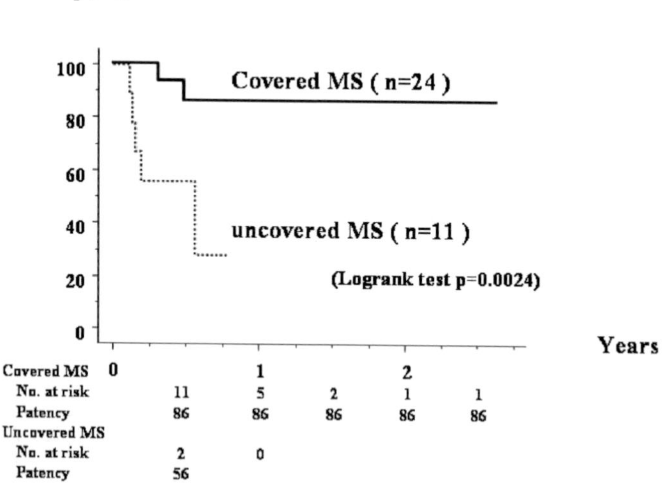

FIG. 3. Cumulative stent patency of metastatic nodes cases. *MS*, metallic stent

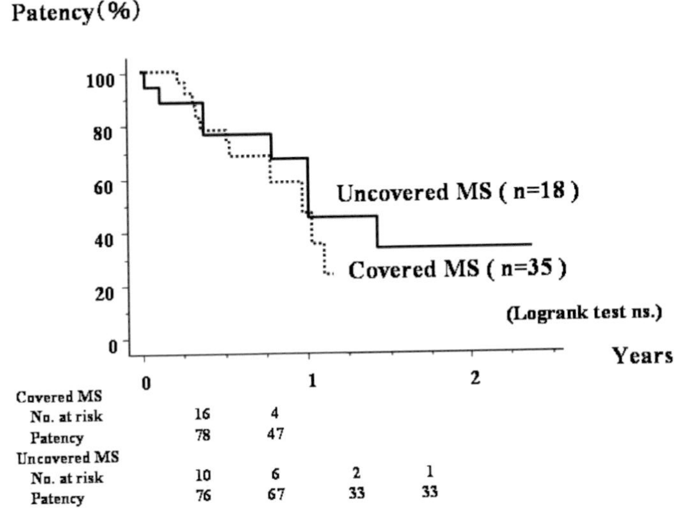

FIG. 4. Cumulative stent patency of bile duct cancer cases. *MS*, metallic stent

Prevention Strategy of Complications of CMS

We should select the CMS first, but have to resolve some problems. From our metallic stent placed in cases for distal malignant biliary obstruction, including RCT cases, CMS showed significantly longer patency, but also showed higher incidence of complications such as migration, pancreatitis, and cholecystitis. We considered that prevention of complications was the most important role.

From our experience, the results of CMS placement in each disease showed a different incidence of some complications (see Table 2). In pancreas cancer cases, high incidences of bile duct kinking, food impaction, sludge, and migration were observed. We reported that the ComVi stent, a newly developed CMS with low axial force, showed a very low incidence of bile duct kinking and migration (Figure 5) [9,10]. For pancreas cancer cases, we recommended ComVi stent placement.

We analyzed cholecystitis cases after metallic stent placement. It was said that obstruction of the orifice of the cystic duct by covered membrane caused cholecystitis. However, we previously reported that the independent risk factor of cholecystitis after metallic stent placement was tumor involvement of the orifice of the cystic duct (OCD), but not the presence of a covered membrane [11]. Table 4 shows the analysis of cholecystitis cases in our experience. OCD involvement cases showed a high incidence with both CMS and UMS; however, those of CMS were higher than UMS. ComVi stent showed a similar incidence rate of cholecystitis to UMS. We thought that the outer uncovered layer of ComVi stent might be effective for prevention of cholecystitis.

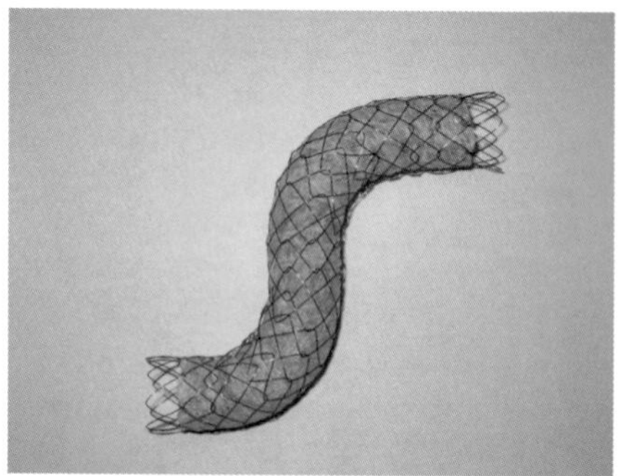

Fig. 5. ComVi stent (Niti-S stent, ComVi type; Taewoong Medical, Seoul, Korea). This stent has very low axial force (makes stent straight)

Table 3. Uni- and multivariate analysis of predicting factor of pancreatitis after CMS placement.

Risk factors	Univariate	Multivariate
Age (>70/<70)	0.2117	—
Sex (M/F)	0.5264	—
Causative disease	0.1540	—
Stricture portion (mid/lower)	>0.9999	—
MPD obstruction/intact	0.0200	0.0142
Covering of orifice of MPD (+/–)	0.6098	—
Insertion route (ERCP/PTBD)	0.4246	—
Across/above papilla	0.2142	—
Types of MS	0.0500	0.9613
Prior procedure for papilla (None/EPBD/EST)	0.0990	—

MPD, main pancreatic duct

Table 4. Analysis of cholecystitis after metallic stent placement.

	Covered MS				Uncovered MS		
	PCD	PCW	SCW	CV	UD	UW	SM
Cases	57	21	133	47	58	32	19
Cholecystitis (%)	3 (5)	1 (5)	7 (5)	1 (2)	1 (2)	0	2 (11)
OCD Involvement (+)	14	3	24	16	14	—	12
Cholecystitis (%)	3 (21)	1 (33)	6 (25)	1 (6)	1 (7)	—	2 (17)

OCD, orifice of cystic duct; PCD, polyurethane-covered Diamond stent; PCW, polyurethane-covered Wallstent; SCW, silicone-covered Wallstent; CV, ComVi stent; UD, uncovered Diamond stent; UW, uncovered Wallstent; SM, SMART stent

Pancreatitis was one of the most severe complications at endoscopic retrograde cholangiopancreatography (ERCP) and its related procedures. The independent risk factor of pancreatitis after CMS placement was absence of tumor obstruction of the main pancreatic duct (MPD) (see Table 3). In the intact MPD cases, the incidence of pancreatitis was 37.5% in no prior procedure cases, 22.7% in endoscopic papillary balloon dilation (EPBD), and 0% in EST cases, respectively. Thus, we recommend EST before CMS placement in intact MPD cases.

Knack of Endoscopic MS Placement

The delivery system of the MS is very stiff and difficult to insert into the papilla. While inserting the MS into the papilla, usage of an up-angle to get near to the papilla and adjust the angle to the bile duct is important. For passing the stricture, the important point is insertion of a stiff guidewire that is as long as possible. Scope manipulation is also important to increase insertion force, such as using an up-angle, twisting the scope to the left, and pulling the scope to get close to the papilla. The MS should be released slowly to place it in a precise position and should be adjusted by scope manipulation.

Indication for Hilar Obstruction Cases

For patients with hilar malignant biliary obstructions, we should select the UMS because of its longer patency compared to a plastic stent. However, there are few articles comparing the metallic stent with a plastic stent for hilar obstructed cases. Wagner et al. reported that UMS was superior to plastic stent by their randomized study [2]. Many articles reported that the patency of the UMS lasted longer than that of a plastic stent but that reintervention was difficult when the UMS had been occluded. We have to resolve this important problem and prove the advantages of the UMS.

Insertion Procedure and Stent Selection

Before ERCP, we should obtain an magnetic resonance cholangiopancreatography (MRCP) to decide the drainage area. Freeman et al. reported that a decision according to MRCP was very useful to avoid cholangitis [12]. We should select an area where the largest part of the liver could be drained and received portal venous flow. Freeman et al. did not use contrast media to select the area but used a guidewire according to previous MRCP. Chen et al. reported that an opacified but undrained area was the highest risk for cholangitis [13]. Thus, we select an adequate area without contrast media using a guidewire according to the previous MRCP.

To select an adequate branch, we use a hydrophilic coated guidewire (Radifocus M; Terumo, Tokyo, Japan). We think that an angle changeable tip catheter (Swing tip catheter; Olympus Medical Systems, Tokyo, Japan) is also useful to select a branch.

Preservation of the sphincter of Oddi is a very important factor for placing the metallic stent for hilar obstruction cases. Refluxed enteric juice may cause cholangitis at the undrained area. Therefore, we do not perform EST but EPBD, because it was reported that the function of sphincter of Oddi that received EPBD could be preserved [14]. We place the metallic stent above the papilla without EST.

What are the requirements for the metallic stent for a hilar lesion? The bile duct may be angled at the hilar lesion, and there are many branches to the upper hilar lesion. We do not select the Wallstent because of its large shortening ratio and strong axial force, which make the stent straight. We ordinary select the laser-cut type nitinol metallic stent with less axial force or a Y-type braided stent (Niti-S stent, Y-type; Taewoong Medical, Seoul, Korea) with a loose mesh portion at the center of the metallic stent. These metallic stents have weak axial force and easy to place as a partial stent in stent style through the mesh.

References

1. Davids PHP, Greon AK, Rauws EAJ, et al (1992) Randomized trial of self-expanding metal stents versus polyethylene stents for distal maliganant biliary obstruction. Lancet 340:1488–1492
2. Wagner HJ, Knyrim K, Vakil N, et al (1993) Plastic versus metallic stents in the palliative treatment of malignant hilar biliary obstruction. A prospective and randomized trial. Endoscopy 25:213–218
3. Isayama H, Komatsu Y, Tsujino T, et al (2002) Polyurethane-covered metal stent for management of distal malignant biliary obstruction. Gastrointest Endosc 55:366–370
4. Nakai Y, Isayama H, Komatsu Y, et al (2005) Efficacy and safety of covered Wallstent in patients with distal malignant biliary obstruction. Gastrointest Endosc 62:742–748
5. Kahaleh M, Tokar J, Conaway MR, et al (2005) Efficacy and complications of covered Wallstents in malignant distal biliary obstruction. Gastrointest Endosc 61:528–533
6. Isayama H, Komatsu Y, Tsujino T, et al (2004) A prospective randomized study of "covered" vs. "uncovered" Diamond stents for the management of distal malignant biliary obstruction. Gut 53:729–734
7. Kahaleh M, Tokar J, Le T, et al (2004) Removal of self-expandable metallic Wallstents. Gastrointest Endosc 40:640–644
8. Wasan SM, Ross WA, Staerkel GA, et al (2005) Use of expandable metallic biliary stents in resectable pancreatic cancer. Am J Gastroenterol 100:2056–2061
9. Isayama H, Nakai Y, Ito Y, et al (2007) A result with newly-developed covered metallic stent, ComVi Stent. Gastrointest Endosc 65:AB221
10. Isayama H, Nakai Y, Toyokawa Y, et al (2006) The investigation of radial and axial force in biliary metallic stent. Gastrointest Endosc 63:AB282
11. Isayama H, Kawabe T, Nakai Y, et al (2006) Cholecystitis after metallic stent placement in patients with malignant distal biliary obstruction. Clin Gastroenterol Hepatol 4:1148–1153
12. Freeman ML, Overby C (2003) Selective MRCP and CT-targeted drainage of malignant hilar biliary obstruction with self-expanding metallic stents. Gastrointest Endosc 58:41–49
13. Chang WH, Kortan P, Haber GB (1998) Outcome in patients with bifurcation tumors who undergo unilateral versus bilateral hepatic duct drainage. Gastrointest Endosc 47:354–362
14. Isayama H, Komatsu Y, Inoue Y, et al (2003) Preserved function of the Oddi sphincter after endoscopic papillary balloon dilation. Hepatogastroenterology 50:1787–1791

Plastic Stent Placement for Unresectable Malignant Extrahepatic Biliary Stricture

Kei Ito, Naotaka Fujita, and Osamu Takasawa

Summary. Endoscopic stent placement is an efficacious treatment for patients with malignant extrahepatic biliary stricture. Metal stents have a significantly longer patency than plastic stents. Furthermore, metal stent placement contributes to cost-effectiveness, shorter duration of hospitalization, and reduction in the frequency of repeated endoscopic retrograde cholangiopancreatography. The indication for plastic stent placement as palliative therapy for unresectable malignant biliary stricture is drainage for patients with an expected survival of less than several months. Because patients who have undergone metal stent placement have a shorter survival period after stent occlusion, additional placement of a plastic stent is acceptable.

Key words. Biliary stent, Malignant biliary obstruction, Plastic stent, Metallic stent, Covered metal stent (CMS)

Introduction

Although preoperative biliary drainage in resectable cases of malignant extrahepatic biliary stricture remains controversial, biliary stenting is generally performed in Japan. Thin stents, i.e., 7 Fr. or 8 Fr., are sufficient to relieve jaundice in this situation. On the other hand, indwelling stents with a larger diameter are preferably employed in patients with unresectable malignant biliary obstruction. Although it is easy to endoscopically replace plastic stents, stent clogging is a major problem. Self-expanding metal stents, which achieve a larger luminal diameter, have been used for the purpose of prolonging stent patency. There are no universally accepted recommendations for plastic stent deployment in cases of unresectable malignant extrahepatic biliary stricture. We herein review the literature and discuss the indications for plastic stent placement in patients with malignant extrahepatic biliary stricture.

Department of Gastroenterology, Sendai City Medical Center, 5-22-1 Tsurugaya, Miyagino-ku, Sendai, Miyagi 983-0824, Japan

Randomized Controlled Trial of Plastic Stent Versus Metal Stent for Malignant Extrahepatic Biliary Obstruction

According to the Medline database, five randomized controlled trials (RCTs) of plastic stents versus metal stents for unresectable malignant extrahepatic biliary stricture had been published by 2006 (Table 1) [1–5]. The plastic stents used in those trials were 10–11.5 Fr. polyethylene stents or Tannenbaum stents. The metal stents used were noncovered/covered Wallstents or Strecker stents.

In the initial report by Davids et al. [1], 105 patients with unresectable malignant biliary stricture were randomly assigned to either the metal stent group ($n = 49$) or the plastic stent group ($n = 56$). Although there was no significant difference between the two groups in survival duration, mean duration of stent patency in the metal stent group was significantly longer than that in the plastic stent group (273 vs. 126 days, $P = 0.006$). Placement of a metal stent instead of a polyethylene stent led to a 28% reduction in number of endoscopic retrograde cholangiopancreatography (ERCP) procedures per patient, which, despite the greater cost for a metal stent, resulted in an overall cost benefit. Knyrim et al. [2] evaluated 62 patients with malignant common bile duct obstruction, consisting of a plastic stent group and a metal stent group, each with 31 patients. Stent occlusion was more common in the plastic stent group (36%) than in the metal stent group (22%). The rate and cost of retreatment were significantly greater in the plastic stent group compared with the metal stent group.

In their RCT, Prat et al. [3] assigned 101 patients with malignant extrahepatic biliary stricture to placement of either an 11.5 Fr. plastic stent to be exchanged on evidence of dysfunction (group 1, $n = 33$), an 11.5 Fr. plastic stent to be exchanged every 3 months (group 2, $n = 34$), or a Wallstent (group 3, $n = 34$). Although the overall survival rate did not differ between the groups, complication-free survival in groups 2 and 3 was longer than that in group 1 ($P < 0.05$). Group 2 required a greater number of ERCPs than group 1. Furthermore, an overall cost advantage was seen in group 3

Table 1. Plastic stent versus metal stent for malignant extrahepatic biliary obstruction.

Year Author	Plastic stent (n) Metal stent (n)	Median survival period	P	Median stent patency	P
1992	10-Fr polyethylene (56)	147 d	0.45	126 d	0.0006
Davids	Wallstent (49)	175 d		237 d	
1993	11.5-Fr polyethylene (31)	n.m.	n.m.	4.6 +/− 0.7 m	
Knyrim	Wall or Strecker stent (31)	n.m.		6.2 +/− 1.9 m	
1998	11.5-Fr polyethylene (33)	4.8 m	n.s.	3.2 m	
Prat	*11.5-Fr polyethylene (34)	5.6 m		—	<0.05
	Wallstent (34)	4.5 m		4.8 m	
2003	10-Fr Tannenbaum (59)	3.3 m	n.s.	5.5 m	0.007
Kaassis	Wallstent (59)	5.1 m		not reached	
2006	10-Fr polyethylene (51)	3.9 m	0.2776	1.8 m	0.0020
Soderlund	Covered Wallstent (49)	5.3 m		3.6 m	

*plastic stent to be exchanged every 3 months; d, day; m, months; n.m., not mentioned; n.s., not significant

as compared with group 1 or group 2. They stated, "Use of a metal stent in patients surviving less than 3 months (37% in their study) is unnecessarily costly. In this subgroup, costs per patient are 15% lower with plastic than with metal prostheses." They concluded that metal stents are advantageous only for the subgroup of patients with an expected survival of more than 6 months (32% in their study). Kaassis et al. [4] conducted a multicenter study comparing the efficacy and cost of a plastic stent and a metal stent in 118 patients with malignant extrahepatic biliary obstruction. There was no significant difference in survival between the two groups. Time to first stent obstruction was longer in the metal stent group ($P = 0.007$). Additional periods of hospitalization, period of antibiotic therapy, and the numbers of ERCPs and transabdominal ultrasonography procedures were significantly longer and higher in the plastic stent group. They concluded that although metal stent placement is the most effective treatment for unresectable malignant extrahepatic biliary obstruction, placement of a plastic stent is justified in patients with liver metastasis because expected survival is shorter.

In spite of the wider caliber of metal stents, occlusion by tumor ingrowth can occur because of their meshwork design. Covered metal stents have been developed to prevent stent occlusion by tumor ingrowth. Isayama et al. [6] carried out an RCT enrolling 112 patients with unresectable malignant biliary obstruction for endoscopic insertion of either a covered diamond stent ($n = 57$) or an uncovered diamond stent ($n = 55$). They reported a higher cumulative patency rate for covered stents (304 versus 161 days). In the study by Soderlung and Linder [5], plastic stents ($n = 51$) had a higher and earlier dysfunction rate compared with covered Wallstents ($n = 49$). Covered Wallstents were deemed to be cost effective in patients with distal malignant obstruction who are expected to survive for a median of 4–5 months post procedure.

Plastic Stent for Malignant Biliary Obstruction

Various plastic biliary stents have been developed in terms of shape, bore, and length. Most endoscopists typically use a 10 Fr. straight polyethylene stent with side flaps at both ends that inhibit stent migration. The mechanism of stent clogging is multifactorial and includes binding of biliary proteins and adherence of bacteria to the inner wall of the stent. In vitro experiments comparing straight stents with and without side holes have shown that sludge formation is usually more prominent near the side holes. Side holes cause local turbulence, resulting in eddy currents that enhance bacterial incrustation and sludge deposition. Binmoeller et al. [7] performed endoscopic placement of Tannenbaum stents without side holes (Wilson-Cook Medical, Winston Salem, NC, USA) in 55 patients with malignant biliary stricture, the median stent patency being 64 weeks. They concluded that the stent patency period of the Tannenbaum-type stent was longer than that of conventional plastic stents with side holes and comparable to that of metal stents. However, in recent RCTs comparing Tannenbaum and polyethylene stents, there were no differences in median duration of patient survival and stent patency between the two stent types (Table 2). Only one RCT comparing polyethylene stents with a new 10 Fr. stent (DoubleLayer Stent) placed endoscopically found a longer stent patency and lower risk of stent occlusion

TABLE 2. Plastic stent for malignant extrahepatic biliary obstruction.

Year Author	10 Fr Stent (n)	Median survival Period (days)	P	Median stent Patency (days)	P
1998	Telfon (42)	165	0.60	83	0.93
Berkel	PE (42)	140		80	
2000	Tannenbaum (65)	115	0.765	181	0.49
England	Cotton-Leung (69)	151		133	
2000	Tannenbaum (29)	88	0.48	96	0.12
Terruzzi	Cotton-Hyubregtse (28)	75.6		75.5	
2002	Tannenbaum (54)	n.m.		91	>0.05
Catalano	Cotton-Leung (52)	n.m.		94	
2002	polymer-coated PU (54)	132	0.25	77	0.04
Berkel	PE (52)	145		105	
2003	Tannenbaum (41)	n.m.	>0.05	58	>0.05
Schilling	polymer-coated PU (40)	n.m.		76	
	PE (39)	n.m.		108	
2003	DoubleLayer (60)	114	>0.05	144	<0.05
Tringali	PE (60)	105		99	

*PE: polyethylene; PU: polyurethane; n.m.: not mentioned

before death with the DoubleLayer Stent [8]. Further RCTs are necessary for precise evaluation of the usefulness of this stent.

It seems likely that multiple plastic stent placement contributes to longer stent patency as a consequence of the increased bore of the drainage route. We conducted a retrospective study involving 58 patients with unresectable malignant distal biliary stricture who had undergone endoscopic stent placement of either two 10-Fr. stents without side holes (DoubleLayer; Olympus Medical Systems, Tokyo, Japan) ($n = 34$) or one such stent ($n = 24$) [9]. There was no significant difference between the two groups in overall patient survival. The median stent patency of the two-stent group was longer than that of the one-stent group (225 ± 22 vs. 155 ± 74 days), although it did not reach statistical significance (log-rank test, $P = 0.470$). Elucidation of the utility of multiple stent placement by prospective RCTs is awaited.

Indication for Plastic Stent Placement in Malignant Extrahepatic Biliary Obstruction

As already mentioned, stent patency was significantly longer in the metal stent group than in the plastic stent group. Moreover, metal stent placement contributes to cost-effectiveness, shorter duration of hospitalization, and reduction in the number of ERCP procedures. In patients with predicted short survival, the benefits of the metal stents with longer patency over plastic stents may not be sufficient to warrant their use. Therefore, the indication for plastic stent placement for unresectable malignant biliary stricture is drainage for patients with an expected survival of less than several months.

Although metal stents have a long patency period, stent occlusion occurs in 19%–33% of the patients after a mean or median of 105–273 days [1–5]. Because such patients have a shorter survival period after stent occlusion, additional placement of a plastic stent is recommended. Davids et al. [1] stated that 14 of 16 patients with stent occlusion underwent placement of 11 Fr. straight plastic stents in the metal stent group and that no stent occlusion occurred (median patient survival after second-stent placement, 85 days). Prat et al. [3] also reported good results of second placement of a plastic stent in their 6 patients. Recently, some authors have reported the feasibility of removal of a covered metal stent [10]. Further study is necessary for establishment of adequate treatment for first stent occlusion.

References

1. Davids PH, Groen AK, Rauws EA, et al (1992) Randomised trial of self-expanding metal stents versus polyethylene stents for distal malignant biliary obstruction. Lancet 340:1488–1492
2. Knyrim K, Wagner HJ, Pausch J, et al (1993) A prospective, randomized, controlled trial of metal stents for malignant obstruction of the common bile duct. Endoscopy 25:207–212
3. Prat F, Chapat O, Ducot B, et al (1998) A randomized trial of endoscopic drainage methods for inoperable malignant strictures of the common bile duct. Gastrointest Endosc 47:1–7
4. Kaassis M, Boyer J, Dumas R, et al (2003) Plastic or metal stents for malignant stricture of the common bile duct? Results of a randomized prospective study. Gastrointest Endosc 57:178–182
5. Soderlund C, Linder S (2006) Covered metal versus plastic stents for malignant common bile duct stenosis: a prospective, randomized, controlled trial. Gastrointest Endosc 63:986–995
6. Isayama H, Komatsu Y, Tsujino T, et al (2004) A prospective randomized study of "covered" versus "uncovered" diamond stents for the management of distal malignant biliary obstruction. Gut 53:729–734
7. Binmoeller KF, Seitz U, Seifert H, et al (1995) The Tannenbaum stent: a new plastic biliary stent without side holes. Am J Gastroenterol 90:1764–1768
8. Tringali A, Mutignani M, Perri V, et al (2003) A prospective, randomized multicenter trial comparing DoubleLayer and polyethylene stents for malignant distal common bile duct strictures. Endoscopy 35:992–997
9. Ito K, Fujita N, Noda Y, et al (2007) Is placement of two 10-Fr. plastic stents (DoubleLayer) superior to single stent placement for the palliation of unresectable malignant biliary stricture? Gastrointest Endosc 65:AB226 (abstract)
10. Familiari P, Bulajic M, Mutignani, M, et al (2005) Endoscopic removal of malfunctioning biliary self-expandable metallic stents Gastrointest Endosc 62:903–910

Indication and Procedure of Pancreatic and Bile Duct Stenting

Yan Zhong, Stefan Groth, and Nib Soehendra

Summary. Stenting is one of the most commonly practiced endoscopic procedures in the management of biliary and pancreatic disorders. Endoscopic stenting is the treatment of choice for biliary and pancreatic duct strictures. It serves as a palliation in patients with inoperable malignant bile duct obstruction to relieve jaundice and pruritus, thus improving quality of life. The self-expandable metallic stent (SEMS) with a 10-mm lumen diameter is preferable to plastic stents because it provides better and longer-lasting drainage. Plastic stents occlude after an average of 3 to 4 months because of bacterial growth and sludge formation. Patients with cholangitis and predicted survival longer than 6 months therefore benefit most from SEMS. A covered SEMS avoiding tumor ingrowth seems to improve drainage results. However, currently available covered SEMS may carry increased risks of cholecystitis and pancreatitis. For benign strictures of both biliary and pancreatic duct, a plastic stent is used because the SEMS is not readily removable. Placement of multiple stents for 6 to 12 months achieves a long-term dilatation of the strictures. In unresectable pancreatic cancer associated with intractable pain, decompression of the distended pancreatic duct may relieve pain. Temporary stent placement in the pancreatic duct following sphincterotomy or other procedures at the papilla is recommended to avoid acute pancreatitis.

Key words. Stenting, Biliary duct, Pancreatic duct

Introduction

Endoscopic stent placement in the biliary duct was introduced in 1979. Since then, there have been several improvements regarding the technique and technology. Today, endoscopic stenting is widely accepted as the first-line treatment of biliary stricture of both benign and unresectable malignant nature and bile duct leaks. Stenting has also become the mainstay in the nonsurgical treatment of chronic and recurring obstructive pancreatitis. Several other indications for pancreatic duct stenting have also been proved to be useful.

Department of Interdisciplinary Endoscopy, University Medical Center Hamburg-Eppendorf, Martinistrasse 52, 20246 Hamburg, Germany

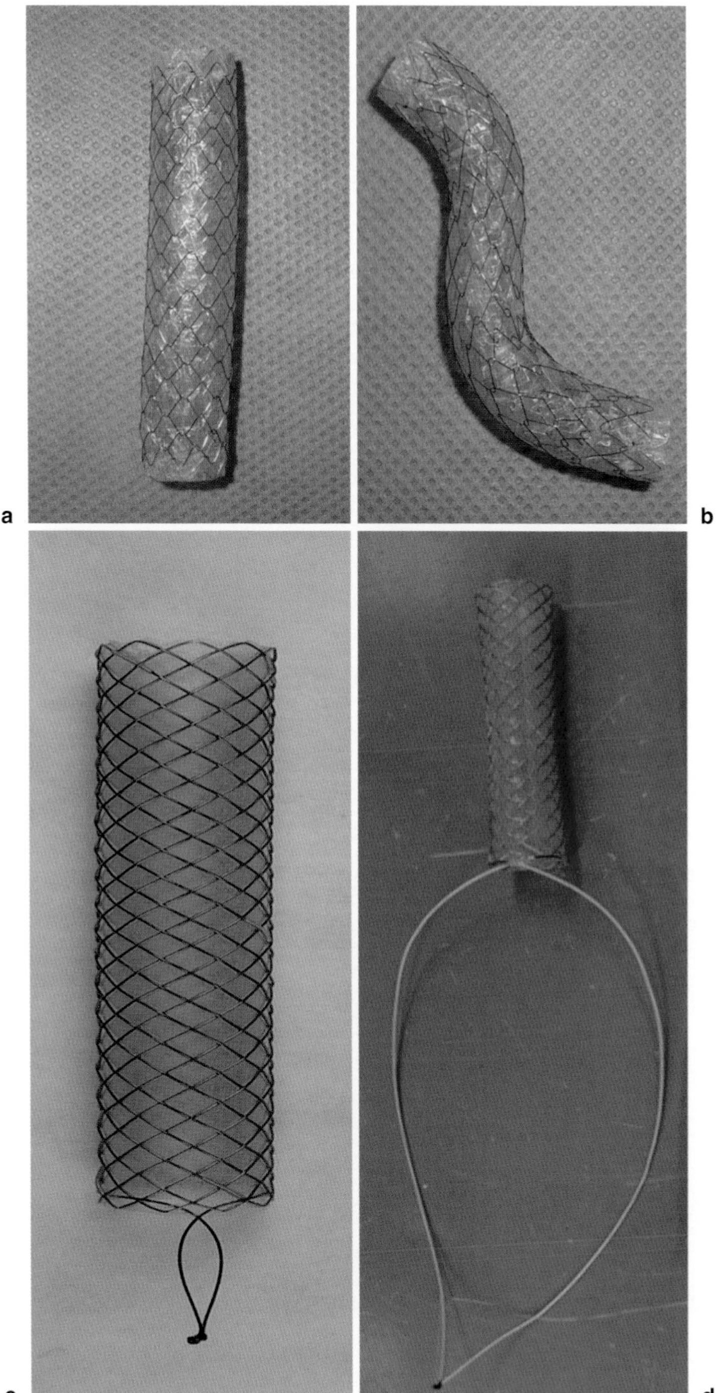

FIG. 1. **a, b** Fully covered self-expandable metallic stent (SEMS) with Teflon coating between two nitinol meshes adaptable to ductal anatomy whereby maintaining the maximum lumen. **c, d** Removable fully silicone-covered nitinol SEMS with retrieval lasso of different lengths for distal and proximal stricture (TaeWoong Medical)

Materials

Plastic stent, guiding catheter, and pusher are made of a radiopaque polyethylene or Teflon catheter. Teflon has a lower friction coefficient and is stiffer than polyethylene. Teflon stents with a tapered tip are therefore more suitable for tight strictures. The guiding catheter used for the insertion of 10 and 11.5 Fr. plastic stents has two metal marking rings at the distal end with a distance of 7 cm to be used for measuring the length of the stricture. The pusher tube is of a different colour from the stent, allowing better differentiation from the stent, hence preventing pushing the stent into the duct.

Biliary SEMS provide a longer patency compared to plastic stents because of their larger lumen, up to 10 mm when fully expanded. Newer SEMS are all made of more flexible nitinol wire, and the covering material is silicone, polyurethane, or Teflon. Some SEMS are partially coated, leaving both ends uncovered to enable better anchoring. Fully coated SEMS are likely have less clogging caused by plant fibres sticking at the distal end and are removable after short-term use, so long as the membrane is intact. Removable SEMS have a retrieval lasso at the distal end to facilitate removal. To prevent dislocation, coating is made at the inner layer of the stent (Fig. 1).

Plastic Stent Design

A variety of straight and curved plastic stents of different lengths and diameters is available (Fig. 2). For the common bile duct (CBD) and intrahepatic duct strictures, curved stents adapted to the ductal anatomy are preferable. Side flaps or pigtails are made at both ends to prevent migration, and side holes improve drainage. Double-pigtail stents are recommended to reduce the risk of perforating the duodenal wall.

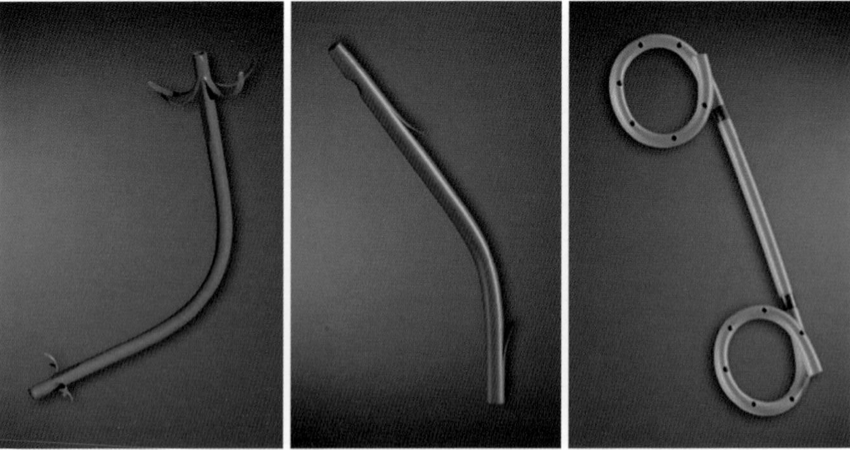

Fig. 2. Commonly used plastic stents made of radiopaque polyethylene or Teflon. **a** Tannenbaum without side holes made of Teflon. **b** Polyethylene stent with side holes and flaps at both ends. **c** Double-pigtail stent with several side holes and marking rings at both ends

Cholangioscopy and Pancreatoscopy

The Role of Peroral Cholangioscopy in the Management of Biliary Tract Diseases

TOSHIO TSUYUGUCHI, TAKESHI ISHIHARA, and OSAMU YOKOSUKA

Summary. Peroral cholangioscopy can allow direct visualization of the bile duct noninvasively. A major role of peroral cholangioscopy is the management of difficult biliary stones which are resistant to conventional endoscopic treatment, including mechanical lithotripsy. Electrohydraulic or laser lithotripsy under strict peroral cholangioscopic guidance may be a safe and effective alternative to surgery. Several clinical studies suggest the utility of peroral cholangioscopy for the management of various bile duct lesions. Cholangioscopic observation, with or without direct biopsy, may be a useful adjunct to endoscopic retrograde cholangiopancreatography (ERCP) for distinguishing malignant from benign bile duct lesions. However, an assessment of its diagnostic accuracy needs further clinical controlled studies. At present, the fragility of the equipment and technical difficulties lessen its popularity. Preliminary data obtained using newly designed cholangioscopes, which provide excellent quality images and improved maneuverability, are encouraging.

Key words. Peroral cholangioscopy, Bile duct stricture, Bile duct stones, Lithotripsy

Introduction

Possible indications for cholangioscopy of the bile duct include direct visual assessment, tissue sampling, and therapeutic interventions. Initially, a percutaneous transhepatic approach was required for cholangioscopy. Subsequently, "mother–baby" systems were developed which permit the introduction of the cholangioscope via the transpapillary approach. Although the "mother–baby" systems were first described in the mid-1970s [1], they were not widely adopted because early prototype cholangioscopes were difficult to use, and the optical fibers were easily fractured during passage over the elevator of the duodenoscope. Images obtained through the use of video adapters may be less than optimal and therefore unsatisfactory. The development of the small-sized charge-coupled device made it possible to produce a video peroral cholangioscope, which provided excellent quality images [2]. Recently, video cholangioscopy using narrow-band imaging (NBI), which made it possible to emphasize

Department of Medicine and Clinical Oncology, Graduate School of Medicine, Chiba University, 1-8-1 Inohana, Chuo-ku, Chiba 260-8677, Japan

the imaging of mucosal structures and microvessels, was developed as a diagnostic modality for better visualization of bile duct lesions [3]. These developments in cholangioscopes will contribute to the clinical utility of peroral cholangioscopy.

Peroral Cholangioscopic Lithotripsy (Table 1)

Standard endoscopic stone removal techniques, including mechanical lithotripsy, fail in 5% to 10% of cases owing to the presence of very large stones. A series of 162 consecutive patients who underwent mechanical lithotripsy was evaluated retrospec-

Table 1. Peroral cholangioscopic lithotripsy for difficult bile duct stones.

Reference	Methods	No. of patients	Stone diameter (mm)	Stone clearance rate	P	Complications[a]
Leung and Chung 1989 [6]	EHL	5	31	100% (5)		0%
Binmoeller et al. 1993 [7]	EHL	65	22	98% (64)		1.5% (1 retroperitoneal leakage)
Adamek et al. 1996 [8]	EHL	46	24.3	74% (34)	NS	6.5% (1 cholangitis, minor bleeding), 2 others
	ESWL	79	27.6	78.5% (62)		6.3% (2 cutaneous hematoma, 2 cholangitis, 1 respiratory arrest), 23 others
Hui et al. 2003 [9]	EHL	17	30	76.5% (13)	NS $P = 0.17$	7.7% (3 bleeding, 2 mucosal laceration, 1 cholecystitis)
	Stent	19	26	100% (19)		5% (1 perforation)
Arya et al. 2004 [10]	EHL	94	NA 81/94 > 20 mm	90% (85)		18% (13 cholangitis, 4 others)
Farrell et al. 2005 [11]	EHL	26	20	100% (26)		0%
Piraka et al. 2007 [12]	EHL	32	12	81% (26)		3.8% (1 cholangitis, 1 hypoxia)
Cotton et al. 1990 [13][b]	Laser	10 (25)	18	80% (20/25)		1 minor bleeding (1/25)
Neuhaus et al. 1998 [14][c]	Laser	30	24.2	97% (29)	<0.05	7% (1 cholangitis, 1 pancreatitis)
	ESWL	30	22.7	73% (22)		17% (1 respiratory failure, 1 cholangitis, 3 others)

[a]Reported complications were mild and the mortality rate was 0

[b]Total number of patients, including 15 patients who were treated via the percutaneous route or under fluoroscopic guidance

[c]Including 27 patients who were treated via the percutaneous route

EHL, electrohydraulic lithotripsy; ESWL, extracorporeal shock wave lithotripsy; NA, not available; NS, not significant

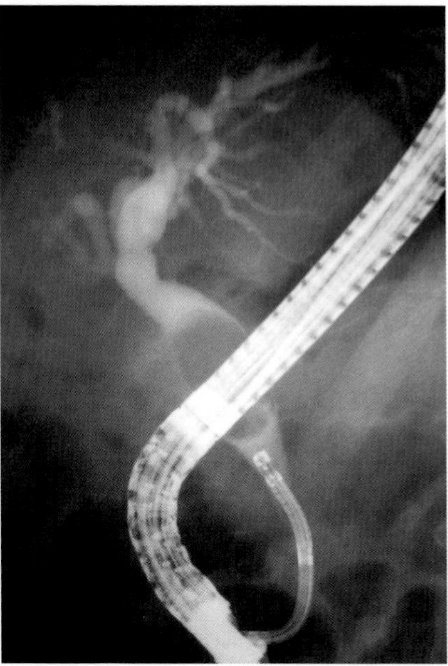

Fig. 1. ERC showing a single large stone in a common bile duct. A peroral cholangioscope is in position for electrohydraulic lithotripsy (EHL)

tively, and a large number of variables were tested for their association with a successful outcome [4]. Univariate and multivariate analyses showed that stone size was the only outcome predictor. The cumulative probability of bile duct clearance ranged from over 90% for stones with a diameter less than 10 mm to 68% for those greater than 28 mm in diameter ($P < 0.02$). Impacted bile duct stones, broken traction wires on the basket, and intrahepatic bile duct stones were other causes of resistance to conventional endoscopic therapy. Siegel et al. [5] performed electrohydraulic lithotripsy (EHL) under fluoroscopic control using an inflatable balloon to center the probe within the bile duct lumen, and found this approach to be safe. However, direct visualization of the target intuitively enhances the success of stone fragmentation and minimizes complications, especially when the bile ducts are tortuous or angulated. A major therapeutic role of peroral cholangioscopy is the management of these difficult bile duct stones noninvasively (Fig. 1, Table 1) [6–14].

Electrohydraulic Lithotripsy (EHL) Under Peroral Cholangioscopic Guidance

In 1989, Leung and Chung [6] reported that peroral EHL was performed with a 3 Fr lithotripsy probe inserted through a cholangioscope under direct vision, and all nine stones (mean maximal diameter 3.1 cm) were successfully fragmented, allowing subsequent extraction with the aid of endoscopy and clearance of the common bile duct. Using peroral EHL in a larger series of 94 patients, difficult stones could be fragmented in 89 patients (96%) and be completely evacuated in 85 patients (90%) [7]. There have been no reported deaths and no significant duct injuries as a result of peroral EHL (Table 1). Although permanent biliary stenting is an alternative method for elderly patients with irretrievable common bile duct stones, late complications occur in many patients and the risk increases proportionally over time. Hui et al. [9] assessed whether peroral EHL compared with stenting alone decreased the risk of cholangitis and mortality for high-risk elderly patients. There was no significant difference in the early postendoscopic retrograde cholangiopancreatography (ERCP) complication rate between the EHL and the stent groups. This indicates that EHL plus further endoscopic attempts at the complete removal of difficult stones can be performed safely even in high-risk patients. Moreover, the long-term outcome revealed that EHL significantly decreased cholangitis mortality rates compared with those of the stent group. Therefore, removing the bile duct stones may be attempted whenever possible, even in elderly patients. An alternative management strategy for difficult bile duct stones is extracorporeal shockwave lithotripsy (ESWL). ESWL is a less invasive method, and was compared with peroral EHL in a comparative study [8]. Although the mean number of EHL procedures was lower than that needed for ESWL, there were no significant differences between EHL and ESWL in the number of procedures or in the stone clearance rates.

Laser Lithotripsy Under Peroral Cholangioscopic Guidance

The pulsed dye laser has been developed as an alternative lithotripsy method for difficult bile duct stones. Neuhaus et al. [14] conducted a prospective randomized study comparing endoscopic laser lithotripsy with ESWL in 60 patients with difficult bile duct stones, and laser lithotripsy appeared to be significantly more effective than ESWL in terms of stone clearance rate and treatment duration (Table 1). However, this study included 27 patients who had laser lithotripsy via the percutaneous route. In contrast to several reports on peroral EHL, experience with peroral laser lithotripsy is still limited. Cotton et al. [13] published a triple-center study on 25 patients who were treated with flash-lamp excited dye laser lithotripsy. Although they performed laser lithotripsy on 10 patients using the "mother–baby" system, they reported difficulties in achieving good targeting of the stones. Furthermore, "mother–baby" systems require two experienced endoscopists, and have remained a time-consuming procedure. To date, there have been few studies on cholangioscopic laser lithotripsy because of the above-mentioned drawbacks. Hence, an automatic stone-tissue detection system (STDS), which made laser lithotripsy possible under fluoroscopic control, has now been developed and adopted [15].

Mirizzi Syndrome

Mirizzi syndrome is a relatively rare complication of gallbladder disease, and endoscopic treatment usually fails because of an inability to access or capture the impacted cystic duct stones. McSherry et al. [16] classified Mirizzi syndrome into two types:

type I consists of external compression of the common hepatic duct by a stone in the cystic duct or gallbladder neck, and type II involves erosion of the stone into the common hepatic duct, with subsequent fistula formation. The standard surgical management of type II is more difficult than that of type I owing to an increased risk of bile duct injury. Although the stones in type I patients are inaccessible to the peroral cholangioscope, type II stones can be successfully treated with peroral cholangioscopic lithotripsy. In a series of 25 patients with Mirizzi syndrome, shock-wave lithotripsy (EHL or dye laser lithotripsy) was performed under direct vision with a "mother–baby" endoscope system [17]. In the two type I patients, the cholangioscopic approach failed and both patients underwent open cholecystectomy. The 23 remaining type II patients were all successfully treated with shock-wave lithotripsy alone. Of the 6 type II patients with large residual gallbladder stones, 4 had acute cholangitis due to stone migration 6, 9, 28, and 34 months, respectively, after endoscopic treatment. This is the largest series of patients with Mirizzi syndrome who have been treated using "mother–baby" endoscope systems, and a favorable long-term outcome depends on the absence of large residual gallbladder stones. Peroral cholangioscopic lithotripsy should be a safe and effective alternative to surgery, especially in patients with type II syndrome.

Intrahepatic Bile Duct Stones

Intrahepatic bile duct stones are prevalent in East Asia, and are a serious and challenging health problem. Percutaneous transhepatic cholangioscopic lithotripsy (PTCSL) is reported to be less invasive than conventional hepatic resection. However, PTCSL needs to take a transhepatic route, which can cause complications such as bleeding or bile leakage. Furthermore, PTCSL is time-consuming because of the need to allow the sinus tract to mature. Peroral cholangioscopic lithotripsy, which is less invasive than PTCSL, may be an effective alternative for intrahepatic bile duct stones. We reported the long-term results of peroral cholangioscopic lithotripsy for 36 patients with intrahepatic stones [18]. Successful stone fragmentation was achieved in 27 (75%) of 36 patients, and subsequent complete stone clearance was achieved in 23 (64%) patients. Although the complete stone removal rate was lower than that with PTCSL, the cumulative recurrence rate for patients in whom complete removal was attained was 21.7% at 164 months after the procedure, which compares favorably with that reported for PTCSL [19].

Cholangioscopic Characterization of Various Bile Duct Lesions

With the exception of biliary strictures which have clearly followed surgery or trauma, such strictures always raise concerns for malignancy. ERCP with or without tissue sampling might be nondiagnostic despite a high clinical suspicion. Cytological brushing of bile duct strictures has a low yield for malignancy of up to 50%–60% by adjunctive techniques such as combination brushing or forceps biopsy [20]. Direct visualization of bile ducts may be a useful adjunct to ERCP for distinguishing between malignant and benign biliary lesions [21–23]. We reported our experience of the diagnostic utility of peroral cholangioscopy in 97 patients who all had diagnoses of unknown biliary diseases (46 malignant lesions, 51 benign lesions) [23]. On the basis of ERCP findings, there were 76 indeterminate strictures and 21 filling defects. The results of ERCP/tissue sampling were as follows: accuracy, 82.2%; sensitivity, 65.2%; negative-predictive value, 68.6%. The addition of peroral cholangioscopy significantly improved the accuracy to 94.8%, the sensitivity to 100%, and the negative-predictive value to 100%. While the accuracy for strictures was 93.5% (71/76), the accuracy of filling defects was as high as 100% (21/21). This was because direct cholangioscopic visualization can reveal at a glance whether a filling defect is a tumor or a stone. If the filling defect proves to be biliary stones, peroral cholangioscopy also allows EHL or laser lithotripsy for the stones under direct guidance.

Since the advent of orthotopic liver transplantation (OLT) as a life-saving procedure for patients with end-stage liver disease, it has been found that various biliary complications may occur after OLT. Peroral cholangioscopy may help in the early diagnosis and correct management of complications such as ischemic-type biliary lesion, anastomotic strictures, and biliary cast [21].

Directed tissue acquisition in biliary strictures by using PTCS provides differentiation between malignant and benign lesions, a definition of proximal and distal cancer extension, and the early detection of small and multiple foci [24]. However, PTCS is invasive and carries a risk of malignant seeding of the tract. On the other hand, peroral cholangioscopy/direct biopsy is safe, but has not been rigorously studied because obtaining adequate samples from the bile duct via the limited maneuverability of the long baby scope and the tiny biopsy forceps presents major challenges. In addition, obtaining samples from bile duct lesions above the hilum is more difficult because of the significant limitations in the retroflexion capability of the baby scope tip. To overcome these limitations, a single-operator peroral cholangiopancreatoscopy system with 4-way deflected steering and dedicated irrigation channels has been developed [25]. A major advance of this system is the incorporation of dedicated irrigation channels, which allow continuous irrigation to keep the cholangioscopic view clear of blood, stone debris, sludge, or pus during visual inspection and biopsy. Although the preliminary report showed excellent results with the new cholangioscope/direct biopsy, further studies are needed.

A definition of proximal cancer extension is possible only when a baby scope passes through the strictures. Therefore, the diagnosis of tumor extensions by using peroral cholangioscopy has not been assessed properly until now. Several case reports have shown that peroral cholangioscopy could facilitate operative planning based on exact knowledge of the extent of a bile duct tumor both proximally and distally [26]. With the increasing availability of suitable instruments, newly designed peroral cholangioscopy may improve our ability to diagnose tumor extensions of a bile duct carcinoma.

Peroral cholangioscopy is useful not only for evaluating the etiology of a stricture, but also for its guidewire assistance. Siddique et al. [21] reported a series of 60 cholangioscopies, and 4 patients with bile duct strictures were treated with cholangioscopy by maneuvering the guide-wire through tortuous strictures followed by stent placement. Our preliminary report also confirmed that peroral cholangioscopy was useful for inserting a guide-wire into tortuous bile duct strictures [27].

Primary Sclerosing Cholangitis (PSC)

It was found by ERCP that nearly half of primary sclerosing cholangitis (PSC) patients had bile duct stones either at the time of diagnosis or that were subsequently discovered. Awadallah et al. [28] assessed the role of peroral cholangioscopy in 41 consecutive patients with PSC. They found that cholangiography missed nearly one out of every three patients with stones, which probably contributed to the chronic inflammation, stricturing, cholestasis, and cholangitis which is seen in PSC patients. Peroral cholangioscopy-directed stone therapy achieved a clinical improvement in the majority of PSC patients with stones. PSC is associated with the development of cholangiocarcinoma (CCA) in up to 10% of patients, and it is of interest that peroral cholangioscopy may help to detect CCA in PSC patients. Although the above-mentioned authors noted that peroral cholangioscopy-directed or -assisted biopsies yielded adequate tissue samples, two cholangiocarcinomas were discovered at the hilum and the right anterior lobe at 1 and 12 months, respectively, following peroral cholangioscopy. On the other hand, a report from Germany showed that peroral cholangioscopy may frequently help to diagnose malignancy in PSC patients with dominant stenoses [29]. In this report, 53 PSC patients with dominant bile duct stenoses were studied. Peroral cholangioscopy was significantly superior to ERCP for detecting malignancy in terms of its sensitivity (92% vs. 66%; $P = 0.25$), specificity (93% vs. 51%; $P < 0.001$), and accuracy (93% vs. 51%; $P < 0.001$). However, intrahepatic CCA was not included in this study. The detection of intrahepatic CCA in patients with PSC remains a challenge.

Peroral Direct Cholangioscopy

Peroral "mother–baby" systems require two experienced endoscopists to carry out, and are therefore a time-consuming procedure. Attempts at peroral direct cholangioscopy have been made in order to overcome these problems. Urakami et al. [30] published the first report of peroral direct cholangioscopy using a routine straight-view endoscope in 1977. In 1987, Liguory et al. [31] described a successful peroral EHL using a pediatric forward-viewing scope in a case of choledochoduodenostomy. However, peroral direct cholangioscopy has not been used because of the lack of adequate endoscopes. Recently, ultra-slim upper endoscopes have been developed for pediatric patients and transnasal applications. These upper endoscopes might make peroral direct cholangioscopy possible [32]. Compared with "mother–baby" systems, direct cholangioscopy has the following advantages: (1) it can be operated by a single endoscopist; (2) a larger working channel allows the use of various probes such as biopsy forceps or EHL probes. However, there are few preliminary reports, and further studies are needed to compare peroral direct cholangioscopy with conventional mother–baby systems.

Conclusion

Peroral cholangioscopy has become a well-established therapeutic method for difficult bile duct stones. However, its diagnostic utility has not yet been properly assessed. The addition of peroral cholangioscopic visualization of the bile duct to ERC may help to diagnose the cause of bile duct lesions. At present, the fragility of the equipment and technical difficulties limit its popularity. Access to small intrahepatic ducts and cholangioscopy-directed forceps biopsies are hindered by the relatively large caliber of current cholangioscopes and by the limitations of two-way tip deflection. Newly designed cholangioscopes may resolve these problems, and further investigations are needed.

References

1. Nakajima M, Akasaka Y, Fukumoto K, et al (1976) Peroral cholangiopancreatoscopy (PCPS) under duodenoscopic guidance. Am J Gastroenterol 66:241–247
2. Kodama T, Tatsumi Y, Sato H, et al (2004) Initial experience with a new peroral electronic pancreatoscope with an accessory channel. Gastrointest Endosc 59:895–900
3. Itoi T, Sofuni A, Itokawa F, et al (2007) Peroral cholangioscopic diagnosis of biliary-tract diseases by using narrow-band imaging (with videos). Gastrointest Endosc 66:730–736
4. Cipolletta L, Costamagna G, Bianco MA, et al (1997) Endoscopic mechanical lithotripsy of difficult common bile duct stones. Br J Surg 84:1407–1409
5. Siegel JH, Ben-Zvi JS, Pullano WE (1990) Endoscopic electrohydraulic lithotripsy. Gastrointest Endosc 36:134–136
6. Leung JW, Chung SS (1989) Electrohydraulic lithotripsy with peroral choledochoscopy. BMJ 299:595–598
7. Binmoeller KF, Bruckner M, Thonke F, et al (1993) Treatment of difficult bile duct stones using mechanical, electrohydraulic and extracorporeal shock wave lithotripsy. Endoscopy 25:201–206
8. Adamek HE, Maier M, Jakobs R, et al (1996) Management of retained bile duct stones: a prospective open trial comparing extracorporeal and intracorporeal lithotripsy. Gastrointest Endosc 44:40–47
9. Hui CK, Lai KC, Ng M, et al (2003) Retained common bile duct stones: a comparison between biliary stenting and complete clearance of stones by electrohydraulic lithotripsy. Aliment Pharmacol Ther 17:289–296
10. Arya N, Nelles SE, Haber GB, et al (2004) Electrohydraulic lithotripsy in 111 patients: a safe and effective therapy for difficult bile duct stones. Am J Gastroenterol 99:2330–2334
11. Farrell JJ, Bounds BC, Al-Shalabi S, et al (2005) Single-operator duodenoscope-assisted cholangioscopy is an effective alternative in the management of choledocholithiasis not removed by conventional methods, including mechanical lithotripsy. Endoscopy 37:542–547
12. Piraka C, Shah RJ, Awadallah NS, et al (2007) Transpapillary cholangioscopy-directed lithotripsy in patients with difficult bile duct stones. Clin Gastroenterol Hepatol 5:1333–1338
13. Cotton PB, Kozarek RA, Schapiro RH, et al (1990) Endoscopic laser lithotripsy of large bile duct stones. Gastroenterology 99:1128–1133
14. Neuhaus H, Zillinger C, Born P, et al (1998) Randomized study of intracorporeal laser lithotripsy versus extracorporeal shock-wave lithotripsy for difficult bile duct stones. Gastrointest Endosc 47:327–334

15. Jakobs R, Adamek HE, Maier M, et al (1997) Fluoroscopically guided laser lithotripsy versus extracorporeal shock wave lithotripsy for retained bile duct stones: a prospective randomised study. Gut 40:678–682
16. McSherry CK, Ferstenberg H, Vishup M (1982) The Mirizzi syndrome: suggested classification and surgical therapy. Surg Gastroenterol 1:219–225
17. Tsuyuguchi T, Saisho H, Ishihara T, et al (2000) Long-term follow-up after treatment of Mirizzi syndrome by peroral cholangioscopy. Gastrointest Endosc 52:639–644
18. Okugawa T, Tsuyuguchi T, Sudhamshu KC, et al (2002) Peroral cholangioscopic treatment of hepatolithiasis: long-term results. Gastrointest Endosc 56:366–371
19. Lee SK, Seo DW, Myung SJ, et al (2001) Percutaneous transhepatic cholangioscopic treatment for hepatolithiasis: an evaluation of long-term results and risk factors for recurrence. Gastrointest Endosc 53:318–323
20. Baillie J, Paulson EK, Vitellas KM (2003) Biliary imaging: a review. Gastroenterology 124:1686–1699
21. Siddique I, Galati J, Ankoma-Sey V, et al (1999) The role of choledochoscopy in the diagnosis and management of the biliary tract diseases. Gastrointest Endosc 50:67–73
22. Shah RJ, Langer DA, Antillon MR, et al (2006) Cholangioscopy and cholangioscopic forceps biopsy in patients with indeterminate pancreaticobiliary pathology. Clin Gastroenterol Hepatol 4:219–225
23. Fukuda Y, Tsuyuguchi T, Sakai Y, et al (2005) Diagnostic utility of peroral cholangioscopy for various bile duct lesions. Gastrointest Endosc 62:374–382
24. Nimura Y (1993) Staging of biliary carcinoma. Endoscopy 25:76–80
25. Chen YK, Pleskow DK (2007) SpyGlass single-operator peroral cholangiopancreatoscopy system for the diagnosis and therapy of bile duct disorders: a clinical feasibility study (with video). Gastrointest Endosc 65:832–841
26. Wakai T, Shirai Y, Hatakeyama K (2005) Peroral cholangioscopy for non-invasive papillary cholangiocarcinoma with extensive superficial ductal spread. World J Gastroenterol 11:6554–6556
27. Saisho H, Tsuyuguchi T, Yamaguchi T, et al (1995) A new therapeutic approach towards balloon dilatation of biliary strictures using a peroral cholangioscope. Dig Endosc 7:50–55
28. Awadallah NS, Chen YK, Piraka C, et al (2006) Is there a role for cholangioscopy in patients with primary sclerosing cholangitis? Am J Gastroenterol 101:284–291
29. Tischendorf JJ, Kruger M, Trautwein C, et al (2006) Cholangioscopic characterization of dominant bile duct stenoses in patients with primary sclerosing cholangitis. Jul 38:665–669
30. Urakami Y, Seifert E, Butke H (1977) Peroral direct cholangioscopy (PDCS) using routine straight-view endoscope: first report. Endoscopy 9:27–30
31. Liguory CL, Bonnel D, Canard J M, et al (1987) Intracorporeal electrohydraulic shock wave lithotripsy of common bile duct stones: preliminary results in 7 cases. Endoscopy 19:237–240
32. Larghi A, Waxman I (2006) Endoscopic direct cholangioscopy by using an ultra-slim upper endoscope: a feasibility study. Gastrointest Endosc 63:853–857

Techniques and Indications of Pancreatoscopy

Koji Uno, Kenjiro Yasuda, and Masatsugu Nakajima

Summary. Peroral pancreatoscopy was developed to gain direct visualization of the pancreatic duct. Since then, various refinements have been made to pancreatoscopes. At present, precise observation is possible by means of electronic pancreatoscopes. Peroral pancreatoscopy is performed under duodenoscopic guidance (mother and baby scope system). Fiberoptic endoscopes, which are about 3 mm in tip diameter, are usually used for pancreatoscopy. In addition, electronic pancreatoscopes, which have a 2.6- or 3.4-mm tip diameter, are commercially available in Japan. Indications for pancreatoscopy include differential diagnosis of stenosis or filling defect in the main pancreatic duct. Diagnosis of surface spreading of tumor in patients with intraductal papillary mucinous neoplasm in the main pancreatic duct is also a diagnostic indication. Treatment of stones in the main pancreatic duct is a therapeutic indication for pancreatoscopy. Future improvements of pancreatoscopes are expected in image quality, insertion tube, and working channel.

Key words. Peroral pancreatoscopy (PPS), Intraductal papillary mucinous neoplasm (IPMN), Pancreatic cancer, Chronic pancreatitis, Endoscopic retrograde cholangiopancreatography (ERCP)

Introduction

Peroral pancreatoscopy (PPS) was developed in the 1970s to visualize the pancreatic duct directly [1,2]. Since then, some refinements of external diameter, distal end bending, working channel, and image resolution have been made for endoscopes [3]. At present, electronic pancreatoscopes, which have higher image resolution than

---

Department of Gastroenterology, Kyoto Second Red Cross Hospital, 355-5 Haruobi-cho, Kamigyo-ku, Kyoto 602-8026, Japan

fiberoptic endoscopes, have become commercially available in Japan [4]. In this chapter, the techniques and indications for pancreatoscopy are described.

Instruments and Examination Technique

A thin pancreatoscope ("baby scope") is inserted into the main pancreatic duct via the duodenal papilla through the working channel of a duodenoscope ("mother scope") by endoscopic retrograde cholangiopancreatography (ERCP) (mother and baby scope system) (Fig. 1). Endoscopic sphincterotomy (EST) is usually performed beforehand to insert the pancreatoscope into the pancreatic duct easily, except for patients with an open papilla of Vater resulting from mucin derived from an intraductal papillary mucinous neoplasm (IPMN).

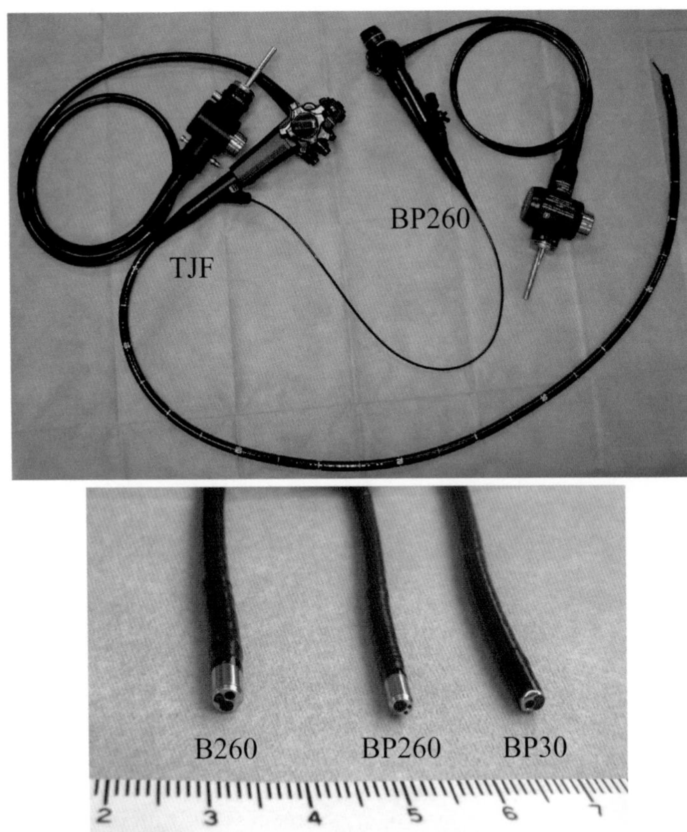

Fig. 1. Pancreatoscopes

TABLE 1. Specifications of pancreatoscopes[a].

	Videoscope		Fiberscope	
	CHF-B260	CHF-BP260	CHF-BP30	PF-8P
Tip diameter (mm)	3.4	2.6	3.1	0.8
External diameter of insertion tube (mm)	3.5–3.9	2.9–3.7	3.4	0.8
Internal diameter of working channel (mm)	1.2	0.5	1.2	None
Bending section up/down (degrees)	70/70	70/70	160/130	None
Field of view (degrees)	90	90	90	75

[a]These endoscopes are manufactured by Olympus Medical Systems, Tokyo, Japan

The fiberoptic endoscope, which is 3.1 mm in tip diameter with a 1.2-mm working channel (CHF-BP30; Olympus Medical Systems, Tokyo, Japan) (Table 1), usually has been used for pancreatoscopy in combination with the therapeutic duodenoscope, which has a 4.2-mm working channel (TJF type; Olympus Medical Systems). The electronic pancreatoscopes, which provide a clearer image, with 2.6- or 3.4-mm tip diameter (CHF-BP260 and CHF-B260, respectively; Olympus Medical Systems), became commercially available in Japan recently. CHF-BP260 and CHF-B260 have 0.5-mm and 1.2-mm working channels, respectively. The ultrathin fiberscope, which has an external diameter of less than 1 mm without a working channel (PF-8P; Olympus Medical Systems), also has been applied for pancreatoscopy (Fig. 2). This scope can be advanced to a target by insertion into a guiding ERCP catheter without EST.

Although pancreatoscopes, except for ultrathin endoscopes, are inserted into the main pancreatic duct directly or along a guidewire after ERCP, an operator must insert a pancreatoscope carefully in combination with both tip angulation of the pancreatoscope and manipulation of the duodenoscope. It is necessary to not raise the elevator of the duodenoscope sharply when inserting the pancreatoscope because the insertion tube of the pancreatoscope is fragile. Pancreatoscopes with a 1.2-mm working channel can be inserted over a guidewire placed into the main pancreatic duct. When pancreatoscopy is performed by means of pancreatoscopes with working channels, lavaging the pancreatic duct with saline to remove mucin is important for visualizing the pancreatic duct clearly. In such cases, to avoid pancreatitis after the examination, it is necessary to not inject excessive saline into the pancreatic duct. Although saline is injected into the guide catheter when using the ultrathin pancreatoscope, it is too narrow to lavage the pancreatic duct sufficiently.

Pancreatoscopes with a 1.2-mm working channel are used for biopsy. These endoscopes are also applied for treatment of stones in the pancreatic duct in combination with electrohydraulic lithotripsy (EHL) or laser under direct vision. On the other hand, biopsy cannot be performed by a pancreatoscope with a 0.5-mm working channel because the working channel is too small.

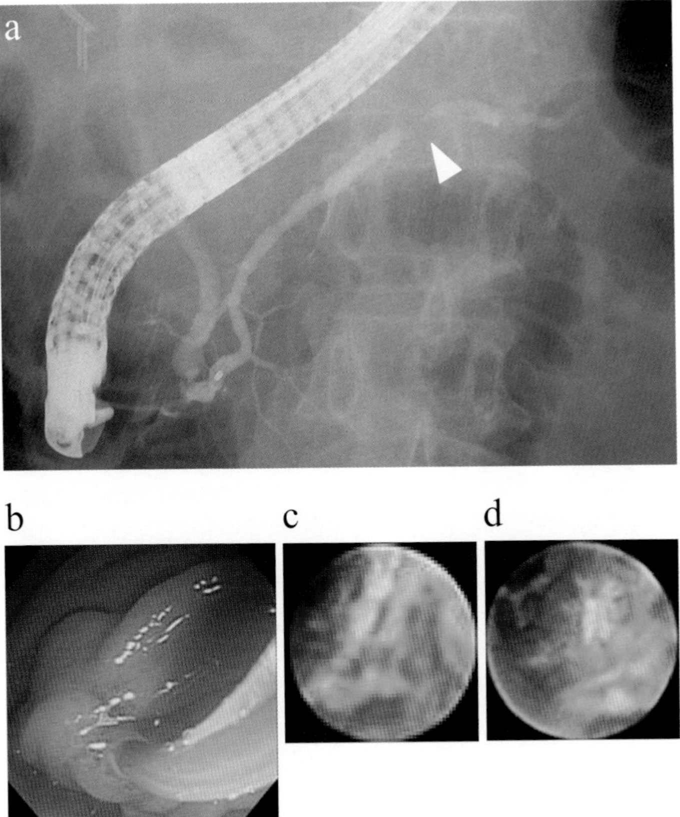

Fig. 2. Adenocarcinoma of the pancreas. **a** Endoscopic retrograde cholangiopancreatography (ERCP) reveals stenosis of the main pancreatic duct in the body of the pancreas (*arrowhead*). **b** Duodenoscopic image reveals the ultrathin pancreatoscope inserted into the main pancreatic duct via the duodenal papilla through a guide catheter. **c, d** Peroral pancreatoscopy (PPS) shows irregular mucosa and dilated vessels of internal surface of the main pancreatic duct in the body of the pancreas

Indications and Clinical Use

Diagnostic indications include differentiation of stenotic lesions and filling defects in the main pancreatic duct. Diagnosis of tumor extension in the main pancreatic duct is also one of the diagnostic indications. However, inserting an endoscope into the main pancreatic duct without dilatation or with a sharp bend is difficult. Successful observation rates reported with thin or ultrathin pancreatoscopes for pancreatic cancer, benign ductal stenosis, and IPMN were 63%, 80%, and 95%, respectively [5]. In this paper, tapering stenosis or obstruction of the main pancreatic duct with asymmetrical deviation was reported as the cause of failing in observation of ductal change in patients with pancreatic cancer.

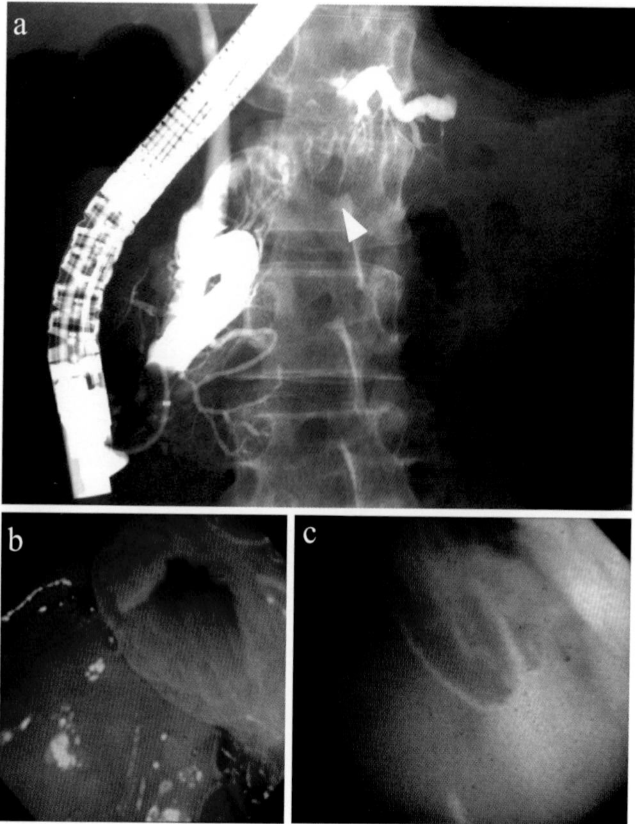

FIG. 3. Intraductal papillary mucinous neoplasm (IPMN) of the pancreas. **a** ERCP reveals a filling defect of the main pancreatic duct in the body of the pancreas (*arrowhead*). **b** Duodenoscopic image shows the opened duodenal papilla. **c** PPS reveals a villous tumor of the main pancreatic duct in the body of the pancreas

Intraductal papillary mucinous neoplasm (IPMN) with a dilated main pancreatic duct caused by excessive mucin is a good indication for pancreatoscopy (Fig. 3). In such a case, differentiation between carcinoma, adenoma, and hyperplasia and diagnosis of extent of tumor in the main pancreatic duct are performed by pancreatoscopy in combination with biopsy or cytology under direct vision [6,7]. Characteristic findings of pancreatoscopy in patients with IPMN in the main pancreatic duct are papillary tumor and fish-egg-like appearance. Especially, a papillary tumor is frequently observed in patients with a malignancy, according to our case series, which is diagnosed histologically after laparotomy. In such malignant cases, the detection rate of redness and proliferation of blood vessels is also high (Table 2). Pancreatoscopy is also applied to determine a resection line in some patients with IPMN in the main pancreatic duct before or during surgery.

Pancreatoscopy is also indicated in differentiation of stenotic lesions in the main pancreatic duct between pancreatic cancer and chronic pancreatitis. In our

Table 2. Pancreatoscopic findings for intraductal papillary mucinous neoplasms (IPMN).

	Adenocarcinoma ($n = 6$)	Adenoma ($n = 16$)	Hyperplasia ($n = 4$)
Papillary tumor	6 (100%)	2 (13%)	
Redness and proliferation of blood vessels	5 (83%)	5 (31%)	
Fish egg-like appearance		5 (31%)	1 (25%)

Table 3. Pancreatoscopic findings for pancreatic cancer and chronic pancreatitis.

	Pancreatic cancer ($n = 27$)	Chronic pancreatitis ($n = 12$)
Irregular mucosa	24 (89%)	
Redness and erosion	24 (89%)	6 (50%)
Scar		8 (67%)
Tumor vessel	20 (74%)	
Proliferation of blood vessels		6 (50%)

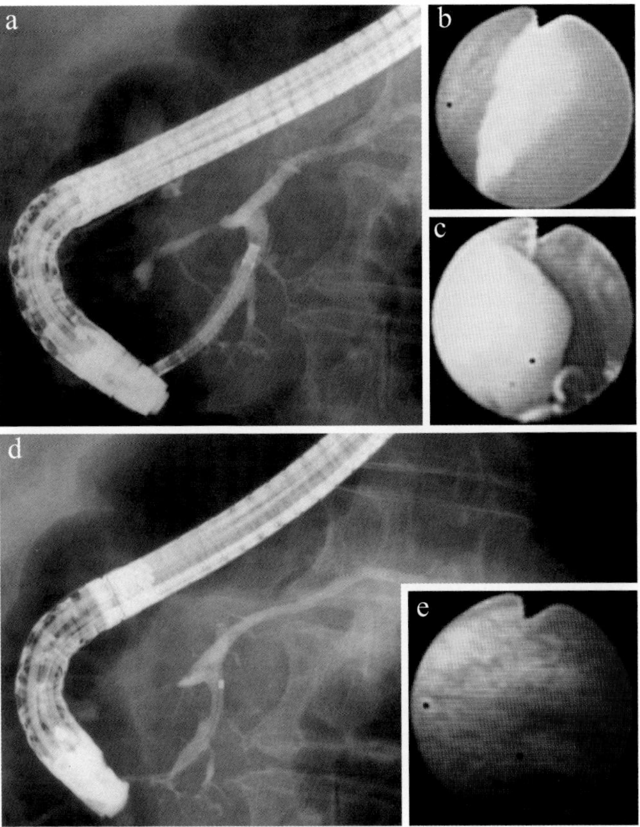

Fig. 4. Stones in the main pancreatic duct. **a–c** PPS reveals stones in the main pancreatic duct. **d, e** ERCP and PPS show no residual stone in the main pancreatic duct after extracorporeal shock wave lithotripsy (ESWL) and endoscopic removal of stones

experience, characteristic findings of pancreatoscopy in patients with pancreatic cancer, which is diagnosed pathologically, are irregular mucosa, redness, erosion, and tumor vessels. In contrast, scar is a characteristic finding of ductal stenosis resulting from chronic pancreatitis, which is confirmed by follow-up for more than 1 year (Table 3). In addition, an attempt at detecting carcinoma in situ in the main pancreatic duct by means of ultrathin pancreatoscopes was reported [8].

Therapeutic indications include treatment of stones in the main pancreatic duct, which can be approached by pancreatoscopes and cannot be treated by other modalities such as extracorporeal shock wave lithotripsy (ESWL). These pancreatic duct stones are treated by electrohydraulic lithotripsy (EHL) or laser under direct vision. Pancreatoscopy is also applied for extraction of stones in the main pancreatic duct with a small wire basket when it is difficult to remove stones in the main pancreatic duct with an ordinary wire basket under fluoroscopy (Fig. 4).

New Technology

Narrow-band imaging (NBI), which depends on the relationship between depth of light penetration and wavelength, has been recently developed. Using NBI, we can emphasize capillary and mucosal pattern by means of the special red-green-blue (RGB) filter. An attempt to apply NBI to differentiation and diagnosing the superficial extent of IPMN was recently reported [9].

On the other hand, development of the pancreatoscope system, which can be performed by a single operator, was reported from the United States [10]. This system is composed of an ultrathin optical probe, which has an external diameter of less than 1 mm, and a delivery catheter with four-way angulation and channels for irrigation, optical probe, and instruments that are 0.6, 0.9, and 1.2 mm in diameter, respectively.

Future Aspects

Although various improvements of pancreatoscopes have been made, some problems remain concerning insertion, observation, treatment, and durability. First, concerning insertion, reducing the external diameter and increasing the range of distal end bending with four-way angulation are needed. Next, concerning observation, improvement of image quality and development of new technologies to improve diagnostic ability, such as NBI, are expected. Furthermore, increasing the internal diameter of the working channel is desirable not only for lavaging the pancreatic duct but for also easy insertion of instruments. Concerning durability, further improvement of the insertion tube is expected, because present pancreatoscopes are still fragile. In, addition, development of a pancreatoscope system that can be used easily is desirable.

On the other hand, concerning treatment, drainage of a pseudocyst that had communicated with the main pancreatic duct, by means of inserting a guidewire under pancreatoscopic guidance, is one of the interesting application attempts.

Conclusion

Although various improvements of pancreatoscopes have already been done, their functionality is still inadequate. The development of smaller endoscopes with a larger working channel and better image quality and durability is needed. In addition, application of pancreatoscopy to the early detection of small malignant lesions in the pancreatic duct and therapeutic endoscopy is also expected.

References

1. Takekoshi T, Maruyama M, Sugiyama N, et al (1975) Retrograde pancreatocholangioscopy (in Japanese). Gastroenterol Endosc 17:676–683
2. Nakajima M, Akasaka Y, Fukumoto K, et al (1976) Peroral cholangiopancreatoscopy (PCPS) under duodenoscopic guidance. Am J Gastroenterol 66:241–247
3. Riemann JF, Kohler B (1993) Endoscopy of the pancreatic duct: value of different endoscope types. Gastrointest Endosc 39:367–370
4. Kodama T, Sato H, Horii Y, et al (1999) Pancreatoscopy for the next generation: development of the peroral electronic pancreatoscope system. Gastrointest Endosc 49:366–371
5. Yamao K, Ohashi K, Nakamura T, et al (2003) Efficacy of peroral pancreatoscopy in the diagnosis of pancreatic diseases. Gastrointest Endosc 57:205–209
6. Yasuda K, Sakata M, Ueda M, et al (2005) The use of pancreatoscopy in the diagnosis of intraductal papillary mucinous tumor lesions of the pancreas. Clin Gastroenterol Hepatol 3:S53–S57
7. Mukai H, Yasuda K, Nakajima M, et al (1998) Differential diagnosis of mucin-producing tumors of the pancreas by intraductal ultrasonography and peroral pancreatoscopy. Endoscopy 30:A99–A102
8. Uehara H, Nakaizumi A, Tatsuta M, et al (1997) Diagnosis of carcinoma in situ of the pancreas by peroral pancreatoscopy and pancreatoscopic cytology. Cancer (Phila) 79:454–461
9. Itoi T, Sofuni A, Itokawa F, et al (2007) Initial experience of peroral pancreatoscopy combined with narrow-band imaging in the diagnosis of intraductal papillary mucinous neoplasms of the pancreas. Gastrointest Endosc 66:793–797
10. Chen YK (2007) Preclinical characterization of Spyglass peroral cholangiopancreatoscopy system for direct access, visualization, and biopsy. Gastrointest Endosc 65:303–311

Diagnosis of Pancreaticobiliary Diseases Using Cholangioscopy and Pancreatoscopy with Narrow-Band Imaging

Takao Itoi, Atsushi Sofuni, and Fumihide Itokawa

Summary. Narrow-band imaging (NBI) makes it possible to emphasize the imaging of certain features such as mucosal structures and mucosal microvessels in gastrointestinal tract diseases. Recently, video peroral cholangioscopy (POCS) and pancreatoscopy (POPS) have been developed as diagnostic endoscopy for better observation of pancreaticobiliary lesions. Herein, we describe the clinical usefulness of POCS/POPS using NBI for the diagnosis of pancreaticobiliary diseases. In all pancreaticobiliary lesions, identification of the surface structure and vessels of the lesions by NBI observation was significantly better than with conventional observation. In conclusion, although maneuverability and fragility of POCS/POPS are limited and the current POCS/POPS is not equipped with magnification, POCS/POPS using NBI may be helpful for the observation of both fine mucosal structures and tumor vessels, resulting in correct target biopsy in patients with pancreaticobiliary diseases.

Key words. Cholangioscopy, Pancreatoscopy, Bile duct cancer, Intraductal papillary mucinous neoplasm

Introduction

Peroral choledochoscopy (POCS) and peroral pancreatoscopy (POPS) were developed three decades ago as diagnostic endoscopy tools for observation of bile duct or pancreatic duct lesions that are difficult to differentiate on endoscopic retrograde cholangiopancreatography and for accurate diagnosis in biopsy [1–6]. To date, furthermore, we have evaluated the observation of biliary tract disease using chromoendoscopy (CE) with methylene blue or autofluorescence imaging (AFI) because of the limitation of white light illumination; however, we did not obtain more informative results [7]. In gastrointestinal tract diseases, narrow-band imaging (NBI) makes it possible to emphasize the imaging of certain features such as mucosal structures and mucosal microvessels [8]. We herein summarize our data [9,10] and evaluate diagnostic cho-

Department of Gastroenterology and Hepatology, Tokyo Medical University, 6-7-1 Nishishinjuku, Shinjuku-ku, Tokyo 160-0023, Japan

ledochoscopy using NBI as a novel diagnostic tool in conjunction with the possibility of POPS.

Methods

Conventional POCS/POPS and NBI Endoscopic System

Endoscopic sphincterotomy (ES) was or had been performed previously before the POCS procedure. In contrast, ES was not performed during the POPS procedure. A video cholangiopancreatoendoscope (CHF-B260; Olympus Medical Systems, Tokyo, Japan) was advanced through the accessory channel of a conventional therapeutic duodenoscope (TJF 200; Olympus Medical Systems) into the bile duct. All endoscopic procedures were performed by conventional POCS/POPS and the newly available NBI system (CV-260SL processor, CVL-260SL light source; Olympus Medical Systems). The bile duct and pancreatic duct were irrigated through an accessory channel with saline solution during endoscopic biliary and pancreatic duct examination. The NBI system used in this study is based on the modification of spectral features with an optical color separation filter narrowing the bandwidth of spectral transmittance. The filter is placed in the optical illumination system. The filter cuts all illumination wavelengths, except two narrow wavelengths. The central wavelengths of each band are 415 and 540 nm. The image is reproduced in the processor with information from two illumination bands. The wavelength of 415 nm provides most information on the capillary and pit patterns of the superficial mucosa, and the wavelength of 540 nm provides information about thicker capillaries in slightly deeper tissues. After inspection with white light endoscopy and NBI, biopsies of all abnormal lesions were performed under direct vision using 3 Fr. ultrathin biopsy forceps (FB-44U-1; Olympus Medical Systems).

To evaluate the feasibility of the NBI system for clinical usage, its ability to identify biliary tract or main pancreatic duct lesions was compared with conventional observation. Biopsies from lesions using POCS/POPS were attempted in all cases. The evaluation points were the delineation of (i) the margin of the lesions distally or proximally if possible and (ii) identification of vessels on the surface of the lesions.

Outcome

POCS Using NBI

Twelve patients, 8 men and 4 women, were enrolled. On the basis of endoscopic retrograde cholangiopancreatography (ERCP) findings, they consisted of 6 strictures and 6 filling defects. All POCS procedures were performed successfully with no procedure-related morbidity or mortality. The findings were 7 extrahepatic bile duct cancers, 2 mucosal hyperplastic lesions in the bile duct, and 3 inflammatory bile duct changes caused by choledocholithiasis. Surgical resection was performed in 5 patients with bile duct cancers. Two patients with mucosal hyperplasia have been followed up for more than 14 months without malignant findings. In 3 patients with inflammatory changes, POCS was performed to distinguish benign and malignant lesions after endoscopic lithotripsy.

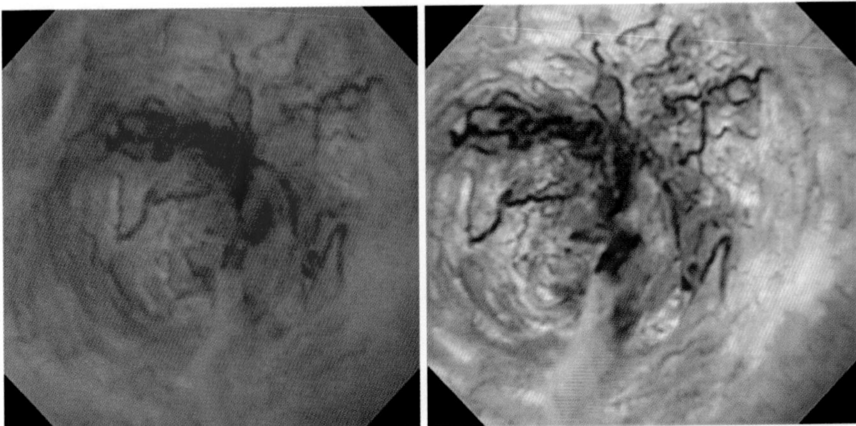

Fig. 1. Bile duct cancer. Conventional cholangioscopy showed biliary stricture and tumor vessels (*left*). Narrow-band imaging (NBI) could clarify tumor vessels (*right*)

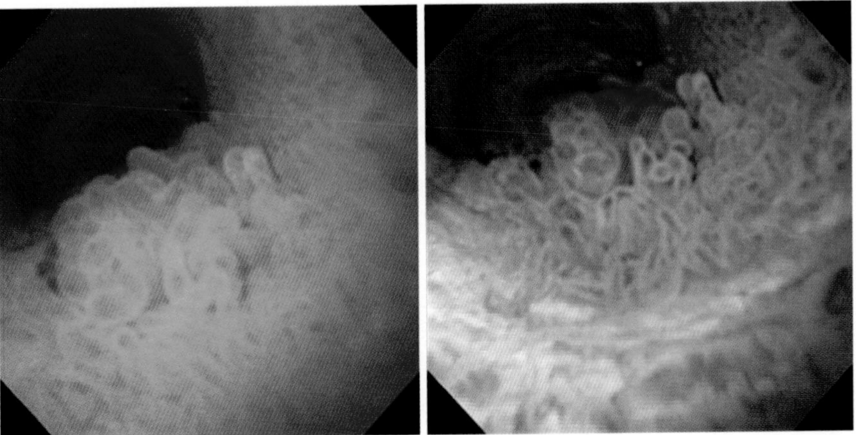

Fig. 2. Benign mucosal hyperplasia. Conventional cholangioscopy shows a low papillary mucosal lesion (*left*). NBI reveals clear margin of the lesion (*right*)

Twenty-one lesions of 12 patients were evaluated using POCS with conventional white light imaging and NBI. In cases of bile duct cancers, the distal portion of the main lesions was observed. In contrast, the proximal portion was evaluated in 2 cases in which POCS could move the tumor to the hepatic side. Regardless of a benign or malignant main lesion, the ability of NBI observation to identify both the surface structure (Figs. 1, 2) and mucosal vessels was as good as or better than conventional observation. In particular, in the portion with superficial cancerous extent, NBI was predisposed to be better than conventional observation. In the case showing intramural cancerous extent, there was no abnormal surface structure or vessels by both conventional and NBI observation.

diagnosis of the tumor's superficial extension within the bile duct mucosa. For this reason, a video PTCS, which is capable of providing detailed observations of the biliary mucosa and any minute changes there, is considered to be highly useful, particularly for diagnosing mucin-producing bile duct tumors [6].

Narrow-band imaging (NBI) is an observation method which enhances the blood vessels and the minute patterns of the mucosa by altering the spectrum of the endoscope. Its utility for the early detection of cancer, and in diagnosing and recognizing its extension in the region of the digestive tract, has been reported. Along with the recent development of cholangioscopy, NBI has been used in the biliary tract and the main pancreatic duct [7]. Here we report on the utility of PTCS for mucin-producing bile duct tumors, and our clinical experiences of NBI observations.

Patients and Methods

We used a CHF-XP260, Olympus Medical Systems, Tokyo, Japan, which is a videoscope with a small diameter, to assess 6 cases of mucin-producing bile duct tumor between April 1998 and October 2007. For those cases which had been treated before the development of the small-diameter videoscope we used an electron bronchial scope by expanding the PTBD fistula to the size of 16 Fr. The outer diameter of the CHF-XP260 is 3.7 mm, which is the same as that of the CHF-XP20, and scope insertion is achieved through a PTBD fistula of 12 Fr. The channel lumen, through which devices for biopsy or stone treatment can be inserted, is 1.2 mm in diameter.

Case Reports

Case 1

Case 1 was a 72-year-old woman with a mucin-producing bile duct tumor. Using ultrasound (US) and computed tomography (CT), a marked dilatation of the bile duct was observed. Endoscopic retrograde cholangiopancreatography (ERCP) revealed a largely opened papilla and the discharge of abundant mucin (Fig. 1). A papillary tumor surrounding the upper bile duct was observed by PTCS (Fig. 2). This was diagnosed as a papillary tumor primarily developed in Bs, and a resection of the extrahepatic bile duct was performed. The postoperative findings were macroscopically a papillary tumor located in Bs (Fig. 3), and pathologically the multiple development of papillary adenoma, presenting the features of papillomatosis (Fig. 4). The papillary tumor had been observed clearly by video PTCS.

Case 2

An abdominal CT showed a cystic tumor and dilatation of the bile duct in S4 of the liver (Fig. 5). Since a mucin-producing bile duct tumor was suspected, a PTBD route was constructed to treat the jaundice and to evaluate the tumor extension. Dilatation of the bile duct was shown by biliary contrast imaging. The bile duct branch in B2 was not imaged. In this case, it was of crucial importance to discover whether or not the tumor had a superficial extension in the biliary mucosa before deciding on the surgical approach. By carrying out PTCS, we found a papillary elevation at the bile

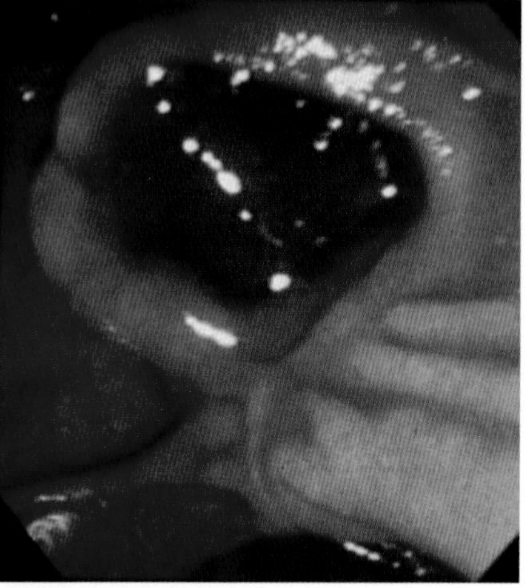

Fig. 1. Endoscopic retrograde cholangiopancreatography (ERCP) revealed a largely opened papilla and the discharge of abundant mucin

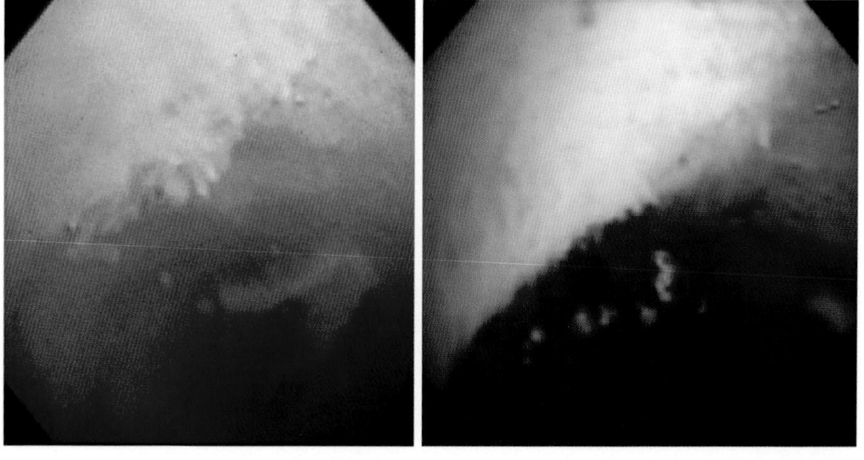

Fig. 2. Percutaneous transhepatic cholangioscopy (PTCS) findings. A papillary tumor surrounding the upper bile duct was observed

duct branch which had a cystic dilatation in B2, and confirmed that the papillary elevation continued into B2/3 (Fig. 6a), Bs (Fig. 6b), and Br (Fig. 6c).

We also applied NBI to this case. By regular optical cholangioscopy, it is possible, to a limited extent, to recognize the papillary elevation in the biliary mucosal surface and the border of normal mucosa. However, the border between the normal mucosa and the tumorous mucosa was more clearly recognized by NBI observations (Fig. 7). In the future, it is possible that the border between a papillary tumor and normal mucosa will be determined more precisely by NBI observations.

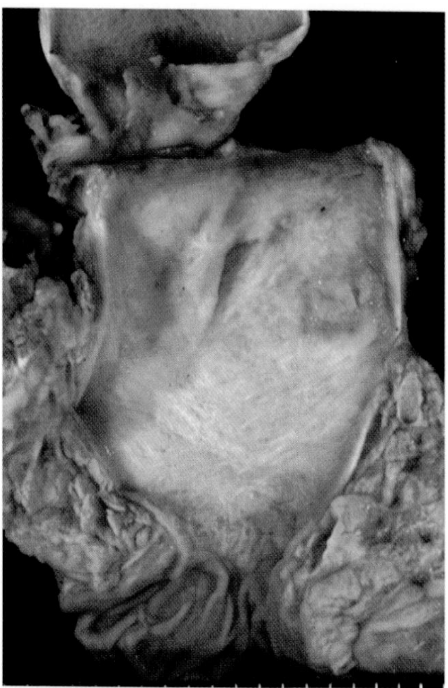

FIG. 3. Macroscopic postoperative findings of a papillary tumor located in the superior part of the bile duct

a

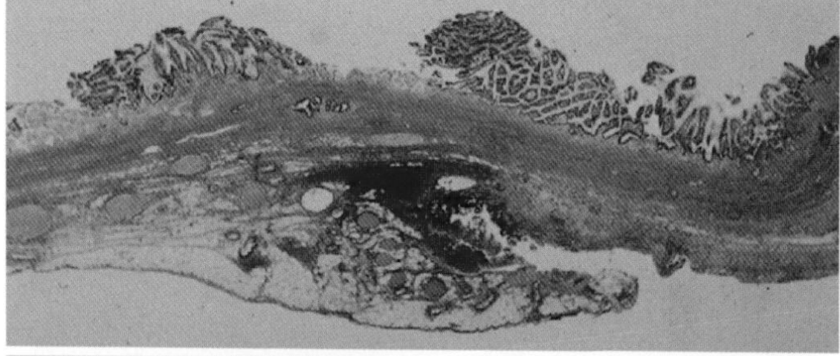

b

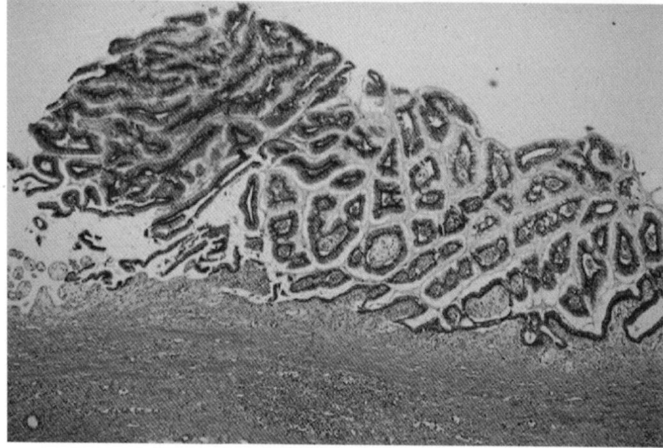

FIG. 4. Pathological findings of the multiple development of a papillary adenoma presenting the feature of papillomatosis

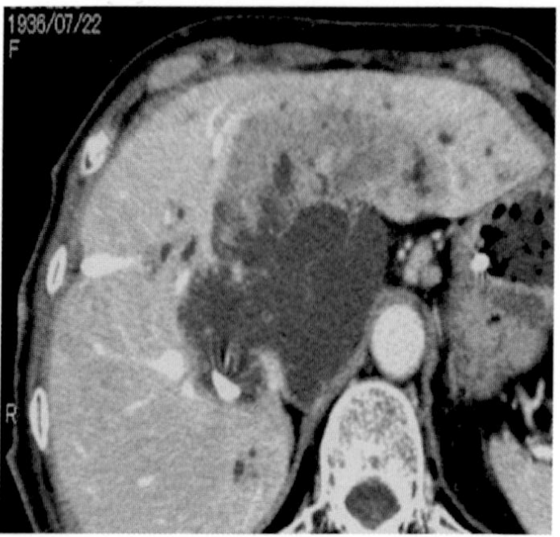

Fig. 5. Abdominal computed tomography (CT) findings. A cystic tumor and dilatation of the bile duct in S4 of the liver

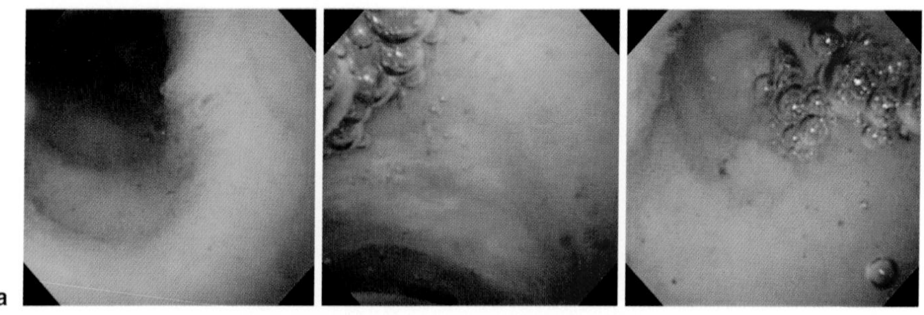

Fig. 6. PTCS findings. Papillary elevation at the bile duct branch. **a** B2/3; **b** Bs; **c** Br

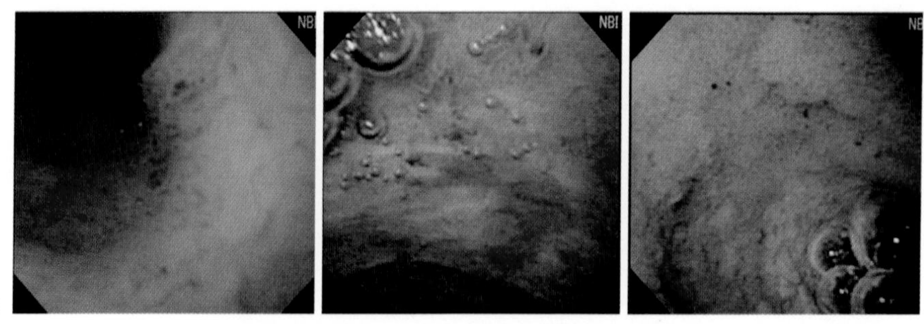

Fig. 7. Narrow-band imaging (NBI) observation. The border between the normal mucosa and the tumorous mucosa is clearly recognizable. **a** B2/3; **b** Bs; **c** Br

Discussion

In mucin-producing bile duct tumors, the existence of a superficial extension in the bile duct mucosa is extremely important for deciding the treatment plan. Our 6 treated cases were observed with video PTCS. In all of them it was possible to observe minute changes in the bile duct mucosa, and these were found to be useful in diagnosing the superficial extension of the tumor.

However, not infrequently we found it difficult to distinguish the tumors from hyperplastic or inflammatory changes of the bile duct mucosa because of the extremely high capability of the videoscope to demonstrate very fine changes in the mucosa. When observing the inside of the bile duct by PTCS, we may sometimes find secondary changes in the bile duct mucosa, such as an artifact brought about by the tube or inflammatory changes caused by cholangitis. Although it is important to observe the continuity of a tumor closely from the main focus when diagnosing a tumor extension, often this evaluation can also be difficult. Therefore, the diagnosis must be made based on comprehensive pathological findings by biopsy as well as newly accumulated endoscopic findings by videoscope.

NBI can also be useful for diagnosing the extent of a tumor. In our experience, we have found that NBI revealed the border between a tumor and normal mucosa very much more clearly than regular optical cholangioscopy. However, the resolution of video PTCS is not particularly high compared with the scopes used for the region of the digestive tract. Therefore, it is difficult to obtain vascular images of high resolution, and NBI observations with a cholangioscope seem only to recognize structural abnormalities. Therefore, it is still uncertain whether it is possible to distinguish between a tumor and a nontumor with PTCS. Experience of a larger number of cases and improvements in the resolution of electron endoscopy should improve the situation.

POCS (Peroral cholangioscopy) is available to replace PTCS. POCS is now also equipped with a video system, and it has been shown that images obtained by video POCS are of as high a resolution as those obtained by video PTCS. However, problems remain with video POCS in scanning, water supply, aeration, and aspiration. In a case such as mucin-producing bile duct cancer in particular, a detailed diagnosis is difficult unless bile containing a considerable amount of mucin is removed. If this is not possible, it is necessary to insert the scope repeatedly into the periphery of the bile duct branches in order to observe the mucosa. In such cases POCS is not suitable, and for an accurate diagnosis PTCS must be carried out after constructing the PTBD route. Considering the burden to the patient and the complications experienced with PTBD, it would naturally be desirable that the examination should be done by POCS. Before that can happen, the further development of improved and effective scopes is eagerly anticipated.

Conclusion

The CHF-XP260 videoscope can obtain high-resolution images. It is also capable of revealing tiny changes in the bile duct mucosa, and is useful for diagnosing bile duct diseases, particularly any superficial mucosal extension of a mucin-producing bile duct tumor.

References

1. Van Steenbergen W, Van Aken L, Van Beckevoort D, et al. (1996) Percutaneous transhepatic cholangioscopy for diagnosis and therapy of biliary diseases in older patients. J Am Geriatr Soc 44:1384–1387
2. Nimura Y, Shionoya S, Hayakawa N, et al. (1988) Value of percutaneous transhepatic cholangioscopy (PTCS). Surg Endosc 2:213–219
3. Nimura Y (1993) Staging of biliary carcinoma: cholangiography and cholangioscopy. Endoscopy 25:76–80
4. Kato M, Nimura Y, Kamiya J, et al. (1997) Carcinoma of the common bile duct with superficial spread to the intrahepatic segmental bile ducts: a case report. Am Surg 63:943–947
5. Kokubo T, Itai Y, Ohtomo K, et al. (1988) Mucin-hypersecreting intrahepatic biliary neoplasm. Radiology 168:609–614
6. Katanuma A, Maguchi H, Itokawa F, et al (2005) Clinical evaluation of the percutaneous transhepatic videocholangioscope with a thin diameter. Dig Endosc 17:S85–S88
7. Itoi T, Sofuni A, Itokawa F, et al. (2007) Initial experience of peroral pancreatoscopy combined with narrow-band imaging in the diagnosis of intraductal papillary mucinous neoplasms of the pancreas (with videos). Gastrointest Endosc 66:793–797

EUS

Standardization of Imaging Techniques in the Pancreatobiliary Region Using Radial Scanning EUS

Hiroyuki Maguchi, Akio Katanuma, Manabu Osanai, and Kuniyuki Takahashi

Summary. Standard imaging techniques in the pancreatobiliary region using radial scanning endoscopic ultrasonography (EUS) were prepared by the Endoscopic Forum Japan (EFJ) Working Group and published in 2003. Among the techniques, the most difficult point for physicians is how to image the pancreatic head region from the descending part of the duodenum. There are two methods, the Pull method and the Push method. The Pull method is the same as the endoscopic retrograde cholangiopancreatography (ERCP) stretch technique, and the Push method is applied when imaging of the bile duct by the Pull method is difficult. Mastering EUS in the pancreatobiliary region requires intensive and long-term training. The standard imaging techniques are highly useful for education. We hope that these standard imaging techniques will be widespread and help to establish effective training and education programs throughout the world.

Key words. Standard imaging technique, EUS, Pancreatobiliary region

Introduction

Endoscopic ultrasonography (EUS) was originally developed in 1980 in Japan for detecting early-stage pancreatobiliary malignancies [1]. Its use has spread for diagnosis of not only pancreatobiliary diseases but also gastrointestinal diseases.

The advantages of EUS are its high resolution and capability of local observation. It is one of the most accurate diagnostic methods, particularly for the pancreatobiliary region, among the various advanced imaging diagnostic methods available today [2–4]. However, the operating techniques are difficult, and also no standard EUS operation has been established for examination of the pancreatobiliary region. In other words, being operator dependent has been a disadvantage of EUS.

With the aim of solving this difficulty, the Endoscopic Forum Japan (EFJ) decided to organize a working group and publish a handbook as a reference of standard techniques in 1999. The members were Kazuo Inui (Fujita Health University), Mitsuhiro Kida (Kitasato University East Hospital), Naotaka Fujita (Sendai City

---

Center for Gastroenterology, Teine-Keijinkai Hospital, 1-jo 12-chome, Maeda, Teine-ku, Sapporo 006-8555, Japan

Medical Center), Kenjiro Yasuda (Kyoto Second Red Cross Hospital), Kenji Yamao (Aichi Cancer Center Hospital), and Hiroyuki Maguchi (Teine-Keijinkai Hospital). After 3 years of fruitful discussion, we issued the handbook *Standard Imaging Techniques in the Pancreatobiliary Region Using Radial Scanning EUS* in 2003, and it was published in the journal *Digestive Endoscopy* in 2004 [5].

Standard Imaging Techniques

This handbook describes the standard imaging methods of the pancreatobiliary region by EUS and shows the indices for localization of organs in the pancreatobiliary region.

The position of the endoscopist and orientation of the handle of the scope are important. In the images in this handbook, the endoscopist is facing the patient and the scope handle is oriented orthogonally to the axis of the patient's body (Fig. 1).

There are three basic scanning positions for pancreatobiliary EUS: the stomach, the duodenal bulb or the gastric antrum, and the descending part of the duodenum (Fig. 2). In the process of publishing the book, the most controversial point was the technique to image the pancreatic head region from the descending part of the duodenum.

Scanning from the Descending Part of the Duodenum

There are two different methods of scanning from the descending part of the duodenum: the Pull method and the Push method. The Pull method is the same as in the endoscopic retrograde cholangiopancreatography (ERCP) stretch technique, and the Push method is applied when imaging of the bile duct by the Pull method is difficult. For observation of the pancreatic head and major papilla, two scanning methods are available depending on the scope angulation at the initial step: the longitudinal method and the transverse method (Fig. 3) [6].

The longitudinal method is to rotate the up/down knob in the "up" direction and perform scanning while withdrawing the scope. This procedure provides a longitudinal view of the pancreatic head, and the scanning goes parallel to the aorta and infe-

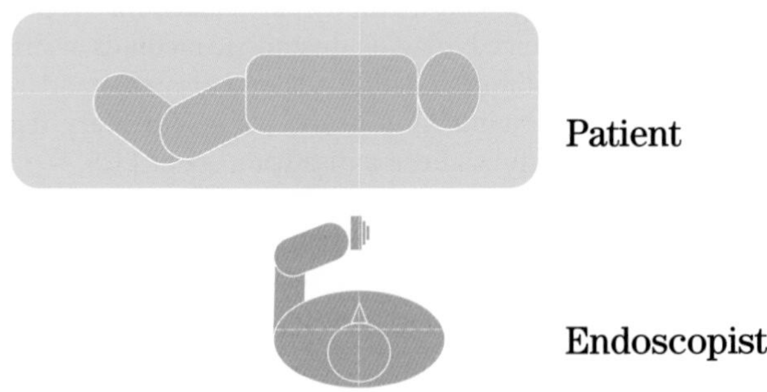

Fig. 1. Position of endoscopist and orientation of handle of scope

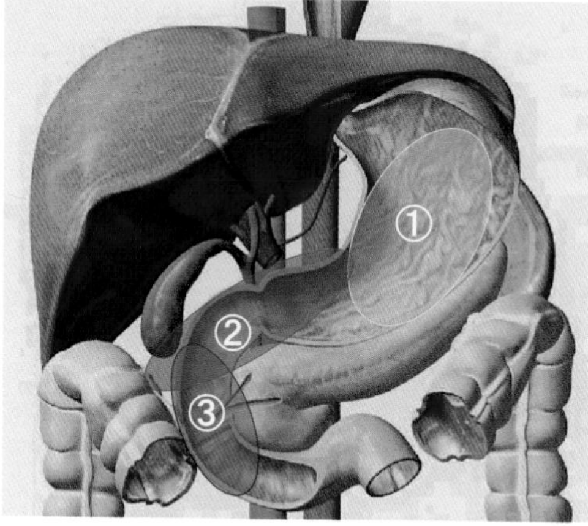

Fig. 2. Scanning position: recommended order of scanning is *1* to *3* to *2* or *3* to *2* to *1*

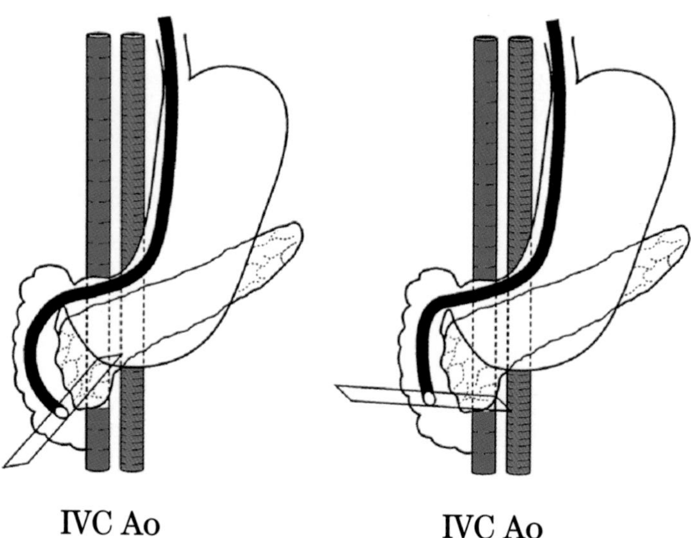

Fig. 3. Schematic illustration of scanning methods: *left*, longitudinal method; *right*, transverse method; *IVC*, inferior vena cava; *Ao*, aorta

rior vena cava. The advantages of this method are that a wide view of the pancreatic head is imaged and that it is easy to delineate the longitudinal view of the common bile duct and main pancreatic duct near the papilla. A disadvantage is that beginners may have difficulty in identifying the major papilla.

The transverse method is to adjust the "up/down" and "right/left" knobs to obtain a cross-sectional view of the aorta and then perform scanning while pulling the scope backward. This procedure provides a transverse view of the pancreatic head, aorta, and inferior vena cava. One of the advantages of this method is that it is easy to identify the major papilla. A disadvantage is that longitudinal images of the common bile duct cannot be obtained in this scope position.

Procedure of the Longitudinal Method

At the start of scanning, the scope approaches the inferior duodenal angle as in the ERCP stretch technique. When the up/down knob is in the neutral position, the aorta (Ao) and inferior vena cava (IVC) should be observed as circular cross-sectional images at the 6- to 9-o'clock position in the ultrasound image (Fig. 4a). Then, the up/down knob is rotated in the "up" direction until the longitudinal view of the Ao and IVC is obtained. The superior mesenteric vein (SMV) can be seen on the opposite side. A portion of the pancreatic head that is surrounded by the Ao, SMV, and the scope is demonstrated in the right half of the image (Fig. 4b).

Withdrawing the scope allows visualization of the triangle region of the lower echogenicity adjacent to the scope: this is the level of the major papilla (Fig. 5a). By withdrawing the scope a little further, the longitudinal view of the bile and pancreatic ducts is obtained. The ductal structure closer to the scope is the bile duct and the other is the pancreatic duct (Fig. 5b).

Use the image rotating function to observe the junction between the pancreatic and bile ducts at a preferred position. After imaging the Ao and IVC as longitudinal structures, rotate the image so that those structures are positioned in the upper half of the image. The pancreatic head can be observed in the lower half of the image (Fig. 6a). When the pancreatic and bile ducts are in the lower half of the image, it is possible to magnify their images by using the lower semicircular display mode (Fig. 6b).

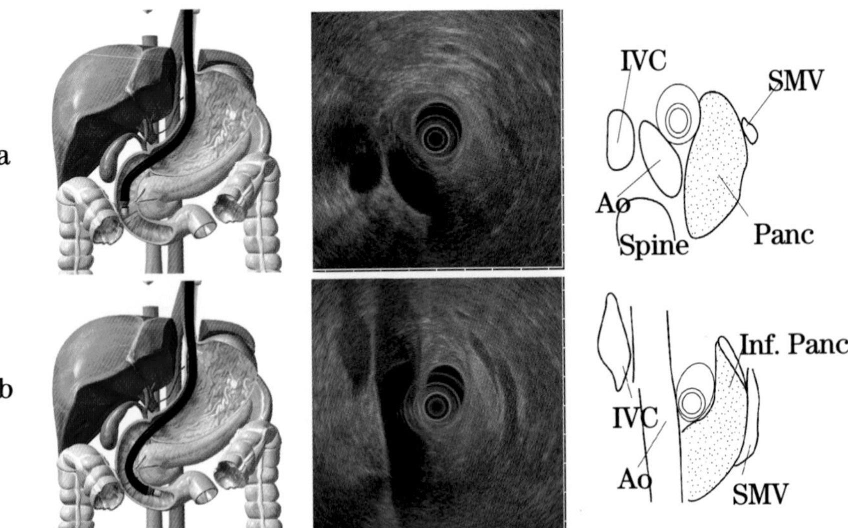

Fig. 4. Longitudinal method (1). *SMV*, superior mesenteric vein; *Inf. Panc*, inferior pancreatic head

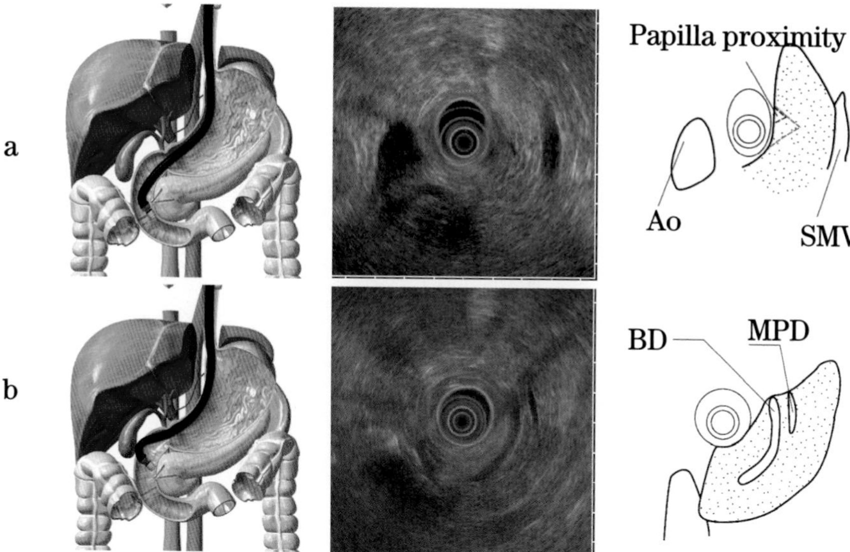

FIG. 5. Longitudinal method (2). *BD*, bile duct; *MPD*, main pancreatic duct

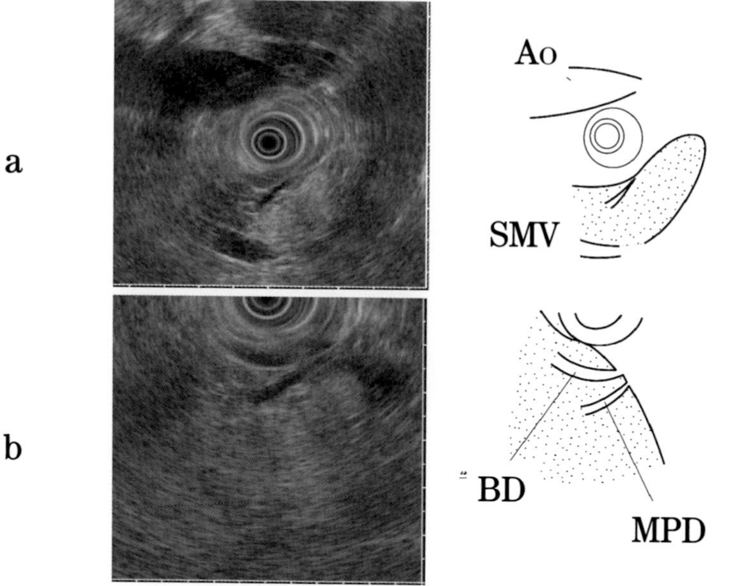

FIG. 6. Using the image rotation function

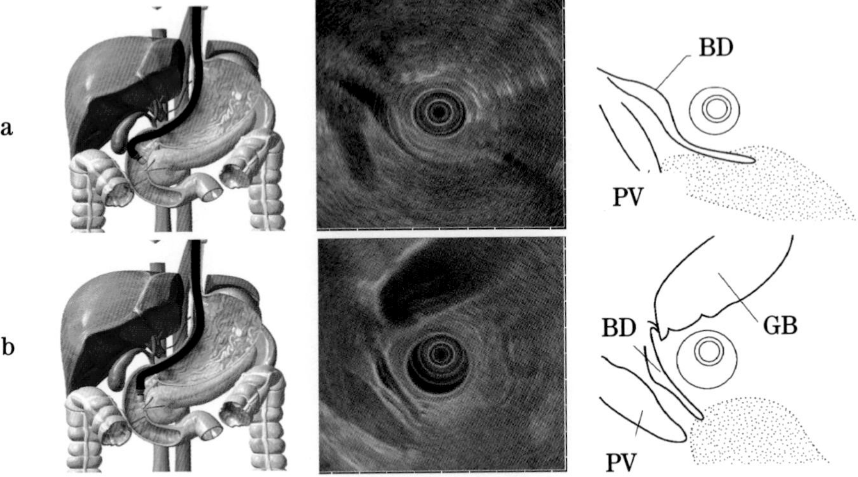

FIG. 7. Longitudinal method (3). *PV*, portal vein; *GB*, gallbladder

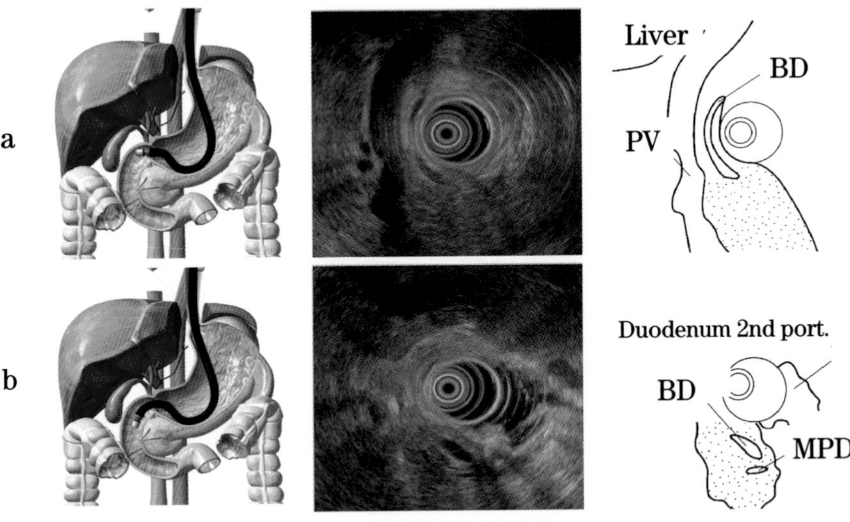

FIG. 8. Push method

After observing the pancreatic head, withdraw and twist the scope counterclockwise; the bile duct will be visualized along its axis (Fig. 7a). As the scope is withdrawn slowly, the neck of the gallbladder will appear on the left side of the image (Fig. 7b). When the bile duct and gallbladder cannot be observed satisfactorily with the Pull method, the Push method is often useful.

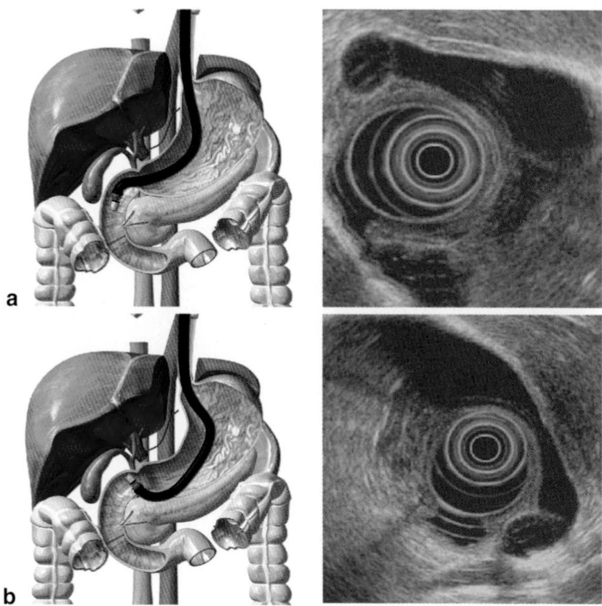

Fig. 9. Notes for understanding images of the gallbladder. **a** Pull method; **b** Push method

Procedure of the Push Method

Reinsert the scope into the duodenal bulb and push the scope to the superior duodenal angle; the portal vein is imaged on the left side of the image and the bile duct is visualized between the portal vein and the scope (Fig. 8a). After the bile duct is visualized, trace it and push the scope; this makes it possible to image the area near the major papilla (Fig. 8b).

Observation of the Gallbladder

Please note the following to understand images of the gallbladder. When the gallbladder is visualized by withdrawing the scope from the descending part of the duodenum with the Pull method, the neck of the gallbladder is located on the left side of the image (Fig. 9a). If we scan by the Push method, the neck appears on the right side of the image (Fig. 9b) because the tip of the scope is oriented upward in the patient when using the Push method whereas it is oriented downward with the Pull method.

Utility of Standard Imaging Techniques in the Pancreatobiliary Region Using Radial Scanning EUS

Mastering EUS in the pancreatobiliary region requires intensive training and a long training period [6]. We have performed EUS examinations for more than 600 cases per year (Fig. 10) according to this standard method, and many young doctors have

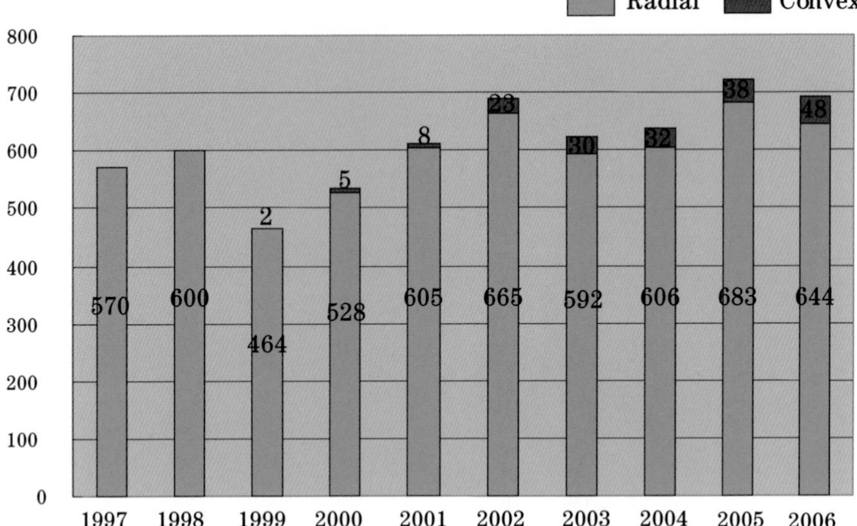

Fig. 10. Numbers of endoscopic ultrasonography (EUS) examinations in the pancreatobiliary region at our institution, 1997–2006

come to our hospital to learn it. We have also held a EUS live demonstration seminar annually in our institute for wide dissemination of the standard imaging techniques. It is necessary to foster skillful EUS operators. We hope that our standard imaging techniques will become widespread and help to establish effective training and education programs throughout the world.

References

1. Yasuda K (2000) The handbook of endoscopic ultrasonography in digestive tract. Blackwell Science, Japan, pp 1–6
2. Maguchi H (2004) The role of endoscopic ultrasonography in the diagnosis of pancreatic tumors. J Hepatobiliary Pancreat Surg 11:1–3
3. Maguchi H, Takahashi K, Osanai M, et al (2006) Small pancreatic lesions: is there need for EUS-FNA preoperatively? What to do with the incidental lesions? Endoscopy 38:S53–S56
4. Maguchi H (2001) Roles of endoscopic and intraductal ultrasonography in the diagnosis of pancreaticobiliary lesions. Dig Endosc 13:S42–S46
5. EFJ working group on standardization of pancreatobiliary EUS (2004) Standard imaging techniques in the pancreatobiliary region using radial scanning endoscopic ultrasonography. Dig Endosc 16:S118–S133
6. Maguchi H (2004) Education and training for endoscopic ultrasonography in Japan. Dig Endosc 16:S148–S152

New Diagnostic Technique of EUS Using Contrast-Enhanced Agents

Yoshiki Hirooka[1], Akihiro Itoh[2], and Hidemi Goto[1,2]

Summary. The analysis of morphology obtained by endoscopic ultrasonography (EUS) has been the main aim of EUS diagnosis. On the other hand, various disorders have their own characteristic vascularities in the digestive organs. The combination of diagnosis with morphology and vascularities is thought to be important and useful. Needless to say, the core function of EUS is ultrasonography, and EUS should follow state-of-the-art technology of ultrasonography. In this chapter, we discuss EUS angiography, contrast-enhanced EUS (CE-EUS) using the first contrast agent (Albunex), the next agent (Levovist), and the latest agent (Sonazoid).

Key words. Contrast-enhanced EUS, Carbon dioxide, Albunex, Levovist, Sonazoid

Introduction

Analysis of morphology obtained by endoscopic ultrasonography (EUS) has been the main aim of EUS diagnosis. On the other hand, various disorders have their own characteristic vascularities in the digestive organs. Abdominal angiography, for example, revealed such characteristic vascularities and was believed to be a useful diagnostic modality. It is not sufficient, however, to diagnose disorders by their vascularities alone; the combination of morphology and vascularity is thought to be much more important and useful. Consequently, diagnostic modalities such as computed tomography (CT) and magnetic resonance imaging (MRI), in which the combination diagnosis of morphology and vascularity is possible, are believed to be the most reliable.

Needless to say, the core function of EUS is ultrasonography, and EUS should follow state-of-the-art technology of ultrasonography. In this chapter, we discuss the past and present of contrast-enhanced EUS (CE-EUS).

---

[1]Department of Endoscopy, Nagoya University Hospital, 65 Tsuruma-cho, Showa-ku, Nagoya, Nagoya 466-8550, Japan
[2]Department of Gastroenterology, Nagoya University Graduate School of Medicine, Nagoya, Japan

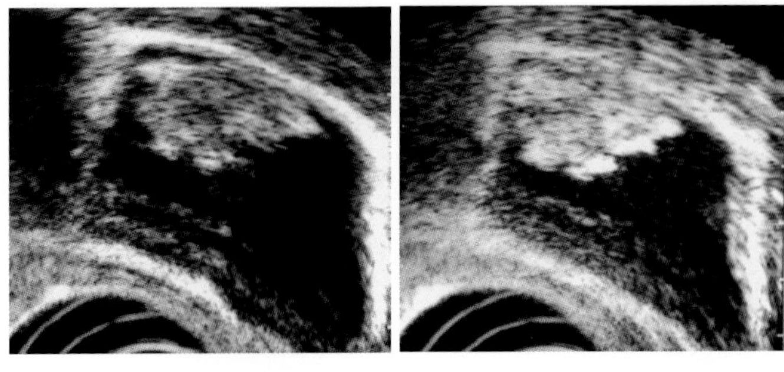

a: plain EUS **b: CE-EUS**

Fig. 1. Gallbladder cancer. **a** A hypo-iso-echoic mass was seen at the body of the gallbladder. Plain endoscopic ultrasonography (EUS). **b** After the injection of carbon dioxide, the echo intensity of the tumor was obviously increased, indicating the hypervascular tumor. Contrast-enhanced EUS (CE-EUS)

EUS Angiography

Matsuda and Yabuuchi [1] gave the first epoch-making report on ultrasonographic angiography (US angiography) in 1986. Ultrasonographic angiography made it possible to observe changes of echo intensity on B-mode US images. The characteristic vascularities of hepatic lesions were clearly demonstrated, and US angiography became the gold standard in their diagnosis. We utilized the technique of US angiography for EUS, namely, EUS angiography [2]. In the procedure of EUS, carbon dioxide was injected into an artery, such as the celiac artery or the common hepatic artery.

Figure 1 shows gallbladder cancer. After injection of carbon dioxide, the echo intensity of the tumor was obviously increased, indicating the hypervascular tumor. Despite its usefulness, EUS angiography had to wait for the advent of a new-generation contrast agent, mainly because of the burden on the patients.

The Advent of Albunex

In 1995, sonicated serum albumin (Albunex; Shionogi, Osaka, Japan) was introduced into the clinical setting in Japan. Albunex injected into a peripheral vein could pass through the pulmonary alveoli and show enhancement in the abdominal organs. The enhancing power of the agent however was weak, so Albunex was mainly used for the enhancement of color/power Doppler flow imaging using transabdominal US. Theoretically, in the B-mode images, the agent or its aggregation was recognized only by at least 10 MHz or more in ultrasonographic frequency; thus, we tried to observe the various targets using 12-MHz frequency EUS. As was expected, enhancement of B-mode EUS images was observed [3–6].

Figure 2 shows a pancreatic endocrine tumor. A clearly delineated hypoechoic mass was observed at the pancreatic head, which was suspected to be an endocrine tumor.

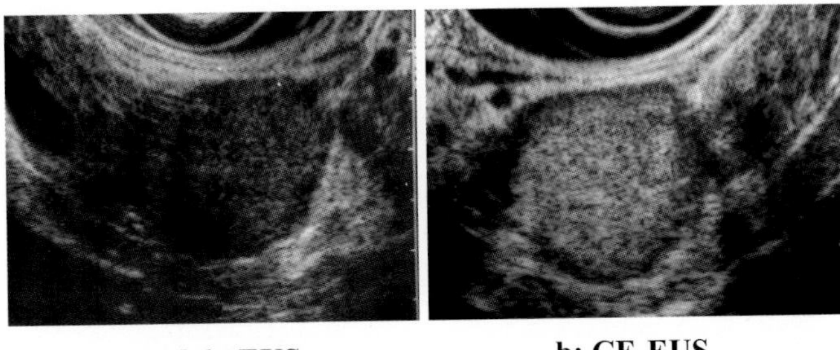

Fig. 2. Pancreatic endocrine tumor. **a** On plain EUS, a clearly delineated hypoechoic mass was observed at the pancreatic head, suspicious of endocrine tumor. **b** A few minutes after injection of Albunex, the echo intensity of the tumor was increased, indicating hypervascularity of the tumor

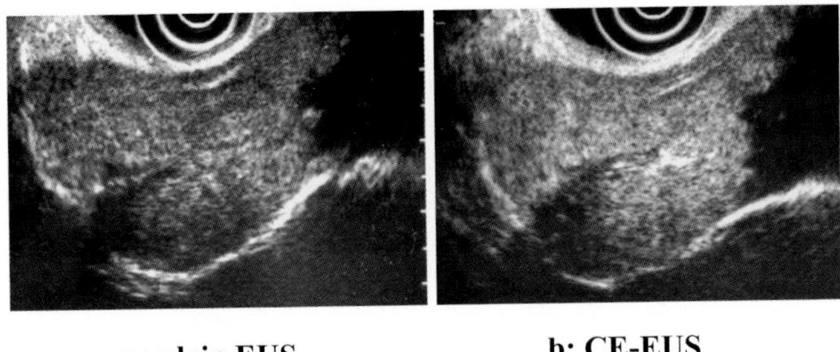

Fig. 3. Gallbladder cancer. **a, b** A massive hypoechoic tumor was seen in the gallbladder, the echo intensity of which was increased after injection of Albunex, indicating hypervascular gallbladder cancer

A few minutes after injection of Albunex, the echo intensity of the tumor was increased indicating the hypervascularity of the tumor. Figure 3 demonstrates gallbladder cancer. A massive hypoechoic tumor was seen in the gallbladder, the echo intensity of which was increased indicating hypervascular gallbladder cancer. Albunex had feasibility and utility as a diagnostic agent but was discarded, partly because the agent was very fragile but mainly because a new agent, Levovist (Nihon Schering, Osaka, Japan), appeared in the clinical setting in Japan.

Progress of Endosonoscope and Appearance of Levovist

Figure 4 demonstrates the recent progress of EUS. The scanning method has been converted from a mechanical scanning method into an electronic scanning method (electronic radial and electronic linear). Using electronic scanning methods, many applications that were already in use in clinical practice in transabdominal ultrasonography could be applied to EUS, such as tissue harmonic imaging (THI),

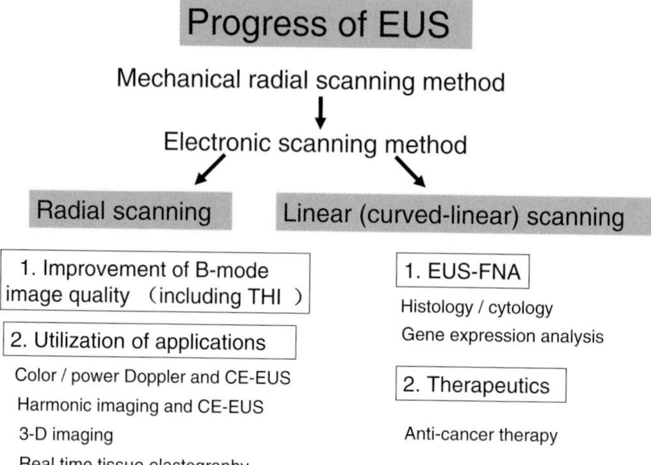

Fig. 4. Progress of EUS. *THI*, tissue harmonic imaging; *CE-EUS*, contrast-enhanced EUS; *3-D*, three-dimensional; *FNA*, fine-needle aspiration

color/power Doppler flow imaging, contrast-harmonic imaging, three-dimensional imaging, and elastography. As for the CE-EUS, color/power Doppler flow imaging and contrast-harmonic imaging were very important.

Levovist provides significant enhancement both for color and for power Doppler flow imaging, but the combination of power Doppler flow imaging and Levovist gave limited utility, mainly because of an artifact called blooming. Power Doppler signals enhanced by Levovist were too radiant and glowing for details to be recognized, resulting in lesser clinical usefulness. For the reason already mentioned, we usually adopt color Doppler flow imaging for CE-EUS, and in addition, contrast-harmonic imaging with Levovist gives minimal and impractical information.

The target lesions were observed by EUS, then the agent (Levovist) was adjusted to 300 mg/ml in concentration, injected intravenously at a rate of 1 ml/s, and the enhancement effect was estimated. The endoscopes and ultrasound systems used were as follows: one set was from Pentax and Hitachi (Fig. 5), and the other was from Olympus Medical Systems and Aloka (Tokyo, Japan) (Fig. 6). Figure 7 shows a pancreatic cancer case. A hypoechoic mass was seen at the pancreatic head, suspected to be pancreatic cancer; the hypoechoic mass was hypovascular, indicating pancreatic cancer by hemodynamics. Figure 8 demonstrates a pancreatic endocrine tumor. Some color signals were seen in the tumor on plain color Doppler flow imaging on CE-EUS, the tumor was filled with numerous color signals, except for the distal part of the EUS probe. Necrosis was proved in the area of no color on the resected specimen. Figure 9 shows invasive carcinoma derived from main duct type intraductal papillary mucinous neoplasm (IPMN). A papillary-like structure was seen at the dilated main pancreatic duct; color signals were seen at the papillary structure, indicating true papillary growth.

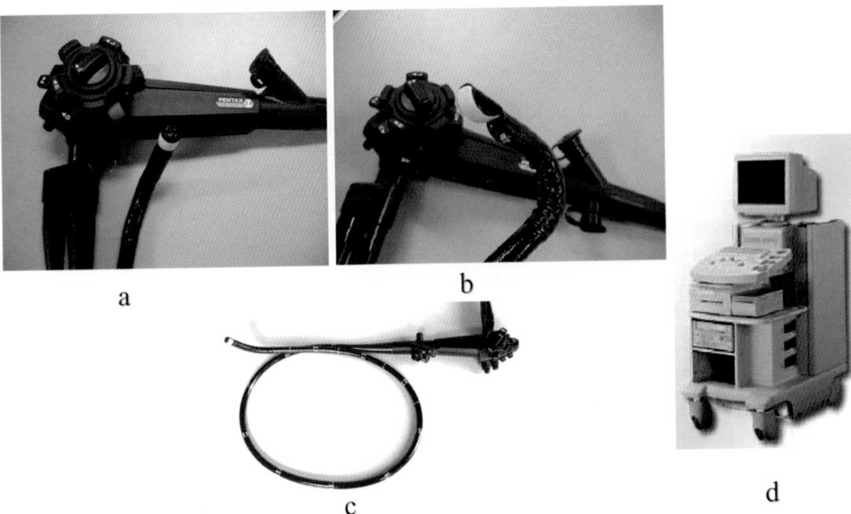

FIG. 5. EUS systems–1. **a** EG-3670URK (electronic radial type; Pentax, Tokyo, Japan). **b** EG-3870UTK (electronic convex type; Pentax). **c** EG-3630UR (electronic radial type; Pentax); **d** EUB-8500 (Hitachi, Tokyo, Japan)

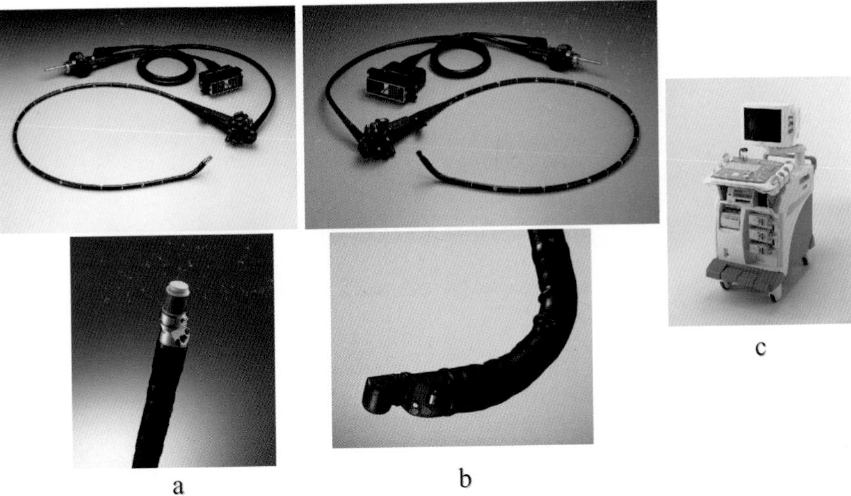

FIG. 6. EUS systems–2. **a** GF-UE260-AL5 (electronic radial type; Olympus Medical Systems, Tokyo, Japan). **b** GF-UCT240 (electronic convex type; Olympus Medical Systems). **c** SSD Prosound α-5 (Aloka, Tokyo, Japan)

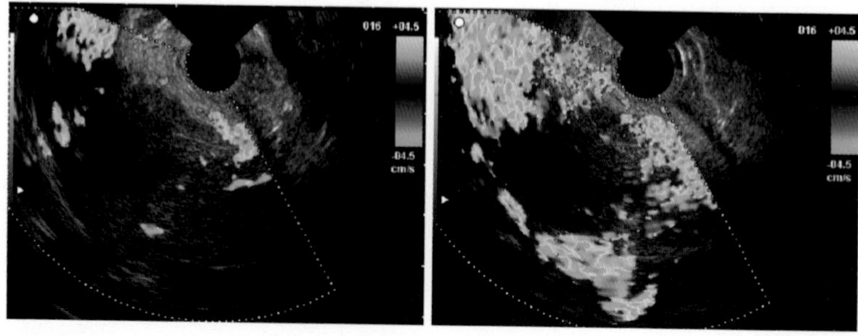

Fig. 7. Pancreatic cancer. **a** A hypoechoic mass was seen at the pancreatic head that was suspected to be pancreatic cancer. **b** On CE-EUS, the hypoechoic mass was hypovascular, indicating pancreatic cancer, as suggested by hemodynamics

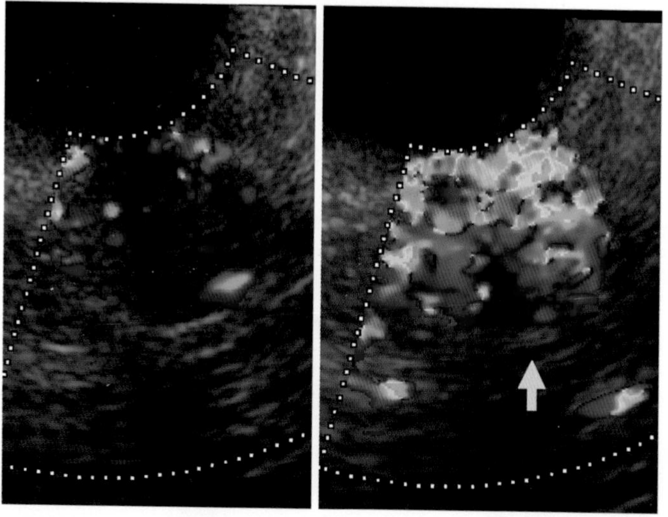

Fig. 8. Pancreatic endocrine tumor. **a** Some color signals were seen in the tumor on plain color Doppler flow imaging. **b** On CE-EUS, the tumor was filled with numerous color signals, except for the distal part (*arrow*) of the EUS probe. Necrosis was proved by the area of no color on the resected specimen

The diagnosis of an enlarged lymph node as benign or malignant is very important for staging [7]. CE-EUS gives useful information for the differential diagnosis of lymph node enlargement. Figure 10 shows benign lymphadenopathy, which was filled with color signals on CE-EUS, whereas a color defect was demonstrated for malignant lymphadenopathy (Fig. 11). The combination study of plain image and contrast-enhanced image produced useful diagnostic information.

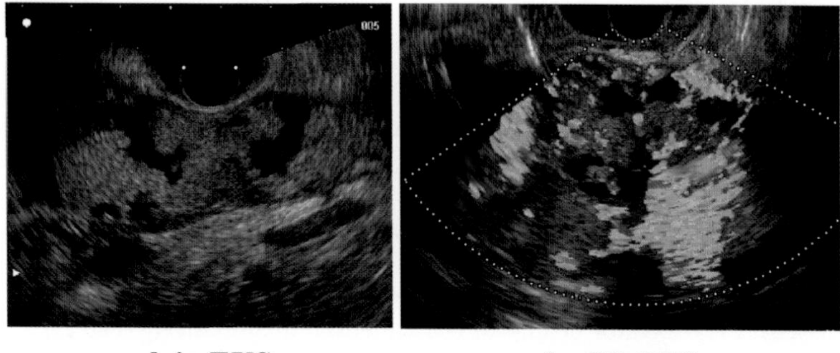

a: plain EUS **b: CE-EUS**

Fig. 9. Intraductal papillary mucinous neoplasm (IPMN). **a** A papillary-like structure was seen at the dilated main pancreatic duct. **b** On CE-EUS, color signals were seen at the papillary structure indicating true papillary growth

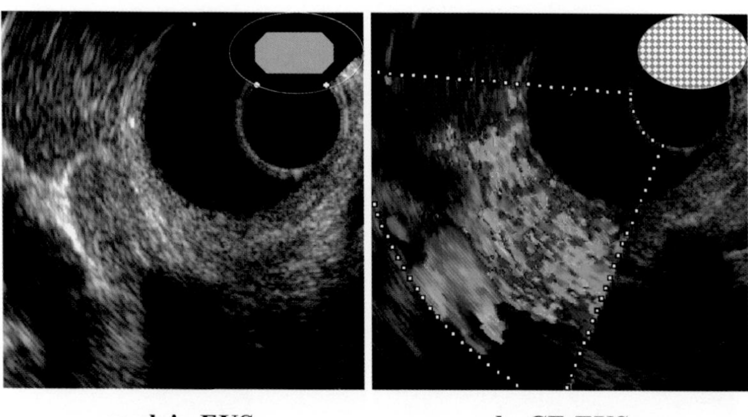

a: plain EUS **b: CE-EUS**

Fig. 10. Benign lymphadenopathy. **a** A hypoechoic enlarged lymph node was seen, 15 mm in diameter. **b** The lymph node was filled with color signals after injection of Levovist

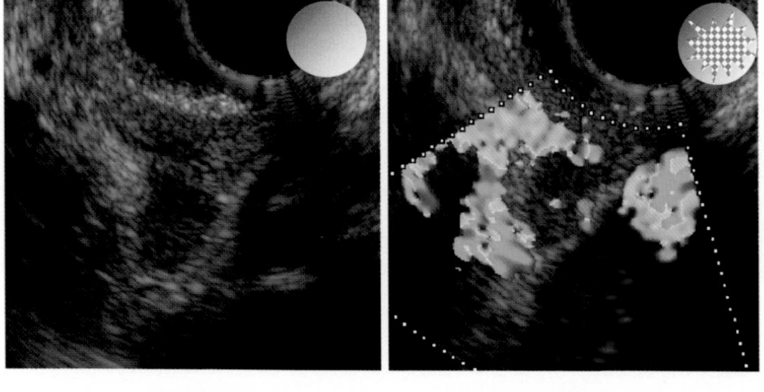

a: plain EUS **b: CE-EUS**

Fig. 11. Malignant lymphadenopathy. **a** A hypoechoic enlarged lymph node. **b** A color perfusion defect was depicted after injection of Levovist

The New-Generation Contrast Agent (Sonazoid)

In 2007, Sonazoid (Daiichi-Sankyo, Tokyo, Japan) was introduced into clinical settings in Japan. Sonazoid consists of perflubutane microbubbles whose median diameter is 2–3 μm. Sonazoid made it possible to enhance the B-mode imaging (contrast-harmonic imaging) and allowed further detailed information.

Figure 12 shows pancreatic cancer. The hypoechoic mass was seen at the pancreatic head; 30 s after the injection of Sonazoid, echo intensity increased to the same degree as in the pancreatic parenchyma and decreased over less than 1 min. The time–intensity curve revealed the change of echo intensity quantitatively (Fig. 13).

Figure 14 shows another case of pancreatic cancer. This image showed the vessel distribution of the lesion; the standard deviation (SD) of vessel distribution was increased (from 9.3 to 11.5) 3 min after Sonazoid injection, indicating the destruction of systemic vessel structure.

As already stated, the hemodynamics of lesions could be analyzed quantitatively. At present, the feasibility of contrast harmonic imaging using Sonazoid is confirmed. We should ascertain the clinical usefulness of CE-EUS with an accumulation of clinical cases.

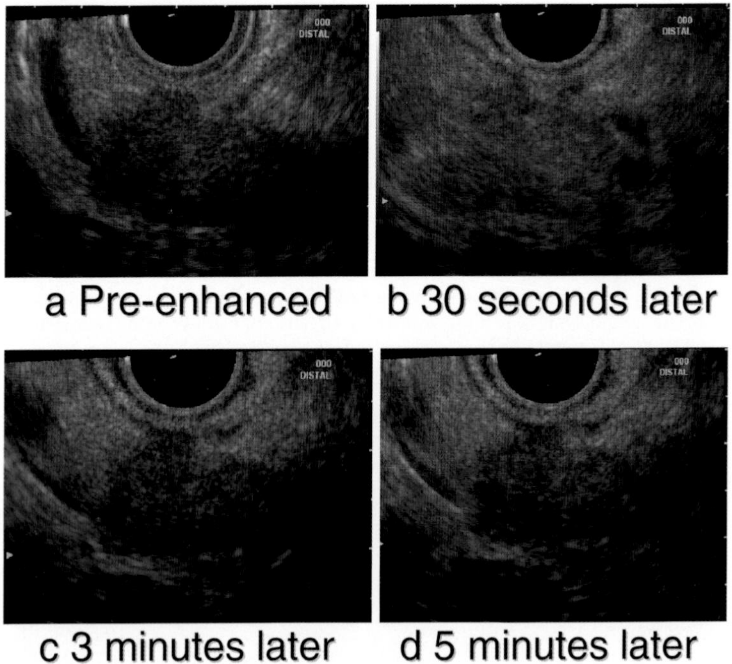

Fig. 12. Pancreatic cancer. A hypoechoic mass was seen at the pancreatic head (**a**, pre-enhanced). At 30 s after the injection of Sonazoid (**b**), echo intensity increased to the same degree as in the pancreatic parenchyma, and decreased over less than 1 min (**c**, **d**)

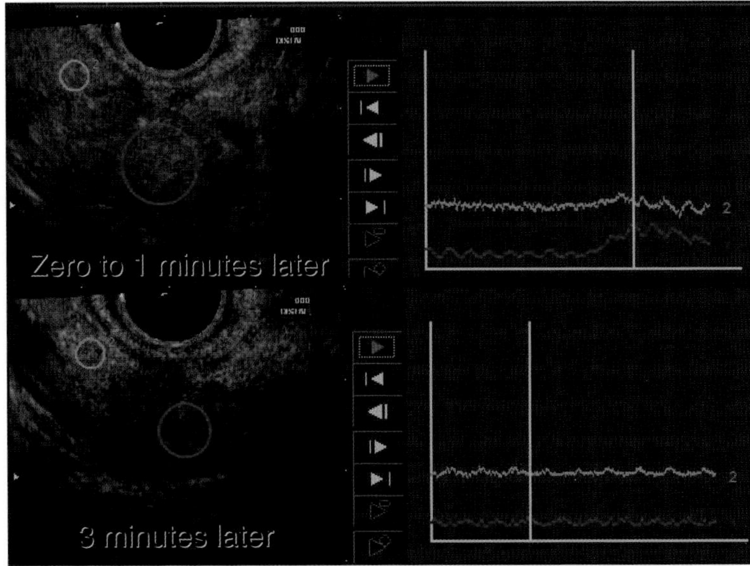

Fig. 13. Pancreatic cancer. The time–intensity curve revealed echo-intensity changes quantitatively, as mentioned in Fig. 12

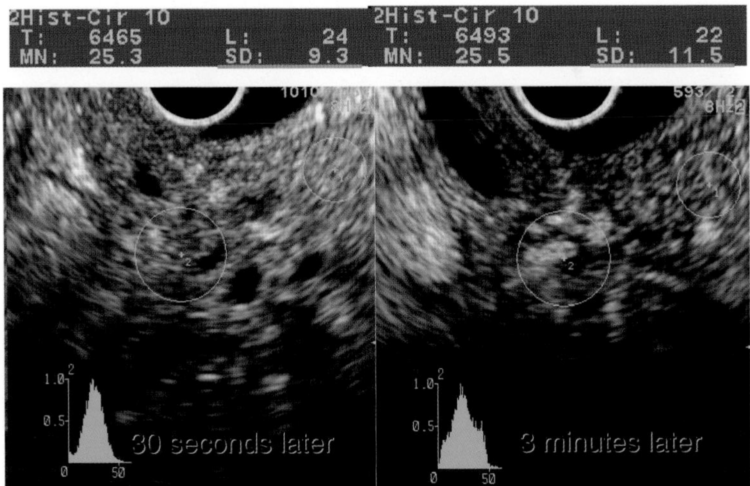

Fig. 14. Pancreatic cancer. This image shows the vessel distribution of the lesion. The standard deviation (SD) of vessel distribution was increased (from 9.3 to 11.5) 3 min after Sonazoid injection, indicating the destruction of the systemic vessel structure

References

1. Matsuda Y, Yabuuchi I (1986) Hepatic tumors: UD contrast enhancement with CO_2 microbubbles. Radiology 161:701–705
2. Kato T, Tsukamoto Y, Naitoh Y, et al (1995) Ultrasonographic and endoscopic ultrasonographic angiography in pancreatic mass lesions. Acta Radiol 36:381–387
3. Hirooka Y, Naitoh Y, Goto H, et al (1997) Usefulness of contrast-enhanced endoscopic ultrasonography with intravenous injection of sonicated serum albumin. Gastrointest Endosc 46:166–169
4. Hirooka Y, Naitoh Y, Goto H, et al (1998) Contrast-enhanced endoscopic ultrasonography in gallbladder diseases. Gastrointest Endosc 48:406–410
5. Hirooka Y, Goto H, Itoh A, et al (1998) Contrast-enhanced endoscopic ultrasonography in pancreatic diseases: a preliminary study. Am J Gastroenterol 93:632–635
6. Nomura N, Goto H, Niwa Y, et al (1999) Usefulness of contrast-enhanced EUS in the diagnosis of upper GI tract diseases. Gastrointest Endosc 50:555–560
7. Kanamori A, Hirooka Y, Itoh A, et al (2006) Usefulness of contrast-enhanced endoscopic ultrasonography in the differentiation between malignant and benign lymphadenopathy. Am J Gastroenterol 101:45–51

Standard Scanning Techniques for EUS Examinations with Curved Linear Array Echoendoscopes

Kenji Yamao,[1] Atsushi Irisawa,[2] and Teruo Kozu[3]

Summary. Standard imaging techniques using a curved array echoendoscope are summarized to facilitate the attainment of expertise in endoscopic ultrasonography and endoscopic ultrasound-guided fine-needle aspiration and to promote the widespread use of this diagnostic and therapeutic tool. Typical images of the mediastinal organs, the biliopancreatic systems and neighboring organs by scanning from the esophagus, stomach, duodenal bulb, and descending portion of the duodenum are shown in a sequential manner.

Key words. Endoscopic ultrasonography, Standard imaging, Scanning method, Convex echoendoscope

Introduction

Endoscopic ultrasonography (EUS) has been widely accepted for more than 20 years as a powerful tool for the diagnosis of gastrointestinal disorders [1]. Endoscopic ultrasound-guided fine-needle aspiration (EUS-FNA) using a curved linear array echoendoscope (convex echoendoscope) has recently begun to be used for pathological diagnosis [2]. It is, however, still an underutilized tool. One of the factors hindering the widespread use of EUS-FNA is the difficulty in understanding ultrasonographic anatomy with a convex echoendoscope. To consider this problem, we formed a committee (Table 1) in May 2004 whose main objective was to establish standard scanning techniques for EUS examinations with the convex echoendoscope. This committee held five meetings and completed and published the guidelines in May 2005.

This chapter shows standard imaging techniques, which were established by this committee, for EUS examinations with convex echoendoscopes. We hope this chapter will help readers acquire a better understanding of techniques for diagnosis and therapy with a convex echoendoscope.

[1]Department of Gastroenterology, Aichi Cancer Center Hospital, 1-1 Kanokoden, Chikusa-ku, Nagoya 464-8681, Japan
[2]Department of Gastroenterology, Fukushima Medical University Hospital, Fukushima, Japan
[3]Department of Endoscopic Diagnostics and Therapeutics, Chiba University Hospital, Chiba, Japan

TABLE 1. EUS-FNA Standardization Committee.

Kenji Yamao	Aichi Cancer Center Hospital
Atsushi Irisawa	Fukushima Medical University
Hiroyuki Inoue	Mie University
Koji Matsuda	Jikei University Aoto Hospital
Mitsuhiro Kida	Kitasato University East Hospital
Shomei Ryozawa	Yamaguchi University
Yoshiki Hirooka	Nagoya University
Teruo Kozu	Chiba University

TABLE 2. Indices for scanning technique.

Scanning Position	Landmarks	Tips
Esophagus	Descending aorta Inferior vena cava (IVC) Azygos vein Right atrium, Left Atrium & left ventricle Ascending aorta Pulmonary artery Tracheal bifurcation Aortic arch	Insert the scope into the stomach past the EG junction, and visualize the liver, hepatic veins and IVC, and then observe the entire image while visualizing each of the indices
Stomach	Hepatic veins Abdominal aorta Celiac artery Splenic artery vein Superior mesenteric artery/vein Liver Pancreas Left kidney Spleen Left adrenal gland Bile duct Gallbladder	Insert the scope till the EG junction. After recognizing the hepatic veins, observe the entire image while imaging each of the indices. Alternately, observe the duodenal region first and then observe other regions while withdrawing the scope toward the oral side.
Duodenal bulb	Portal vein Superior mesenteric artery/vein Splenic vein IVC Abdominal aorta Gallbladder Bile duct Pancreatic head Pancreatic body	Insert the scope as far as the duodenal bulb and observe using the push technique
Descending part of duodenum	Abdominal aorta IVC Superior mesenteric artery/vein Pancreatic head Papilla of Vater Bile duct Right Kidney	Straighten the scope in the same way as ERCP (pull technique), and then observe while withdrawing from the distal to proximal duodenum.

Standard Scanning Techniques

Indices for Scanning Technique

The scanning target positions are divided into four regions for standard techniques for imaging with the convex echoendoscope. Table 2 shows the landmark structures observed from each scanning position including esophagus, stomach, duodenal bulb, and descending part of duodenum.

Positioning of the Endoscopist and Orientation of the Echoendoscope

The orientation of the images is with the endoscopist facing the patient, and with the scope handle oriented orthogonally to the patient's body.

Rotating the Curved Linear Array Echoendoscope

To correctly identify the position relationships of the surrounding organs, observation should generally be performed while the scope is straight. In the stretched condition, the transducer is oriented toward the direction opposite to the universal cord. Rotation of the curved linear array echoendoscope is the key maneuver for complete imaging of targets. When the transducer is oriented anteriorly toward the abdominal wall, rotate the scope clockwise to observe the right side of the body or counterclockwise to observe the left side. When the transducer is oriented toward the back, rotate the scope clockwise to observe the left side of the body or counterclockwise to observe the right side.

View of Ultrasound Images and Procedure

Scanning from the Esophagus

When the scope is inserted into the stomach past the esophageal gastric (EG) junction with the control free, the left lobe of the liver is visible on the screen below the scope. Now rotate the scope clockwise to visualize the hepatic vein and the inferior vena cava (IVC). After observing the liver, rotate the scope clockwise to observe the abdominal aorta. Then advance the scope slightly until the celiac artery bifurcation and superior mesenteric artery are recognized. Observe the lymph nodes around the celiac artery from this position.

While observing the aorta, withdraw the scope slightly, while rotating it counterclockwise, until a long triangular hypoechoic structure is seen in front of the aorta. This is the crus of the diaphragm, which is an important landmark for defining the boundary between the abdominal cavity and mediastinum (Fig. 1a). After evaluating this region, withdraw the scope while viewing the aorta to observe the surroundings of the thoracic aorta.

After observing the IVC, withdraw the scope to observe the right atrium. Rotate the scope clockwise to observe the entire surroundings of the esophagus. Then withdraw the scope slightly until the azygos vein is identified. Trace the azygos vein in

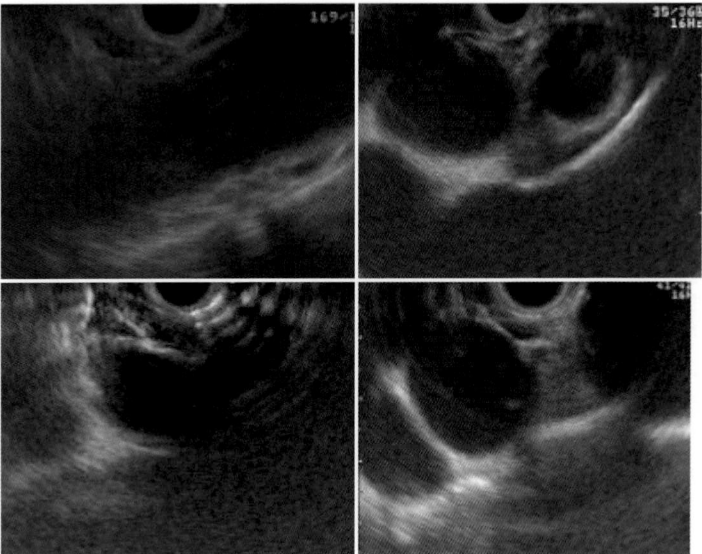

FIG. 1. Scanning from the esophagus

both longitudinal directions toward the caudal and oral sides, and look for any adjacent lymph nodes. Rotate the scope further clockwise to observe the descending aorta also. Trace the descending aorta longitudinally toward both the caudal and oral directions, and look for any adjacent lymph nodes. Rotate the scope counterclockwise to return to the positioning in displaying the right atrium, and withdraw the scope while rotating it further counterclockwise to visualize the left atrium, left ventricle, ascending aorta, and right pulmonary artery (Fig. 1b). While watching the right pulmonary artery, withdraw the scope while rotating it slightly counterclockwise to visualize the trachea or main bronchi. The point toward the oral side (right in the image), where the multiple-echo lines end, is the tracheal bifurcation into the left and right main bronchi (Fig. 1c). If imaging of this point is difficult, trace the multiple-echo lines from the oral side to the point where these are interrupted. Visualize the right pulmonary artery again, and withdraw the scope while rotating it counterclockwise to visualize the right pulmonary artery on the left side in the image and the cross section of the aortic arch on the right side. The region between the two blood vessels is the aortopulmonary window (AP window) (Fig. 1d). While observing the aortic arch, withdraw the scope while rotating it counterclockwise to visualize the left subclavian artery and left common carotid artery. Rotating the scope further counterclockwise at this level makes it possible to observe the brachiocephalic artery.

Scanning from the Stomach

With the patient lying in the left lateral position, the left lobe of the liver is imaged after the scope has passed the diaphragm. The transducer is now oriented anteriorly toward the abdominal wall of the patient. The left hepatic vein is also observed from

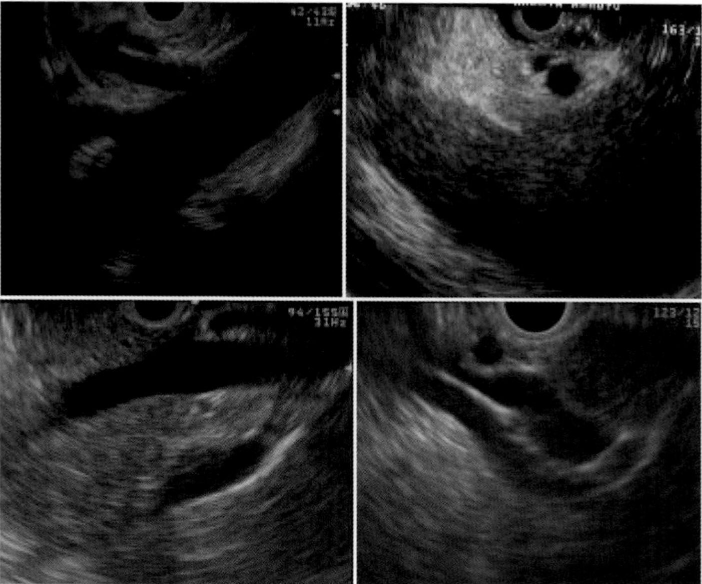

Fig. 2. Scanning from the stomach

this position. Rotate the scope clockwise to visualize the abdominal aorta. When the scope is advanced caudally from this position along the abdominal aorta, the celiac artery and superior mesenteric artery are imaged (Fig. 2a). Note that the celiac artery and superior mesenteric artery are not always imaged simultaneously; the celiac artery is usually easier to image. It is therefore recommended to visualize the celiac artery first and then rotate the scope slightly clockwise or counterclockwise to identify the superior mesenteric artery. Advance the scope slightly and rotate it clockwise to visualize the pancreatic body and tail. In general, the splenic artery is imaged nearer and splenic vein farther from the transducer. The splenic artery and vein can be discriminated by means of color and pulse Doppler. While imaging the spleen by using the splenic vein as the landmark, rotate the scope to visualize the pancreatic tail and left kidney. Rotate the scope further to observe the pancreas until the splenic hilum (Fig. 2b). From the previous position, advance the scope to observe the left adrenal gland, which is located between the abdominal aorta and upper pole of the left kidney.

When the splenic vein is traced, the confluence between the superior mesenteric vein and portal vein can be observed (Fig. 2c). In this position, part of the pancreatic head is also imaged. When the scope is rotated counterclockwise at the portal confluence, the junction between the pancreatic head and body, the main pancreatic duct, and the bile duct can also be observed. After imaging the superior mesenteric artery from the gastric body, rotate the scope counterclockwise to visualize the superior mesenteric vein that is running parallel to the superior mesenteric artery. Manipulate the scope to visualize the superior mesenteric vein in the longitudinal direction, and then withdraw the scope gradually to observe its junction with the main trunk of the portal vein. After imaging the main trunk of the portal vein, withdraw the scope to trace the portal vein toward the liver. This step makes it possible to observe the hilum of the liver (Fig. 2d).

When the scope is pushed in, the gallbladder can be imaged from the antrum.

Scanning from the Duodenal Bulb

Insert the scope into the duodenal bulb and rotate the scope counterclockwise to visualize the gallbladder. The neck lies on the left side of image and the fundus lies on the right side. Rotate the scope clockwise to visualize three luminal structures. The portal vein, bile duct, and common hepatic artery can be identified using Doppler as required. Advance the scope slightly from this position and rotate it counterclockwise to visualize the portal vein, bile duct, and right hepatic artery (Fig. 3a). At this time, the transducer is directed cranially. While rotating the scope clockwise, trace the imaged bile duct toward the papilla to visualize the bile duct and main pancreatic duct near the papilla (Fig. 3b). Continue imaging along the portal vein to visualize the confluence between the portal vein, splenic vein, and superior mesenteric vein. The pancreatic head and body can also be observed from the duodenal side. Rotate the scope counterclockwise to visualize the pancreatic head and body.

Scanning from the Descending Part of the Duodenum

Insert the scope into the descending part of the duodenum and straighten it before starting observation. Rotate the scope clockwise to visualize the aorta and IVC. While imaging the aorta, withdraw the scope slowly to visualize the lower part of the pancreatic head. The aorta gradually lines up parallel with the image, and the pancreatic

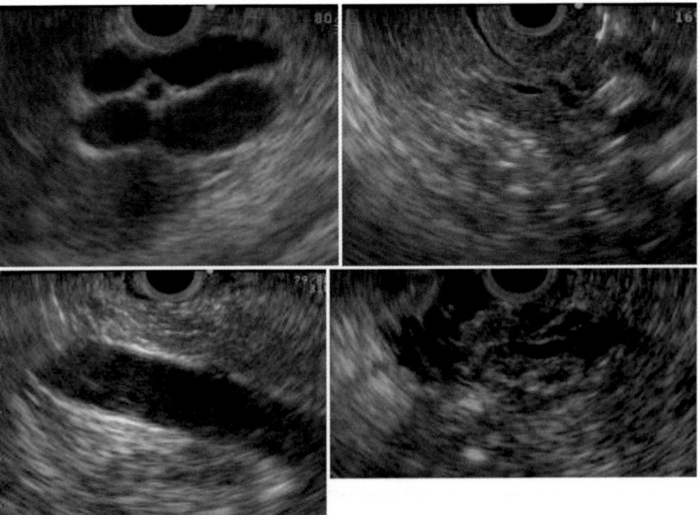

Fig. 3. Scanning from the duodenum

head will be imaged between the aorta and transducer (Fig. 3c). While observing the pancreatic parenchyma, withdraw the scope slowly to image a low-echo region near the transducer. Rotate the scope slightly clockwise and counterclockwise to identify two luminal structures in the low-echo region (Fig. 3d). The bile duct is imaged near the transducer, and the main pancreatic duct is imaged at a further point. The right kidney may sometimes be imaged from the descending part of the duodenum.

Conclusion

Standard imaging techniques using a convex echoendoscope are summarized to facilitate the attainment of expertise in endoscopic ultrasonography, and in endoscopic ultrasound-guided fine-needle aspiration, and to promote the widespread use of this diagnostic and therapeutic tool.

Acknowledgments. The authors thank Akio Katanuma (Teine Keijinkai Hospital), Masayuki Kitano (Kinki University), Tatsuya Nagakawa (Sapporo-Kosei General Hospital), Soji Ozawa (Fujita Health University 2nd Hospital), Taketo Yamaguchi (Chiba University), and Ichiro Yasuda (Gifu University) for their technical advice for this manuscript and Vikram Bhatia (All India Institute of Medical Sciences, New Delhi) for advice in preparing the English version of this manuscript. We also deeply appreciate the support of Olympus Medical Systems for this project.

Present Status and Future Perspectives of Endoscopic Ultrasonography-Guided Fine-Needle Aspiration

Mitsuhiro Kida, Masao Araki, and Katsunori Saigenji

Summary. Since endoscopic ultrasonography (EUS) for gastroenterological diseases was first reported in 1980, EUS has widened its indications and has become an indispensable examination in the clinical field. However, it had been necessary to obtain cytology or histology also because of unsatisfactory EUS diagnostic accuracy. Then, the first report of EUS-FNA (fine-needle aspiration) was made by Vilmann and Grimm in 1992. After its introduction, EUS-FNA has widened its indication with high accuracy and a low complication rate in the clinical field. Also, the EUS-FNA technique has been improved as to the size of the needle, stroke, number of passes, and negative aspiration pressure. Furthermore, pseudocyst drainage, celiac trunk neurolysis, etc., have been established and immunotherapy such as dendritic cell injection and gene therapy has been applied. EUS-FNA seems to be a promising technique and will improve day by day.

Key words. Endoscopic ultrasonography (EUS), Fine-needle aspiration (FNA), Fine-needle injection (FNI), Fine-needle therapy (FNT), Future perspectives

History and Review of Literature of Endoscopic Ultrasonography-Guided Fine-Needle Aspiration (EUS-FNA)

Since endoscopic ultrasonography (EUS) for gastroenterological diseases was first reported in 1980, EUS has widened its indications and has become an indispensable examination in the clinical field. Although characteristic findings of malignancy for metastatic lymph node and gastrointestinal stromal tumor (GIST), etc., have been reported, its accuracy was still only 70%–80%. To improve its accuracy, it seemed to be necessary to obtain histology or cytology studies. There was no imaging diagnostic examination that was more accurate than histology and cytology. Then, the first reports about endoscopic ultrasonography-guided fine-needle aspiration (EUS-FNA),

Department of Gastroenterology, Kitasato University East Hospital, 2-1-1 Asamizodai, Sagamihara, Kanagawa 228-8520, Japan in which Vilmann et al. reported fine-needle aspiration cytology of pancreas cancer and Grimm et al. treated pseudocysts by the EUS-FNA technique, were made in 1992 [1,2]. After that, EUS-FNA became popular in the clinical field, especially in Western countries. According to the literature, the accuracy of EUS-FNA has been 76%–90% in pancreas diseases, 82%–100% in lymph node and mediastinal diseases, and 38%–100% in gastrointestinal diseases such as submucosal tumor (Table 1) [3–5].

EUS-FNA then assumed an indispensable role in examination and widened its applications, such as cytology, pseudocyst drainage, celiac plexus neurolysis, biliary drainage, botulinus toxin injection for achalasia, ethanol injection therapy, immunotherapy, and gene therapy. On the other hand, concerning complications of EUS-FNA, a complication rate of 0%–2.6% has been reported, although a rate of 7.4% was seen in the drainage of pancreas pseudocysts (Table 2) [6,7]. However, it has been accepted that the complication rate seems to be relatively low.

TABLE 1. Sampling, diagnostic rate of EUS guided FNA.

Author	Year	n	Sampling rate	Pancreas	LN	GI tract	TOTAL
Wiersema	1994	19		82%	100%	100%	84%
Giovannini	1995	141		79%	82%	60%	79%
Chang	1997	61	95%	88%	88%		88%
Gress	1997	133 (Lineal)	91%	86%	95%		90%
		75 (Radial)		81%	95%		81%
Wiersema	1997	457		90%	92%	67%	82% (MC study)
Williams	1999	327	98%	76%	89%	38%	82%

LN: Lymph node including mediastinal tumor; GI: Gastrointestinal; MC: multicenter

TABLE 2. Complications of EUS guided FNA.

Author	Year	Aim	n	needle (G)	Complications (%)	Remarks
Wiersema MJ (2)	1994	FNAB	26	25	0	
Chang KJ (3)	1994	FNAB	38	22	0	
Bohnnacker S (4)	1996	Drainage	27	?	7.4	bleeding (2) (surgery (1))
Wiersema MJ (5)	1996	CPN	30	23	10	diarrhea (3)
Hoffman BJ (6)	1997	BTI	4	23	0	
Chang KJ (7)	1997	FNAB	44	23, 22	2.2	infection (1) (panc mass with cyst)
Gress FG (8)	1997	FNAB	208	22, 23	2 (0.8% linea array) (4% radial scan)	pancreatitis (2) bleeding (2)
Wiersema MJ (9)	1997	FNAB	457	21~25	1.1 (0.5% in solid) (14% in cystic)	infection (2), bleeding (1) perforation (2)
Williams DB (10)	1999	FNAB	333	23, 22	0.3	sepsis (1) (pancreatic cyst)
Sahai AV (11)	1999	FNAB	152	?	0	multicenter (GF-UM30P)
Arima K (12)	1999	FNAB	76	22, 21	2.6	bleeding (1), infection (1)
O'Toole (13)	2001	FNAB	322	22	1.6	pancreatitis (3), pneumonia (2)

Recent Indications for EUS-FNA

A fundamental principle in establishing the indication for EUS-FNA is a determination whether the information obtained has potential in choosing patient treatment, and that it is easier and safer than other options to treat a disease (Table 3). Of course, the puncture route between convex endosonography and its target has to be established to avoid vascular structures, and informed consent should be obtained before the procedure. Thus, if the information cannot affect patient treatment, for example, in a case of a lesion that has been already decided to be treated surgically, the procedure should not be performed. Furthermore, bleeding tendency and the possibility of malignant cell seeding must always be considered. The current standard indications of EUS-FNA are shown in Table 4.

At first, submucosal tumor, which cannot be diagnosed by other examinations such as conventional EUS, seemed to be the ordinary target of EUS-FNA in Japan, whereas lymph nodes (LN) or pancreas masses are the targets in Western countries. Its main role is to diagnose gastrointestinal stromal tumor. However, it is practicably difficult to perform EUS-FNA in a lesion less than about 2 cm in diameter because of

TABLE 3. Fundamental principle for EUS guided FNA.

1. EUS guided FNA is a determination as to whether or not its information obtained has the potential in the choice of patient treatment, and is to treat a disease easier and safer than other options.
2. Puncturing route between convex endosonography and its target has to be established without vascular structure.
3. Informed consensus should be obtained before its procedure.

TABLE 4. Recent Indication of EUS-FNA & Related Techniques.

Diagnostic
Pancreas mass
Submucosal tumor
Lymph node swelling around gastrointestinal tumor
Mediastinal tumor
Intra-abdominal or intrapleural fluid
etc.

Therapeutic
Pseudocyst drainage (clinical level)
Celiac plexus neurolysis (clinical level)
Biliary drainage (clinical level)
Pancreatic duct drainage (clinical level)
Botulinus toxin injection for achalsia (clinical level)
Ethanol injection therapy (case report level)
Immunotherapy (under investigation)
Gene therapy or Biological cell injection (under investigation)
etc.

its mobility, whereas a pancreas tumor and lymph nodes more than 1.0 cm can be punctured.

Concerning pancreas tumor, EUS-FNA for operable pancreas cancer is still controversial, especially in cases of neoplastic pancreas cystic tumor such as intraductal papillary mucinous tumor (IPMT) and mucinous cystic tumor. These cases are contraindications for EUS-FNA in Japan at present, because there is a reported case with neoplastic pancreas cystic tumor that had EUS-guided FNA, with peritonitis carcinomatosa confirmed at the time of the surgical operation. Concerning operable pancreas solid cancer, tumors located in the body or tail are still controversial for EUS-FNA; however, tumors in the pancreas head, in which the needle passage way will be removed by the subsequent surgical operation, may have indication. Furthermore, for a case in which it is difficult to differentiate cancer from inflammation, and in cases requiring histological evidence before chemotherapy, etc., there is good indication for EUS-FNA.

Mediastinal tumor, metastatic lymph node of lung cancer, and abdominal lymphoma are good indications for EUS-FNA. However, lymph nodes just behind the gastrointestinal main tumor, which will be removed at the surgical operation, seem not to be punctured. On the other hand, a swollen lymph node after operation, which cannot be confirmed except for reoperation, is a good indication.

Fine-needle therapy (FNT), such as for pseudocyst drainage or celiac plexus neurolysis, seems to be popular in Japan. Several investigations have reported complications of infection with aspiration of pseudocysts; therefore, it is recommended to avoid EUS aspiration of pseudocysts unless subsequent drainage will be performed.

Gene therapy or biological cell or agent injection is still under investigation. However, these techniques have future promise. We are looking forward to developing a new agent or cell with high efficacy and without side effects.

Normal Anatomy by Convex EUS

To perform EUS-FNA, it is important to know the normal anatomy of the biliopancreas systems first. Although standardization of the normal biliopancreas system with radial EUS has been established, it has not yet been established with convex EUS [8,9].

From the Esophagocardiac Junction

When we insert the scope up to the esophagocardiac junction, the left lobe is generally revealed (Fig. 1). We turn the scope up to 180°; then the aorta is revealed, and we follow it up to the celiac trunk. The pancreas body is revealed in between the celiac trunk and the scope (Figs. 2, 3). We should follow the pancreas up to the splenic hilum and left kidney (Fig. 4). The left adrenal gland is revealed in between the pancreas tail and the kidney (Fig. 5). Then, we push the scope up to the angle of the stomach, and follow the portal vein and bile duct up to the liver hilum.

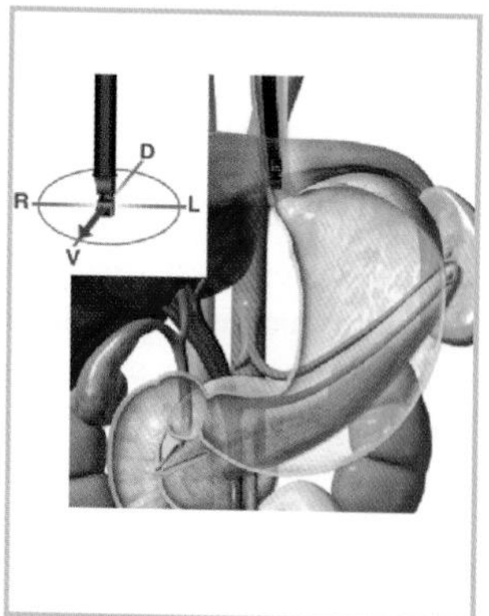

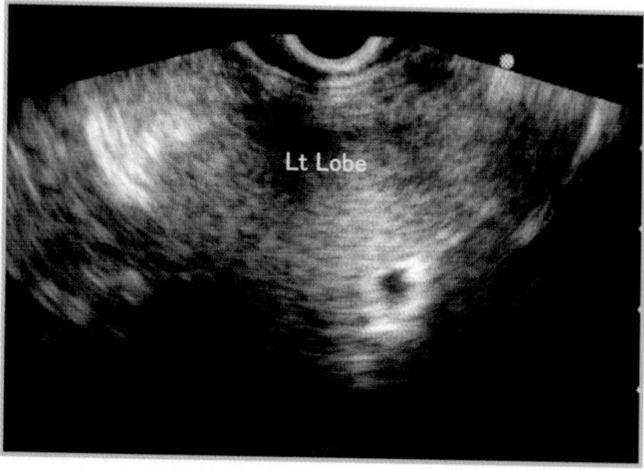

FIG. 1. When the echoendoscope inserted up to esophagocardiac (EG) junction, the left lobe of liver is naturally revealed

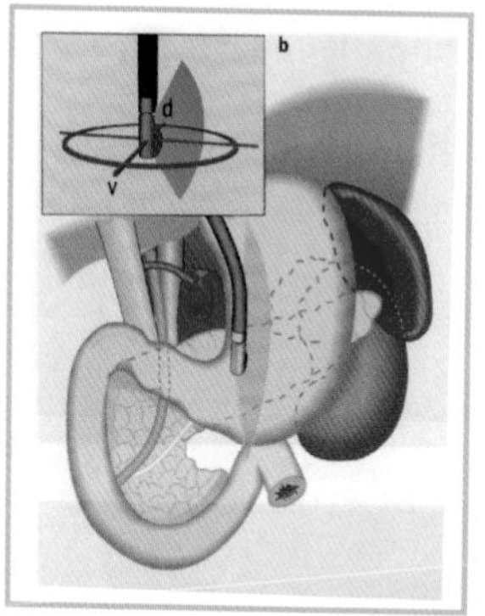

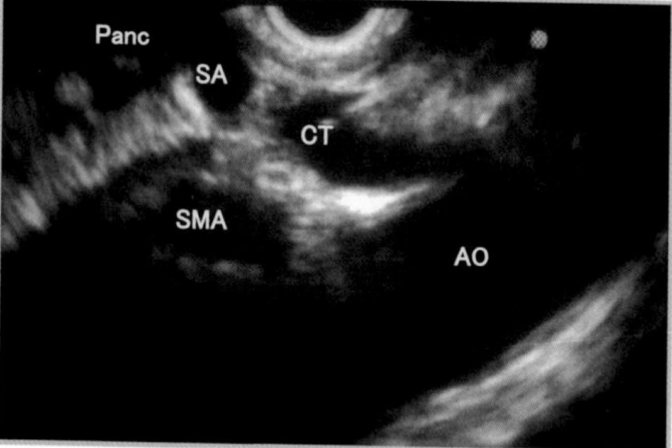

FIG. 2. View from the stomach. *Panc*, pancreas; *SMA*, Superior mesenteric artery; *SA*, splenic artery; *CT*, celiac trunk; *AO*, aorta

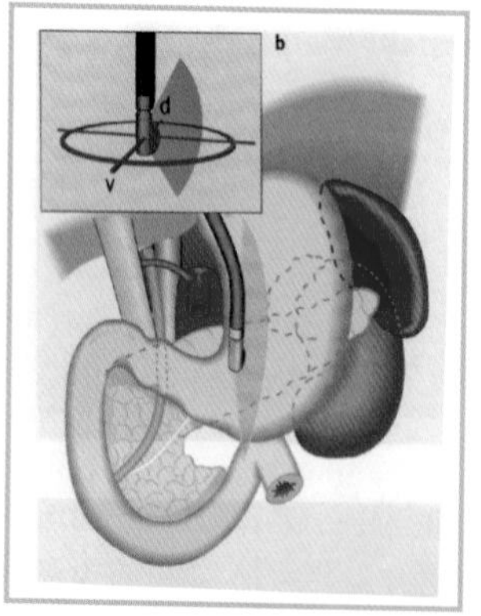

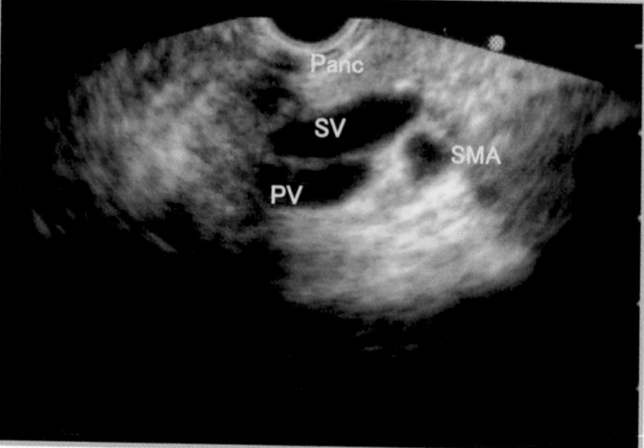

FIG. 3. Another view from the stomach. *SV*, splenic vein; *PV*, portal vein

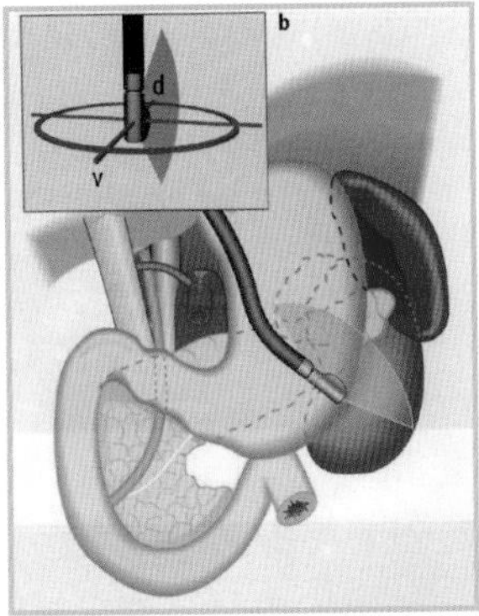

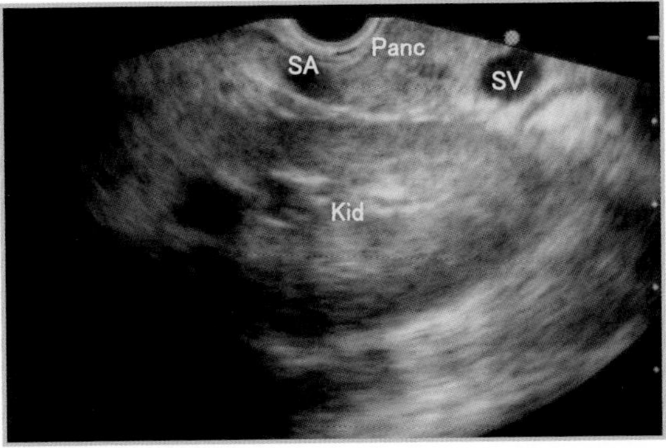

FIG. 4. A further view from the stomach. *Kid*, kidney

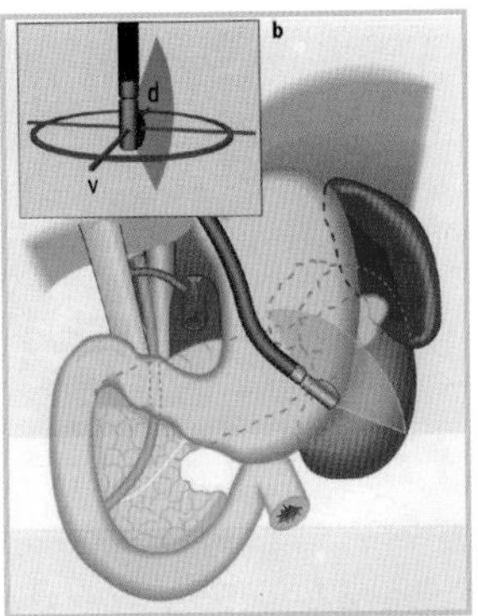

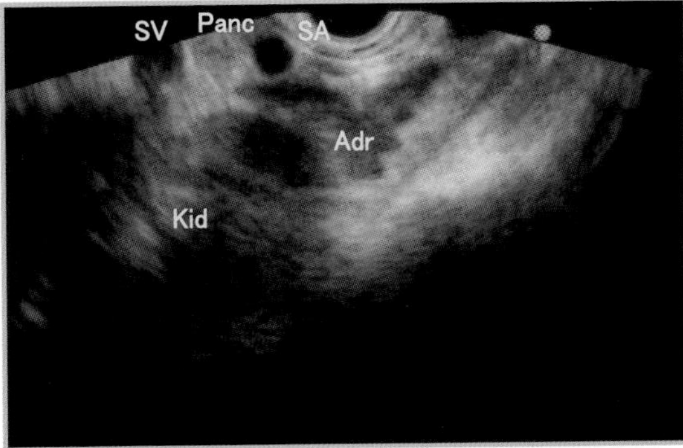

FIG. 5. Seen from the stomach: pancreas (*Panc*), adrenal gland (*Adr*), kidney (*Kid*)

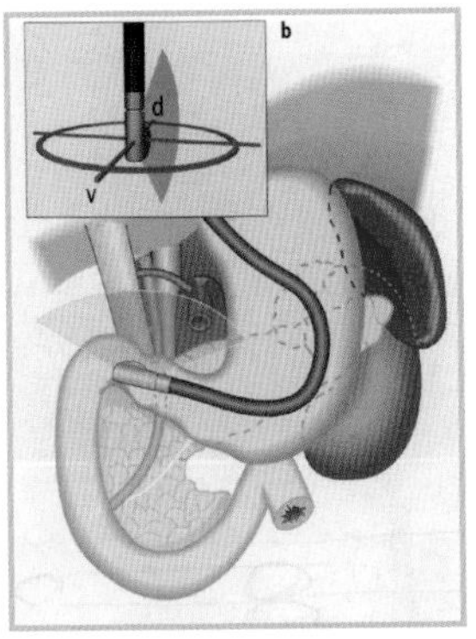

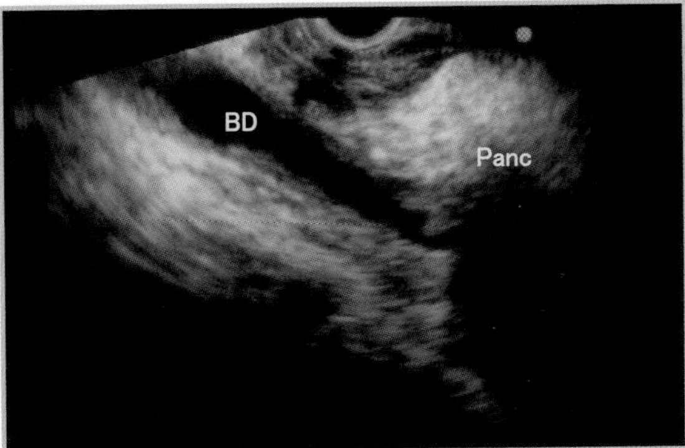

FIG. 6. From the duodenal bulb. *BD*, bile duct

From the Duodenal Bulb

When we push the scope into the duodenal bulb, we can find the transitional part of the pancreas head and body; the portal vein and bile duct will be revealed by rotating the scope (Fig. 6). We then follow the bile duct up to the papilla as in radial scanning.

From the Inferior Duodenal Angle

Using the stretch technique, the convex scope reaches to the inferior duodenal angle; we should aspirate air from the duodenal lumen and fill it with 50–100 ml deaerated water, if necessary. At this point, there are two large transverse ductal structures in the lower half, which are the aorta and vena cava (Fig. 7). Then, we pull the scope gradually after doing an up-angle to the lesser curvature of the duodenum and find the thickening of the duodenal wall (papilla) and two ductal structures (bile duct and main pancreatic duct) that arise from the papilla (Fig. 8). However, using this pulling

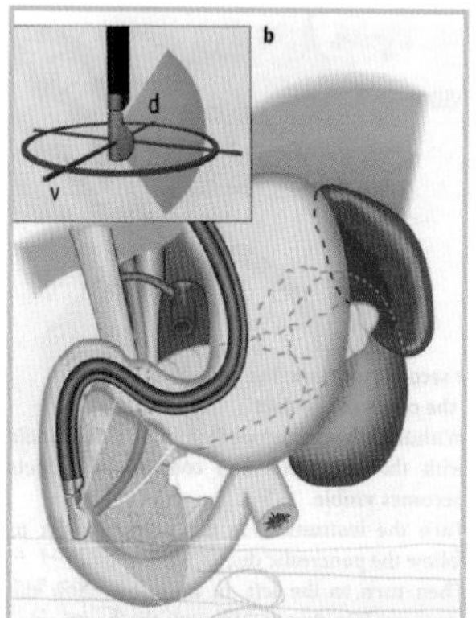

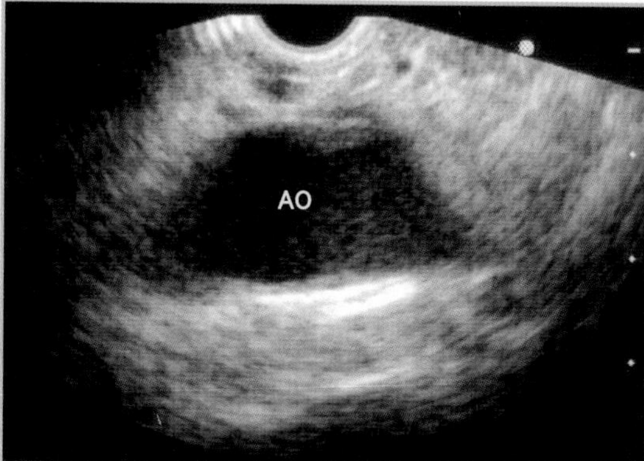

FIG. 7. From the inferior duodenal angle. *AO*, aorta

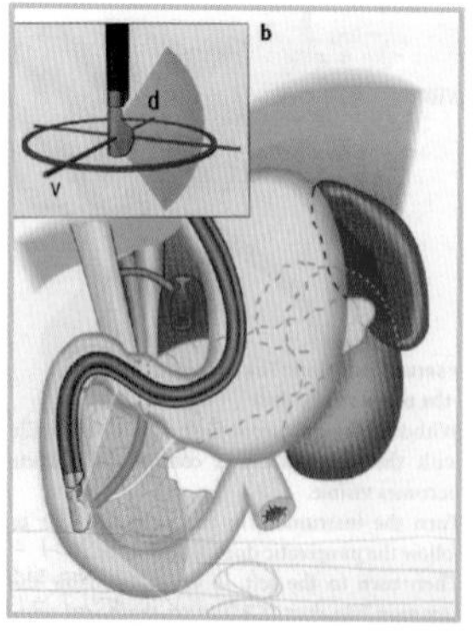

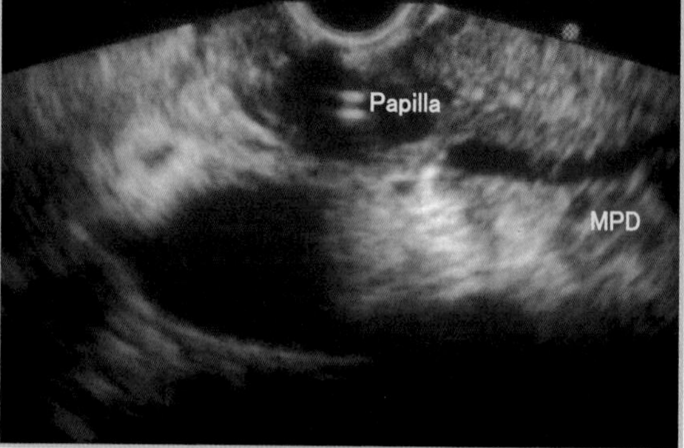

FIG. 8. From the inferior duodenal angle, starting from papilla. *MPD*, main pancreatic duct

method, it is difficult to visualize the transitional part of the pancreas head–body, because the scope can slip out easily.

Technical Consideration of EUS-FNA

To detect and perform EUS-FNA, first it is important to understand convex or linear EUS anatomy. After detecting the target lesion and ruling out vascular structures between EUS and the target lesion with color Doppler function, the target lesion is punctured by a needle. Then, after removing the needle stylet and attaching a negative-pressure syringe, the needle is moved back and forth ten strokes or more in the target lesion. Finally, tissue samples are obtained and checked histologically.

Needle Size for EUS-FNA

Basic in vitro study with pig liver and uterus determined that a larger sample of tissue was obtained by a larger needle. Concerning the range of fine-needle biopsies (19, 22, or 25 gauge, G), the choice of needle size also influences cytology results. As the size of needle increases, a larger amount of tissue might be obtained; however, it becomes rather difficult to perform EUS-FNA. There are several reports about 19 G, true cut, and 22 G needles, and it has been concluded that there is not a significant difference between 19 G and 22 G, except for Levy's report (Table 5). Recently, a 25 G needle has been frequently employed because specific evaluation of diagnostic adequacy of the 25 G needle showed that 92% of pulmonary aspirations were performed with a 25 G needle, with a definitive diagnosis in 88% of cases. Of course, diagnosis with a 25 G needle is made by cytology, and a smaller needle size decreases potential complications such as bleeding. However, a 22 G needle for EUS-guided FNA is commonly employed in the clinical field at the moment.

Table 5. 19G EUS-FNA vs 19G EUS-TNB vs 22G EUS-FNA.

2002	MJ. Wiersema Rochester, USA	N = 78, Dx accuracy TNB 78%: FNA 95% NS Adequate Sample TNB 35%: FNA 45% NS 22G FNA compl. 1 Pancreatitis, 1 Bacteremia
2004	A. Larghi NY, USA	N = 23, TNB Sampling rate 74% (17/23) TNB Dx accuracy 61%, No complications
2004	S. Varadarajulu Charlston, USA	N = 18, Dx accuracy TNB 78%: FNA 89% NS TNB Compl. 1 Mediastinitis (Emerg ope), 1 bleeding
2004	MJ. Levy Rochester, USA	No of pass TNB 2.21 (1–8) vs FNA 3.62 (1–12) $p < 0.05$ Dx accuracy TNB 85% (40/47), 62% (29/47) $p < 0.05$

Number of Punctures and Strokes of Passes

Concerning the times of puncture, it is optimal that EUS-FNA is repeated sufficiently to obtain enough tissue and to be confirmed histologically by the onsite pathologist. However, it is generally confirmed by macroscopic view whether enough tissue has been obtained. LeBlanc et al. concluded that the optimal number of EUS-FNA passes seems to be seven times for pancreatic masses with a sensitivity and specificity of 83% and 100%, and five times for lymph nodes, etc., with a sensitivity and specificity of 77% and 100% (Fig. 9) [10]. It is reported that two or three punctures were sufficient for mediastinal lymph nodes, that four punctures have produced a diagnosis in 95% of cases, and all cases were diagnosed by a sixth puncture.

Second, the number of needle passes back and forth in the lesion comprises ten or more needle strokes, and the pass of each stroke should be also changed (Fig. 10). It has been believed that changing the pass way is one of the most important factors to obtain tissue, because the center of the lesion sometimes becomes necrotic. However, it is practicably impossible to change the pass way in the puncture of a small lymph node. Generally, it is rather difficult to puncture a submucosal tumor because of its mobility, compared to other targets such as pancreas cancer. At this point, we recommend a shotgun needle be employed (NA-11J-KB; Olympus Medical Systems). Furthermore, it is really difficult to puncture target lesions in or near the cardia, greater curvature of the stomach body, lesser curvature of the antrum, and uncinate process of the pancreas, etc.

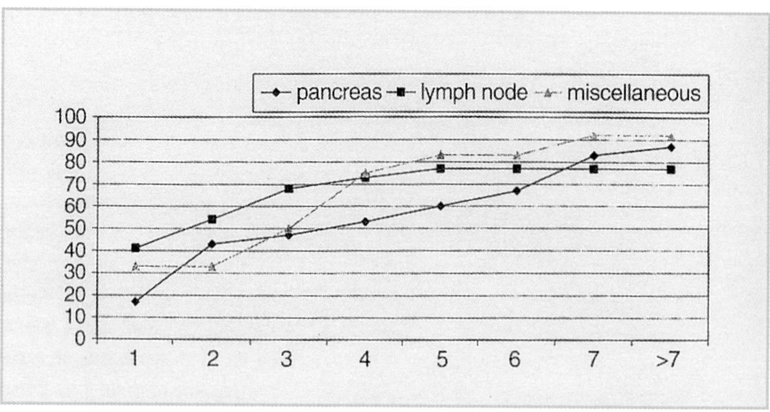

Fig. 9. Sensitivity of EUS-FNA with each fine-needle pass. The sensitivity and specificity for seven passes from the pancreas are 83% and 100%, respectively; the sensitivity and specificity for five passes from a lymph node are 77% and 100%, respectively. (From LeBlanc et al. Gastrointest Endosc 2004;59:475 [10])

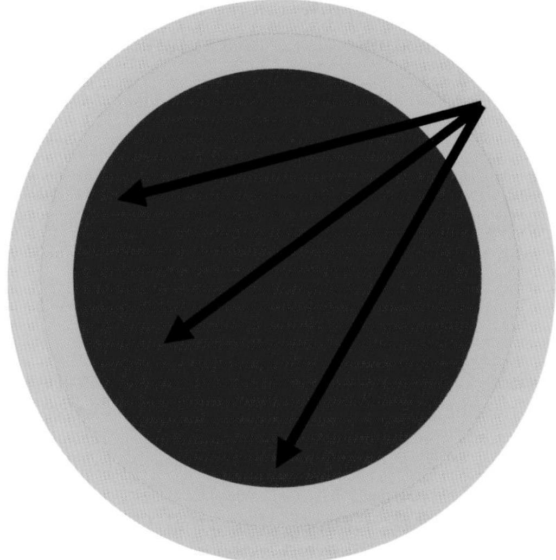

Fig. 10. Changing the way of passing of each stroke in fine-needle aspiration (FNA)

Negative Pressure by Suction

Negative pressure by suction with a 20-ml syringe has been used in most institutions. The purpose of suction is not to draw the cells into the needle, but to hold the tissue against the cutting edge of needle. Suction is turned off before withdrawing the needle. Concerning negative pressure, Wallace et al. found no difference in suction versus no suction in terms of overall diagnostic yield for lymph nodes, but noted excess blood in the specimens to which suction was applied. In general, applying suction to the needle increases cellular yield but potentially increases artifact and blood, especially in vascular lesions.

Future Perspectives

Recently, there have been several reports about immunological treatment and gene therapy with the EUS-fine-needle injection (EUS-FNI) technique, which includes dendritic cell injection, Onix, TNFerade, etc. Irisawa et al. reported that inoperable pancreatic cancers have been treated by dendritic cell injection and minor response had been obtained. Chang et al. also reported about the efficacy of TNFerade, which is a sensitive gene for radiation therapy; they injected adenovirus with TNFerade into pancreatic cancer, integrated this gene, and treated with chemoradiation. EUS-FNI is also employed for anticancer agents such as OncoGel. Furthermore, customized therapy for pancreatic cancer with EUS-FNA has been applied, in which resistance and sensitive genes for some agents such as Gemcitabine have been checked and an appropriate agent has been chosen in vitro before treatment.

Nevertheless, EUS-FNA or EUS-FNI has many possibilities of diagnosis and treatment and will widen its applications in the near future.

Conclusions

EUS-FNA seems to be difficult; however, its complications are quite low, and its clinical efficacy is quite high. To make the optimal diagnosis and treatment, we must employ EUS-FNA, which has many possibilities for diagnosis and treatment.

References

1. Vilmann P, Jacobsen GK, Henriksen FW, et al (1992) Endoscopic ultrasonography with guided fine needle aspiration biopsy in pancreas disease. Gastrointest Endosc 38:172–173
2. Grimm H, Binmoeller K, Soehendra N (1992) Endosonography-guided drainage of a pancreas pseudocyst. Gastrointest Endosc 38:170
3. Wiersema MJ, Kochman ML, Cramer HM, et al (1994) Endosonography-guided real-time fine-needle aspiration biopsy. Gastrointest Endosc 40:700–707
4. Grees FG, Hawes RH, Savides TJ, et al (1997) Endoscopic ultrasound-guided fine-needle aspiration using linear array and radial scanning endosonography. Gastrointest Endosc 45:243–250
5. Willams DB, Sahai AV, Aabakken L, et al (1999) Endoscopic ultrasound guided fine needle aspiration biopsy: a large single centre experience. Gut 44:720–726
6. Bohnnacker S, Binmoeller KF, Seifert K, et al (1996) EUS-guided transmural drainage of pancreatic pseudocysts in 27 patients. Gastrointest Endosc 43:416
7. O'Toole D, Palazzo L, Arotcarena R, et al (2001) Assessment of complications of EUS-guided fine-needle aspiration. Gastrointest Endosc 53:470–474
8. Kida M (2002) Endoscopic ultrasonography in Japan: present status and standardization. Dig Endosc 14:s24–s29
9. Yamao K, Irisawa A, Inoue H, et al (2007) Standard imaging techniques of EUS-guided FNA using a curved linear array echoendoscope. Digest Endosc 19(S1):S180–S205
10. LeBlanc JK, Ciaccia D, Al-Assi MT, et al (2004) Optimal number of EUS-FNA passes. Gastrointest Endosc 59:475
11. Wallace MB, Kennedy T, Durkalski V, et al (2001) Randomized controlled trial of EUS-FNA technique for the detection of malignant lymphadenopathy. Gastrointest Endosc 4:441–447
12. Chang KJ (2006) EUS-guided fine needle injection (FNI) and anti-tumor therapy Endoscopy 38(S1):S88–S93

Instruments

We have used a 3D-IDUS system, developed by Olympus Medical Systems, Tokyo, Japan, [an ultrasound image processing unit, EU-IP; a 3-D ultrasonic probe, UM-3D-2R (12 MHz) or UM-3D-3R (20 MHz), with a diameter of 3.4 mm; and a probe driving unit, MAJ-355] since 1995. These components were connected to an endoscopic ultrasonic observation unit (EU-M30). Since 2000, we have used an endoscopic ultrasound center, EU-M2000, including an ultrasound image processing unit, EU-IP2, and a probe driving unit, MAJ-2000. The 3-D ultrasonic probe consists of an external tube as an outer sheath and the probe itself with a diameter of 2.4 mm and a 12- or 20-MHz radial scan transducer at its tip. Now, we usually use a 3-D ultrasonic probe, UM-DG20-35R, with a frequency of 20 MHz, with a diameter of 2.5 mm, developed by Olympus Medical Systems. Using a ropeway system with a guidewire in the transpapillary approach, for bile duct scanning, the rate of success was increased.

Ultrasonography was performed while the ultrasonic probe in the outer sheath was withdrawn automatically. During the scanning time, the outer sheath did not move. Linear reconstruction images were produced from integrating 40 to 118 serial radial images. The length of the longitudinal images can be set at 10, 20, 30, or 40 mm, and in pitches of 0.25, 0.5, 0.75, or 1.0 mm. After taking radial images, reconstruction images, such as longitudinal or oblique reconstruction images, were made at real time by the ultrasound image processing unit, the EU-IP2 viewer (Fig. 1).

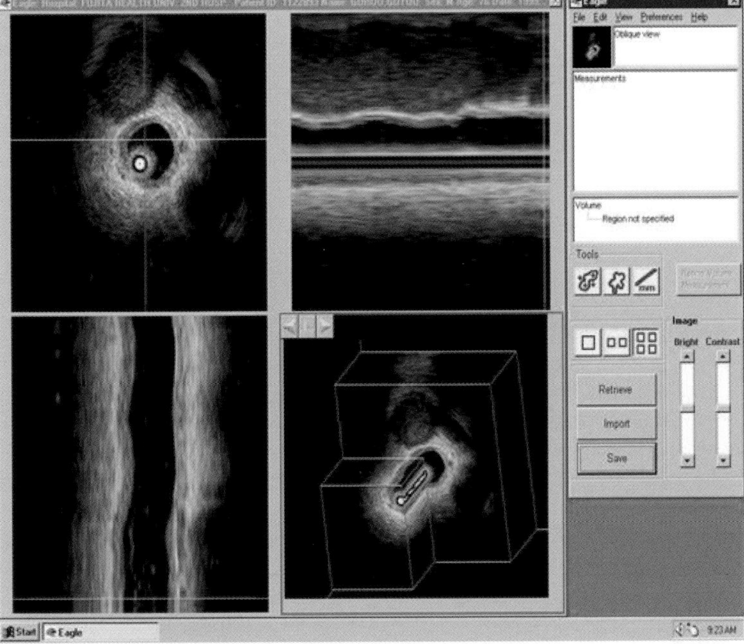

Fig. 1. Screen of the ultrasound image processing unit, EU-IP2 viewer. After taking radial images, reconstruction images, such as longitudinal or oblique reconstruction images, were made in real time

Methods

When we performed 3D-IDUS in patients with biliary diseases, there are two approaches for 3D-IDUS, transpapillary and the percutaneous transhepatic approach. In both approaches, 3D-IDUS was performed and the area observed by the probe was confirmed by fluoroscopy.

In the percutaneous transhepatic approach, an ultrasonic probe was inserted into the stenosis of the bile duct through a percutaneous transhepatic biliary drainage catheter, 16 Fr. in diameter. In the transpapillary approach, we inserted an ultrasonic probe into the stenosis of the bile duct through the biopsy channel of a duodenoscope. After endoscopic retrograde pancreatocholangiography, the ultrasonic probe was inserted into the common bile duct.

Functions of 3D-IDUS

We could produce longitudinal reconstruction images using the functions of the 3D-IDUS systems, dual-plane reconstruction (DPR) images, including radial and longitudinal reconstruction images and oblique reconstruction images. DPR and oblique reconstruction images are useful to assess the tumor extension and the relationship with surrounding organs. Especially, an oblique reconstruction image is useful to assess the relationship with the left hepatic duct and cystic duct in a patient with biliary carcinoma with invasion to the subserosal layers (Fig. 2).

We could calculate the tumor volumes using the traced areas of the serial radial images. When the whole outline of the tumor could be visualized, we could measure the tumor volumes.

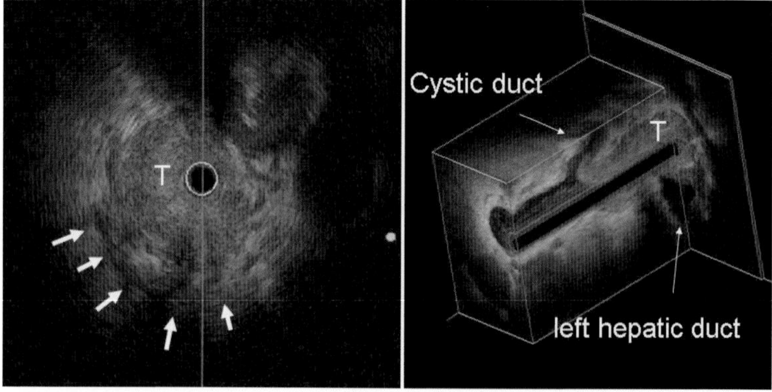

Fig. 2. Radial and oblique images in case of bile duct cancer with invasion to the subserosal layers. The oblique reconstruction image is useful to assess the relationship with the left hepatic duct and cystic duct. *T*, tumor; *white arrows*, invasion to the subserosa

Diagnosis of Bile Duct Carcinoma

Depth of Tumor Invasion

We could observe the bile duct wall as having two to three layers. In contrast, IDUS showed a carcinoma as a hypoechoic area of irregular thickness. When the tumor in an ultrasonogram reached the hyperechoic layer of the bile duct, we could diagnose that the tumor had invaded the subserosa. The results of 3D-IDUS and pathological studies for tumor extension in 25 patients with bile duct carcinoma were investigated. Overall accuracy for depth of tumor invasion was 88%. Accuracy of EUS was 83.3%. Accuracy of 3D-IDUS was higher than one of EUS diagnosis.

Invasion to the Portal Vein

When the tumor echogram reached the high echoic wall of the portal vein, it could be diagnosed that the portal vein had been invaded. In the case of bile duct cancer without invasion to the portal vein, an oblique reconstruction image is useful to assess the relationship with the right hepatic artery and portal vein. In cases of bile duct cancer with invasion to the portal vein, a longitudinal scanning image is useful to assess the extent of cancer invasion to the portal vein. The results of 3D-IDUS and pathological studies for tumor extension in 25 patients with bile duct carcinoma were investigated. Overall accuracy for tumor invasion to the portal vein was 92%, and accuracy of EUS was 91.7%. The accuracy of 3D-IDUS was almost the same as that of EUS diagnosis.

Invasion to the Pancreas

When the tumor echogram reached the parenchyma of the pancreas, it could be diagnosed that the pancreas had been invaded. The important finding to diagnose tumor invasion to the pancreas is a high echoic layer between the bile duct and the pancreas. In cases of bile duct carcinoma without invasion to the pancreas, oblique reconstruction images reveal easily the relationship between the tumor and the pancreas. In bile duct carcinoma with invasion to the pancreas, longitudinal scanning images reveal comprehensively the extent of cancer invasion to the pancreas. The results of 3D-IDUS and pathological studies for tumor extension in 25 patients with bile duct carcinoma were investigated. Overall accuracy for tumor invasion to the pancreas was 84%. Accuracy of EUS was 75.0%. Accuracy of 3D-IDUS was higher than that of EUS diagnosis.

Intraductal Spreading of Tumor

Intraductal spreading of tumor is known as one of the characteristics of tumor extension of extrahepatic bile duct carcinoma. It is difficult to diagnose precisely. We have tried to diagnose cancer spreading along the bile duct superficially with wall thickness by using 3D-IDUS.

The shape of wall thickness at the upper part of the main lesion was divided into three types (Fig. 3). Type 1 is without wall thickness, type 2 is a regular wall thickness of the bile duct, and type 3 has an irregular thickness. In type 1, there were no patients

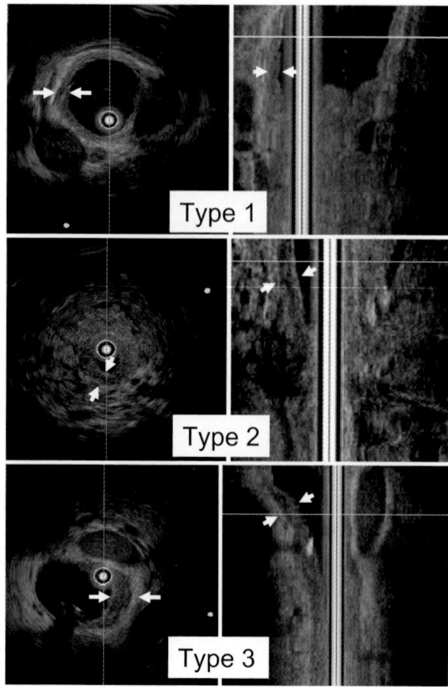

Fig. 3. The shape of wall thickness at the upper part of the main lesion in bile duct carcinoma. *Type* 1 is without wall thickness (top), *type* 2 is the regular wall thickness of the bile duct (middle), and *type* 3 has an irregular thickness (bottom). *White arrows*, bile duct wall thickness

with ductal spreading; in type 2, two of four patients had ductal spreading; and in type 3, three of four had ductal spreading.

When diagnosed as type 3 with ductal spread, accuracy was 70.0%, sensitivity 60%, and specificity 80%. The result was not satisfactory, as Tamada et al. [7] reported the limitation of 3D-IDUS in the assessment of longitudinal spread in 2000.

Discussion

Accurate assessment of cancer extent is necessary to plan adequate surgical procedures. When US has detected extrahepatic obstruction as the cause of jaundice, choice of the next examination has become an issue. EUS is considered the best procedure for diagnosis of biliary obstruction, and it is the most precise and accurate way to identify a lesion that is causing extrahepatic obstruction and to stage biliary tract cancers [8].

We investigated the accuracy of EUS for T staging in 12 patients with cancer of the middle and distal segment of the bile duct in our institute. Accuracy of diagnosis of invasion to the duct wall was 83.3%, to the portal vein was 91.7%, and to the duodenum was 100%, which were relatively high. However, that of invasion to the pancreas and lymph nodes was 75.0%.

Menzel and Dosmschke [9] reported the usefulness of IDUS for diagnosis of bile duct cancers, with tumor extent determined correctly in 76.8% of cases using IDUS but only 53.6% of those using EUS. Tamada et al. [10] reported that the accuracy of IDUS in assessing pancreatic parenchyma invasion was 100%, compared with 78% for EUS.

EUS has limitations in diagnosing and staging hepatic hilum tumors, but 3D-IDUS is accurate for staging. 3D-IDUS clearly demonstrates invasion of the pancreas or portal vein. The advantage of 3D-IDUS is that the time required for the examinations is reduced compared with that required for conventional IDUS, because conventional IDUS needs to clarify the relationship between lesions and surrounding organs and vessels. However, 3D-IDUS could not detect subsequently demonstrated histological infiltration of fibrous layer of perimuscular loose connective tissue that was macroscopically limited in T1 tumors. Another problem of 3D-IDUS for diagnosis of bile duct cancer is the limitation in diagnosis of lymph node metastasis. We have to continue to study and develop 3D-IDUS systems to resolve these problems.

References

1. Palazzo L (1997) Which test for common bile duct stones? Endoscopic and intraductal ultrasonography. Endoscopy 29:655–665
2. Tamada K, Inui K, Menzel J (2001) Intraductal ultrasonography of the bile duct system. Endoscopy 33:878–885
3. Inui K, Nakazawa S, Yoshino J, et al (1998) Mucin-producing tumor of the pancreas: intraductal ultrasonography. Hepato-Gastroenterology 45:1996–2000
4. Kanemaki N, Nakazawa S, Inui K, et al (1997) Three-dimensional intraductal ultrasonography: preliminary results of a new technique for the diagnosis of diseases of the pancreatobiliary system. Endoscopy 29:726–731
5. Inui K, Nakazawa S, Yoshino J, et al (1998) Ultrasound probes for biliary lesions. Endoscopy 30(suppl 1):A120–A123
6. Inui K, Miyoshi H (2004) Cholangiocarcinoma and intraductal sonography. Gastrointest Endosc N Am 15:143–155
7. Tamada K, Yasuda Y, Nagai H, et al (2000) Limitations of three-dimensional intraductal ultrasonography in the assessment of longitudinal spread of extrahepatic bile duct carcinoma. J Gastroenterol 35:919–923
8. Fujita N, Noda Y, Kobayashi G, et al (1998) Staging of bile duct carcinoma by EUS and IDUS. Endoscopy 30(suppl 1):A132–A134
9. Menzel J, Dosmschke W (1999) Intraductal ultrasonography (IDUS) of the pancreatobiliary duct system. Personal experience and review of literature. Eur J Ultrasound 10:105–109
10. Tamada K, Kanai N, Ueno N, et al (1997) Limitations of intraductal ultrasonography in differentiating between bile duct cancer in stage T1 and stage T2: in-vitro and in-vivo studies. Endoscopy 29:721–725

Future of EUS Technology

Kenji Hirooka

Summary. The development of endoscopic ultrasound (EUS) originated in 1978 as an imaging diagnostic device to detect early pancreatic cancers. Over the last 30 years, several technical evolutions have taken place, such as the electronic radial transducer, which was developed recently and provides a paradigm shift in the scanning method of radial EUS from mechanical scanning to electronic scanning.

In the early 1990s, a curvilinear array (CLA) echoendoscope was developed, which established EUS-guided fine-needle aspiration (EUS–FNA). Along with the development of CLA scopes, EUS applications have been expanded from image diagnosis to tissue acquisition and therapeutic interventions.

This chapter describes imaging EUS, interventional EUS, utilizing technology from other fields, and education and training.

Contrast harmonic imaging (CHI) will be the next trend in imaging EUS, and a new concept of CLA scopes dedicated to interventional EUS is described. Olympus Medical Systems Co. (Tokyo, Japan) also developed endobronchial ultrasonography (EBUS), which allows Transbronchial Needle Aspiration (TBNA) to be performed under EBUS guidance (EBUS–TBNA). The EBUS–TBNA scope can go through strictures in the gastrointestinal (GI) tract because of its small diameter.

Education and training are very important to the expansion of EUS, so Olympus Medical Systems has been working to develop training tools. The role of the EUS navigation system and the Rob and Koji (R-K) model will be described.

Key words. EUS–FNA, Interventional EUS, Bi-plane EUS, EBUS-TBNA, EUS navigation system

Introduction

The development of endoscopic ultrasound (EUS) originated in 1978 as an image diagnostic device for the purpose of detecting early pancreatic cancer. Ever since the first prototype of the mechanical radial EUS was produced in 1980, it has evolved as

---

Olympus Medical Systems Co., Research and Development Division 2, Ultrasound Technology Department, 2951 Ishikawa-cho, Hachioji-shi, Tokyo 192-8507, Japan

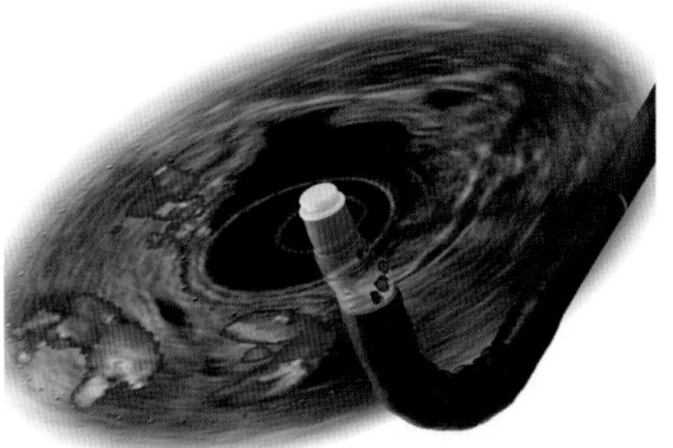

Fig. 1. GF-UE160-AL5/GF-UE260-AL5

follows: dual transducer (GF-UM3); waterproofing (GF-UM20); videoizing (GF-UM200/GF-UM130); broadbanding (GF-UM160/GF-UM2000). The latest evolution is the paradigm shift in radial EUS scanning methods from mechanical to electronic (Fig. 1).

A catheter-type ultrasound probe (UM-1W), which passes through the instrument channels of regular endoscopes, was developed in 1990. Thereafter, ultrasound probes of various frequencies (12, 20, and 30 MHz) and sizes (1.8–3.2 mm in diameter) were developed. Functional progress has also resulted in a guidewire-port-equipped system for intraductal ultrasonography (IDUS) and a three-dimensional scanning ultrasound probe.

In order to provide a curved linear array (CLA) type, an electronic CLA–EUS was developed in the early 1990s. This development enabled physicians to perform EUS-guided fine-needle aspiration (EUS–FNA) and changed EUS to a tool not only for imaging, but also for tissue acquisition.

In this chapter the future of EUS technologies, including imaging EUS, interventional EUS, utilizing the technology of other fields, and education and training, will be described from the EUS research and development point of view.

Imaging EUS

EUS was developed by applying abdominal ultrasound technologies to an intraluminal cavity. By actively adopting several technical innovations in abdominal ultrasound, EUS will be advanced based on the intraluminal ultrasound technology that has long been well established for EUS.

Recently, X-ray computed tomography (CT) has been dramatically improved, but the spatial resolution and contrast resolution are still not at the level of EUS. Intraluminal EUS scanning offers absolute advantages over other imaging modalities, so a target can be visualized very closely, and moreover there is no risk of X-ray exposure.

Mechanical radial-type systems (probes/scopes) can offer high-resolution imaging by using a high-frequency transducer in a way that cannot be achieved by abdominal ultrasound probes. Electronic scanning-type systems can provide physicians with additional information over the ultrasound image, such as color Doppler imaging and tissue harmonic imaging (THI).

Contrast harmonic imaging (CHI) utilizing a second-generation ultrasound contrast agent is now under investigation for EUS applications. A second-generation ultrasound contrast agent named Sonazoid was approved in Japan, for the first time in the world, in October 2006. Microbubbles of Sonazoid pass through the capillaries and enhance the blood vessel by the reflection and diffusion of ultrasound. Sonazoid produces enhancement at a lower acoustic power than Revovist, which is a first-generation ultrasound contrast agent with a relatively long enhancement duration. This is a very important feature, since EUS produces limited acoustic power, which is lower than that from an abdominal ultrasound probe, depending on the size of the transducer. From the limited number of trials to date, CHI–EUS with Sonazoid seems to be promising.

In order to perform CHI, the transducer should have a broadband frequency range and be sensitive enough to sense harmonic ultrasound waves from the tissue. Therefore, we are working on the development of a new transducer with new materials and the establishment of appropriate production processes. In addition to the broadband and sensitized transducer, a transmitting/receiving process and flexibility in parameter settings are important, and these greatly depend on the performance of the ultrasound processor.

Aloka ProSound Alpha10 (Fig. 2) is a flagship ultrasound machine. CHI and THI have already been applied with Aloka abdominal ultrasound probes. Although Alpha10 has been introduced for EUS in some markets (including Japan), at present, the compatibility between Alpha10 and the new EUS transducer is under

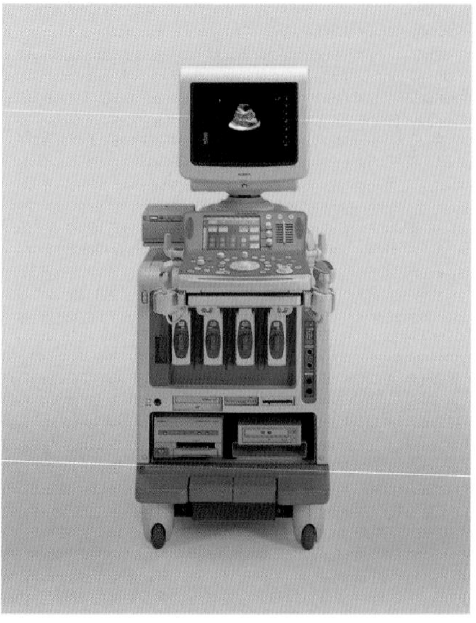

Fig. 2. Aloka SSD-Alfa10

development. Enhancement of the detection of early pancreatic cancer is expected by means of CHI–EUS, which would provide vivid high-quality ultrasound images with higher directivity.

Interventional EUS

To date, EUS-guided pancreatic pseudocyst drainage, celiac plexus neurolysis, and injection against tumors have been performed as interventional EUS procedures. More advanced procedures, such as the treatment of jaundice (i.e., choledochoduodenostomy [1]) in cases of difficult transpapillary stenting and EUS-guided suturing, are being considered.

In order to perform these advanced interventional procedures, not only suitable endotherapeutic devices but also suitable EUS scopes are required. The conventional CLA–EUS scopes have a curvilinear array transducer at the distal end, oblique optics, and an instrument channel with some angles at the exit (Fig. 3).

The following requests have been received for a conventional CLA configuration.

1. The distal end should be shortened so that the maneuverability can be improved to perform advanced interventional EUS procedures.
2. The insertability of endotherapeutic devices should be improved since the exit of the instrument channel is not straight and endotherapeutic devices can be bent, which generates resistance when endotherapeutic devices are inserted.
3. Endotherapeutic devices should protrude straight to get a better approach route to a target in an intervention.

To comply with these requests, a forward-viewing CLA prototype EUS scope was developed, and its applications are now under investigation (Fig. 4). A miniaturized CLA transducer is installed at the distal end, and end-fire scanning has been achieved. Forward-viewing optics have been adopted, and the direction in which the device protrudes is straight, which is the same as in regular endoscopes. The inner diameter of the instrument channel is 3.7 mm. A water-jet function is included to obtain clear endoscopic and ultrasonic views in an interventional procedure. The main characteristics of this scope are (Fig. 5):

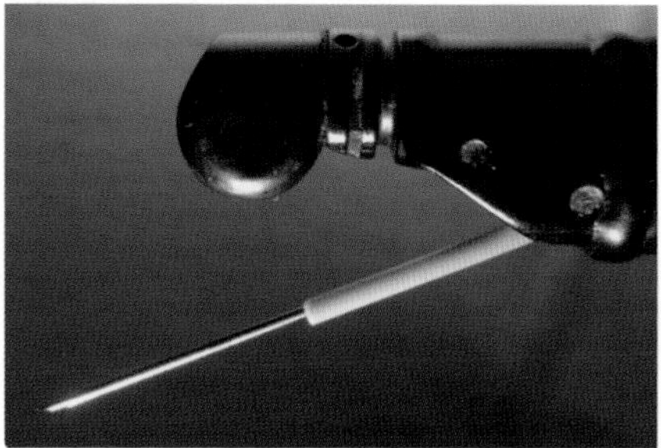

Fig. 3. Conventional CLA EUS

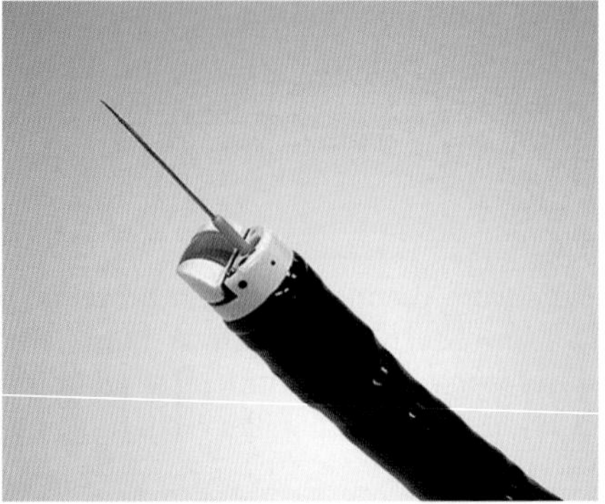

Fig. 4. Forward-viewing CLA EUS

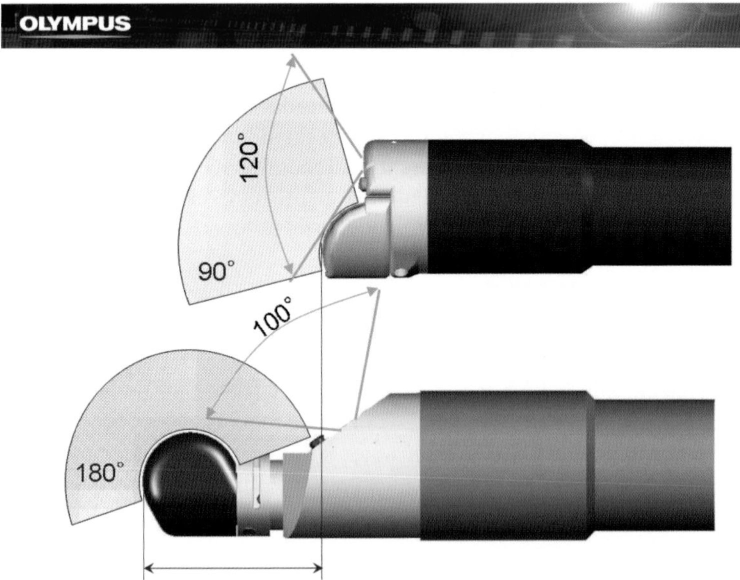

Fig. 5. Comparison of distal end section

1. a short rigid distal end, which allows a turn to be made in a small radius;
2. better endotherapeutic device insertability with a straight instrument channel.

This scope has shown good performance for EUS-guided pancreatic pseudocyst drainage by achieving better insertion of endotherapeutic devices and easier access to targets. This is a performance which even conventional CLA cannot reach, and which offers more possibilities for interventional EUS. Despite the fact that the forward-viewing CLA scope has a 3.7-mm channel, it is easier to insert than endotherapeutic devices owing to its straight instrument channel, which also allows

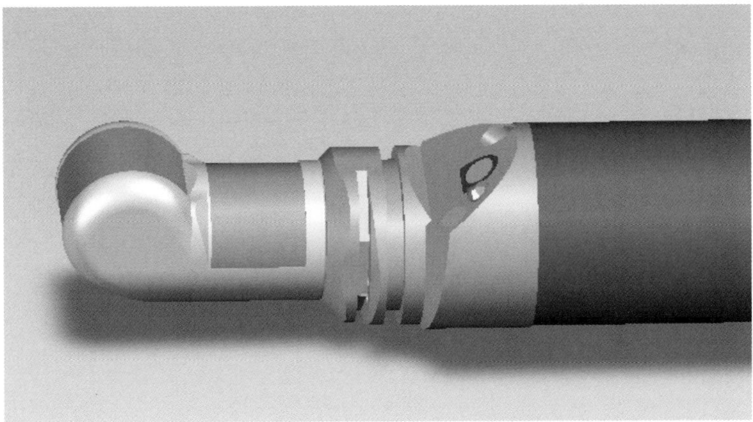

Fig. 6. Bi-plane EUS

physicians to use more varieties of therapeutic device. Olympus Medical Systems hopes to contribute to interventional EUS by collaborating with physicians to improve both scopes and devices.

As described above, the mainstream use for EUS is interventional EUS, and new devices are now under development to explore the possibilities. We have had many requests from physicians for a scope that covers all needs from diagnosis to intervention. One idea for this is a biplane EUS scope (Fig. 6) that can offer both cross-sectional and longitudinal planes. However, it will require improvements or innovations in EUS technology to achieve such a scope without having a longer distal end and a larger diameter, since both radial and curvilinear characteristics should be built into it. The evolution from a biplane EUS to a multiplane EUS to provide an arbitrary scanning plane will be our aim in the future.

Utilizing Technology from Other Fields

Many transesophageal EUS–FNA performed in mediastinum in order to perform lung cancer staging or to diagnose lymphadenopathy have been reported. However, the transesophageal approach cannot reach the anterior side, which was a big problem. Olympus Medical Systems resolved this issue by developing and commercializing a new miniaturized CLA–EUS scope (Fig. 7) for a respiratory field in 2005.

This scope was developed for endobronchial ultrasound-guided transbronchial needle aspiration (EBUS–TBNA [2]). The outer diameter of the distal end of the scope is 6.9 mm, which is almost half that of conventional CLA–EUS scopes. The inner diameter of the instrument channel is 2.0 mm, which is compatible with a dedicated 22-gauge needle (Fig. 8). Since this is a miniaturized EUS scope, it is expected to allow physicians to perform transesophageal EUS–FNA for stenotic cases in a gastrointestinal (GI) tract.

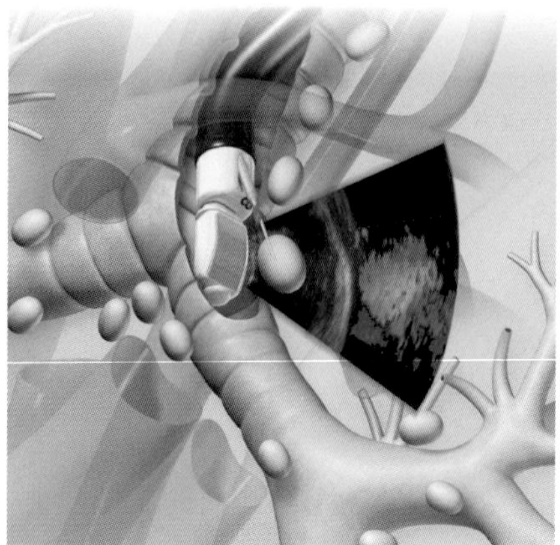

Fig. 7. BF-UC160F-OL8/BF-UC260F

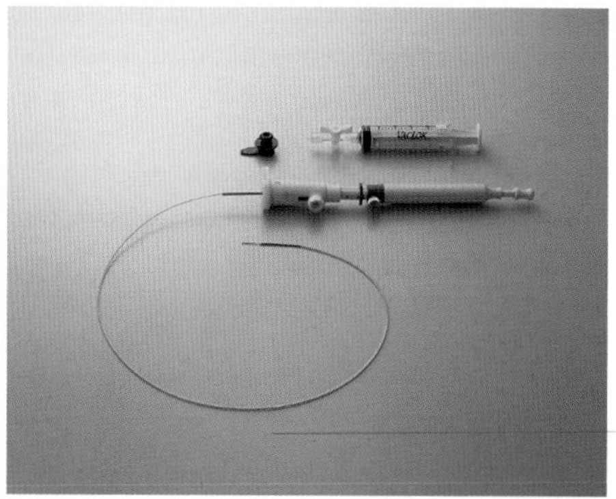

Fig. 8. NA-201SX-4022

Education and Training

EUS is a low-invasive procedure that can offer guidance for interventions and high-resolution images. However, difficulties with EUS operation and interpretation remain a big problem [3], especially in pancreatobiliary procedures, which is a main indication for EUS.

To provide a solution, we are working on an EUS navigation system that displays guide images showing the relationship between preoperative X-ray CT image data and an EUS image (Fig. 9). By building position sensors in an EUS scope (radial), the preoperative X-ray CT data can be displayed on a screen linked to a real-time EUS image (Fig. 10).

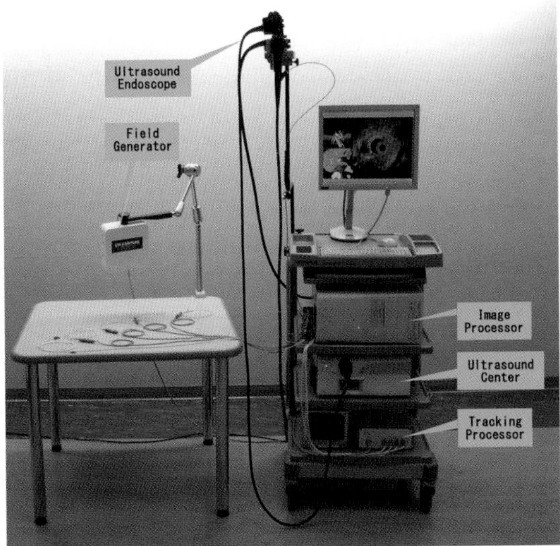

Fig. 9. EUS navigation system

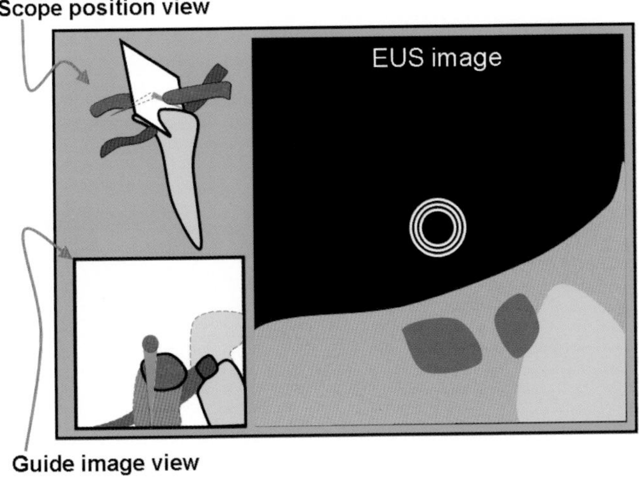

Fig. 10. Navigation screen

As can be seen in Fig. 10, two guide images are shown on the left-hand side displaying the information from three-dimensional X-ray CT and/or magnetic resonance imaging (MRI) data. Thus the targets can be seen in advance, with colors identifying the organs. The top-left image provides a three-dimensional wide-range view, and the bottom-left image provides a detailed cross-sectional guide cut with an ultrasound plane.

At first, the physician can refer to the wide-range guide image and move a scope to a target area so that the target can be shown on the ultrasound image. Then the physician can be supported by the detailed guide image to obtain the EUS interpretation in order to get a better anatomical understanding of the target and its relationship to surrounding organs. These guide images follow the physician's operation in real time. An oral presentation of clinical experiences with the EUS navigation system has already been made [4], and the necessary improvements for its practical use are now under development. To maximize the advantages of the system, applications in interventional EUS should also be investigated, and this should be done with a CLA-EUS scope with built-in sensors.

In order to promote interventional EUS procedures, Olympus Medical Systems has supported many training opportunities to provide education in curvilinear EUS with a realistic phantom along with the EUS equipment. As a body-simulating phantom, we developed an EUS paracentesis support system by working cooperatively with Dr. Koji Matsuda, Jikei University, and others. This system has a pig esophagus, stomach, and duodenum in the correct positions, and many grapes to represent lymph nodes in a lower attenuation polyurethane elastomer container stabilized with jelly (Figs. 11 and 12).

This model was used for training at the 13th to 15th EUS International Symposia held in the years 2002, 2004, and 2006, and highly praised by both trainers and trainees. However, it takes 4–6 h to prepare and lasts for approximately 2 days, which means that it cannot be used very often. In order to be able to conduct effective training, we have substituted artificial materials for pig organs, and expanded the interventional EUS training in addition to the EUS–FNA training.

We will proceed with the development of training tools which will be synchronized with the development of devices that will explore new indications/applications for interventional EUS in the future.

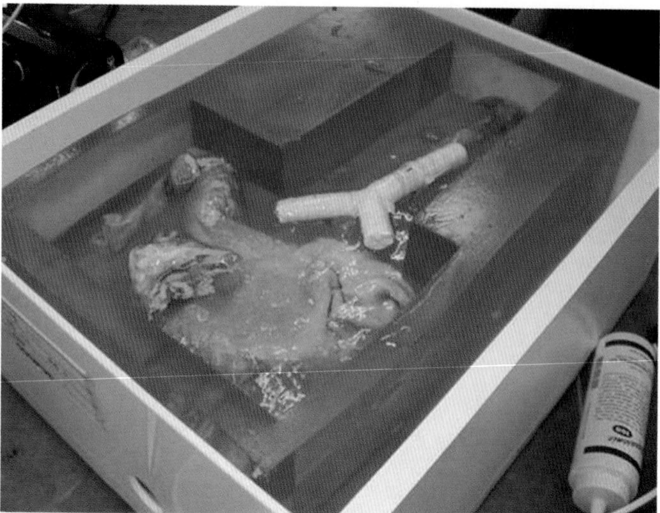

Fig. 11. Pre-completed model (R-K model)

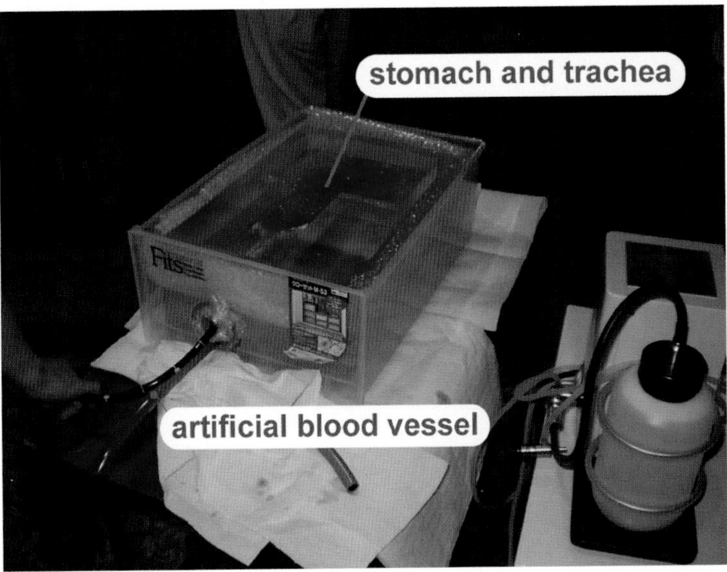

Fig. 12. Completed model (R-K model)

Conclusion

When we look back at the history of the endoscope, we see that its use has expanded to applications from diagnosis to treatment (intervention). The key for device development in the history of the endoscope has been collaboration with doctors and healthcare professionals, which is the key for the EUS as well. We hope for more progress in complex educational–industrial activities in order to develop a highly effective EUS system based on an understanding of the medical benefits and patient safety.

I would like to express my cordial gratitude for the guidance and cooperation provided by many physicians in the development and expansion of EUS.

References

1. Yamao K, Sawaki A, Takahashi K, et al. (2006) EUS-guided choledochoduodenostomy for palliative biliary drainage in cases of papillary obstruction: report of 2 cases. Gastrointest Endosc 64:663–667
2. Yasufuku K, Chiyo M, Sekine Y, et al. (2004) Real-time endobronchial ultrasound-guided transbronchial needle aspiration of mediastinal and hilar lymph nodes. Chest 126:122–128
3. EFJ Working Group on Standardization of Pancreatobiliary EUS (2004) Standard imaging techniques in the pancreatobiliary region using radial scanning endoscopic ultrasonography. Dig Endosc 16:S118–S133
4. Kida M, Moriki H, Kikuchi H, et al. (2006) Navigation system for endoscopic ultrasonography. Endoscopy 38:5

Appendix

Memories of the Establishment of Endoscopy Forum Japan (EFJ)

Masatsugu Nakajima

It is a great pleasure to me that the Endoscopy Forum Japan (EFJ), established in 1999, celebrates its 10th anniversary this year. As one of the members who were engaged in the establishment of EFJ and who have watched its development closely, I would like to look back upon its progress once more for the record.

Beginning of EFJ

It is not an exaggeration to say that the establishment of the EFJ began with the 10th Mt. Hiei symposium entitled "Digestive Endoscopy: the Forefront of Diagnosis and Treatment," which was held in March 1995. This symposium, with the name of Mt. Hiei, symbolizing Kyoto, had been held every other year since 1973 by Prof. Keiichi Kawai, Department of Preventive Medicine, Kyoto Prefectural University of Medicine. The symposium had been held at the Mt. Hiei Hotel, discussed the most important areas of gastroenterology each time, and invited the most advanced researchers in each subject from the whole country. The participants stayed at the hotel from the day before the conference and discussed and exchanged views from early morning until evening, and at night, they had pleasant chats and enjoyed meals and drinks. This type of informal communication was also an aim of these meetings.

As the main subject of the 10th Mt. Hiei symposium was digestive endoscopy, with the support of Olympus Medical Systems, Dr. Masahiro Tada (Department of Gastroenterology, Kyoto First Red Cross Hospital) and I (Department of Gastroenterology, Kyoto Second Red Cross Hospital) took charge of all the planning, managing, and moderating of the symposium. In particular, for this symposium, we invited the young rising researchers in digestive endoscopy, which was meaningful not only from the point of view of fruitful discussion, but also for promoting communication. We received very favorable comments on this meeting from the participants, which indicated that such an opportunity was very hard to find at the usual conventional conference. We also had many requests from the guests to continue this kind of meeting. Together with the staff of Olympus Medical Systems, we were pleased with the success of this symposium, and discussed the possibility of its continuance in the near future.

Chairman of the First-Term Organizing Committee of EFJ

Establishment of EFJ

In the summer of 1997, I was asked by Olympus Medical Systems to establish a new endoscopic conference which was to be modeled on the 10th Mt. Hiei symposium. In the United States, a worldwide conference on digestive endoscopy, which had a limited membership and was called the Endoscopy Master Forum (EMF), had already been held in Orlando, Florida, with the support of Olympus Medical Systems, and Olympus Medical Systems wanted to establish a similar forum in Japan. I approved of this idea, but an organization called the Japanese Promotion Liaison of Digestive Endoscopy had already been established in 1935 by endoscopists and Olympus Medical Systems. Therefore, the name, the significance, and the state and position of the new forum had to be discussed. After the discussion with Olympus Medical Systems, we came to the following decisions and agreed to start immediately.

1. The forum will be named the Endoscopic Forum Japan (EFJ), and is to be positioned as a subordinate organization of the Japanese Promotion Liaison of Digestive Endoscopy. It will be held every summer with the support of Olympus Medical Systems.
2. The prospectus of the establishment of the EFJ is as follows: to contribute to the research and development of Japanese digestive endoscopy; to aim at the standardization of endoscopic techniques through collaborative research; to publish books or journals in English to make available the academic results to the rest of the world.
3. The management of the EFJ will be carried out by the organizing committee (Chairman Masatsugu Nakajima) whose members are changed every 5 years.
4. There will be about 50 participants, and they must all be under 50 years of age. About one-third of the participants will be changed every year. The participants are required to speak English in the lectures and discussions, and write articles in English after the forum.

After these procedures had been carried out, the first EFJ conference was held at the Kiroro Resort in Hokkaido on August 4 and 5, 1999. The details and the history of the EFJ are mentioned in the preface by Prof. Hisao Tajiri and in the appendix by Dr. Kenjiro Yasuda. At present, as the EFJ is celebrating its 10th memorial year, the total number of participants exceeds 180, and most of the presentations and discussions are given in English. The academic achievements of the forum have been published every year as a supplement to Digestive Endoscopy (DEN), the official English journal of the Japan Gastroenterological Endoscopy Society. More than 5000 issues have been distributed worldwide every year, and they have been highly evaluated. This development of the EFJ is very exciting to me since I have worked hard for the establishment of the forum from the beginning, and I expect further developments and success in the future.

References

1. Kawai K, Nakajima M, Tada M (1996) Digestive endoscopy: in the forefront of diagnosis and treatment—The Therapeutic Research Symposium Series No. 493, Life Science Publishing
2. Nakajima M (2000) Preface. Dig Endosc. 12 (Suppl.):1

Endoscopy Forum Japan (EFJ)—History and Contents of the Meetings

KENJIRO YASUDA, M.D. (Secretary General)

MASATSUGU NAKAJIMA, M.D. (Chairman of first term of EFJ, 1999–2003)

HISAO TAJIRI, M.D. (Chairman of second term of EFJ, 2004–2008)

Endoscopy Forum Japan (EFJ) was started in 1999 for the purpose of the development of diagnostic and therapeutic endoscopy procedures, unconstrained discussion with younger generation of endoscopists, internationalization of Japanese endoscopists, and the world wide distribution of scholarly achievements of Japanese endoscopists.

Once a year, we gathered at the hotel in the rural district for discussion and communication.

The meeting was held for 2days at the weekend in summer.

The first memorial forum was held August 7th and 8th in the Hokkaido Kiroro Hotel Piano, with 54 participants from all over Japan. Scientific meetings on endoscopy were held in the daytime, and a long and enjoyable evening meeting was also held with all participants from the daytime meetings. Exchanging opinions and impressions among doctors from different specialties, and engaging in fervent discussions where doctors who had met for the first time talked about their dreams and hopes for the future as well as about current problems made it the most unusual meeting we had ever had. We were glad we did not have to go home at night, and we could not go out for drinks as the hotel was on a mountainside far from Otaru City.

About the participants, almost one third of the member was changed depending on the topic and theme of the meeting year by year. In addition, the members are limited under 50 years old except for organizing committee members.

I will describe the program of the successive meetings, but at first I report the place, date, and number of participants.

First EFJ meeting, Hokkaido Kiroro Hotel Piano, August 7, 8, 1999, 54 endoscopists
2nd meeting, Hokkaido Kiroro Hotel Piano, August 5, 6, 2000, 52 endoscopists
3rd meeting, Hokkaido Kiroro Hotel Piano, August 4, 5, 2001, 52 endoscopists including 2 foreign guests
4th meeting, International Conference Hall, Awaji-Yumebutai, July 27, 28, 2002, 62 endoscopists including 3 foreign guests
5th meeting, International Conference Hall, Awaji-Yumebutai, August 8, 10, 2003, 61 endoscopists including 2 foreign guests

6th meeting, Hakone Prince Hotel, July 31, August 1, 2004, 67 endoscopists including 4 foreign guests
7th meeting, Hakone Prince Hotel, July 30, 31, 2005, 68 endoscopists including 4 foreign guests
8th meeting, Hakone Prince Hotel, July 30, 31, 2006, 63 endoscopists including 3 foreign guests
9th meeting, Otaru Hilton Hotel, August 4, 5, 2007, 60 endoscopists including 6 foreign guests
10th meeting, Otaru Hilton Hotel, August 2, 3, 2008, 57 endoscopists including 7 foreign guests

Facility: The chairman decided the place for meeting. It should make the participants feel relaxed, far from the city, and the good accommodation for scientific meeting. Hokkaido was a good place to have a meeting in summer season, but in 2001, it was incredibly hot. Chairman Nakajima decided to move the meeting place to Awaji, Hyogo, where is his hometown. Facility was better than Kiroro Hotel but it was hotter than Hokkaido. From the 2nd term, chairman, Prof. Tajiri changed the place to Hakone Prince Hotel, which was also good place located at the center of Japan and convenient to gather from all over Japan. Of course, it was also far from the center of city.

Members: Participants are selected from the young leaders of each area, who have many cases and experience of diagnostic and therapeutic endoscopic procedures. We expected them the role of international activities of this field.

The organizing committee members are listed at the end of the paper.

Main theme and topic: By the big effort of organizing committee members, we could decide the programs of the meeting according to the new trend of gastroenterological endoscopy. Basically, we divide the session into two categories, one is clinical session held in the first day and the other is technology session on the new and developing instruments and devices held in the 2nd day.

Inviting foreign guests and official language of the meeting: As internalization of Japanese endoscopists was one of the biggest aims of EFJ, we invited several foreign endoscopist and gastroenterologist from Asian counties, EU or USA. Number of foreign guests is increasing, according to the level up of our English communication ability. When we started EFJ, we presented the paper in Japanese. However, since when we invited foreign guests, official language of EFJ became English. In the beginning, we had a strange feeling and some communication difficulties, but gradually English presentation and discussion became naturally.

Contents of the meeting—Main theme and topic:

1st meeting (1999);
1. Spread of the indication of endoscopic treatments of upper and GI tract
2. Endoscopic stenting for bilio-pancreatic lesions
3. Indication and limitation of Endoscopic balloon dilatation
4. Indication of magnifying endoscopy and EUS for tumorous lesions of colon
5. Developments of EUS (FNA. 3D-EUS)

2nd meeting (2000);
1. What should we do for better diagnosis of colon cancer expansion
2. Future aspects of magnifying endoscopy in upper GI lesions

3. Role of EUS and IDUS in bilio-pancraetic lesions
4. Wide-spreading of indication of EUS-FNA

3rd meeting (2001);

1. Important factor for the standalization of endoscopic treatments
2. Standalization of EUS in Asian countries
3. Future view of colonoscopy (IHb enhancement)
4. Future view of gastric endsocopy (magnification and color enhancement)

4th meeting (2002);

1. EMR (endoscopic mucosal resection) for gastric cancer
2. EMR for esophageal cancer
3. Indication and problems of endoscopic papillectomy
4. EMR for colon lesion

5th meeting (2003);

1. Endoscopic treatments for upper Gi tract stenosis
2. Endoscopic treatments for bilio-pancreatic duct stricture
3. Endoscopic treatments for lower GI stenosis
4. Development of device for EMR and ESD (endoscopic submucosal dissection) of upper GI lesions
5. Development of device for EMR of lowerGI lesions
6. Development of device for EUS-FNA

6th meeting (2004)

1. Significance of magnification endoscopy for upper GI tract
2. Significance of magnification endoscopy for ulcerative colitis
3. Role of per-oral cholangioscopy
4. Clinical possibility of multi-bending scope
5. Screening of colon lesion by NBI (narrow band imaging)
6. Future of cholangio-pancreatoscopy

7th meeting (2005);

1. Endoscopic diagnosis of degree of dysplasia in pharyngo-esophageal lesions
2. Endoscopic diagnosis of degree of dysplasia in colon lesions
3. Diagnostic and therapeutic strategy of IPMN
4. Trans-papillary biliary drainage
5. Control of bleeding in ESD

8th meeting (2006);

1. Risk managements in ESD
2. Risk managements of EMR and ESD in colon
3. Risk managements of endoscopic treatments of biliary stones
4. NBI in cholangio-pancreatoscopy
5. AFI (auto fluorescent imaging) in lower GI tract
6. Possibility of ECS (endoscopic cytoscopy)

9th meeting (2007);

1. Role of endoscopy in early diagnosis of gastric cancer
2. Colonoscopy as the 2nd screening study
3. Screening study of early diagnosis of bilio-pancreatic malignancy
4. Possibility of NBI in bile duct cancer
5. Method and device in endoscopic treatment of colon lesions

10th meeting (2008);

1. Towards the global standardization of ESD-Proposal for 10 year from now
2. Current status and future perspective of endoscopic treatment for colorectal neoplasia
3. Current status and future perspective of Interventional EUS

These main theme were taking the lead in world endoscopy stream, as this meeting was held by the sponsorship of Olympus medical systems, world leading company of endoscopy. About the style of session, we desided the highly important rules, that is, slides are presented by English and a session with foreign guests should be discussed by in English. The level of English session was remarkable improved and excellent comparing with the first few years during the past 9 years.

In addition, Special lectures on the historical story of endsocopic procedures or present status in their special fields were presented by outstanding doctors as follows; 1st meeting by Prof. H Niwa, 2nd meeting by Prof. S Nakazawa, 3rd by Prof. R Fujita, 4th by Prof. K Kawai and Prof. N Soehendra, 5th by Prof. H Suzuki, 6th by Prof. T Yamakawa, 7th by Prof. W SC Chao, 8th by Prof. M Schoeman, 9th by Prof. JF Rey, and 10th by Dr. M Nakajima.

Outcome of EFJ: One of the most important purposes of EFJ is to publish and dispatch our achievements in English. We are able to publish our English papers, as a supplement of Digestive Endsocopy, Official Journal of the Japan Gastroenterological Endoscopy Society and Asian Pacific Society for Digestive Endoscopy year by year to accomplish the issue before the next year EFJ meeting.

Organizing Committee members of EFJ

Name	Institute	Position	Term
M Nakajima	Kyoto Second Red Cross Hosp.	Chairman	1999–2003
		Advisory committee	2004–2008
H Tajiri	The Jikei University School of Medicine	Steering committee	1999–2003
		Editorial committee	1999–2003
		Chairman	2004–2008
K Yasuda	Kyoto Second Red Cross Hospital	Secretary general	1999–2008
M Igarashi	Cancer Institute Ariake Hosp.	Steering committee	1999–2003
H Inoue	Showa Univ. Yokohama Northern Hosp.	Steering committee	1999–2003
N Fujita	Sendai City Medical Center	Steering committee	1999–2003
K Yao	Fukuoka University Chikushi Hospital	Steering committee	1999–2003
S Tanaka	Hiroshima Univ.	Steering committee	2001–2005
K Maguchi	Teine Keijin-kai Hosp	Steering committee	2001–2005
T Mine	Tokai Univ. School of Medicine	Editorial committee	1999–2008
Y Igarashi	Toho Univ. Omori Medical Center	Steering committee	2004–2008
M Kida	Kitasato Univ. East Hosp.	Steering committee	2004–2008
Y Saito	Asahikawa City Hosp.	Steering committee	2004–2008
N Yahagi	Toranomon Hosp.	Steering committee	2004–2008
M Muto	Natinal Cancer Center East Hosp.	Steering committee	2006–2008
H Yamano	Akita Red Cross Hosp.	Steering committee	2006–2008
K Inui	Fujita Health Univ. of School of Medicine	Editorial committee	2004–2008
H Niwa	President of JGES	Advisory committee	1999–2008
R Fujita	President of Foundation of endosc research	Advisory committee	1999–2008

In the EFJ meetings, some of new trials such as multi-center studies and establishment of the standalization of endsocopic diagnosis, treatments, and endoscopy manipulation, have been born.

However, the most valuable outcome of EFJ is a communication of the leaders of Japanese endoscopists in the different situation from JGES meeting easygoing and informally.

Looking back on EFJ history, I realize not only the progress of endoscopic techniques and instruments but also the growth of the international mind of Japanese endoscopists. I believe that international spirit is the most important element for Japanese endoscopists to lead the world endoscopic activities and not to be isolated in the world.

Acknowledgement. I really appreciate the big support of Olympus Medical Systems Co. for Endoscopy Forum Japan.

Subject Index